Surgical Disorders of the Peripheral Nerves

Verachtet mir die Meister nicht!
(Hans Sachs to Walther von Stolzing)

Technical note

The magnifications given within the figure legends are the original magnifications used when the original photograph was taken.

Surgical Disorders of the Peripheral Nerves

Rolfe Birch MChir FRCS
Orthopaedic Surgeon, Royal National Orthopaedic Hospital,
Peripheral Nerve Unit, Stanmore, Middlesex, UK;
Honorary Orthopaedic Surgeon, The Royal London Hospital,
and to the University of Shanghai, People's Republic of China;
Honorary Orthopaedic Surgeon to the Royal Navy

George Bonney MS
Formerly Orthopaedic Surgeon, St Mary's Hospital,
Paddington, London, UK

C B Wynn Parry MBE, DM, FRCP, FRCS
Formerly Director of Rehabilitation, Royal National Orthopaedic Hospital,
London and Stanmore, UK; Consultant in Rehabilitation Medicine,
Devonshire Hospital, London.

With one chapter on Electrodiagnosis by
Shelagh J M Smith BSc MB ChB FRCP
Consultant Neurophysiologist, The National Hospital
for Neurology and Neurosurgery, London, UK;
Honorary Consultant at The Royal National Orthopaedic Hospital, UK.

Illustrated by
Patrick Elliott BA(Hons) ATC MMAA AIMA RMIP

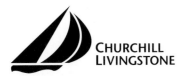
CHURCHILL
LIVINGSTONE

EDINBURGH LONDON NEW YORK PHILADELPHIA SAN FRANCISCO SYDNEY TORONTO 1998

CHURCHILL LIVINGSTONE
A division of Harcourt Brace & Co Ltd

ISBN 0 443 04443 0

British Library Cataloguing in Publication Data
A catalogue record for this book is available from the British Library.

Library of Congress Cataloging in Publication Data
A catalog record for this book is available from the Library of Congress.

Medical knowledge is constantly changing. As new information
becomes available, changes in treatment, procedures, equipment and
the use of drugs become necessary. The editors/authors/contributors
and the publishers have, as far as it is possible, taken care to ensure
that the information given in the text is accurate and up to date.
However, readers are strongly advised to confirm that the information,
especially with regard to drug usage, complies with latest legislation
and standards of practice.

The
publisher's
policy is to use
**paper manufactured
from sustainable forests**

Printed in Hong Kong

Contents

Introduction   vii

Plate Section after page xi

1. The peripheral nervous system   1

2. The microscopic structure of the nervous system   17

3. The motor and sensory pathways   27

4. Reactions to injury   37

5. Regeneration   57

6. Clinical aspects of nerve injury   71

7. Operating on peripheral nerves   87

8. Compound nerve injury   123

9. Traumatic lesions of the brachial plexus   157

10. Birth lesions of the brachial plexus   209

11. Results   235

12. Entrapment neuropathy   245

13. Iatropathic injury   293

14. The peripheral nervous system and neoplastic disease   335

15. Pain   373

16. Recovery of sensibility after nerve repair   405

17. Reconstruction   415

18. Rehabilitation   451

19. Electrodiagnosis   467

References   491

Index   529

Introduction

The work and achievements of Seddon and his colleagues in Oxford and in London; the advantages of segregation; advances in peripheral neurology; rise of obstetric and iatropathic lesions; the aims and scope of the present work; acknowledgements and apologies.

"Opportunity comes to the mind prepared." Opportunity came in full measure to H. J. Seddon with his appointment as surgeon in charge of the Medical Research Council's (MRC) Peripheral Nerve Injury Unit in Oxford during the Second World War (1939–1945). It was after all in the Oxford of those days that J. Z. Young was doing the work on the nervous system that was to be the beginning of so many of the later developments in neuroanatomy and neurophysiology. The rewards of the MRC's far sighted planning were abundant: to Seddon in particular was due that happy result. He was, however, the first to acknowledge the fortunate circumstances that enabled him to undertake the work in the company of so many doctors and scientists distinguished in the fields of anatomy, physiology and pathology of the peripheral nerves. He acknowledged too his debt to two great colleagues in clinical medicine: Hugh Cairns and George Riddoch. It was also fortunate that the Oxford unit was not allowed to die away at the end of the War, and that Seddon was able to continue at the Royal National Orthopaedic Hospital and the Institute of Orthopaedics the work that had begun and flourished at Oxford. After Seddon's retirement his close colleague Donal Brooks and others developed and extended his work in London, while in other centres those who had worked with these men made their own contributions.

Sadly, the bright hope that with introduction of the National Health Service the planning that contributed so much to the earlier success would be continued, has withered and died. Seddon's belief that "the necessity for this segregation, this concentration of cases" would be recognised has been proved wrong. The hope may finally have been extinguished in this country by the introduction through the National Health Service Act of 1990 of an artificial internal market in health care, with competition between "providers of health care" and by the necessary corollary of the forced *Gleichschaltung* of the medical profession.

Seddon's firmness of purpose, clarity of thought, immense capacity for sustained hard work and powers of organisation were shown in 'Peripheral Nerve Injuries' (1954) presented by the Nerve Injuries Committee of the Medical Research Council under his chairmanship. These characteristics were complemented by the qualities of those who collaborated in the work at Oxford. In the preface to the first edition of *Surgical Disorders*, Seddon paid generous tribute to J. Z. Young, P. B. Medawar, Graham Weddell and others. A special prominence was accorded to the contribution made by Donal Brooks. One who knew and worked with both has recorded the view that even that recognition was inadequate. He has made the disrespectful comparison of Brooks and Seddon with Jeeves and Wooster, and others who shared that experience may recognise the origins of that impious thought. Seddon's character was of course the antithesis of that of Wooster, but those who saw these men at work cannot doubt that the calm guidance from the Irish Jeeves greatly influenced Seddon's work and actions.

Both editions of Surgical Disorders bear the mark of Seddon's personality: the ordered thought; the meticulous observation and recording; the awareness of the ambient scientific field; the occasional dogmatic assertion; the love of tabulation. No one can read the book and not admire its depth and scope; no one can read it without astonishment at the comprehensive manner in which the subject is treated. One finds in it flashes of insight which, thought by the reader to have originated with him or her, turn out to be the subliminal origins of that thought.

Some may consider it too bold an undertaking to attempt the revision of a work which is a classic of British clinical science and an abiding monument to Seddon's work and leadership. However, things have moved on since 1975. Advances have been made in this country in the field of disorders of peripheral nerves by Eames, Fullerton, Gamble, Gilliatt, Thomas, Urich and others. In continental Europe the work of Brunelli, Carlstedt, Gilbert, Hagbarth, Landi, Lundborg, Millesi, Morelli, Narakas, Slooff, Torebjörk, Wallin and others has opened new possibilities and destroyed old certainties. In the USA, Gelberman, Kline, Leffert, Omer, Spinner, Terzis, Wilbourn and many others have made massive contributions. In Canada, Hudson and Mackinnon have made great clinical and experimental contributions. In Australia, the doctrine of primary repair of injuries in the upper limb and hand was developed by Rank, O'Brien and others. In China, where the feasibility of "replantation" was first demonstrated, Professor Gu of Shanghai has made and continues to make advances in the field. The development of neurotisation was largely due to work in Japan, where Nagano and Sugioka and many others continue that and other work. In particular, ideas about all types of lesion of the brachial plexus have changed; conceptions of pain mechanisms have developed, and much enlightenment has come to the understanding of the pathology of tumours. Lastly, and most sadly, the incidence of "iatrogenic" lesions has greatly increased, though in this connection great advances have been made in the treatment of birth injuries of the brachial plexus.

The authors of the present work hope that they may have succeeded in restoring *Surgical Disorders* to its place as the British text on the present state of affairs in the field. George Bonney had the privilege and pleasure and occasional pain, of working with Seddon; Christopher Wynn Parry came to the Royal National Orthopaedic Hospital at the time of its Renaissance under the leadership of Lipmann Kessel when new fields in neurophysiology, in the treatment of pain and in the surgery of the brachial plexus were being explored; Rolfe Birch came to the field at St Mary's and the Royal National Orthopaedic Hospitals armed with experience in microsurgery, and in histological and electron-microscopic techniques. Most of the work on the results of which we have drawn was done at St Mary's and the Royal National Orthopaedic Hospitals.

The original layout of the book has largely been retained, but the text has been entirely rewritten. Chapters on "iatrogenic" lesions, on birth injuries of the brachial plexus and on recovery of sensibility after repair have been added. The subjects of pain and of tumours are considered in more depth than formerly. The subject of electro-physiological examination is considered by an expert in the field, Dr Shelagh Smith. Rather more attention is given to anatomical considerations than was formerly the case. As Last (1949) remarked with some asperity "restatement of the facts appears to be warranted by the misconceptions shown by many postgraduate students." Not just by students. Evidently, we have tried to keep abreast of continuing advances in this developing field, but we shall inevitably be overtaken by the march of events. One does what one can.

As was shown by his magisterial reorganisation of a then famous London medical library, Seddon saw a clear separation between "medicine" and "surgery". As the title of this book suggests, we have aimed to deal mainly with disorders which are generally amenable to treatment by operation, and with the appropriate techniques of operation. However, we maintain a belief in the unity of medicine. The book is aimed at surgeons in training and in practice, at physicians in general and at neurologists in particular.

We even hope that undergraduates will come to no great harm through reading it. The aim has been determined by observation over the years in the clinic and in the courts of a general lack of knowledge and want of interest in conditions of peripheral nerves. These defects in medical education have generally been unhelpful to patients: injuries of nerves have been "missed" in accident departments; the delay so produced is compounded by a lack of appreciation of the urgency of the situation and of the possibilities of repair; tumours of nerves too often go unrecognised until at operation a junior practitioner is confronted by a tumour occupying, or in close proximity to, a major nerve. We hope that this book may help in stimulating interest in conditions affecting peripheral nerves, that it may aid in enhancing the quality of treatment of such lesions, and that it may bring the field of study to the notice of clinicians highly placed in surviving teaching institutions. Lesions of peripheral nerves are indeed very useful in teaching the interpretation of physical signs, which is after all the main business of the clinician. It has not been possible to treat exhaustively every aspect of the now large subject, but we hope that sufficient and sufficiently well chosen references have been given to open avenues for further reading. We had hoped to include a chapter on disorders of selected cranial nerves, and in particular of the facial nerve. That hope was, alas, born to die: we have in the event restricted the cranial nerve study to one which is really a spinal nerve – the spinal accessory – and to some aspects of damage to the fifth, seventh, tenth and twelfth nerves.

Rashly, perhaps, we have proposed one or two new terms for varieties of nerve injury and for pain arising from the nerve injury. We have also revived an old suggestion for a term to replace that commonly used to designate injury inflicted by doctors. We do not hope to escape criticism for this presumption, but we hope that, at least, our derivations will be found by classicists to be correct. We hope that those derivations do no discredit to the august institution where their principles were imparted.

All who work in this field owe a debt of gratitude to the late Sir Herbert Seddon, and to the late Sir Sydney Sunderland. The extent of their contribution is overwhelming: no list of references, however long, can indicate its magnitude. Any book on this subject must draw heavily on *Peripheral Neuropathy*, and in particular on the third edition (1993). We are glad to acknowledge our debt to the editors of and authors contributing to that majestic work. The late Professor Roger Gilliatt was foremost amongst those who after the Second World War made advances in the field and stimulated the interest of his colleagues and juniors at Queen Square and in other centres. No-one contributed more to the study and treatment of lesions of the brachial plexus than did the late Professor Algimàntas Narakas of Lausanne. We gratefully acknowledge the contribution of these two men and the lasting influence of their work.

ACKNOWLEDGEMENTS

In the preparation of this book we have received help from so many friends and colleagues that we despair of acknowledging adequately their contribution. Some will perhaps repine because we have failed to acknowledge their assistance; equally, others, having read the book, may regret the exposure of their connection with it. To both groups we apologise sincerely: omission arises not from ingratitude but from incompetence; the faults of the book are not in any way the faults of the contributors. We name in particular the following:

Mrs Margaret Taggart (Research Co-ordinator of the Peripheral Nerve Injury Unit, RNOHT), not only provided the analyses and the basis for analysis of much of the work that forms the substance of this book; she also devised and maintained the prospective programme of measurement of outcome in cases of injury of the brachial plexus, initiated work on pain, rehabilitation and the birth injury of the plexus, and found time to record, store, edit and type all the manuscript. First of the first, thus we pronounce Pompilia.

For help in the development of microsurgical work we thank Peter French and Charles Gallanaugh, orthopaedic surgeons to St George's Hospital, and Liam Murphy, orthopaedic surgeon to St Peter's Hospital; for help in the experimental work, John Hynd, Philip Perry and John Fish, of St George's Hospital Medical School. The electron microscopic section owes most to Stephen Gschmeissner of the Royal College of Surgeons, and Stephen Griffiths and Jeremy Rees of the Institute of Orthopaedics, supported by Professor Yusuf Ali. Stephanie Wilson, Arthur Boylston, Jean Pringle and Anne Sandison made a large and essential contribution with histological work and with immuno staining techniques. Our guides and friends in the whole field of "imaging" were David Sutton, Mohammed Al-Kutoubi, Witold Gedroyc and John Stevens of St Mary's Hospital, Denis Stoker, Nan Mitchell and Asif Saifuddin of the Royal National Orthopaedic Hospital and Brian Kendall of the National Hospital, Queen Square. Shelagh Smith, Nicholas Murray and José Payan were our generous mentors in neurophysiology. We have had much help from neurologists at the Royal Free and National Hospitals: Peter Thomas, Gareth Llewellyn, Christopher Earl, John Morgan-Hughes, Richard Hughes, Dafydd Thomas, Geoffrey Schott and Roman Kocen: from neurosurgeons, in particular Lindsay Symon, Alan Crockard, Robert Bradford, David Thomas and Maurice Williams, and from plastic surgeons, Roy Sanders and David Evans in particular. We gratefully acknowledge help received from Averil Mansfield, Felix Eastcott, John Wolfe and Andreas Nicolaides, all, of course, of St Mary's Hospital; vascular surgeons all.

The experience, which we think is unique, that is narrated here was possible only because of referral of patients and, in particular, of patients in the acute stage, by colleagues in orthopaedic and general surgery. For this we thank Frank Horan, Stephen Copeland, Robert Marshall, Arthur Themen, John Strachan, Michael Laurence, Peter Baird, Leslie Klenerman, Christopher McCullough, David Jameson Evans, Nicholas Geary, Dalton Boot, John Fixsen, Margaret McQueen, Charles Court-Brown, Nicholas Clarke, David Halpin, Anthony Jenkins and many others. Angus Jamieson made at least one seminal observation whilst working with us at St Mary's Hospital: he noted that, in one case at least, roots were not "avulsed" but ruptured just proud of the surface of the spinal cord. He made many other contributions then and later. Campbell Semple gave much useful information from his own experience. Colleagues in continental Europe, China and Japan have illuminated areas which were dark for us: Thomas Carlstedt, of Stockholm, now, happily, past the transitional zone and in Stanmore; Alain Gilbert and Laurent Sedel, of Paris; Yves Allieu, of Montpellier; Piero Raimondi of Legnano; Professor Akira Nagano and Dr Sugioka, of Tokyo; Dr Liang Chen, of Shanghai. Dr Chen worked with us at Stanmore, and contributed greatly in thought about and discussion of problems. His coming owes much to the foresight of Professor Ivan Roitt, Chairman of the Board of Clinical Studies at the Royal National Orthopaedic Hospital. Perhaps co-operation between colleagues in competition against disease and disability is a better strategy than is competition between colleagues and hospitals in search of a place in the "League Tables"?

Charles Dewhurst, formerly of Hempsons, now head of the legal department of the Medical Defence Union, gave valuable help. Michael Saunders, now Chief Executive, and Suzanne Collinge, formerly General Manager, Operations, of the Union, provided very useful information.

We thank all nurse colleagues, particularly Evelyn Hunter and her staff and Moira Nurse, head of the rehabilitation ward. In dealing with physiotherapy and occupational therapy we have had much help from Alison Somek and her staff at the Royal National Orthopaedic Hospital: Jane Taylor, Annette Leong and Lydia Dean. In the same institution Miss Pam Barsby and Miss Janet Laverty and their colleagues gave us much help in the matters of transcutaneous stimulation and splint work; in the days at St Mary's Hospital Pat Clifton helped greatly in the whole field of physiotherapy.

We owe most of the photographic work to Emrys Sparks, Rachel Hann and Bernie Tallon of the former St Mary's Hospital Medical School, and to Uta Boundy and Dirk De Camp and their colleagues in the Photographic Department of the Institute of Orthopaedics. Dr Peter Smith, Librarian at the Institute of Orthopaedics, gave much help with the references. At the library of the Royal Society of Medicine, Robert Greenwood, Librarian, and Helen Rivett, Senior Library Assistant, gave much help over many years. Mr Peter Cozens, Employment Advisor at the Royal National Orthopaedic Hospital, gave freely of his knowledge of all aspects in the field of disability and employment legislation.

We thank those who were our juniors over the years during which the evidence presented here was accumulated, for their work, help and advice. We thank our patients who endured and co-operated.

Patrick Elliott did all the art work for this book, patiently translating our ideas into intelligible images. We are glad to acknowledge the magnitude of his work and to thank him for it. We have drawn heavily on the work of others as models for the illustrations. We think that the attribution has in all cases been acknowledged, but we express here our gratitude to authors, illustrators and publishers. All those at Churchill Livingstone involved in this work have been very helpful. We thank Nora Naughton, in particular, for her great contribution.

Last, and very particularly, we thank Professor Ruth Bowden, for help in assessment of sensibility; Dr Praveen Anand, of the Royal London Hospital, and Dr Giorgio Terenghi, of the Blond-McIndoe Institute, for all we know about nerve growth factors, and Dr Jonathan Berman, for releasing to us much of his unpublished work on pain mechanisms. We have been very fortunate that so many have given so freely of their time and knowledge to help in the preparation of this book.

Figs 2.4 and 2.5 Sensory cells in a posterior root ganglion avulsed from the spinal cord with its spinal root.

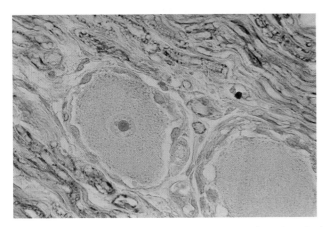

Fig. 2.4 Dorsal root ganglion 6 months after avulsion from the spinal cord. Solochrome cyanin × 960.

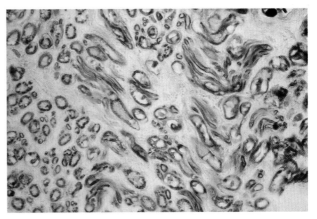

Fig. 2.5 Specimen showing myelinated fibres. Solochrome cyanin × 960.

Figs 5.10 to 5.13 Neurotrophic factors visualised through immunoreactivity. (Micrographs courtesy of Dr Praveen Anand and colleagues.)

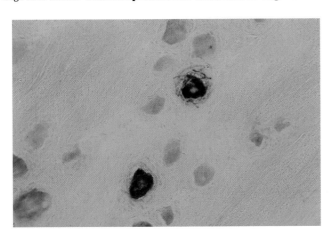

Fig. 5.10 Brain derived neurotrophic factor (BDNF) immunoreactivity in medium-sized neuronal cell bodies and associated axons in human dorsal root ganglion after avulsion of spinal root. × 150.

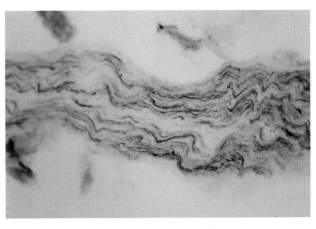

Fig. 5.11 Glial derived neurotrophic factor (GDNF) immunoreactivity in Schwann cell of healthy human sural nerve. × 150.

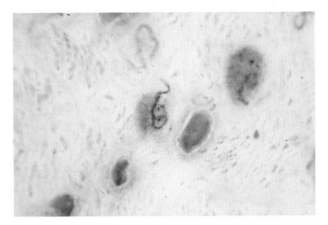

Fig. 5.12 GDNF immunoreactivity in neuronal cell bodies and adjacent axons in human dorsal root ganglion after avulsion of spinal root. × 150.

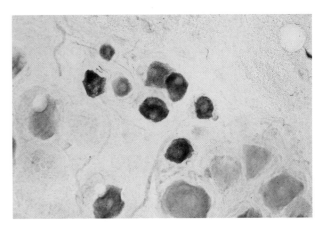

Fig. 5.13 GDNF receptor C ret immunoreactivity in neuronal cell bodies of human dorsal root ganglion after avulsion of spinal roots. × 150.

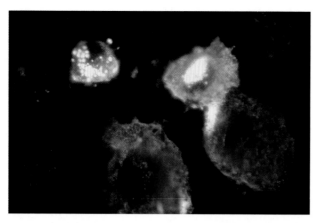

Fig. 5.24 NGF immuno-reactivity in primary sensory neurones in human dorsal root ganglion, which was avulsed from spinal cord six weeks earlier. Immuno-reactivity, identified by green fluorescent staining, is localised to cells of the small type. The yellow intracellular granules are lipofuchsin deposits which exhibit auto-fluorescence. Indirect immuno fluorescence method × 50.

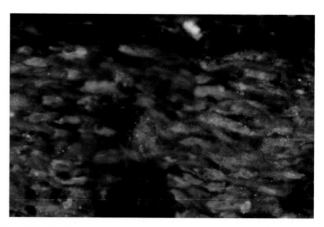

Fig. 5.25 NGF immuon-reactivity localised to most of the Schwann cells in the distal stump of a human common peripheral nerve. Indirect immuno fluorescence method × 50.

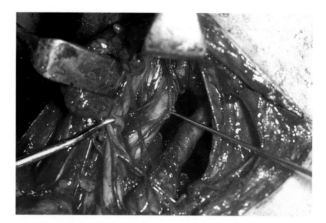

Fig. 12.26 Recent thrombosis of the subclavian artery. Note the periarteritis and post-stenotic dilation. Successful endarterectomy.

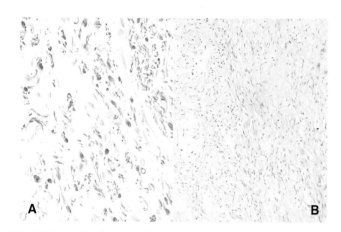

Fig. 14.2 a and b S-100 positive staining of Schwann cells in an intact fascicle within a plexiform neurofibroma; the myelinated nerve fibres are demonstrated by solochrome cyanin. A × 400, B × 160. (Courtesy of Dr Jean Pringle.)

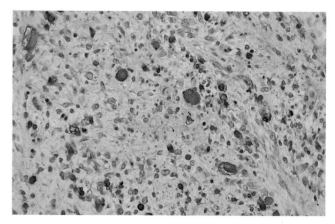

Fig. 14.4 MPNST in a patient with NF1, arising from the brachial plexus. A proportion of the tumour cells are expressing myoglobin, in particular, larger cells (triton tumour). × 400. (Courtesy of Dr Kim Suvarna.)

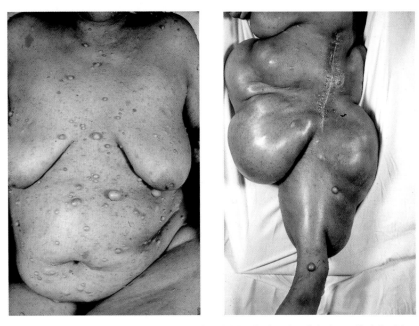

Fig. 14.5 (Left) A 48-year-old woman with NF1. (Right) Deformity of the lower limb in this case.

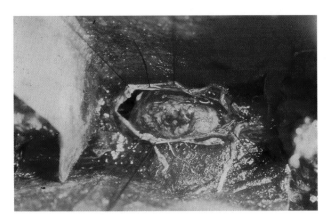

Fig. 14.9 Intradural extramedullary schwannoma exposed at operation. The patient presented with back pain.

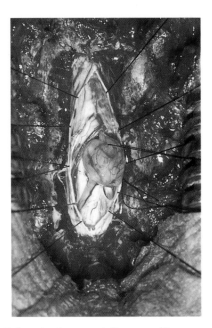

Fig. 14.10 Intradural extramedullary neurofibroma exposed at operation. The patient presented with back pain and paraparesis.

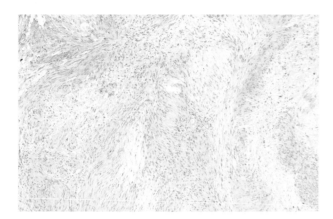

Fig. 14.14 Schwannoma, showing Antoni A and B tissue, palisading and Verocay bodies. Haematoxylin and eosin, × 250. (Courtesy of Dr Jean Pringle.)

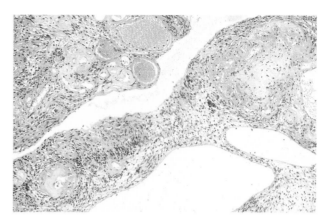

Fig. 14.15 Ancient changes in schwannoma. There is hyalinisation of the walls of the small blood vessels, haemorrhage, haemosiderin pigment and cystic change. Haematoxylin and eosin, × 250. (Courtesy of Dr Jean Pringle.)

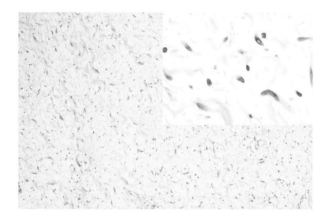

Fig. 14.19 Solitary benign neurofibroma. The matrix is fibrillary and there are comma-shaped nuclei. Haematoxylin and eosin, × 250 and × 960 (Inset). (Courtesy of Dr Jean Pringle.)

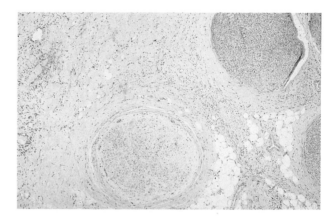

Fig. 14.32 MPNST in the medial cord of the brachial plexus in a patient with NF1. A biopsy of C8, 15 cm proximal to the main tumour mass, shows one bundle completely replaced by tumour and some degenerative changes in adjacent bundles. Haematoxylin and eosin, × 160. (Courtesy of Dr Jean Pringle.)

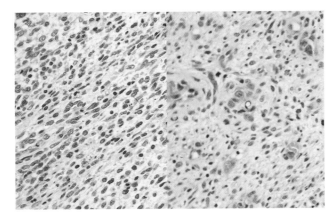

Fig. 14.36 MPNST. The tumour is densely cellular with moderate pleomorphism and high mitotic index. Haematoxylin and eosin, × 400. (Courtesy of Dr Jean Pringle.)

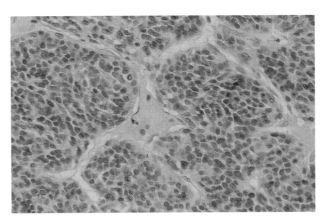

Fig. 14.37 Haemangiopericytoma of the common peroneal nerve showing the characteristic stag horn pattern of the vessels. Haematoxylin and eosin, × 400 (Courtesy of Dr Jean Pringle.)

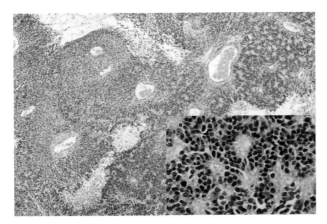

Fig. 14.41 Neuroepithelioma arising from the sciatic nerve in a 14-year-old boy with NF1. There is focal necrosis; viable tissue surrounding the blood vessels. There are areas of rosette formation. Haematoxylin and eosin, × 160 (left) and × 400 (right). (Courtesy of Dr Jean Pringle.)

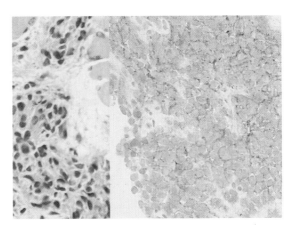

Fig. 14.42 Primitive neuroectodermal tumour arising from the median nerve. The tumour is infiltrating muscle and there is positive staining for MIC 2. Haematoxylin and eosin, left (inset) × 400 and right × 400. (Courtesy of Dr Jean Pringle.)

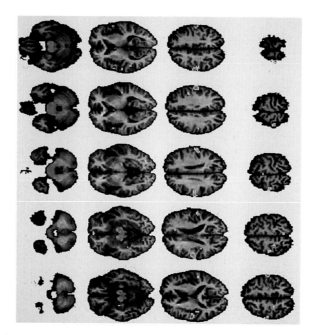

Fig. 15.4 Echo-planar functional magnetic resonance image using a 1.5 Tesla system showing the effects of repetitive stimulation of the left palm of a right-handed volunteer. The yellow areas indicate increased local oxygen concentration, a result of local increase in cerebral activity. There are several areas of activity; the bilateral anterior parietal activation probably represents somato-sensory cortex (by courtesy of Dr Jonathan Berman). Jonathan Berman permits us to refer to other findings as yet unpublished. In one patient with continuing pain, cerebral activity was seen in the midline, in the region of the cingulate cortex. In another case, in which pain disappeared with the return of muscular activity, cerebral activity was much less prominent in the cingulate cortex area.

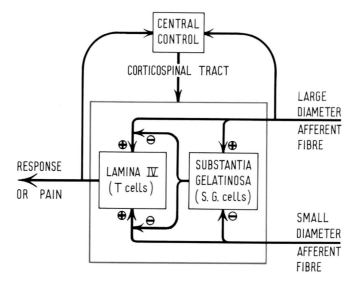

Fig. 15.6 The sensory "gate" mechanism as originally proposed by R. Melzack and P.D. Wall for the modus operandi of the dorsal laminae of grey matter of the spinal cord. See text for a discussion of the effects of an imbalance in the sensory inflow along the large and small diameter afferent fibres. (From an illustration in Melzack and Wall (1965), with permission of the authors and publishers.)

1. The peripheral nervous system

Definition of the nervous system; separation of the central and peripheral nervous systems; gross anatomy of the peripheral nervous system, including cranial and spinal nerves and the autonomic nervous system.

The nervous system is the mechanism through which the organism is kept in touch with its internal structures and external environments and reacts to changes in them. The *central nervous system* – the brain and its caudal prolongation the spinal cord – is connected to the periphery by the *peripheral nervous system*. The latter includes the cranial nerves, the spinal nerves with their roots and rami, the peripheral nerves and the peripheral components of the autonomic nervous system (Gardner & Bunge 1993). The peripheral nerves contain motor fibres (to end plates in skeletal muscle), sensory fibres (from organs and endings in skin, muscle, tendon and joint), and autonomic fibres (to blood vessels, sweat glands and arrectores pilarum muscles). In no other system is so much functional capacity concentrated in so small a volume of tissue. The cervical spinal cord, with a width of about 2 cm and a depth of about 1.5 cm, contains all the apparatus transmitting control of somatic function from the neck down, together with that of control of much visceral function. Because of their greater content of connective tissue, the peripheral nerves have proportionately a lesser functional content, yet severance in an adult's arm of the median nerve of 5 mm diameter effectively ruins the function of the hand and forearm.

The cranial and spinal nerves. Twelve pairs of cranial nerves arise from the brain and brain stem. The second of these, the optic nerves, are in fact prolongations of the central nervous system. Thirty-one pairs of spinal nerves – eight cervical, twelve thoracic, five lumbar, five sacral and one coccygeal – arise from the spinal cord. Each spinal nerve leaves or enters the cord by an anterior, largely motor, root, and a posterior, sensory root (Figs 1.1. and 1.2). Each sensory root splits into several rootlets as it approaches the spinal cord; these enter the cord along the line of the postero-lateral sulcus. The division of the anterior roots into rootlets is less obvious and takes place nearer the cord. Because in the adult the spinal cord extends caudally only so far as the first lumbar vertebral level, the obliquity of the emerging and entering roots in the theca increases from above downwards (Figs 1.3 to 1.5). The theca below the first lumbar level is occupied by the lumbar and sacral roots forming a leash, the appearance of which has been likened to that of a horse's tail (cauda equina).

The nerve cells of the fibres forming the anterior roots are mostly situated in the anterior horn of the grey matter of the spinal cord; those of the fibres of the posterior root are in the root ganglion, situated in or near the intervertebral foramen (see Fig. 1.2). As they approach the foramen, the two roots join to form the nerve, which outside the foramen divides into anterior and posterior *primary rami* (Fig. 1.6). It is with the anterior primary rami and their branches that this study is chiefly concerned.

The autonomic nervous system. Two divisions of the autonomic nervous system – the sympathetic and the parasympathetic – are usually described. In each, preganglionic fibres arise from cells in the brainstem or spinal cord. These relay in ganglia to postganglionic fibres innervating viscera, blood vessels, sweat glands and arrectores pilarum.

The cranial nerves

The first nerve, the olfactory, mediates the sense of smell; the second, the optic, mediates that of sight. The latter nerve is clearly a prolongation of the central nervous system. The third, fourth and sixth nerves control the muscles concerned with movement of the eye. The fifth (trigeminal) nerve has an extensive motor and sensory function, controlling the muscles of the jaw and conveying sensation from the skin of the face and the mucosa of the mouth and nose, and probably from the superficial muscles of the face. Its lingual branch, conveying sensation from the tongue and buccal mucosa, was known to past generations of medical students for provoking critical comment from the duct of the submandibular salivary gland concerning the close relationship of the two structures. The seventh (facial) nerve innervates the superficial muscles of the face and neck. It is remarkable for its vulnerability to damage in each of the three parts of its course – intracranial, intraosseous (in the petrous part of the temporal bone) and extratemporal. The eighth (auditory) nerve mediates the senses of hearing and of balance. The

Figs 1.1 and 1.2 The formation of the spinal nerve.

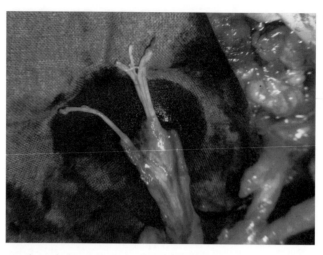

Fig. 1.1 The seventh cervical nerve roots avulsed from the spinal cord. Note the anterior root (left) and the posterior rootlets (right), the posterior root ganglion, the dural sleeve merging into the epineurium, and the spinal nerve itself. The small pieces of tissue on the proximal ends of the anterior root and on one of the posterior rootlets are probably portions of spinal cord.

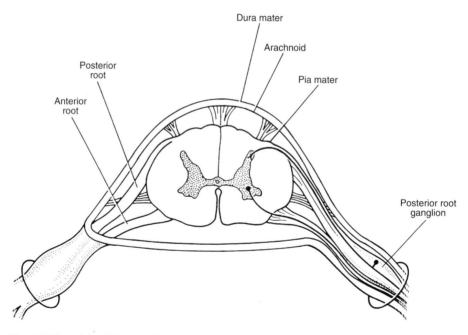

Fig. 1.2 The origin of the roots from the cord, their junction just distal to the posterior root ganglion, and the emergence of the nerve from the spinal canal.

Figs 1.3 to 1.5 The relation of the nerve roots to the spinal cord.

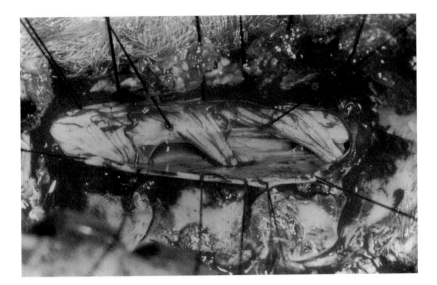

Fig. 1.3 The left side of the spinal cord exposed by hemilaminectomy. The cord has temporarily been rotated by stays passed through the denticulate ligaments. The uppermost roots (left) are those of the fifth cervical nerve: they emerge at an angle of about 45° to the cord. The lowest roots (right) are those of the seventh cervical nerve, emerging at a very oblique angle to the cord.

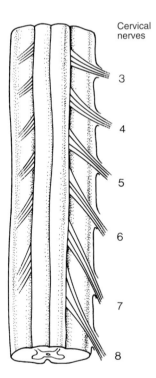

Cervical nerves

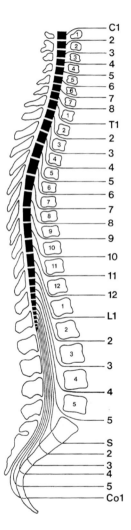

Fig. 1.4 Drawing showing the increasing obliquity of the cervical roots from above down.

Fig. 1.5 Drawing showing the increasing obliquity of the roots in relation to the spinal cord from above down. Below the first lumbar level the spinal canal is occupied by the cauda equina.

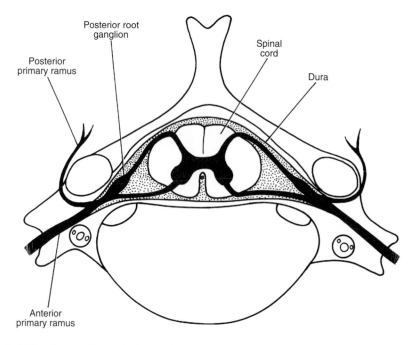

Fig. 1.6 The division of the spinal nerve (cervical region) into anterior and posterior primary rami.

ninth (glossopharyngeal) nerve conveys sensibility from the pharynx and from the back of the tongue and has a small motor function. The tenth (vagus) nerve has, as its name suggests, wide ranging branches and functions, most of the latter being parasympathetic. Motor branches innervate the muscles of the larynx, and sensory branches convey sensation from it. Its recurrent laryngeal branch is in the ascending part of its course in close relationship with the trachea and oesophagus and with the thyroid and parathyroid glands.

The *spinal* part of the eleventh (accessory) nerve arises from cells in the accessory nucleus, "a column of cells of the somatic efferent type, extending from the second to the 5th and 6th cervical segment of the cord" (Brodal 1981a). These cells are in the dorsolateral part of the anterior horn of the grey matter. The fibres emerge segmentally from each side of the cord, to unite to form on each side a nerve which passes rostrally, posterior to the denticulate ligament, into the cranial cavity through the foramen magnum. In the cranial cavity the nerve unites briefly with its cranial part, derived mainly from the nucleus ambiguus, before passing out of the skull with it through the jugular foramen (Fig. 1.7). Outside the skull the two parts separate, the cranial portion going to join the vagus nerve and the spinal part passing obliquely down the neck to innervate the sternocleidomastoid and trapezius muscles.

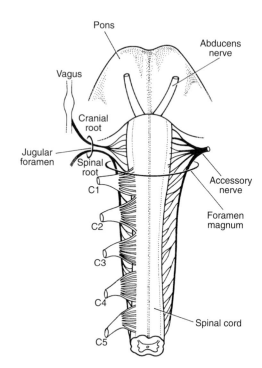

Fig. 1.7 The formation of the eleventh cranial (cranial and spinal accessory) nerve. Note the temporary "cranialisation" of the spinal component of the nerve.

The twelfth (hypoglossal) nerve leaves the skull through the hypoglossal canal in the occipital bone to supply the intrinsic and extrinsic muscles of the tongue. Although there are receptor organs in the muscles of the human tongue (Cooper 1953), it is likely that most of the impulses from them travel in the lingual nerve (Weddell et al 1940). In the upper part of the neck the hypoglossal nerve is joined by fibres from the anterior rami of the uppermost two cervical nerves. These soon leave the nerve to form the *ansa hypoglossi,* from which the infrahyoid muscles are supplied.

THE SPINAL NERVES

The anterior (ventral) primary rami

The anterior primary rami of the uppermost four cervical nerves unite and branch to form the *cervical plexus,* through which the skin of the neck and part of the face and some of the muscles of the neck are innervated (Fig. 1.8). A branch of the fourth cervical anterior ramus, with contributions from the third and fifth rami, passes caudally into the thorax as the phrenic nerve, to supply motor fibres to the diaphragm and sensory fibres to the related pleura and peritoneum (Fig. 1.9).

The anterior primary rami of the lowest four cervical nerves and most of that of the first thoracic nerve unite and branch to form the *brachial plexus* in the lower part of the neck and behind the clavicle (Figs 1.10 and 1.11). The upper limb receives its innervation through the branches of this important plexus. The most proximal muscles are supplied by branches from the rami, the intermediate muscles by branches from the *trunks* and *cords,* and the muscles of the limb itself by branches from the main terminal nerves – the median, ulnar, musculocutaneous, radial and circumflex (Figs 1.12 to 1.16). There is a segmental pattern to this innervation: the most proximal muscles are supplied by branches of the uppermost rami; the most

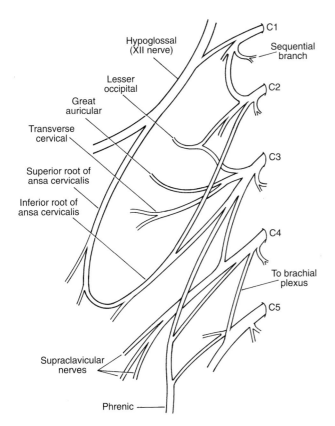

Fig. 1.8 The cervical plexus and its (mainly sensory) branches.

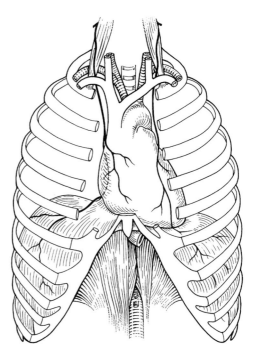

Fig. 1.9 The course of the phrenic nerve. Note the small branch to the pericardium.

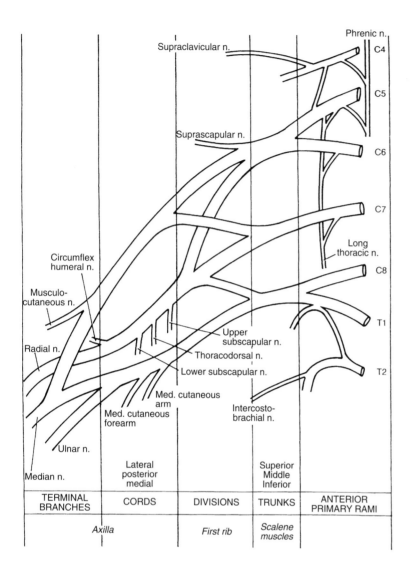

TERMINAL BRANCHES	CORDS	DIVISIONS	TRUNKS	ANTERIOR PRIMARY RAMI
	Lateral posterior medial		Superior Middle Inferior	
Axilla		*First rib*	*Scalene muscles*	

Fig. 1.10 The brachial plexus. Note the sequence: the anterior primary rami; trunks; divisions; cords; nerves. Note that the trunks are upper, middle and lower, and that the cords are lateral, medial and posterior (from their position in relation to the axillary artery).

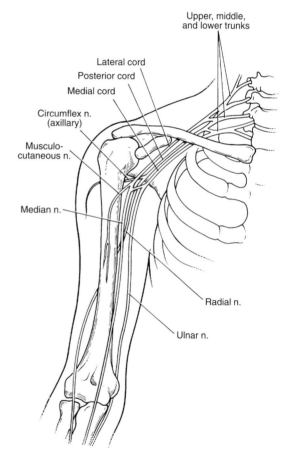

Fig. 1.11 The relation of the brachial plexus to the axial skeleton, the forequarter and the arm.

distal muscles are supplied by branches derived from the eighth cervical and first thoracic nerves. The segmental pattern of innervation is shown more clearly in the cutaneous supply (Fig. 1.17). The cervical root supply has been, as it were, extruded from the supply to the trunk. Thus, in the transition of innervation from the skin of the neck to that of the trunk there is anteriorly a change from the fourth cervical to the second thoracic segment; posteriorly, there is a change from the fifth cervical to the first thoracic segment. The supply of the skin of the hand is divided between the median, ulnar and radial nerves. The first two supply the palmar aspect; all supply the dorsal aspect. The median nerve supplies the skin of the radial side of the palm, the palmar aspects of the thumb, index and middle fingers and of the radial part of the ring finger, and the terminal parts of the dorsal aspect

Figs 1.12 to 1.16 The nerves of the upper limb.
Figs 1.12 to 1.15 Motor distribution.

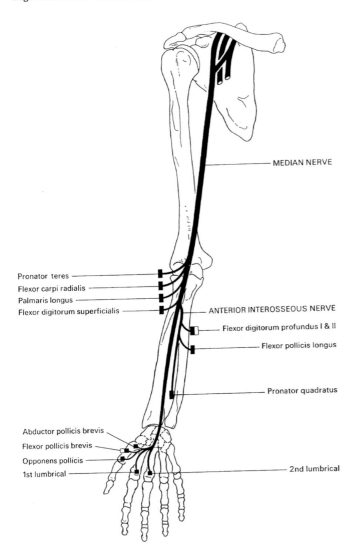

Fig. 1.12 The median nerve.

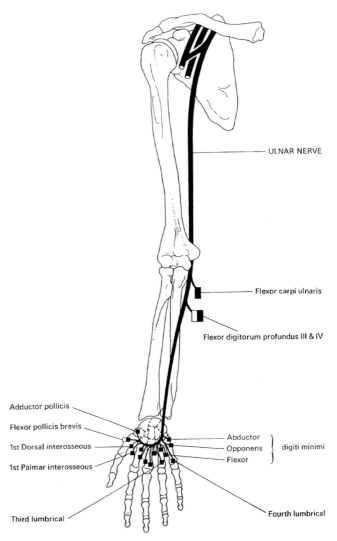

Fig. 1.13 The ulnar nerve.

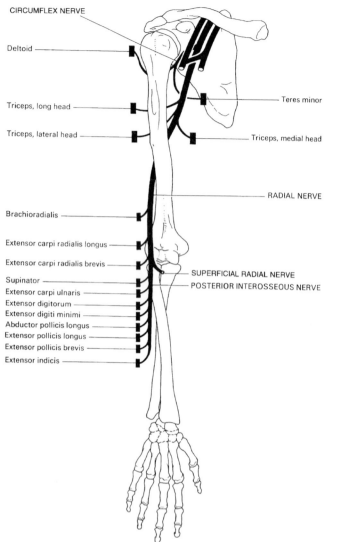

Fig. 1.14 The radial nerve.

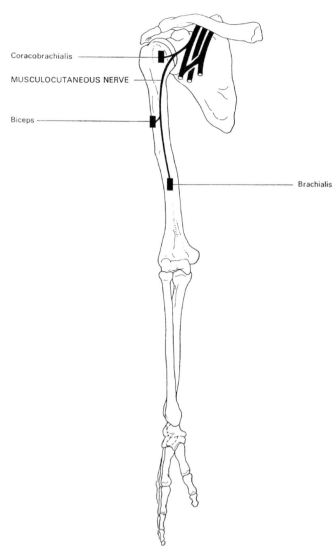

Fig. 1.15 The musculocutaneous nerve.

of these digits. The ulnar nerve supplies the skin of the ulnar side of the palm, the palmar aspects of the little finger and the ulnar part of the ring finger, and the dorsal aspect of the ulnar half of the hand, the little and ring fingers and the ulnar side of the proximal part of the middle finger. The radial nerve supplies the radial side of the dorsum of the hand, of the proximal parts of the thumb and index fingers and of the radial side of the middle finger (Figs 1.18 and 1.19).

An important anatomical and functional differentiation of the plexus takes place with the division of the trunks into anterior and posterior *divisions* (see Fig. 1.10). From the anterior divisions the lateral and medial cords are formed; from the posterior divisions the posterior cord is formed. The lateral and medial cords innervate *pre-axial* (flexor) musculature; the posterior cord innervates *post-axial* (extensor) musculature.

The plexus and the distribution of its nerves vary considerably from one individual to another: the contributions made by the component nerves vary; the origin and method of formation of the main nerves vary; in some cases the contribution of the fifth nerve is large and that of the first thoracic nerve is small, while in others the reverse is the case. The truly autonomous area of cutaneous

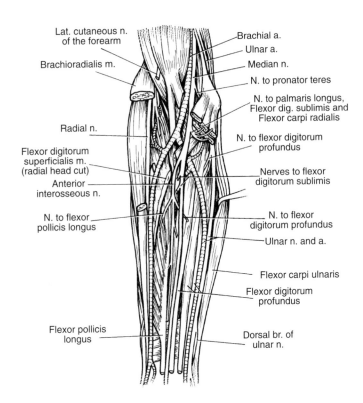

Fig. 1.16 The main nerves at the elbow and in the upper part of the forearm. Note the relation of the deep origin of the pronator teres to the median nerve and the ulnar artery.

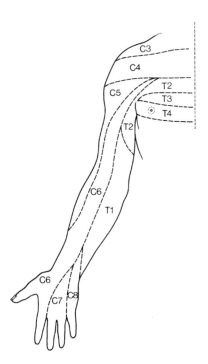

Fig. 1.17 The segmental supply of the skin of the neck, upper chest and upper limb.

supply of each main component nerve is small and variable in extent and location. The contributions made by the fourth cervical and second thoracic nerves vary: usually their contributions are small, but occasionally the fourth cervical nerve makes an important contribution to the innervation of scapulohumeral muscles. An important anomaly affects the median and ulnar nerves in the forearm. This is the "Martin–Gruber" anastomosis. Gruber (1870), having dissected the forearm of 125 cadavers, reported an incidence of 15.2%. Most commonly, a branch runs from the anterior interosseous branch of the median nerve to the ulnar nerve, but Srinivasan and Rhodes (1981) recognise six varieties of anomaly (Fig. 1.20). These workers dissected 24 "normal" and 30 congenitally abnormal fetuses, and reckoned that the anomaly occurred in about 15% of the population. It occurred bilaterally in all eight of the foetuses with trisomy 21 examined. The presence of a Martin–Gruber anastomosis produces particular findings on electromyographic examination in cases of carpal tunnel syndrome (Guttmann 1977).

Figs 1.18 and 1.19 The nerve supply of the skin of the hand.

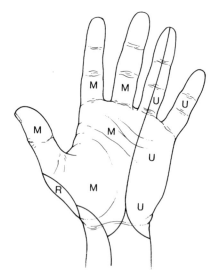

Fig. 1.18 Palmar aspect.

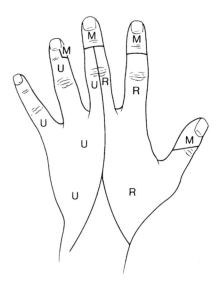

Fig. 1.19 Dorsal aspect.

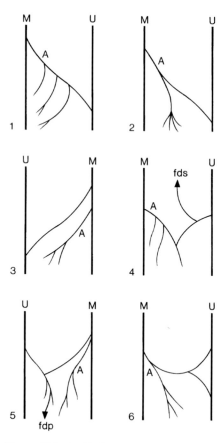

Fig. 1.20 Types of Martin–Gruber anastomosis. M, median nerve; U, ulnar nerve; A, anterior interosseous nerve; fdp, flexor digitorum profundus; fds, flexor digitorum superficialis. (After Srinavasan R, Rhodes J 1981 Archives of Neurology 38: 418–419.)

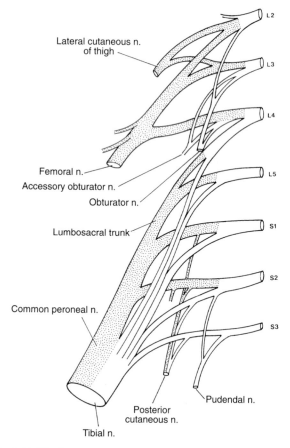

Fig. 1.21 The femoral and sacral plexus. The dorsal divisions are shaded.

Thoracic anterior primary rami

The second to the sixth thoracic anterior primary rami innervate the intercostal muscles and the skin of the chest. Most of the first nerve goes to join the brachial plexus; most of the second goes as the intercostobrachial nerve to innervate the skin of the axilla and of the medial side of the arm. The lower six thoracic anterior rami continue from the intercostal spaces to the anterior wall of the abdomen, innervating its skin and muscles. The lowest nerves supply sensory fibres to the diaphragm. The lowest (twelfth) thoracic ventral ramus, sometimes called the subcostal nerve, is larger than the others and connects with the iliohypogastric branch of the first lumbar nerve.

Lumbar and sacral anterior primary rami

The first lumbar anterior primary ramus gives rise to two mainly cutaneous nerves and part of a third. The iliohypogastric, ilioinguinal and genitofemoral nerves supply, respectively, the skin of part of the buttock, of the groin and external genitalia.

The second, third and fourth lumbar anterior rami unite and branch to form the *lumbar plexus* (Fig. 1.21) from which arise the nerves innervating the skin of the thigh and its anterior and medial muscles. The plexus is in the anterior part of the psoas major muscle, in the posterior wall of the abdomen. Its terminal branches lie under the parietal peritoneum. Some of these emerge lateral and some medial to the psoas major (Fig. 1.22). The most important terminal branch is the femoral nerve, which passes, lateral to the psoas major and femoral vessels, under the inguinal ligament to reach the upper part of the thigh. Through its anterior and posterior divisions it supplies the skin of the anterior surface of the thigh and the quadriceps and sartorius muscles. The saphenous branch of the posterior division descends with the femoral artery to emerge from the femoral canal above the knee

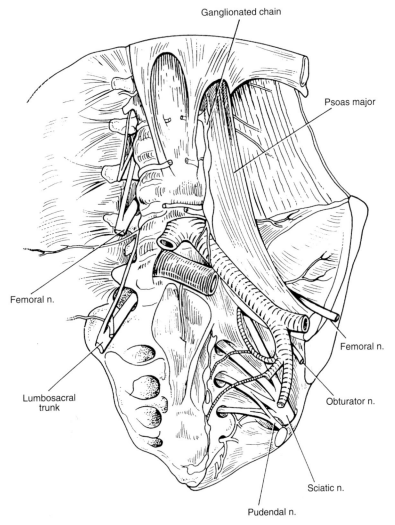

Ganglionated chain

Psoas major

Femoral n.

Femoral n.

Lumbosacral trunk

Obturator n.

Sciatic n.

Pudendal n.

Fig. 1.22 The relations of the lumbar and sacral plexus. Note the lumbosacral trunk entering the upper part of the sacral plexus. (After Frazer J E 1920. The Anatomy of the Human Skeleton. J & A Churchill)

and supply the skin of the medial side of the leg and foot. The obturator nerve emerges medial to the psoas major and, passing along the lateral wall of the pelvis, emerges into the thigh through the obturator foramen. Through anterior and posterior branches the adductor muscles and the skin of the medial side of the thigh are supplied.

Part of the fourth lumbar ramus and all the fifth ventral ramus join to form the *lumbosacral trunk*, which emerges medial to the psoas major to enter the pelvis and join the first, second and third sacral nerves to form the *sacral plexus* on the posterolateral wall of the pelvis (Figs 1.21 and 1.22). The innervation of the perineum and most of the lower limb is derived from the branches of this plexus. The sciatic nerve, the largest in the body, leaves the pelvis

through the greater sciatic foramen and passes behind the hip joint into the back of the thigh, where it innervates the hamstring muscles (Fig. 1.23). Its tibial branch descends in the midline through the popliteal fossa into the back of the leg, to supply its superficial and deep muscles (Fig. 1.24). Its important and frequently useful branch, the sural nerve, arises in the upper part of the popliteal fossa, descends between the two heads of gastrocnemius and pierces the deep fascia in the proximal part of the leg. Usually, a branch from the common peroneal nerve joins the sural nerve; at times, it is larger than the contribution from the tibial nerve. Rarely, the sural nerve arises wholly from the common peroneal division. The nerve then descends to pass lateral to the tendo calcaneus to supply

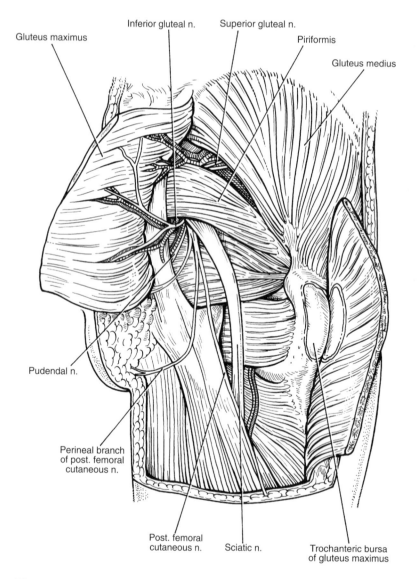

Fig. 1.23 The right sciatic nerve emerging from the pelvis and entering the buttock.

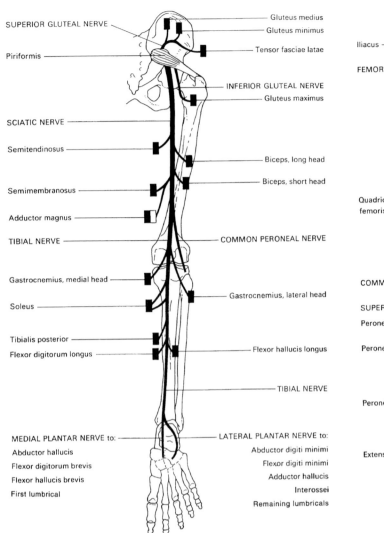

Fig. 1.24 The course and motor distribution of the sciatic and tibial nerves.

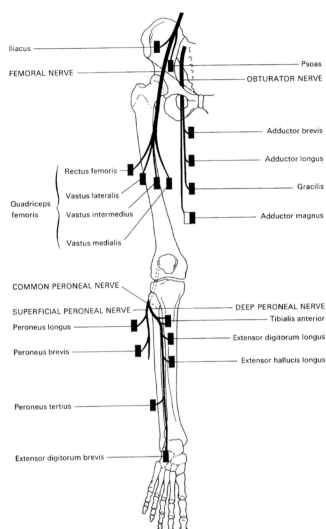

Fig. 1.25 The course and distribution of the femoral and common peroneal nerves.

the skin on the lateral side of the foot. The tibial nerve continues into the foot behind the medial malleolus, and through its terminal medial and lateral plantar branches supplies the intrinsic muscles of the foot and the skin of the sole. The common peroneal nerve diverges laterally from the midline to pass behind the head of the fibula and lateral to its neck (Fig. 1.25). Here it divides into deep and superficial peroneal nerves. The former (anterior tibial) passes into the anterior compartment of the leg to innervate the anterior muscles, and finally to supply the extensor digitorum brevis and the skin of the dorsum of the first interdigital space. The superficial peroneal (musculocutaneous) nerve passes deep to the upper part of the peroneus longus muscle to supply both peronei. Its

continuation pierces the deep fascia in the distal part of the leg to supply the skin of the dorsum of the foot and anterolateral part of the ankle.

The more proximal branches of the sacral plexus supply the gluteal muscles and the skin and muscles of the perineum. The superior gluteal nerve, emerging above the piriformis muscle (Fig. 1.23) supplies the short gluteal muscles and the tensor fasciae latae. The inferior gluteal nerve, emerging below the piriformis muscle (Fig. 1.23), supplies the gluteus maximus muscle. The pudendal nerve leaves the pelvis through the greater sciatic foramen and, entering the pudendal canal through the lesser sciatic foramen, passes into the perineum to innervate its skin and muscles. As in the case of the upper limb, there is a

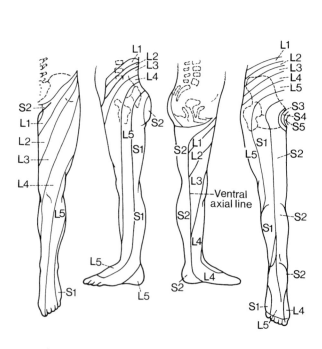

Fig. 1.26 Segmental innervation of the skin of the lower limb.

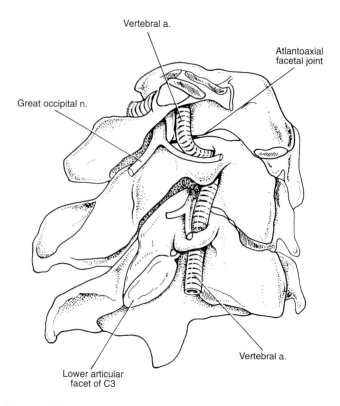

Fig. 1.27 The uppermost three cervical vertebrae and the great occipital nerve.

segmental innervation of the muscles and, more easily seen, of the skin. Again, the segments innervating the limb have been extruded from the innervation of the trunk and perineum, so that in the transition from trunk to perineum there is posteriorly a segmental change from the third lumbar to the third sacral dermatome (Gardner and Bunge 1993). Brodal (1981e) gives an alternative view (Fig. 1.26). The skin of the foot is supplied by all the main nerves of the lower limb save the obturator. The plantar surface is supplied by the tibial nerve, through its plantar branches; the medial side is supplied by the saphenous branch of the femoral nerve, the lateral side by the sural branch of the tibial nerve, and the dorsum by the superficial peroneal and anterior tibial branches of the common peroneal nerve.

The posterior primary rami

The posterior primary rami are usually smaller than the anterior ones. They run posteriorly. Most divide into medial and lateral branches to supply the muscles and skin of the posterior part of the neck and trunk. They do not enter the limbs.

The posterior primary rami of the uppermost three spinal nerves differ from those of the lowest five in extending their supply to the back of the head. The posterior ramus of the first nerve, actually larger than the anterior ramus, chiefly supplies muscles between the atlas and occiput. The posterior ramus of the second cervical nerve, the ganglion of which is extruded, is the largest of the cervical posterior rami and larger than its anterior ramus. Emerging between the posterior arch of the atlas and the lamina of the axis, it divides into a large medial and a smaller lateral branch. The former goes on as the great occipital nerve to innervate the skin of the back of the scalp. At its beginning, it is in close relationship with the back of the atlantoaxial joint (Fig. 1.27). The third cervical posterior ramus provides a *third occipital* branch. The posterior rami of the lowest five cervical nerves innervate the posterior vertebral muscles; the medial branches of the fourth and fifth rami reach the skin.

The thoracic posterior primary rami similarly pass posteriorly close to the posterolateral (zygapophyseal) intervertebral joints to supply posterior vertebral muscles and the skin of the back of the chest. The lumbar posterior rami are similarly disposed, but only the uppermost three reach the skin. The sacral posterior rami are small, having a small distribution to muscle and to the skin of the back of the sacrum.

THE AUTONOMIC NERVOUS SYSTEM

Conventionally, the autonomic nervous system is divided into two parts – the sympathetic and the parasympathetic nervous systems. Langley (1926) proposed the *enteric* nervous system as a third component. Indeed, the complexity and extent of the innervation of the viscera are such as to make this further division attractive (Furness & Costa 1980). Both systems are characterised by having relays between their cells of origin and their terminations: in the case of the sympathetic system the relays are in paravertebral or axial ganglia; in the case of the parasympathetic system they are in or near the organs innervated.

The sympathetic system

The preganglionic cells of the efferent fibres of the sympathetic system are in the lateral part of the grey matter of the spinal cord from the first thoracic to the second lumbar level. The ganglia are in the paravertebral sympathetic chains extending from the top to the bottom of the spinal column. Usually there are on each side two cervical, one cervicothoracic (stellate), eleven thoracic, four lumbar and five sacral or pelvic ganglia. Preganglionic fibres enter the cervicothoracic, thoracic and upper two lumbar ganglia in *white rami* from the first thoracic to the second lumbar

spinal nerve. These fibres relay in the corresponding ganglia or proceed up or down the chain to relay in other ganglia of the chain or in one of the ganglia of the autonomic plexuses. The distribution to the spinal nerves is by way of *grey rami* from the corresponding paravertebral ganglia (Fig. 1.28). Fibres pass directly from the visceral plexuses to their destinations. Afferent fibres have their cells in the posterior root ganglia; their sites of relay are not clearly identified; indeed, they may not relay at all.

The sympathetic supply to the head and neck arises mainly from the uppermost three thoracic segments, passes cranially, and relays in the cervical ganglia to be distributed to vessels and sweat glands and, in particular, to the dilator of the pupil, and the orbitales and levator palpebrae superioris muscles. Most of the supply to these muscles of the eye arises from the first thoracic segment.

The sympathetic supply to the upper limb arises principally from the second to the sixth thoracic segments. Fibres pass up the chain to the middle cervical and cervicothoracic stellate ganglia, where they relay to be distributed by grey rami to the nerves of origin of the brachial plexus (Fig. 1.29).

The sympathetic supply to the lower limbs arises from the lowest three thoracic and uppermost two lumbar segments. Fibres enter the first and second lumbar ganglia by white rami, descend in the chain, relay and are distributed by grey rami to the lumbar and sacral nerves.

The main visceral plexuses are the cardiac, oesophageal, coeliac, mesenteric and hypogastric. They are fed from the cervical and cervicothoracic ganglia, from the middle and

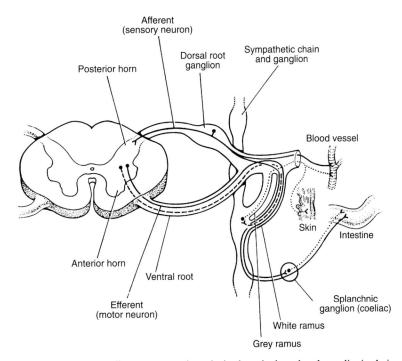

Fig. 1.28 Efferent and afferent autonomic paths in the spinal cord and ganglionic chain.

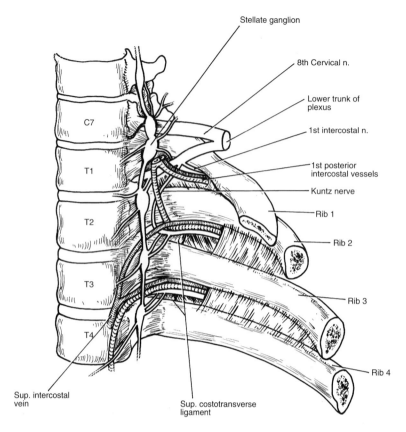

Fig. 1.29 The relations of the cervicothoracic (stellate) ganglion.

lower thoracic ganglia (the splanchnic nerves), from the lumbar ganglia (the lumbar splanchnic nerves) and from the sacral ganglia. Both sympathetic and parasympathetic systems contribute to these plexuses, the vagus (tenth cranial) nerve being the principal source of parasympathetic fibres. The effect of efferent sympathetic activity is to cause sweating, to constrict small vessels and to cause contraction of the arrectores pilarum muscles. The visceral actions are to stimulate the action of the heart and to cause sphincteric contraction.

The parasympathetic nervous system

The efferent outflow of the parasympathetic nervous system arises from nuclei in the midbrain, the hindbrain, the brainstem and the sacral part of the spinal cord. The preganglionic fibres are distributed by the third, seventh, ninth and tenth cranial nerves and by the second to the fourth sacral spinal nerves. From the last arise the *pelvic splanchnic nerves*. The ganglia in which the preganglionic fibres relay are in or near the organs supplied. The effect of parasympathetic activity is inhibitory in the heart, motor to the muscle of the bladder and bowel and dilator in small vessels. The central control of both sympathetic

and parasympathetic function is exercised from nuclei in the hypothalamus, which themselves receive input from higher centres. The fibres from the hypothalamus almost certainly descend in a column in the lateral part of the white matter of the spinal cord (Nathan & Smith 1987).

Afferent autonomic pathways

Autonomic afferent fibres have their cells of origin in the posterior root ganglia and in some cranial ganglia. Their peripheral processes run with efferent fibres, terminating in receptor endings in the walls of viscera and vessels. Impulses from these endings do not necessarily obtrude on consciousness, but evidently mediate sensations such as hunger, distension of the bladder and, perhaps, pain. Most, presumably, are concerned with the initiation of visceral reflexes. Schott (1994) has recently re-examined the role of afferent autonomic pathways in the transmission of painful impulses, and has proposed a return to Langley's (1903) concept of the unitary nature of the sensory system. In particular, he proposes the inclusion of autonomic afferents from the peripheral organs, such as blood vessels, with those from organs in the head, neck, thorax and abdomen under the general heading "visceral afferents".

2. The microscopic structure of the nervous system

The microscopic structure of the peripheral nervous system: the transitional zone; the neuron; the axon–myelin sheath–Schwann cell complex; conduction and the myelin sheath; axonal transport; blood supply; changes with ageing.

The essential component of the system is the cell body with its dendrites and its prolongation, the axon (Figs 2.1 and 2.2). Young (1945) characterised the nerve cell as "a very long cylinder of a semi fluid nature". It is a column of neuronal cytoplasm, the *axoplasm*, enclosed by a cell membrane, the axolemma. Thomas et al (1993a) described the axoplasm a "fluid cytosol in which are suspended formed elements". The most conspicuous of the latter is the cytoskeleton consisting of microtubules, neurofilaments and matrix. In addition, there are mitochondria, axoplasmic reticulum, lamellar and multivesicular bodies, and membranous cisterns, tubes and vesicles. It is the cytoskeleton that provides the apparatus for axoplasmic transport (Hollenbeck 1989). The axon consists of a column of cytoplasm, which has a viscosity about five times that of water (Haak et al 1976), enclosed by its cell membrane, the axolemma.

In *Neuron Theory or Reticular Theory*?, Ramon y Cajal (1954) asserts that "the neuron, a nerve cell with its processes, is the structural unit of nervous tissue, and the neurons are the only elements in the nervous system which conduct nervous impulses" (Brodal 1981b). There is no continuity between nerve cells; the termination of the axon on a cell is no more than a contact. Brodal (1981b) goes on: "not only is the neuron a structural unit; it also, in most cases, behaves as a trophic unit…".

In the central nervous system the neurons are supported in a network of oligodendrocyte and astrocyte processes, with very little extracellular space. The structure of peripheral nervous tissue is one of nerve fibres (axons – Schwann cell units) suspended in a collagen-rich extracellular space (Berthold et al 1993). The transition from central to peripheral nervous structure takes place in the rootlets or, less often, in the roots of the spinal nerves. This is the *transitional region* or *transitional zone*. The extension of the central nervous system structure into the base of the rootlet is cone-shaped (Fig. 2.3). Thus, "each transitional region can be subdivided into an axial central nervous system compartment and a surrounding peripheral nervous system compartment" (Berthold et al 1993). The axons traverse this zone, but the blood vessels of the nerves do not accompany them into the central tissues. Most of the fibres of the anterior roots have their cells in the anterior horn of the grey matter. They can, perhaps, be regarded as outposts of the peripheral system in the central system. The fibres of the posterior roots have their cells in the posterior root ganglion: possibly, outposts of the central in the peripheral nervous system? These neurons are "pseudo-unipolar in form with a single axon and no true dendrites" (Thomas et al 1993c) (Figs 2.4 and 2.5; see also Plate section). Each axon bifurcates into peripherally and centrally directed axons after leaving the cell body at a variable distance from the cell. The centrally directed branch is of smaller calibre than the peripheral one. The central processes enter the spinal cord along the postero-lateral sulcus. In the cord the fibres bifurcate into ascending and descending branches. The branches of the smaller fibres in the lateral part of the root reach the posterior horn of the grey matter, where they soon terminate having traversed between three and five segments. The branches of the larger fibres in the medial part of the root, mostly myelinated, similarly bifurcate after entering the white matter just medial to the posterior horn. Some ascending fibres reach as high as the gracile and cuneate nuclei in the caudal part of the medulla. Other fibres of this group have short ascending and descending branches, which enter the grey matter of the posterior horn to establish synapses with nerve cells in its different laminae (Fig. 2.6).

Unmyelinated afferent fibres certainly enter the spinal cord in the anterior roots (Coggeshall et al 1974). They may be concerned with the transmission of painful impulses (Clifton et al 1976), though White and Sweet (1969) failed to produce pain in man by stimulation of anterior roots. Our own observations are recorded in Chapter 3.

In the peripheral nervous system the axons are closely associated with the Schwann cells (Schwann 1839) or *lemmocytes* (Greek λεμμα {lemma} a rind or husk). The larger axons are enwrapped along their length by a continuous series of contiguous Schwann cells into which they are invaginated (Fig. 2.7). The *nodes of Ranvier* represent

Figs 2.1 and 2.2 The nerve cell unit.

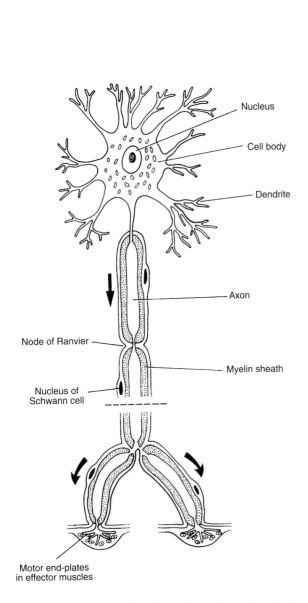

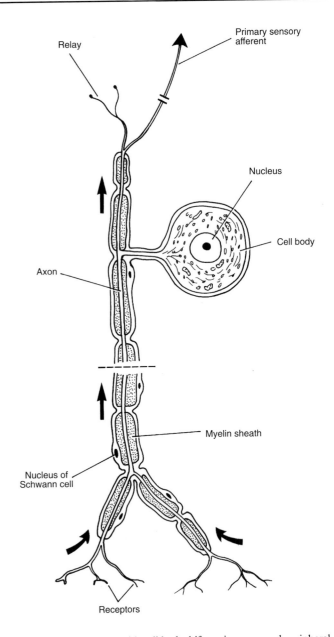

Fig. 2.1 A motor unit, with cell body (perikaryon), dendrites, axon, myelin sheath, Schwann cells, nodes of Ranvier and end plates.

Fig. 2.2 A sensory unit, with cell body, bifurcating axon and peripheral and central connections.

the points of contiguity of adjacent Schwann cells (Figs 2.8 and 2.9). The fibre is contained within a basal lamina or basement membrane. The smaller fibres are contained in bundles by similar columns of Schwann cells (Fig. 2.10). Eames and Gamble (1970) showed the ensheathing arrangement of successive Schwann cells which overlapped and interdigitated.

It is probably the diameter of the axon that determines whether the Schwann cells will lay down a myelin sheath around it. The sheath is laid down in spiral layers by the Schwann cell, or part of its surface, moving around the axon (Webster 1993). The multilamellar sheath has a high lipid content and some protein components. Of the latter, the major component is the Po glycoprotein (Greenfield et

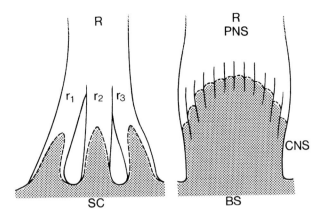

Fig. 2.3 The transitional zone between the central and peripheral nervous systems. R, root; r_1-r_3, rootlets; SC, spinal cord; BS, brainstem; PNS, peripheral nervous system; CNS, central nervous system. (After Berthold et al 1993.)

Figs 2.4 and 2.5 Sensory cells in a posterior root ganglion avulsed from the spinal cord with its spinal root.

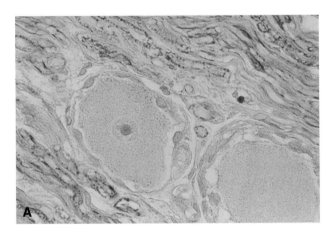
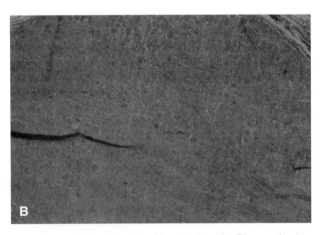

Fig. 2.4 Dorsal root ganglion 6 months after avulsion from the spinal cord. Solochrome cyanin, (a) × 960; (b) × 200 (see also Plate section.)

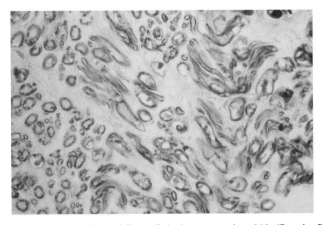

Fig. 2.5 Specimen showing myelinated fibres. Solochrome cyanin × 960. (See also Plate section.)

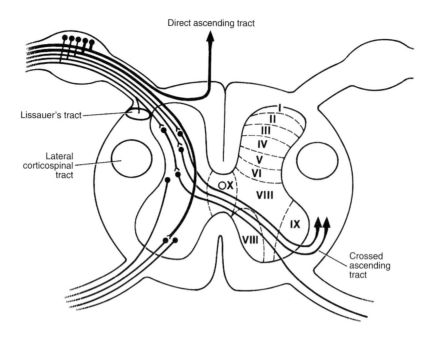

Fig. 2.6 The paths of the afferent fibres entering and efferent fibres leaving the spinal cord. Note (right) the laminae of the grey matter.

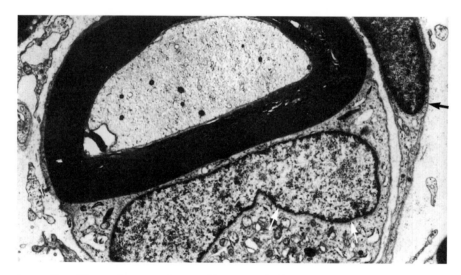

Fig. 2.7 A large myelinated nerve fibre. The axoplasm contains neurofilaments and a few neurotubules. The light arrows mark Schwann cell nuclei. The Schwann cell cytoplasm contains many mitochondria. Heavy arrow indicates fibroblast. × 9350.

al 1973, Linington & Brostoff 1993). The myelin sheath is traversed by cytoplasmic channels – the incisures of Schmidt–Lanterman.

The axon–myelin sheath–Schwann cell complexes are arranged in bundles. In so small a nerve as the fourth cranial there may be as many as 3400 fibres. In the roots inside the spinal canal endoneurial collagen is scanty, in contrast with the abundant content in the nerves outside the foramen (Eames & Gamble 1964, Gamble 1964) (Fig. 2.11). The surgeon who has had dealings with nerves inside and outside the spinal canal will appreciate the distinction: the spinal roots and rootlets are fine and fragile and very susceptible to trauma; the peripheral nerves are strong and have much greater resistance to the trauma of handling.

Figs 2.8 and 2.9 The node of Ranvier.

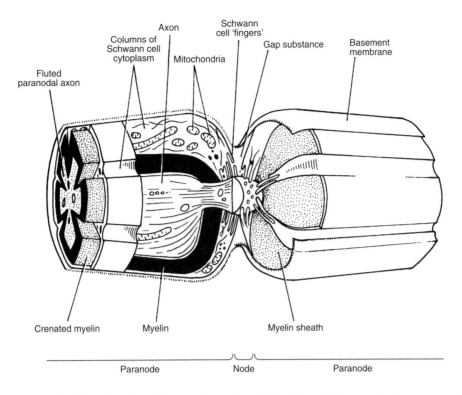

Fig. 2.8 An expanded view of a node of Ranvier of a myelinated fibre. Note the "garlic-bulb" appearance of a fibre at the node and the Schwann cell basement membrane.

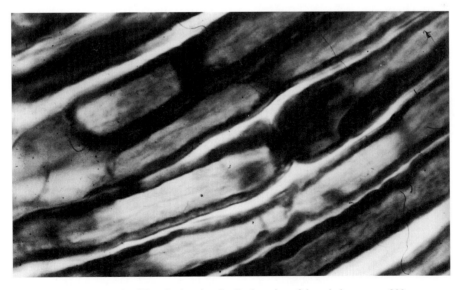

Fig. 2.9 A node of Ranvier in a longitudinal section of the sciatic nerve. × 800.

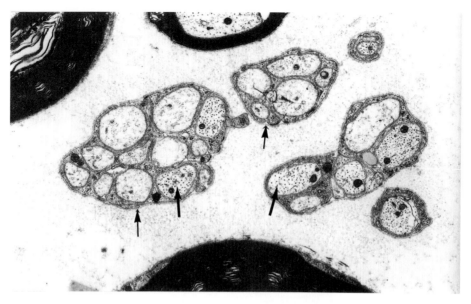

Fig. 2.10 Cluster of unmyelinated nerve fibres (bold arrows), enveloped by Schwann cell cytoplasm. Light arrows indicate basement membrane of Schwann cells. × 26 220.

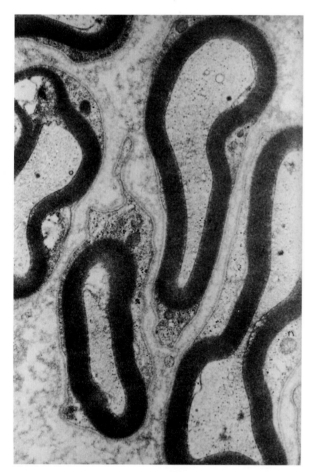

Fig. 2.11 Myelinated nerve fibres in the posterior root (electron micrograph). Note the sparsity of the endoneurial tissue and, in particular, the well-marked basement membranes of the Schwann cells. × 5500.

Outside the intervertebral foramina the three supporting structures, the epi-, peri- and endoneurium, are clearly established (Fig. 2.12). The *epineurium*, in effect the prolongation of the dural sleeve of the nerve roots, is composed of longitudinally directed collagen fibres and fibroblasts (Gamble & Eames 1964). The *perineurium* which ensheaths the bundles, is composed of flattened cell processes alternating with layers of collagen (Gamble and Eames 1964). It provides a barrier to diffusion (Thomas 1963). In the *endoneurium*, supporting the fibres themselves, there is a return to longitudinal direction of cells and fibres; there are abundant collagen fibrils, and some pockets of collagen are invaginated into Schwann cells (Thomas 1963; Gamble and Eames 1964). Thomas (1963) has estimated that 45% of nuclei seen in transverse sections of nerves are those of fibroblasts. Sunderland (1968) mapped the arrangement of bundles along the course of nerve trunks, showing branching, fusion, and changes in number. He and Bradley (Sunderland and Bradley 1949) further showed that the cross-sectional area of the nerve occupied by connective tissue was variable, ranging from 60% to 85%.

These findings, especially those concerning rearrangement of bundles, have been used to cast doubt on the feasibility of achieving accurate co-aptation of the ends of divided nerves. However, in his studies of the median and ulnar nerves, Sunderland (1965) acknowledged that there was a degree of topographical segregation of nerve fibres according to function over considerable lengths of the trunks. Microneurographic studies (Torebjörk & Ochoa 1980) confirmed these findings. Specific organisation (aggregation) of sensory and motor fibres occurs in the

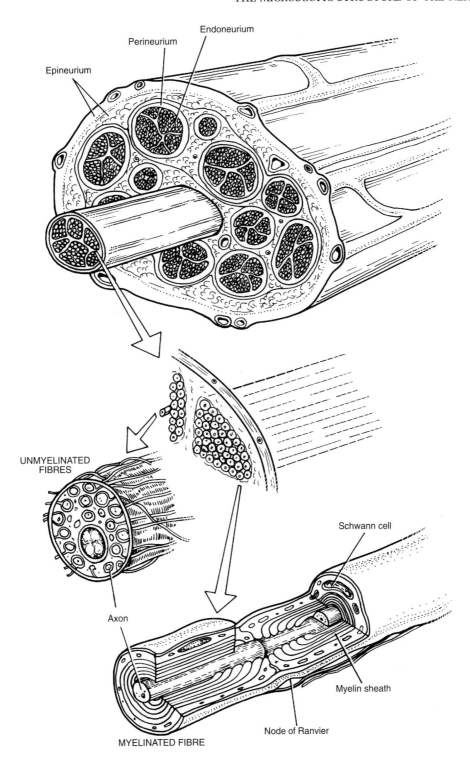

Fig. 2.12 Fascicular arrangement of nerve fibres; supporting structures; and Schwann cell apparatus in myelinated and unmyelinated fibres. (After Lundborg 1988b.)

median nerve in the arm. This segregation permits transfers such as Oberlin's (Oberlin et al 1995), in which one bundle of the ulnar nerve is anastomosed to the nerve to the biceps. Stimulation of individual bundles, the number of which ranges from six to twelve, permits separation of those passing to the flexor muscles of the wrist and fingers from those passing to the small muscles of the hand.

The calibre of myelinated axons varies from 0.4 to 1.25 μm (Gasser 1955); that of myelinated fibres varies from 2 to 22 μm (Ranson 1915, Greenfield & Carmichael 1935, Sunderland et al 1949). The largest, fastest conducting elements are the myelinated fibres of around 20 μm diameter concerned with somatic afferent and efferent activity; the smallest and slowest conducting are the fibres of around I μm diameter that subserve autonomic activity and delayed pain sensibility. The special property of the nerve fibres is that of conducting a signal in the form of a propagated action potential (Landon 1985). In the unmyelinated fibre, a wave of depolarisation spreads continuously along the axon, attenuated by the large capacitance of the axolemma, which limits the velocity of conduction to about 1 m/s. In the myelinated fibre the insulating property of myelin restricts electrical activity to the nodes of Ranvier, so that the impulse has to travel in leaps from one node to the next – the so-called saltatory conduction of Huxley and Stämpfli (1949). Speed of conduction is much increased by this mechanism. Rasminsky (1985) thinks of myelination as an evolutionary response to the need for rapid increase in conduction velocity, which otherwise would require large increases in axonal diameter. Evidently, demyelination is bound to lead to decrease of conduction velocity (McDonald 1963, McDonald & Sears 1970) and eventually to conduction block.

Axonal transport

Young (1993) describes the genesis of the idea of axonal transport, and his part in its discovery. The axon functions as part of the neuron as a whole in transporting materials to and from the cell body. Lasek (1982) goes further than this: "neurons exhibit a remarkable form of locomotion when they extend axons over great distances without moving the cell body. This capacity of neurons to extend axons independently of the movement of the perikaryon is one of the distinctive properties of the neuronal linkage, because it distinguishes neurons from other migratory cell types". Lasek (1982) further proposes that the unusual feature of neurons – their ability to translocate the axonal skeleton independently of the perikaryon – is accomplished by the continuous addition of cytoskeletal proteins at the proximal end of the cytoskeleton in the perikaryon. So, the neuron is able to extend its process "without towing the cell body along". Two forms of transport, fast and slow,

are recognised (Ochs and Brimijoin 1993). The former may be orthograde (centrifugal) or retrograde (centripetal) (Fig. 2.13). Membranous elements are conveyed centrifugally from the cell to the terminal in the form of membrane proteins, secretory proteins and peptides. They resupply the neurotransmitter release system at the end of the axons. "The retrograde fast component recovers membranes from the terminal by endocytosis and conveys this material in the form of multivesicular bodies to the lysosomal system in the cell body" (Lasek 1982). The rates of fast transport are from 200 to 400 mm/day. Landon (1985) puts it this way: fast transport "is concerned with the orthograde transport of particular constituents of the axoplasm and materials such as some transmitter-synthesizing enzymes, glycoproteins and membrane components, and the retrograde transport of membranous prelysosomal structures, and extra cellular materials such as nerve growth factor ingested at the axon terminal." The process is sensitive to temperature; it is sensitive to deprivation of oxygen. Doubtless, the failure of conduction produced by even transient ischaemia is caused by interference with this mechanism. Fast transport may continue briefly after axonotomy (Brady et al 1982); action potentials are not involved in its regulation.

Slow transport is unidirectional, orthograde (centrifugal). Rates of transport are from 1 to 4 mm/day; it is concerned with the transport of the neurotubule–neurofilament network of the cytoskeleton (Hollenbeck 1989). The mechanisms have been examined by Wilson and Stone (1979) and others. The rate of transport is, of course, about the

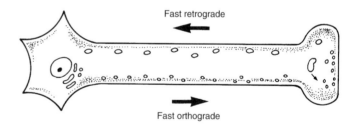

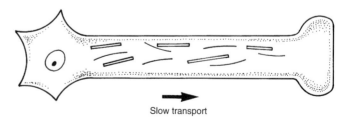

Fig. 2.13 Diagram of axonal transport. (After Lasek 1982.)

same as the rate of peripheral regeneration after axonotomy. The significance of axonal transport in disorders of peripheral nerves is plain: interference with the process is likely to lead to defect or cessation of conduction, and at length to degeneration of the nerve cell.

The blood supply of nerves

Nerves have a very good blood supply: they need it. The surgeon notes the segmental blood supply from without and the axial vessels within the nerve. There are indeed (Lundborg 1988b) *intrinsic* epineurial, perineurial and endoneurial plexuses, and *extrinsic* regional vessels in the "paraneurium" (Figs 2.14 and 2.15). These form "separate but extensively interconnected microvascular systems", providing a wide margin of safety. As McManis et al (1993) remark: "these anastomotic vessels confer a resistance to ischaemia in peripheral nerves so that nerve suffers functional or structural changes only when there is widespread vascular or microvascular damage". Seddon (1975b) commented on the extent to which it was permissible to mobilise the nerve in order to facilitate suture. His rather sanguine views of the effect on the blood supply are not confirmed by the later injection studies of Bell and Weddell (1984); indeed, later clinical experience has shown that it is preferable to bridge a gap by interposition, rather than by mobilisation.

The nervi nervorum

Curiously, but perhaps predictably, nerves have their own nerve supply in the shape of the nervi nervorum, derived from their own fibres. There are free endings in the epi-, peri- and endoneurium, and some encapsulated endings of Pacinian type in the endoneurium (Hromada 1963).

Changes in nerves with ageing

Corbin and Gardner (1937) examined the dorsal and ventral roots of the eighth and ninth thoracic spinal nerves of 34 cadavers whose ages ranged from 1 day to 84 (or possibly 89) years. The highest number of myelinated fibres, found in persons in their second and third decades, was 187% larger than that found in the nerves of a 1-day-old infant. They found that after the third decade there was a gradual loss of myelinated fibres, up to 32% for the person aged 89 years. Cottrell (1940) examined the medium, femoral, sciatic and common peroneal nerves of 30 persons coming to necropsy at ages ranging from 3 hours to 81 years. She found changes in the vessels and the connective tissue, with "alteration and loss of the nerve fibers". Ochoa and Mair (1969) examined portions of the sural nerves of seven volunteers aged 5 to 59 years, and were the first to show that active destruction of

unmyelinated fibres starts early in life, whereas loss of myelinated fibres was found only in the 59 year old.

Tohgi and colleagues (1977) examined the sural nerves of 79 persons coming to necropsy after "acute death", whose ages ranged from 1 week to 88 years. The average density of small myelinated fibres decreased rapidly from the age of 1 week (26 300/mm^2) to the second decade (9560/mm^2), and continued to decrease gradually with age, to reach at the eighth decade an average of 74% of that at the second decade. Large myelinated fibres appeared first in an infant aged 3 months. Their density increased rapidly, to reach at 3 years the level found in the young adult. The average of the third decade was 6480/mm^2; at the ninth decade it was 3480/mm^2. In this extensive study there is mention of the ageing changes in the vasa nervorum and the perineurium. Jacobs and Love (1985) made a qualitative and quantitative study of 27 sural nerves obtained within 24 hours of death from human subjects without history of disease or of ingestion of drugs known to affect the peripheral nerves. Densities of myelinated and unmyelinated fibres decreased from birth to the end of the eighth decade, because of increasing size and separation of fibres during the first decade, and an increase in endoneurial collagen in the older persons. Also, the slope of a plot of internodal length versus fibre diameter increased progressively during the first decade, but then remained virtually constant until the age of 60 years. Then, degeneration, regeneration, demyelination and remyelination caused increasing variation in internodal length. Thomas et al (1993b), summarising previous findings, refer to "mild peripheral neuropathy" of older humans.

Norris et al (1953) examined age changes in the maximum conduction velocity of motor fibres of the ulnar nerves of 175 ambulatory male patients, employees and staff members of the Baltimore City Hospitals. There was steady reduction in conduction velocity from the third to the ninth decade. These workers canvassed possible causes for this regression. Taylor (1984) studied effects of age on conduction and amplitude in motor and sensory fibres of adult nerves. He indicated that tables of normal data of the rise and fall of conduction and amplitude could be constructed for use in clinical investigation. Kimura (1993) stated that "nerve conduction velocities are roughly half the adult value in full-term infants, but increase rapidly, reflecting the process of myelination, to the adult value at age 3–5 years". He noted the slow decline of conduction velocity after the fourth decade, and drew attention to the contemporaneous increase of the latencies of the F wave and somatosensory evoked potentials. These changes must evidently concern clinicians treating the very young and the rather old: in the former, they may have a bearing on diagnosis; in the latter, they may be relevant to the susceptibility of a nerve or nerves to damage by pressure or traction.

Figs 2.14 and 2.15 The blood supply of nerves.

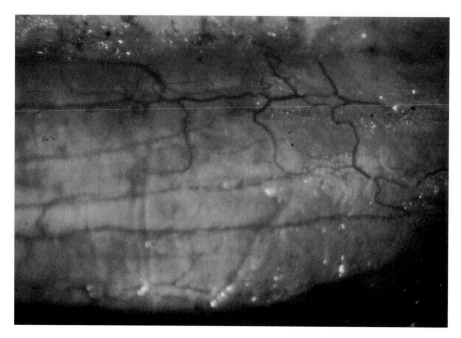

Fig. 2.14 The epineurial vessels of the ulnar nerve. × 40.

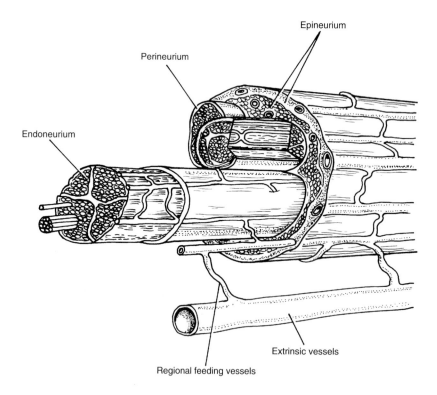

Fig. 2.15 The vascular systems of the peripheral nerve. (After Lundborg G 1988b.)

3. The motor and sensory pathways

The motor and sensory systems: motor path with central and peripheral connections; sympathetic outflow; sensory path with superficial and deep peripheral connections and with central connections; the role of visceral afferents; neurotransmitters.

THE SOMATIC MOTOR SYSTEM

The motor pathway begins in the cells in the precentral gyrus of the cerebral cortex. Their axons pass by the *internal capsule* to the midbrain and to the *pyramids* of the medulla. From each side most fibres cross the midline at the decussation of the pyramids to descend in the lateral part of the white matter of the cord as the lateral cortico-spinal tract. At various segmental levels impulses from this tract activate, through internuncial neurons, the motor cells in the anterior part of the grey matter (Fig. 3.1). "Extrapyramidal" tracts from the red nucleus, the vestibular nuclei and the reticular formation also influence the activity of the anterior horn cells. Brodal (1981c) prefers to discard the designation "extrapyramidal", on the grounds that "those cortical regions which give rise to fibres in the pyramidal tract also give rise to fibres to a number of nuclei which project further caudally...".

The cell bodies of the motor neurons are in lamina IX (Rexed 1954) of the anterior horn of the grey matter. There are large (α) and small (γ) cells. They are acted on by primary sensory fibres and by fibres descending from the cortex and from nuclei in the brainstem. The axons from the large cells are destined for the extrafusal fibres. By correlating the distribution of paralysis with the sites of loss of cells in the ventral horn, Sharrard (1955) was able to show how the cells were grouped in the grey matter. Broadly, the medial group supply the muscles of the trunk and neck; the lateral group supply the muscles of the limbs. Thus, cells of the latter group are present chiefly in the cervical and lumbar enlargements, whereas those of the medial group are found throughout the length of the cord.

The axons pass ventrally to leave the cord in the anterior roots and later to join those of the sensory root to form the peripheral nerve. Contact with, and transmission to, muscle is effected through the motor end-plates. There are two components of each end-plate: neural and muscular. They are separated by a cleft of about 30 nm. The muscular *sole plate* contains a number of muscle cell nuclei; it is not itself contractile. There are two types of neural ending: the *en plaque* terminal on extrafusal (α nerve fibre) muscle

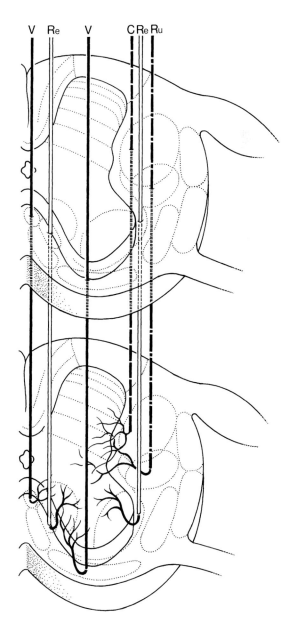

Fig. 3.1 The major descending tracts in the spinal cord, and their overlapping zones of termination in the grey matter. C, corticospinal; V, vestibulospinal; Re, reticulospinal; Ru, rubrospinal.

fibres, and the *plate* endings on intrafusal (γ nerve fibres) muscle fibres (Figs 3.2 and 3.3). Transmission at en plaque endings initiates action potentials which are rapidly conducted to all parts of the muscle fibres, whereas transmission at plate endings of "trail" and "en grappe" types excites the fibres at several points. Acetylcholine released at the nerve ending interacts with receptors to produce depolarisation of the muscle membrane and triggers the action potential in the muscle (Garrett 1991).

The anterior roots from the first thoracic to the second lumbar contain also the efferent (preganglionic) fibres of the sympathetic nervous system: those of the second to fourth sacral nerves contain the efferent pelvic parasympathetic outflow. In addition, as Sherrington (1894) showed, the anterior roots contain a number of afferent fibres arising from cells in the posterior root ganglion or in the anterior roots. Most of these fibres are unmyelinated. The role of unmyelinated afferents in the anterior roots of cats was further examined by Clifton et al (1976). They found that one-third of these fibres had receptive fields in

somatic structures (skin and deep tissues), while two-thirds had receptive fields in viscera. Many of these fibres, especially those with cutaneous receptive fields, had high thresholds. Clifton et al speculated that the fibres might participate in nociception. Maynard et al (1977) examined the central connections of these fibres.

We were able to take advantage of the opportunity offered by intradural damage to nerves of the brachial plexus to demonstrate the presence of afferent fibres in the anterior roots of Man. Stephen Gschmeissner (personal communication, 1996) examined by electron microscopy the anterior root of the eighth cervical nerve "avulsed" with its posterior root and found with it at operation for exploration of the plexus in the posterior triangle of the neck. He found several surviving myelinated and unmyelinated axons (Figs 3.4 and 3.5). Clearly, the cell bodies of these axons must have been in the nerve or in the posterior root ganglion; the fibres must have belonged to the afferent system. We plan later to investigate the site of the receptors that feed these fibres.

Figs 3.2 and 3.3   The motor end-plate.

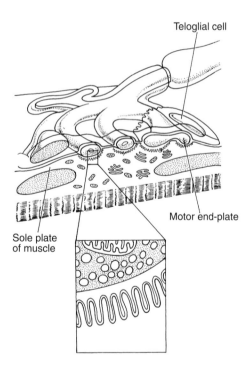

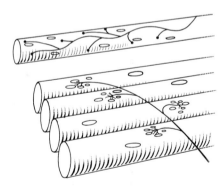

Fig. 3.2 "En plaque" junction, showing the relation of the terminal to the sole plate.

Fig. 3.3 "En plaque" terminals (below) contrasted with "plate" endings (above).

Figs 3.4 and 3.5 Afferent and efferent fibres in the anterior root.

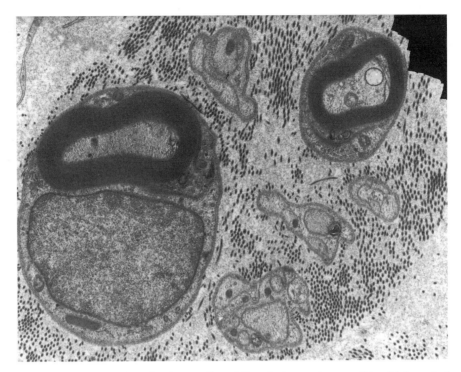

Fig. 3.4 Large healthy myelinated and unmyelinated fibres in the anterior root of the eighth cervical nerve avulsed from the spinal cord 6 weeks previously. There is much abnormal collagenisation. × 9750. (Electron microscopic study by Mr Stephen Gschmeissner.)

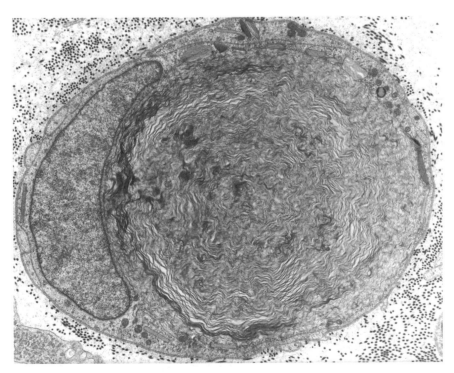

Fig. 3.5 A Schwann cell with a degenerate myelinated (efferent) fibre in the same root. × 7500. (Electron microscopic studies by Mr Stephen Gschmeissner.)

THE SOMATIC SENSORY SYSTEM

The somatic sensory system serves superficial (cutaneous) and deep (muscular and tendinous) receptors.

Cutaneous sensibility. The long debate about the mechanism of cutaneous sensibility begun by Blix (1884) and Goldscheider (1884), and continued by von Frey (1894, 1896), Head et al (1905), Head and Sherrin (1905), Head (1920), Walshe (1942), Weddell (1941), Sinclair (1955) and many others, is now drawing to its close. Von Frey's concept is, in effect, accepted: as Iggo (1985) remarks "the long-standing argument of 'specificity' versus 'pattern' in the operation of cutaneous receptors has been settled in favour of the 'specificity' hypothesis". Or (Iggo 1986), "The long debate concerning sensory functions of the nerves innervating the skin can now be regarded as settled." That this has come about is largely due to the work with microelectrodes and with intraneural microstimulation done by, among others, Vallbo and Hagbarth (1968), Hallin and Torebjörk (1973, 1974), Torebjörk and Hallin (1973), Vallbo et al (1979), Torebjörk and Ochoa (1980, 1983a,b), Hallin et al (1981), Vallbo and Hulliger (1981), Hagbarth (1983), Ochoa and Torebjörk (1983, 1989) and Hagbarth et al (1993). Three types of cutaneous receptor are defined: low threshold mechanoreceptors, thermoreceptors and nociceptors.

Low threshold mechanoreceptors. The distinction is made between slowly adapting receptors responding to sustained displacement such as continuous pressure; rapidly adapting receptors responding to the beginning or withdrawal of a stimulus or by a moving stimulus; and receptors responding to brief mechanical disturbances such as vibration and tapping.

The first group includes the Merkel cells; the second includes the Meissner corpuscles; and the third includes the Pacinian corpuscles. Most are innervated by large and medium-sized fibres conducting at rates of 20–90 m/s. A few morphologically unidentified receptors responding to very slow displacement of hair or skin are innervated by small slowly conducting C fibres. The principal mechanoreceptor in hairy skin is the hair follicle receptor; in hairless (glabrous) skin the two principal types are the Meissner's corpuscle, rapidly adapting, and the Merkel's receptor, slowly adapting. Beneath the skin the rapidly adapting organ is the Pacinian corpuscle; the slowly reacting organ is the Ruffini's corpuscle (Fig. 3.6).

Thermoreceptors

As long ago as 1884, Blix postulated that there were two types of thermoreceptor in the human skin: one for cooling and one for warming. Cooling receptors are served by unmyelinated and fine myelinated fibres, usually serving receptor fields about 100 μm in diameter (Light & Perl 1993). They are very sensitive to decrease in skin temperature from the normal or "neutral" level of 30–35°C. Fowler et al (1988) indicate a conduction velocity of up to 2.1 m/s. The receptor itself may consist of unmyelinated terminal branches of a small myelinated parent, lying near the basal lamina of the epidermis (Hensel et al 1974).

Warming receptors, less common than cooling receptors, have receptive fields of less than 1 mm in diameter. They are excited by rises in skin temperature in the range 30–46°C. Most are served by unmyelinated fibres; in primates, some are served by small myelinated fibres (Light & Perl 1993). Fowler et al (1988) indicate a conduction velocity of 0.5 m/s. The units themselves have not yet been identified. Yarnitsky and Ochoa (1991) indicate mediation of warm sensation by unmyelinated primary afferents and of cold sensation by small myelinated afferents.

Nociceptors

The term is applied to primary afferent units that "uniquely signal stimuli intense enough to threaten physical damage to the tissue" (Light & Perl 1993). Some respond to intense mechanical stimuli, some to strong thermal stimulation, and some are polymodal. Impulses travel in myelinated fibres in the Aδ to Aβ ranges and in unmyelinated C fibres.

Nociceptors innervated by myelinated fibres have receptive fields of up to 50 spots of 50–180 μm in diameter. Each spot responds only to mechanical stimuli of noxious or near-noxious intensity (Light & Perl 1993). Some spots respond to noxious heat. Others respond in a graded fashion: some, after previous sensitisation by damaging heat.

The common type of cutaneous nociceptor innervated by unmyelinated C fibres responds to a variety of noxious stimuli: mechanical, thermal and chemical. It is, in fact, polymodal. Sato and Perl (1991) have shown sensitisation to noradrenaline of such receptors after partial injury of the parent nerve. Impulses are conducted at rates of less than 0.7 m/s.

Deep sensibility

Sensation is conveyed from muscles, ligaments and tendons from specialised receptors and from free nerve endings in those structures. The receptor organs are: in muscle, *muscle spindles and free nerve endings;* in tendons, the *Golgi organs;* and, in capsules and ligaments, various endings, some similar to Ruffini endings, Pacinian corpuscles and Golgi organs, while others supply plexuses of unmyelinated fibres (Figs 3.7 to 3.9).

The muscle spindles. It is over 100 years since Sherrington (1894) demonstrated by anterior root section that "in a muscular nerve-trunk from one-third to one-half of the myelinated fibres are from cells of the spinal

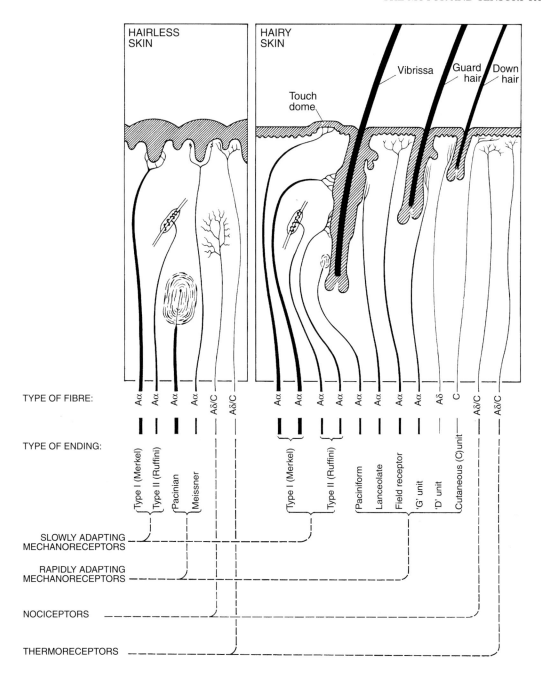

Fig. 3.6 Cutaneous sensory receptors, with fibre sizes. (Left) Glabrous skin; (right) hairy skin.

root-ganglion". The size of these fibres was from 1.5–20 μm; they were not the largest fibres in the nerve – the largest came from the anterior root. On the other hand, the largest of these fibres were larger than any fibres in the cutaneous nerves. Sherrington found too that "the smallest myelinated fibres in the muscular nerve are for the most part, perhaps entirely, root ganglion fibres". Sherrington further showed that there were "recurrent" (afferent) fibres in the anterior roots. He identified the special end-organs of the afferent fibres in the muscle spindles (*muskel-spindeln*) of Kühne (1864). Ruffini (1897), in his observations on sensory nerve endings in muscles, defined the "sensorial" end-organs of muscle as: (1) the muscle spindles; (2) the tendon organs (Golgi organs); and (3) the Pacinian corpuscles. He concluded "in my opinion it is upon these three levels of sense organ that

Figs 3.7 to 3.9 Deep sensory receptors.

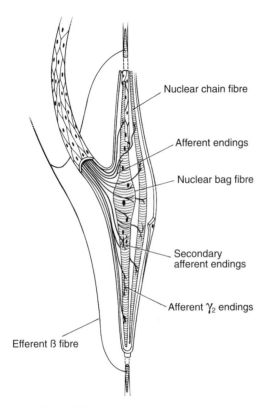

Nuclear chain fibre

Afferent endings

Nuclear bag fibre

Secondary
afferent endings

Afferent γ_2 endings

Efferent ß fibre

Fig. 3.7 Simplified view of a muscle spindle.

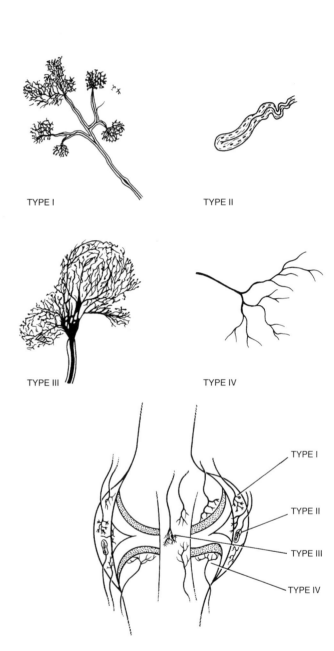

TYPE I

TYPE II

TYPE III

TYPE IV

Fig. 3.9 Receptors in joint capsule. (After Brodal (1981).)

TYPE I

TYPE II

TYPE III

TYPE IV

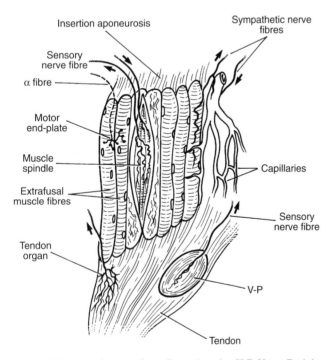

Insertion aponeurosis

Sympathetic nerve
fibres

Sensory
nerve fibre

α fibre

Motor
end-plate

Muscle
spindle

Extrafusal
muscle fibres

Tendon
organ

Capillaries

Sensory
nerve fibre

V-P

Tendon

Fig. 3.8 Receptors in musculotendinous junction V-P, Vater–Pacinian corpuscle. (After Brodal (1981).)

physiology must turn its attention if it will resolve the problem of the muscular sense". Batten (1897), who quoted the observations of Golgi (1882), further examined the muscle spindle and its behaviour in various pathological conditions, including injury to the brachial plexus. Horsley (1897) noted their "preservation in conditions of extreme muscular atrophy".

Since Sherrington's time, a very great deal of work has been done on the structure and function of the muscle spindles (Merton 1953, Boyd 1962, 1966, 1976, 1983, Cooper & Daniel 1963, Goodwin et al 1972, Swash & Fox 1974, Matthews 1981, Banks et al 1982), on their behaviour after nerve injury, and on their regeneration (Tower 1932, Patel et al 1968, De Reuck 1974, Schröder 1974a,b; Sahgal & Morgen 1976, Schröder et al 1979, Barker et al 1986, 1990, Myles & Glasby 1992).

Boyd and Smith (1984) state that: "The whole human body must contain about 20 000 spindles, each of them a marvel of micro-engineering." Most spindles lie deep in muscle near branches of their nerve or blood vessels. Each contains small muscle fibres (intrafusal fibres) within a cellular and connective tissue capsule. Two types of intrafusal fibre are described: the *nuclear bag fibres*, with a central accumulation of nuclei; and *nuclear chain fibres*, smaller and with a single row of nuclei. The spindles vary in length from a few millimetres to a centimetre. Each spindle receives up to 25 terminal branches of motor and sensory axons, together with autonomic innervation. The motor axons are the β and γ axons of the anterior root; the sensory axons are myelinated fibres of groups I and II. The combination of motor and sensory innervation is reflected in the complexity of the function of the spindles. The conception of a servo action is evidently too simple; rather, it is evident that the spindles play several roles in the "feedback" mechanism for regulating muscle contraction and for appreciation of body position.

The other afferent terminals in skeletal muscle are free endings innervated by unmyelinated and small myelinated fibres. Iggo (1961) found that these responded to sustained pressure, but not to stretch or contraction. They responded to hypertonic saline, but that stimulus was sufficient to excite the spindles too. Other studies of these organs and their afferent fibres were made by Iggo (1961), Mense and Schmidt (1974), Mense (1977) and Mense and Meyer (1981), who studied the response to chemical noxious stimulation by single fibre recording. Pomeranz et al (1968) traced fine myelinated afferents from viscera, muscle and skin to lamina V of the posterior horn.

Up to now, most clinical work on sensation and on recovery of sensibility after nerve injury and repair has been directed to cutaneous sensibility. Yet, function such as stereognosis and proprioception must depend principally on signals from endings in muscle, tendons and ligaments. It is perhaps inadequately appreciated that there may be good recovery of sensory function of the hand with very imperfect cutaneous reinnervation, and that pain is just as likely to follow damage to a "purely motor" nerve as it is to follow damage to a "mixed" or "sensory" nerve. There is in fact no such entity as a "purely motor" nerve, except perhaps for the hypoglossal or facial. The signals from the muscles supplied by those nerves probably proceed by other cranial nerves: the lingual in the case of the hypoglossal nerve, and the trigeminal in the case of the facial nerve. Stacey (1969) reckoned that in a "motor" nerve of the cat the distribution of fibres was: one-third myelinated motor, one-third myelinated sensory and one-third unmyelinated sensory. There are indeed a few peripheral nerves with no cutaneous sensory component: the spinal accessory; the phrenic; the anterior and posterior interosseous; the deep branch of the ulnar; and the suprascapular. The content of afferent fibres in all such nerves is about 30%. Laviano (1992/93), in his thesis on "spinal accessory nerve for the suprascapular in avulsions of the brachial plexus", shows electron micrographs of portions of the suprascapular nerve taken at operation as long as 94 days after injury. There are numerous medium-sized and small myelinated fibres in good condition: evidently, the distal processes of posterior root ganglia. Our work along the same lines also suggests a proportion of myelinated afferent fibres in the "motor" nerve of around 30%. Their sizes are probably Aβ and Aδ. Laviano's work confirms the earlier supposition (Bonney 1959) that the posterior root ganglion cells survive for a long time the interruption of their central processes. As to the last, in a case of extensive intradural damage to the plexus we examined a specimen of nerve taken at the time of "neurotisation" well after the period required for degeneration, and found that it contained not less than 30% of myelinated fibres (Fig. 3.10). It is perhaps best to drop the terms "purely motor" and "purely sensory", and even the term "mixed", as applied to nerves with both motor and cutaneous sensory components. The terms "nerves with motor and cutaneous sensory components" and "nerves without somatic motor components" are, unfortunately, cumbersome, but they do say what they mean.

Central connections

The great array of sensory receptors in the skin and deep tissues send back to the centre the signals of the stimuli received. Most afferent fibres, with their cells in the posterior root ganglia, enter the cord by the posterior roots. Others, with cells in the posterior root ganglia or actually in the anterior roots, enter the cord by the latter.

The first analysis of incoming signals takes place in the spinal cord and medulla where all fibres terminate. Most of the large myelinated fibres ascending in the posterior columns terminate in the gracile and cuneate nuclei in the medulla. Some smaller fibres of the dorsal columns terminate and relay in the cord: these are the *propriospinal* fibres.

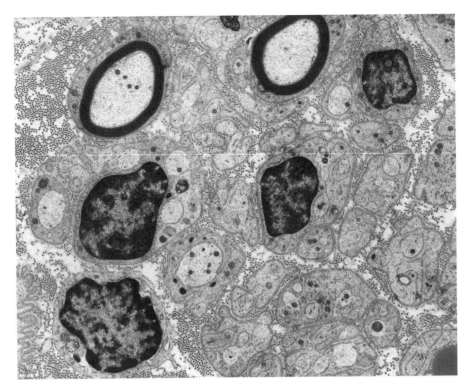

Fig. 3.10 Intact (afferent) myelinated and unmyelinated fibres in the suprascapular ("purely motor") nerve after avulsion lesion of the brachial plexus. Specimen taken 6 weeks after injury, when efferent fibres had degenerated. There is much collagenisation. ×6600. (Electron microscopic study by Mr Stephen Gschmeissner.)

Although the classical view of the function of the posterior columns has been challenged (Wall 1970), it is broadly true that, as Brodal (1981d) states, they "mediate sensory signals necessary for rather complex discrimination tasks".

Other afferent fibres terminate and relay in the grey matter of the posterior horn (Fig. 3.11). Each lamina (Rexed 1952, 1954, Price & Meyer 1974) of the grey matter receives afferents of specific functional modalities; each has a particular neuronal structure. Small myelinated nociceptor and thermoreceptor fibres terminate in lamina I; C fibres, nociceptors, thermoreceptors and mechanoreceptors terminate in lamina II (substantia gelatinosa). Larger mechanoreceptor fibres terminate in laminae III and IV. These relay to cells the axons of which either ascend in the posterior columns or reach the dorsal column nuclei by the dorsolateral fasciculus. Some fibres pass through the posterior horn to relay with the large cells in the motor apparatus in lamina IX. Some unmyelinated and small myelinated fibres enter the dorsolateral fasciculus (Lissauer's tract) just lateral to the tip of the posterior horn to join fibres from cells in the substantia gelatinosa. Some fibres cross the midline to terminate in laminae I and V of the contralateral posterior horn. There is a complex network of interconnecting fibres in the posterior horn, and in the substantia gelatinosa in particular.

Sensory input is first analysed and modified here. Secondary neurons in the posterior horn give rise to fibres which ascend or descend for a few segments in the cord. They give rise principally to the fibres that, crossing the midline, ascend in the long tracts in the anterolateral segment of the spinal cord (Fig. 3.12).

The transmission of impulses from the nuclei of the posterior column is influenced by fibres descending from the sensory motor cortex (Gordon & Jukes 1964). This influence is predominantly inhibitory. The ascending fibres of those nuclei form the *medial lemniscus* of the brainstem, crossing the midline in the medulla to end in the thalamus. The final resolution of sensory impulses takes place in the somatosensory areas of the cerebral cortex (see Fig. 3.12). Not even in this last analysis are afferent functions separated completely from motor function: stimulation of any of these areas produces motor effects (Woolsey 1964). It is doubtful whether pain is perceived at this final level: stimulation of the postcentral gyrus in man does not seem to cause pain (Penfield & Boldrey 1937, Penfield & Rasmussen 1950).

Schott's (1994) principal proposition was that "sympathetically determined" pain was so determined because the afferent pathways were in the autonomic nerves. He noted the finding by Varro et al (1988) of calcitonin

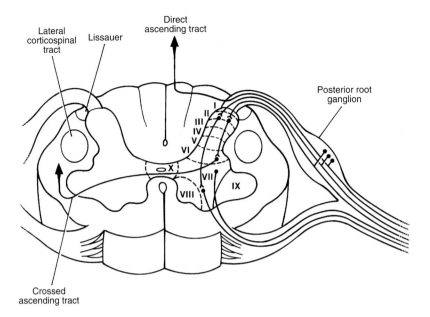

Fig. 3.11 The laminae of the grey matter, with direct ascending, crossed ascending and internuncial tracts.

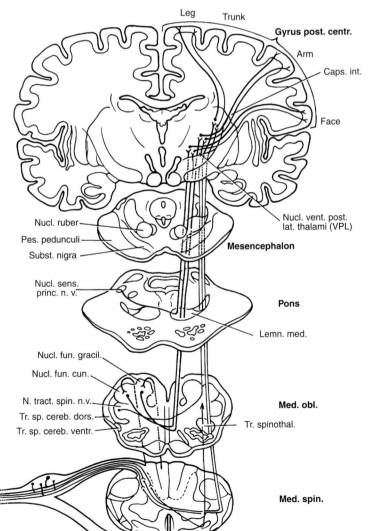

Fig. 3.12 Ascending tracts in the cord, brainstem, and cortex. Note the relay of the direct ascending tracts in the gracile and cuneate nuclei in the medulla. (After Brodal 1981.)

gene-related peptide (CGRP) in visceral afferents, admitting that selective histochemical markers for specifically pain-serving afferents were not available. In developing his thesis, Schott reverted to the concept of a system of visceral afferents, which comprised not only fibres from organs generally classed as "viscera", but also afferents from blood vessels. The evidence for the presence of a system for conveying from all viscera sensations both perceived and unperceived rests largely on indirect observations: the truly autonomic functioning of viscera; the production of pain by mechanical stimulation of peripheral arteries and veins; the operation of "referred pain" mechanisms; pain after operations on the sympathetic chain; and the lack of "visceral sensibility" when the function of visceral afferents is impaired by age. There is evidence from the work of Sugiura et al (1989) that visceral afferents terminate in laminae IV, V and X of the dorsal horn, as well as in laminae I and II. They were also traced up and down in the cord and crossing the midline. In their final "conclusion", Sugiura et al (1989) proposed that their morphological observations suggested that "the somato-visceral convergence could occur in the superficial dorsal horn of the spinal cord", and that "the scattered and extensive distribution of the terminal fields of single visceral C-afferent fibres may be one basis for the poor localisation of visceral sensation". These concepts are further explored in Chapter 16.

Conduction of impulses

Rasminsky (1985) opens the subject thus: "Nerve fibres are specialised processes of nerve cells that have the unique property to propagate action potentials, the *currency of information* in the nervous system." In an unmyelinated fibre a wave of depolarisation passes continuously down the fibre. The velocity of conduction depends on the diameter of the fibre. In the myelinated fibre the myelin sheath acts as a capacitor and limits radial resistance at the internode, so that most of the current flows axially along the fibre. It is, says Bostock (1993) "powered by inward 'kicks' of inward membrane current at the nodes of Ranvier". This method of "saltatory" conduction was so named by Tasaki and Takeuchi (1941, 1942), and further confirmed by Huxley and Stämpfli (1949). The myelin sheath thus enables the fibre to conduct rapidly without the necessity for a very large increase in axonal diameter.

Conduction velocity ranges from about 0.7 m/s in small unmyelinated fibres to about 80 m/s in the largest myelinated fibres. Omer (1980b) gives a range of 40–75 m/s in large myelinated fibres. The electrical changes associated with the wave of depolarisation can be measured through electrodes placed on the skin over the nerve, on the nerve, in the nerve or in individual fibres. These reactions form the basis for electrophysiological examination and for microneurography.

The transmission of impulses at synapses is chemical, by the release of *neurotransmitters* causing a change in the permeability and hence the electrical polarisation of the postsynaptic membrane (Williams et al 1989). Such changes may be excitatory or inhibitory; they are usually short lived, because of early inactivation of the neurotransmitter. This is not, of course, the whole process: the effect of some neurotransmitters may be more prolonged or even permanent; release of certain of them into the cerebrospinal fluid or into intercellular spaces of the central nervous system may lead to diffuse effects on neurons. In addition, some substances released at synapses may simply modify the response of the postsynaptic membrane to neurotransmitters. The general term "neuromediators" has been applied to substances released at synaptic endings; "neurotransmission" implies a direct effect on postsynaptic membrane; "neuromodulation" implies alteration of its response to a neuromediator.

The best-known mediator and the one that has been known longest is, of course, acetylcholine, which is synthesised by motor neurons and released at the motor terminals in skeletal muscle and at the synapses in sympathetic and parasympathetic ganglia. The other well-known mediators belong to the monoamine group: they are noradrenalin, adrenaline, dopamine, serotonin and histamine. Noradrenaline is the chief transmitter at the endings of sympathetic ganglionic neurons. Adrenaline too is present in peripheral neural pathways. The other monoamines are chiefly present in the central nervous system. The range of *neuropeptide* modulators is very wide, including those associated with the function of the hypothalamus and hypophysis, corticotrophin, β-endorphins, the enkephalins, calcitonin-related gene peptide and nerve growth factor. In the field of peripheral nerves, the last is of great and growing importance; the β-endorphins and enkephalins are important in the consideration of the mechanism and treatment of pain.

4. Reactions to injury

Reactions to injury: the reaction of the nerve cell and myelin–Schwann cell complex; differential reaction of fibres of different sizes; two main types of nerve injury – degenerative and nondegenerative; Wallerian degeneration; the special case of the brachial plexus; reactions to various physical agents; the effects of denervation.

Nerves can be damaged in a number of ways:

- ischaemia
- physical agents such as traction, pressure, stretching, distortion, cold, heat, severance, electric shock, injection of noxious substances, ionising radiation
- infection and inflammatory processes
- ingestion of drugs and metals
- infiltration by or pressure from tumours
- the effects of systemic disease.

The damage to the nerve may be "closed", or "open" through a wound of the skin. Damage may be acute or chronic; and single, repeated or continuing. The lesion may affect the whole nerve or only part of it. The *depth* of effect may vary from fibre to fibre or from one part of the nerve to another. The nerve affected may be entirely healthy or may be the subject of a neuropathy from hereditary or systemic causes, or from a more proximal affection. Nerve injury may be associated with damage to one or more important structures: artery, vein, viscus bone, muscle or ligament.

In the mildest form of damage – that produced by transient ischaemia – there is transient failure of conduction affecting principally the large myelinated fibres. Lewis et al (1931a) described this form of centripetal paralysis produced by the application round the arm of a cuff inflated to suprasystolic pressure. First, there is loss of superficial sensibility. This is succeeded by a gradual loss of motor power. The first pain response is lost soon after superficial sensibility fails, but the delayed pain response can still be elicited after 40 minutes of ischaemia. Pilomotor and vasomotor functions are scarcely affected. This differential paralysis reflects, of course, the differing reactions of the fibres of different sizes. Large myelinated fibres are first affected; C fibres and efferent autonomic fibres escape. Recovery of all modalities occurs within a few minutes of release of the cuff. By a simple but ingenious method, Lewis et al demonstrated that the lesion was caused by ischaemia of the segments of the nerves underlying the cuff. Mackinnon and Dellon

(1988a) rightly suggest that all those intending to take up peripheral nerve work should try this experiment on themselves. The experience gives a very clear indication of what is meant by the *depth* of a nerve injury. That knowledge is certain to be important in clinical practice. Further, the experience of the unpleasant quality of the residual delayed pain sensation gives good insight into the feelings of patients affected by dysaesthesia.

With severe and prolonged pressure there is local demyelination and more prolonged conduction block (Fowler et al 1972, Harrison 1976, Gilliatt 1981). The pressures used by Gilliatt could not reasonably be used in experiments on human subjects. The myelin is squeezed proximally and distally from underneath the tourniquet so as to invaginate into the proximal and distal sheaths of the nodes of Ranvier (Fig. 4.1). A conduction block which may last for weeks or months results. If in the clinical situation the cause of the local demyelination persists in the form of, say, a bony projection causing pressure and distortion or of external pressure by haematoma, the block persists. This was so in the three cases reported by Birch and St Clair Strange (1990): in these, removal of the external pressure was rapidly followed by recovery in lesions which had persisted for up to 3 years. The bestowal of the name *axonamonosis* on this type of lesion by Birch and St Clair Strange, abetted by Bonney, was sharply

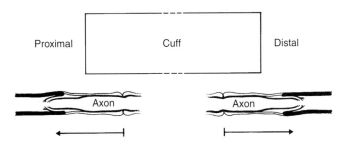

Fig. 4.1 Effect of pressure on nerve: squeezing of myelin with invagination at the node of Ranvier. (After Ochon J, Fowler T J, Gilliat R W 1972)

criticised by Gilliatt in a communication which he was kind enough to keep private. In the experimental situation, conduction recovers and motor and sensory functions are restored, though not necessarily in an orderly manner. In this type of paralysis, the autonomic fibres are usually spared, though not necessarily so. We have seen a lesion of the tibial and common peroneal nerves produced by prolonged pressure during an attempt at suicide, in which there was prolonged vasomotor and sudomotor paralysis.

As Lewis et al (1931a) noted, the differential response of nerve fibres is reversed in the conduction block produced by infiltration of local anaesthetic agent. Here, the first sign of developing paralysis is the drying and warming of the extremity. It is probable that the conduction block is caused by interference with axonal conduction: so, the small unmyelinated fibres are the most susceptible and the first to succumb. Compression of nerves by haematoma or aneurysm produces a characteristic pattern: autonomic paralysis is early and deep; loss of power extends over hours or days; and deep position sense and limited joint position sense persist.

All these forms of paralysis are examples of *neurapraxia* (Seddon 1943); all are examples of the *nondegenerative*
lesion. Seddon gave the credit for the naming of his three types of nerve lesion to Sir Henry Cohen, later Lord Cohen of Birkenhead. "Neurapraxia" is perhaps the most admirable, but potentially the most misleading, of the three: derived from νευρον (neuron – nerve or tendon) and ἀπραξια (apraxia – nonfunction), it signifies loss of nerve function – no more and no less. It will not do as a diagnosis unless the clinician using it is aware that it never signifies a degenerative lesion. The use of the negating "a" (α) is, or should be, familiar to clinicians, since it occurs in terms in common use such as aphasia, aphonia, astigmatism, anorexia, amyotrophy and so on. It is all the sadder that declining standards of literacy have combined with rising looseness of thought to render the use of the term *neuropraxia* a commonplace, even in formerly reputable journals and textbooks. Punishment should be reserved for clinicians using this meaningless neologism; lawyers using it should lose their fees; classicists using it should suffer an appropriate loss; publishers permitting its use should be imprisoned *sine die*.

The situation is wholly different when the lesion is serious enough to cause interruption of the axon. Then follow the changes of a *degenerative* lesion, caused by

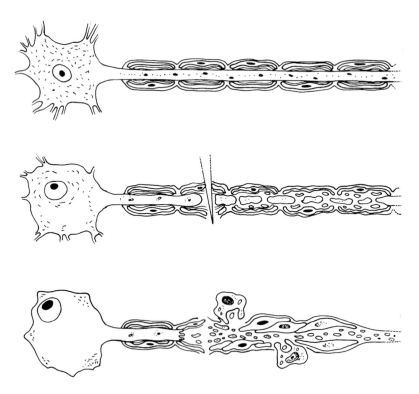

Fig. 4.2 Wallerian degeneration. (Top) Healthy cell body and axon. (Centre) Section through all elements, with early changes proximal and distal to the point of damage. (Bottom) Changes in the cell body and proximal axon: degeneration of distal axon and myelin sheath; macrophage invasion. (After Lundborg 1988.)

the damage to the neuron itself. The changes were first described by Waller (1850), and have since that time been known as those of Wallerian degeneration. We know now that they affect not only the axon but also the cell body; not only the neuron but also its Schwann cell ensheathment and its myelin sheath. There are changes too in the endoneurial cells and, over longer periods of time, in the motor and sensory end-organs. Distal to the site of injury the axon degenerates; there is a granular disintegration of the cytoskeleton and axoplasm, which are converted over succeeding days into amorphous debris (Figs 4.2 to 4.6). Although Adrian (1916, 1917) and Pollock et al (1946) thought that peripheral neural conduction might survive for up to a month after nerve section in humans, Landau (1953) found that the motor response after section

persisted for a much shorter period. The interval between injury and the last observation of a neuromuscular response ranged from 66 to 121 hours. Gilliatt and Taylor (1959) investigated motor response after section of the facial nerve in humans, and found that visible twitch in response to stimulation disappeared within 3–4 days; though an electrical response persisted for a further 48–72 hours. Our own observations on motor conductivity after preganglionic injury to the brachial plexus suggest that the motor response ceases about 3 days after injury. Conduction may cease first in the most proximal part of the fibres. Gilliatt and Hjorth (1972) studied the matter in baboons. The motor response to stimulation disappeared after 4–5 days, but ascending nerve potentials could be recorded for a further 2–3 days. Evidently, failure of

---

Figs 4.3 to 4.6 Changes in the distal stump of an ulnar nerve damaged 3 weeks previously.

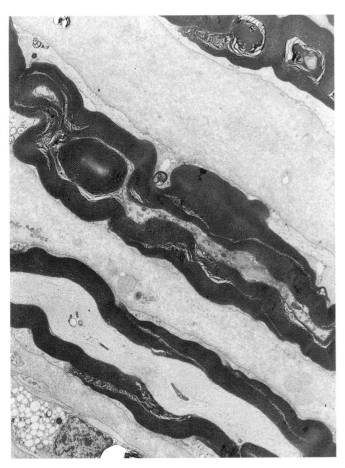

Fig. 4.3 Collapse of myelin sheaths; opening of Schmidt–Lanterman incisures. Axoplasm and neurofilaments are seen in the lower fibre. × 2210.

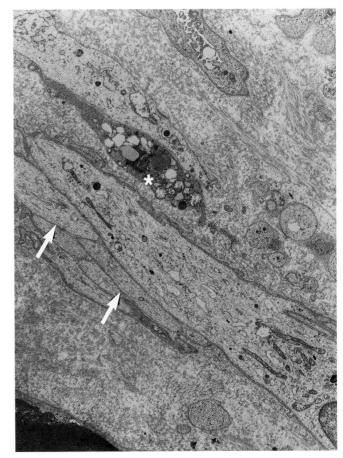

Fig. 4.4 Another part of the same specimen. Numerous Schwann cell processes (arrows). Extensive endoneurial collagen. Myelin debris with a macrophage (asterisk). × 5525.

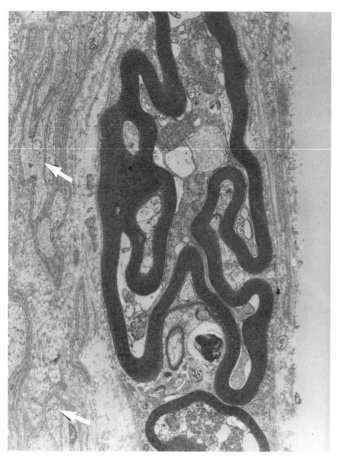

Fig. 4.5 Another part of the same specimen. Collapsed myelinated fibre; fragmentation of axoplasm; Schwann cell processes (arrows). × 11 700.

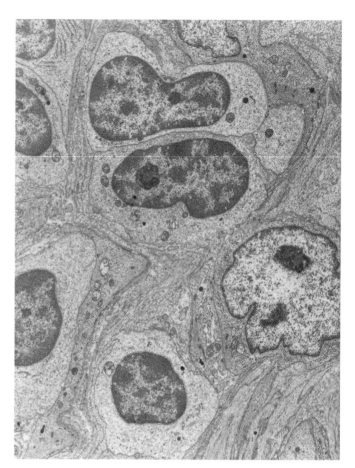

Fig. 4.6 Many Schwann cells, some with active nuclei. × 5525.

transmission at the neuromuscular junction precedes failure of conduction along the degenerating axon.

Landau (1953) made the perceptive comment that "the distinction between complete Wallerian degeneration and less severe injury can be made on the basis of the disappearance of excitability in the peripheral nerve segment at this time"; that is, the time of disappearance of neuromuscular function. Many misdiagnoses of "neurapraxia" could have been and could be avoided if this simple procedure were more widely used.

The cell body and proximal stump

Proximal to the lesion, changes occur in the internal structure of the nerve cell and in the distal part of the myelin sheath. Within a few days there is a reduction in the calibre of the proximal axon; there may be atrophy of the whole axonal "shaft". In the body itself there is chromatolysis and retraction of dendrites. These processes

may continue to actual dissolution of the cell body. They are seen not only in the anterior horn cells after transection of their axons, but also in the cells of the posterior root ganglion after transection of their peripheral axonal processes. Curiously enough, transection of the central branches going to the central nervous system does not produce clear-cut changes in the cell bodies in the posterior root ganglia. These central changes, and those in the distal stump, doubtless reflect interruption of axoplasmic transport, leading to defective synthesis of neurofilament proteins (Griffin & Hoffman 1993). The changes in nerve fibres proximal to axonal section were studied by Gutmann and Sanders (1943). Romanes (1946) observed the changes in the anterior horn cells of mice after permanent *axonotomy*[1] by amputation. Cragg and Thomas

---

[1] The common usage is, of course, *axotomy*, but we believe that *axonotomy* is the more correct term.

(1961) compared conduction velocity and fibre size in the peroneal nerves of rabbits subjected to various types of lesion. Dyck et al (1984) examined the sequence of events after permanent axonotomy in the adult cat produced by amputation of the hind limb at the hip. They showed that axonotomy produced, sequentially, "myelin wrinkling, segmental demyelination and remyelination, and finally axonal degeneration into myelin ovoids and balls". The changes began and were more severe distally, but affected even the proximal segmental nerve. Dyck et al (1984) were able to study the effect of permanent axonotomy on the spinal cords of two patients who had undergone, respectively, partial and total amputation of a lower limb. They found that "loss of target tissue by axotomy leads to atrophy and then loss of motor neurons". The significance of these findings will not be lost on the clinician treating patients with nerve injuries.

The distal stump

The changes in the myelin sheath of the distal nerve stump are rapid and profound after the loss of the axon. The breakdown of the myelin evokes a macrophage reaction, so that within 6 weeks most of the fragments have been removed. Schwann cells in the distal nerve, both in myelinated and unmyelinated fibres, begin a process of proliferation (Figs 4.7 to 4.11). The fact that the Schwann cells of undamaged unmyelinated fibres seem to share the proliferation of Schwann cells of damaged myelinated fibres suggests that diffusible, humoral factors are the stimulants for this proliferation (Archer & Griffin 1993, Griffin & Hoffman 1993). The denervated Schwann cell bands lie within the original basal lamina. There is proliferation too of endoneurial fibroblasts in the distal nerve. These may produce nerve growth factor (Heumann et al 1987). The last important feature is the proliferation of macrophages; some derived from "resident" cells, others "recruited from the circulation" (Stoll et al 1989, Griffin and Hoffman 1993). These are involved in:

- the clearance of the debris of myelin and axoplasm
- the stimulation of the Schwann cells to produce nerve growth factor.

So long as the lesion is not severe enough to interrupt the continuity of the Schwann cell basal lamina from proximal to distal segment, the original pathways for regrowth of axons remain (Young 1949, Causey & Palmer 1952, Thomas 1964, Haftek & Thomas 1967, 1968). As Gutmann and Sanders (1943) noted in their experimental work, "only after crushing (as opposed to section) was the nerve fully reconstituted". It is the difference between preservation and destruction of continuity that underlies the division of degenerative lesions into those with the potential for complete spontaneous recovery and those

that will not recover unless action is taken and even then are unlikely fully to recover. Seddon (1943) named the first axonotmesis, from ἀξων (axono – shaft, or axon) and Τμησις (tmesis – cutting) (Fig. 4.12). That term is still valuable, indicating as it does the vital element of the degenerative lesion: the interruption of the axon and the consequent damage to the neuron. Seddon (1943) named lesions in which interruption of the axon was associated with interruption of the basal lamina, neurotmesis. He, of course, derived the term from νευρον (neuron – nerve, or tendon) and Τμησις (tmesis – cutting). It rightly indicates interruption of continuity of all elements of the nerve. As time goes by, the basal lamina itself is broken down, as Giannini and Dyck informed Griffin and Hoffman (1993).

Sunderland (1951) introduced a rather more elaborate system of classifying injury. Five degrees of severity were named, ranging from simple conduction block to loss of continuity. The views of this pioneer in the field command respect; it may well be that some clinicians find Sunderland's classification an improvement on Seddon's and of more practical use than the earlier method. We, on the contrary, have tended towards a further simplification: to classification as "degenerative" and "nondegenerative". This, we think, is the manner in which clinicians should regard nerve injuries: the first question to be asked is: Is this lesion degenerative or nondegenerative?

Thomas and Holdorff (1993) elaborate this conception of "degenerative" and "nondegenerative" lesions in a manner helpful to clinicians and experimentalists. We reproduce here their table, in which the subdivisions of "focal conduction block" and "axonal degeneration" are set out (Table 4.1). We think that the question mark placed against "axonal constriction" is removed by the case shown to one of us by Campbell Semple (personal communication). In that case of hourglass constriction of a main nerve trunk, which was followed by early and complete recovery, there must have been axonal constriction

Table 4.1 Classification of focal mechanical nerve injury

I. Focal conduction block
  Transient:
    Ischaemic
    Other
  More persistent:
    Demyelinating
    Axonal constriction

II. Axonal degeneration
  With preservation of basal laminal sheaths of nerve fibres
  With partial section of nerve
  With complete transection of nerve

From Thomas P K, Holdorff B 1993 Neuropathy due to physical agents. In: Dyck P J, Thomas P K, Griffin J W, Low P A, Poduslo J F (eds) Peripheral neuropathy, 3rd edn. W B Saunders, London, p 991. With permission.

Figs 4.7 and 4.8 Wallerian degeneration in the anterior root of the eighth cervical nerve root 6 weeks after avulsion from the spinal cord. (Electron microscopic studies by Mr Stephen Gschmeissner.)

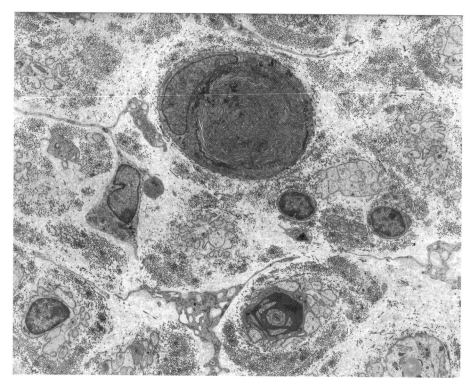

Fig. 4.7 Degeneration of a large myelinated efferent fibre and of unmyelinated efferent fibres. × 2850.

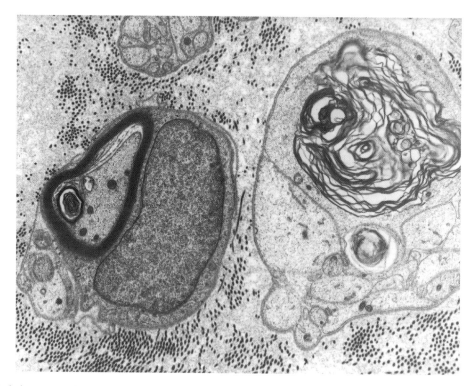

Fig. 4.8 A degenerate efferent myelinated fibre (right) compared with a healthy myelinated afferent fibre (left). × 11 115.

Figs 4.9 and 4.10 The late changes of degeneration.

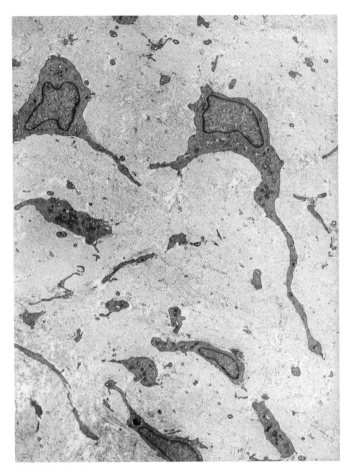

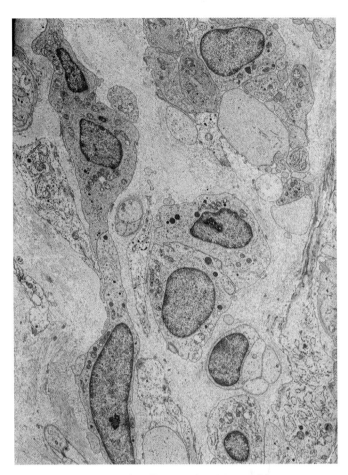

Fig. 4.9 Distal stump of median nerve destroyed by entrapment in supracondylar fracture in a 9-year-old boy. Eight months after injury. In effect, no neural elements are present. × 3245.

Fig. 4.10 Distal stump of median nerve in a 25-year-old man, transected 6 months previously by bullet from military rifle. Schwann cells and some axonal sprouts. × 3245.

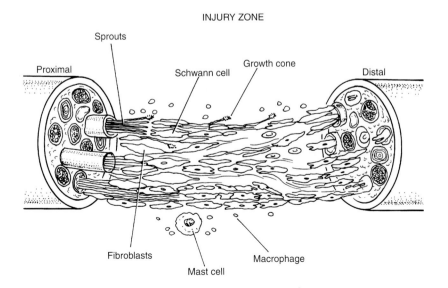

Fig. 4.11 The Schwann cell proliferation in the distal and proximal stumps, with axonal sprouting. (After Lundborg 1988.)

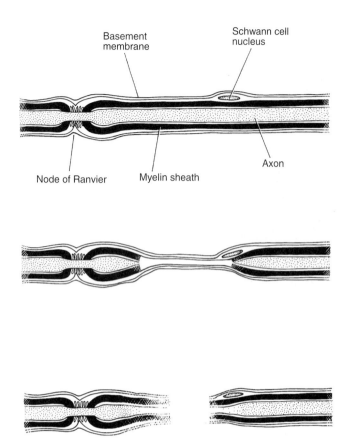

Fig. 4.12 Axonotmesis (centre) and neurotmesis (bottom) at the moment of injury. Note the preservation of the Schwann cell basement membrane in axonotmesis.

(Fig. 4.13). Very recently, Nagano et al (1996) studied "spontaneous" paralysis of the anterior interosseous nerve. They found that, during interfascicular neurolysis of the median nerve, there was "hourglass" constriction of the fascicles belonging to the anterior interosseous nerve. There was no external compression. Recovery after interfascicular neurolysis alone was "generally good".

The special case of the brachial plexus. A wholly different system of thought has to be employed in lesions of the brachial plexus, or for that matter of the lumbosacral plexus, in which there is intradural damage to the roots. In spite of the damage to the proximal branches, the axons whose cells of origin are outside the cord, in the posterior root ganglion, remain healthy for a long time when they are avulsed from the cord or ruptured intradurally. Such axons include all those in the posterior root; also, of course, many "recurrent" fibres in the anterior root, the cells of origin of which are in the posterior root ganglion. These axons, their Schwann cells, and myelin sheaths remain intact and functional, detached not only from central connection but also from Seddon's, Sunderland's, Thomas', Holdorff's and even our systems of classification. This is, in fact, insofar as afferent neurons are concerned, a lesion of the central nervous system. Somatic efferent fibres undergo degeneration; being separated from their cells, postganglionic autonomic efferent fibres also degenerate, because of damage to their grey rami communicantes (Figs 4.14 to 4.16). We did think of applying the term *neuradetosis* (from νευρον {neuron} nerve, and αδετοξ {adetos} unbound, loose, free) to the

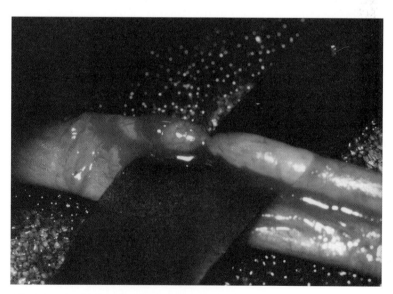

Fig. 4.13 Hourglass "constriction" of the lateral root of the median nerve, the result of traction injury. There was full spontaneous recovery. (Mr Campbell Semple's case.)

Figs 4.14 to 4.16 Intradural damage to nerve roots (neuradetosis). (Electron microscopic studies by Mr Stephen Gschmeissner.)

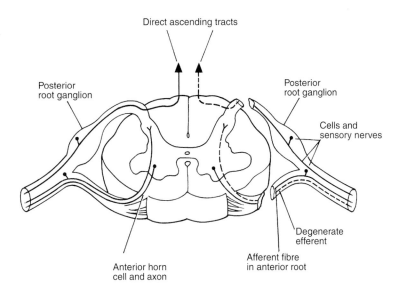

Fig. 4.14 The nerve and roots detached from the spinal cord. Note the intact posterior root ganglion cell, with healthy axons in the detached parts of the roots, and the degeneration of the efferent fibre in the anterior root.

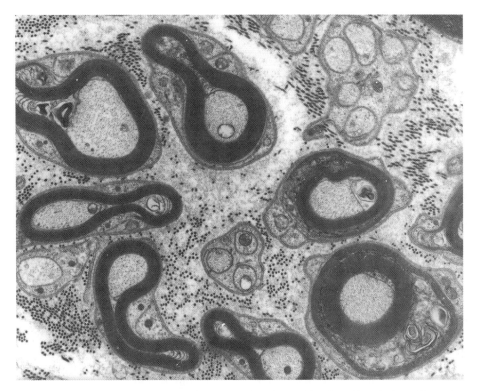

Fig. 4.15 Posterior root of the seventh cervical nerve 6 weeks after avulsion from the spinal cord. Note the healthy myelinated and unmyelinated fibres. × 10 530.

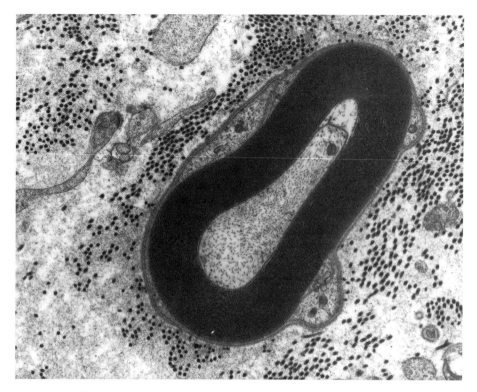

Fig. 4.16 An intact myelinated nerve fibre in the same root. × 16 200.

lesion of the afferent fibres in avulsion of the plexus. However, we suffered so severe a mauling from the late Roger Gilliatt in connection with our previous attempt at naming, that we have decided not to press the point. Once more, we yield the field to Wykehamists.

TYPES OF LESION PRODUCED BY DIFFERENT PHYSICAL AGENTS

Acute nerve compression

Reversible conduction block of the type described by Lewis et al (1931a) has been discussed. It is interesting to note Merrington and Nathan's (1949) observation that the paraesthesia occurring during recovery arises not from the periphery but from the nerve trunks recovering from ischaemia. Acute demyelinating conduction block has also been described, as has the associated differential affection of fibres of different sizes.

Thomas and Holdorff (1993) consider crush and percussion separately. It is likely that in the latter type of injury the lesion is localised – a mixture of demyelination and axonal interruption (Richardson & Thomas 1979). The mechanism of acute conduction block from

demyelination has been considered on page 37. With more severe pressure there is axonal interruption, but that interruption is within the Schwann cell basal laminal tubes. Thomas and Holdorff show a figure which well illustrates this point.

Chronic nerve compression

Entrapment syndromes (see Ch. 12) provide most of the examples of chronic nerve compression, though the latter is one of the causes of neuropathy after ionising radiation (see Ch. 13) and in other conditions in which a nerve is deformed over a tumour or bony abnormality. Clearly, there are a number of mechanisms. Episodic ischaemia clearly accounts for the nocturnal paraesthesiae in "carpal tunnel syndrome", and possibly continued ischaemia accounts for the continuous symptoms (Hongell & Mattson 1971). Evidence on the size of fibres affected comes from Thomas and Fullerton (1963), and on segmental demyelination from Neary and Eames (1975). The systematic studies of Mackinnon and her colleagues (Mackinnon et al 1984, 1985, 1986, Mackinnon & Dellon 1986, Dellon & Mackinnon 1988) showed that the earliest changes occurred in the small vessels of the endo- and perineurium. The presence of numerous Renaut corpuscles (Renaut 1881a,b, Asbury et al 1972, Jefferson et al 1981) was also observed. Later, there is perineurial and epineurial fibrosis, followed by loss of fibres and thinning of myelin sheaths. At the end of the process there is damage to unmyelinated fibres.

Stretch injury

Peripheral nerves outside the spinal canal have considerable tensile strength, but their function is damaged by an elongation of 12% or more, the extent of damage varying with the length of time during which that elongation is maintained. Lundborg and Rydevik (1973) showed that venous flow was blocked when a nerve was stretched by 8% of its resting length, and that stretching by 15% produced ischaemia. At first, elongation is permitted by the elongation of the epineurium and the straightening of the irregular course of the fibres within the fascicles (Haftek 1970, Clarke & Bearn 1972). The latter drew attention to the significance of the "spiral bands of Fontana", confirming the latter's conclusion that the banding appearance of the peripheral nerve is due to the wave-like alignment of its individual nerve fibres (Fig. 4.17). As the fibres are straightened, the banding disappears. Haftek (1970) added the observation that "before rupture of the epineurium the damage to the nerve fibres is either neurapraxia or axonotmesis, because the endoneurial sheaths and Schwann fibres remain intact". Next, the calibre of the fibres is diminished, endoneurial space is diminished and myelin is disrupted (Chalk & Dyck 1993). Then rupture starts: first the epineurium, and last the nerve fibres. The longitudinal extent of damage is considerable (Figs 4.18 to 4.20). The process of damage by a bullet passing through soft tissue near a nerve is comparable, though with a jacketed missile passing through without tumbling rupture is rare. Such lesions are usually conduction blocks.

Acute ischaemia

It is hard to separate the effects of acute ischaemia from those of other physical agents. We have seen that the transient ischaemia of a short period of pressure produces transient failure of conduction. Such a mechanism probably operates when ischaemia is produced by traction. Lundborg (1988a) showed that 8% elongation of a segment of nerve could cause impairment of vascular flow, and that an elongation of 10–15% could arrest all blood flow. Relaxation within 30 minutes would in most cases lead to restoration of flow and conductivity. Acute and persisting ischaemia leads to early loss of axons, and eventually to necrosis of the whole substance of the nerve in the area of affection. Nerve tolerates ischaemia better than does muscle, which cannot tolerate severe ischaemia of longer than 6–8 hours' duration. No nerve escapes unscathed from ischaemia of longer than 8 hours. Hess et al (1979) produced ischaemia of the sciatic nerves of rabbits by ligation of iliac arteries and aorta. These ligations produced ischaemia in six out of seven animals. There was clinical paralysis, with later recovery in two animals which were allowed to survive. Necrosis of muscle occurred, but it was not general, and was not regular in its occurrence or severity. The main nerves showed Wallerian degeneration and paranodal demyelination. "The upper level of nerve damage was characterised by the presence of fibres with normally myelinated internodes proximally and degeneration distally" (Hess et al 1979). Actual infarction of fasciculi with complete necrosis of neural and connective tissue elements was seen in small intramuscular branches only when extensive necrosis of muscle was also present. In the main nerves the central part of the fascicles were the most severely affected. In general, the unmyelinated fibres were spared, but in one case they too were affected. These changes are similar to those seen in human nerves in cases in which ischaemia has been produced by interruption of a main artery or by obstruction of flow by pressure within fascial compartments (Parkes 1945). Indeed, the earlier work of Dyck et al (1972) in cases of ischaemia from necrotising angiopathic neuropathy produced results in the human rather similar to those obtained by Hess et al (1979) in the rat.

The vascular arrangements of nerves are such that injuries of main arteries are more likely to produce infarction of muscle than necrosis of nerve trunks. Even when ischaemic degeneration of myelinated fibres was produced by multiple arterial ligation (Hess et al 1979), Schwann cells and fibroblasts survived and provided the conditions for recovery. Rarely, occlusion of a main artery can cause in man a lesion of nerve without an important degree of muscle infarction (Wilbourn & Hulley 1977).

Case report. In October 1993, a man, then aged 73 years, underwent an injection of steroid into the right forearm. There was instant severe pain and loss of function in the distribution of the right ulnar nerve. Persistence of pain and alteration of sensibility, combined with failure to detect sensory nerve action potentials, led to exploration (August 1995). There were slight localised changes in the flexor carpi ulnaris muscle. The ulnar nerve appeared healthy, but the ulnar artery was tortuous, calcified and distally occluded. Evidently, steroid had been injected into the ulnar artery, which at this point was the principal nutrient of the ulnar nerve. An ischaemic nerve lesion had followed, with very little and very much circumscribed affect on the muscle.

The clinical evidence is distorted by the circumstance that ischaemia is rarely complete. Even nerves that have been seriously ischaemic for 36 hours have been seen to

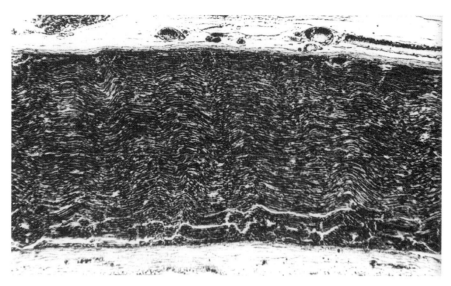

Fig. 4.17 Longitudinal section of the sciatic nerve, showing the undulating paths of fibres. × 140.

Figs 4.18 to 4.20 The results of rupture complicated by sepsis. Electron microscopic study of serial (2-cm intervals) biopsies of proximal stump of sciatic nerve of 34-year-old man 8 months after rupture by fracture, and subsequent sepsis.

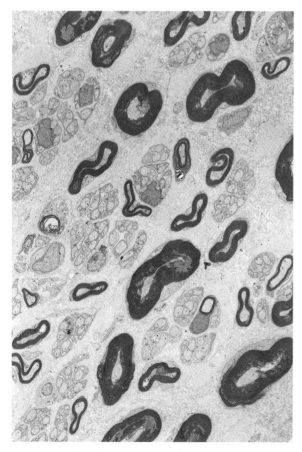

Fig. 4.18 Proximal section. × 1500.

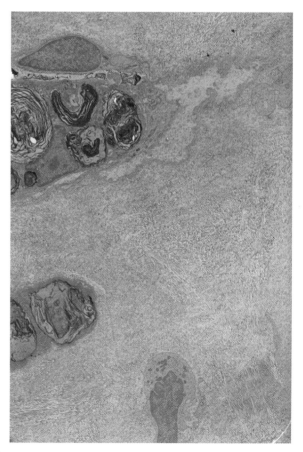

Fig. 4.19 Distal section. × 2340.

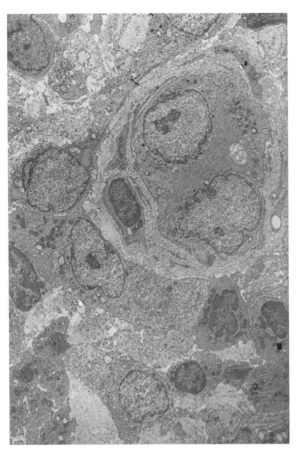

Fig. 4.20 Intermediate section. × 3000.

recover adequate function. In one case of ischaemia after supracondylar fracture of the humerus complicated by thrombosis of the brachial artery, the median nerve was seen at operation to lack all vascular pedicles from elbow to wrist. It lay in the middle of the completely infarcted flexor muscles of the forearm. Three years later there was recovery of sweating and of impaired sensation in its area of distribution.

Evidently there are extremes of effect of ischaemia. At one end there is the transient conduction block of temporary ischaemia; at the other, the effective neurotmesis of infarction of the nerve with destruction of conducting tissue, Schwann cell–myelin structure and connective tissue. In between there must be mixtures and varieties of lesions, some of which are recoverable.

Chronic ischaemia

Eames and Lange (1967) studied clinically and by light and electron microscopy of biopsy specimens the effect of chronic ischaemia on the nerves of 30 patients with arteriosclerotic obliterative disease and two with Buerger's disease. There was a good correlation between the severity of the arterial disease and the incidence of neuropathy. The incidence of neuropathy was high (87.5%). Eames and Lange found extensive segmental demyelination and remyelination, in addition to Wallerian degeneration and regeneration. In all cases – not only in those with Buerger's disease – there were marked occlusive changes in the small arterial vessels of the epineurium. The relation of these changes to "ischaemic pain" and "trophic" changes in the skin was canvassed.

Thermal injury

The effects of cold have been studied extensively (Bickford 1939, Webster et al 1942, White & Scoville 1945, Lundberg 1948, Dodt 1953, Douglas & Malcolm 1955, Franz & Iggo 1968). Bickford (1939), cooling the ulnar nerve, found a sequential loss of the different modalities of sensation: first, appreciation of cold; and last, sensibility to pain, touch and warmth. As Thomas and Holdorff (1993) remark: "observations on non-freezing cold injury of nerve have largely stemmed from the exigencies of war". In the First World War, "trench foot" was a common cause of disablement; in the Second World War, "immersion foot" was a more common occurrence (Ungley & Blackwood 1942, Ungley et al 1945, White & Scoville 1945).

Irwin et al (1997) had the opportunity of investigating the neural damage in a case of "trench foot" or "non-freezing cold injury". A 40-year-old Asian man, homeless in the UK through the operation of Thatcherite principles, was subjected to exposure lasting 19 days, during 8 of which the ambient temperature was below 0°C. He lost all function and sensibility in his feet, and, ultimately, several toes. Sensory nerve function was carefully measured and recorded; at the time of removal of dead tissue, 4 weeks after admission, a biopsy of viable skin was taken from the plantar surface of the right great toe. There was evidence of damage to both myelinated and unmyelinated nerve fibres, possibly, the authors speculate, "in a cycle of ischaemia and reperfusion".

In civil practice at the present time, it is rather the effects of heat that concern the clinician, principally because of damage to the sciatic nerve by the heat of polymerising cement during arthroplasty of the hip. The effects of heat seem to have received little attention. Nerves can of course be destroyed by extremes of heat, or, for instance, by diathermy during operation. Sunderland (1978b) mentions the hazard of damage by heat, and Bremer and Titica (1948b) made some observations on its effect in animals. Hoogeveen et al (1991) investigated the effect of heating a 5-mm segment of the sciatic nerve of the rat for 30 minutes at 45°C. They found that this produced swelling of the endothelium of the neural blood vessels and Wallerian degeneration of all the nerve fibres. There was of course total loss of motor function. The process in the nerves was, however, reversible: regeneration occurred over 4–5 weeks. The vascular changes were not apparently reversible. Xu and Pollock (1994) examined physiologically and morphologically the effect of heat ranging from 47°C to 58°C on rat sciatic nerve. Unmyelinated fibres showed a greater direct vulnerability to hyperthermia, which was first manifested as a reversible conduction block and at higher temperatures by immediate and selective axonal degeneration. Lower grade thermal injury caused a delayed selective loss of myelinated fibres. Xu and Pollock remark in relation to the latter effect: "Evidence from this study suggests that this is secondary to a heat-induced angiopathy, immediately and diffusely manifest in the vasa nervorum and giving rise to a progressive and ultimately severe reduction in nerve blood flow." The relative sparing of unmyelinated fibres was attributed to their greater resistance to ischaemia. It is necessary in considering risk to the sciatic nerve in operation for hip replacement to recall that the temperature of polymerising cement rises to 95° Celsius about 15 minutes after mixing, and remains above 70°C for another 12 minutes. Birch et al (1992) had the opportunity of examining a length of sciatic nerve damaged by the heat of polymerising cement. They later took the opportunity of studying the effect of the heat of polymerising cement on the median nerve of an arm recently amputated because of a complete preganglionic injury of the brachial plexus. The remarkable feature was the localised nature of the lesion: although at the site of burning there was destruction of axoplasm and disruption of myelin, a normal pattern of myelinated and unmyelinated fibres was found 10 mm from the margin of cement (Figs 4.21 to 4.23).

Electric shock

Earl (personal communication, 1988) reports conduction block from electric shock. The severest electrical burn clearly produces destruction of tissue, including nerves. Di Vincenti et al (1969), reviewing 65 cases, reported spotty necrosis of peripheral nerve in cases of severe electrical injury. The fact that these lesions are clinically incomplete indicates a potential for recovery.

Percussion injury

Richardson and Thomas (1979) studied the effects of percussion injury. The clinical application in the peripheral nerve field is perhaps slight, but the authors indicate that their results could give some indication of events in injury of the spinal cord, in spite of the difference in structure between central and peripheral nervous tissue. The lesion appears principally to be a localised axonal interruption with later degeneration and with rather short-lived changes in the myelin sheath. Richardson and Thomas noted that their findings did nothing to explain the transient interruption of nerve function after percussive injury described by Denny-Brown and Brenner (1944).

Radiation

The statement by Janzen and Warren (1942) that "nerve tissue is extremely resistant to radiation" is, alas, true only insofar as the function of conducting an impulse is concerned, and insofar as doses up to 10 000 R (100 Gy) "do not cause overt damage to this normally static cell population" (Janzen & Warren 1942). Cavanagh (1968a,b) investigated in rats the extent to which irradiation impaired the capacity of the Schwann cells to proliferate in response to injury. He found that the capacity to proliferate in response to crushing was seriously impaired if the

Figs 4.21 to 4.23 Thermal damage to the median nerve after exposure to the heat of setting cement, showing the limited longitudinal extent of the neural lesion. (Electron microscopic studies by Mr Stephen Gschmeissner.)

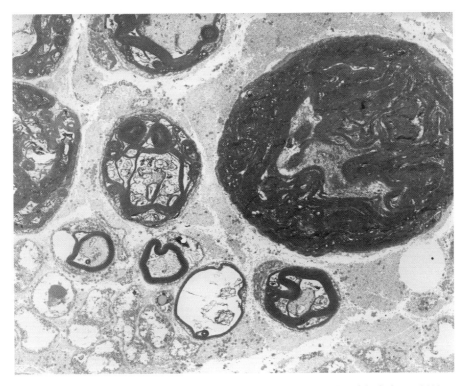

Fig. 4.21 Virtual destruction of axoplasm and cellular elements at the site of the lesion. × 3600.

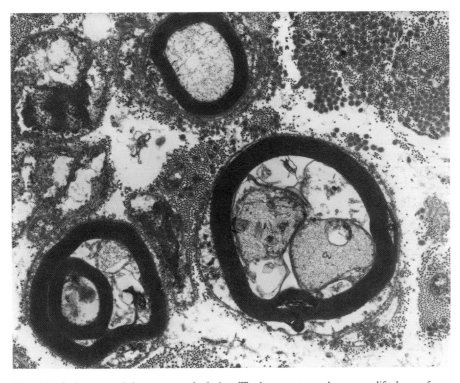

Fig. 4.22 Serious axonal damage near the lesion. The basement membranes are lifted away from the Schwann cell processes. Coagulation of endoneural collagen. × 9000.

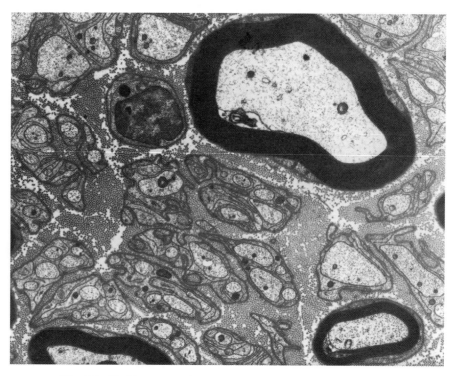

Fig. 4.23 Healthy axons and collagen 10 mm from site of injury. × 9000.

limb had previously been irradiated with 1000 R (10 Gy). Of special interest is his further finding that the effect was no different whether the nerve had been irradiated 3 weeks or 9 months before crushing. The lesion is perhaps best considered as:

- a lesion from external compression exerted by fibrosis of soft tissue in particular the pectoralis minor muscle
- an intrinsic lesion of the nerve.

The latter affects first the axon and then the myelin sheath; it is associated with vasculitis, which leads eventually to fibrosis (Spiess 1972) (Figs 4.24 and 4.25). The effect may extend to the main vessel (Butler et al 1980, Barros D'Sa 1992a). It seems likely that the dose of radiation tolerated by neural tissue depends broadly on the total dose and the period of time for which it is given, but evidently these are individual variations and there may indeed be individual susceptibilities. Thomas and Holdorff (1993) reproduce from Notter and Turesson (1975) a chart showing dose–time relationships in radiation lesions of the brachial plexus. There is room for further study of the relation between time and dose on the one hand, and the incidence of neuropathy on the other, but the difficulties are formidable.

Ultrasound

Young and Henneman (1961), working on the sciatic nerves of large green frogs, made the singular discovery that focused ultrasound would abolish conduction of impulses completely and irreversibly if a sufficiently long pulse width (over 1 second) and train length (over 20 pulses) were used. With shorter pulse widths and lower train lengths effects on conduction of intermediate severity could be produced. It seemed that there was an inverse relation between fibre size and vulnerability to ultrasound. Lele (1963) cast doubt on the interpretation of these findings, considering that the effects attributed to the irradiation were caused by local heating.

Envenomation

In the single case reported by Laing and Harrison (1991), a young man's right ulnar nerve was affected by the venom expressed from the tentacle of a box jellyfish (*Chironex fleckeri*), and presumably conveyed transcutaneously. The nerve was explored and found to be oedematous, but the period elapsing between injury and exploration is not related. There was spontaneous recovery. The case evokes

Figs 4.24 and 4.25 Radiation neuropathy. Biopsy from the lateral cord of brachial plexus.

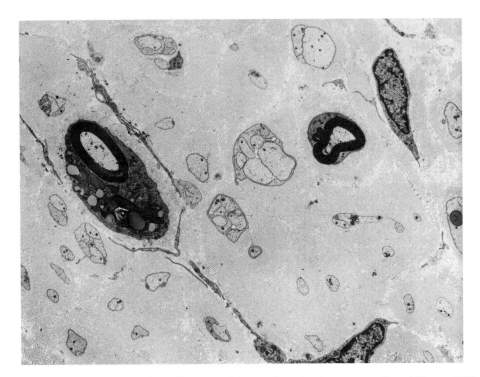

Fig. 4.24 Extensive collagenisation, with two surviving myelinated and some unmyelinated fibres. × 5950.

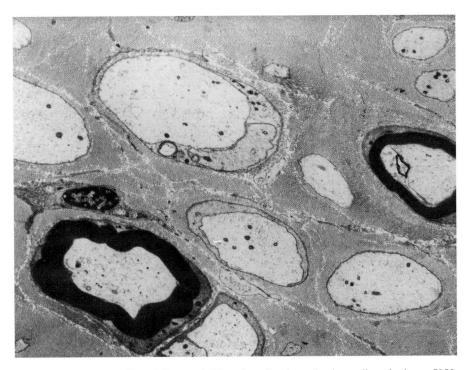

Fig. 4.25 Surviving myelinated fibres; wrinkling of myelin; demyelination; collagenisation. × 5950.

echoes of that of the Lion's Mane (1909), but because of the absence of Dr Watson from the latter we are condemned to remain in the dark about the presence of neuropathy in the surviving victim of *Cyanea capillata*.

The peripheral effects of denervation

These effects follow degenerative lesions in which recovery fails or is long delayed. If regeneration of axons into the distal stump fails, changes, which over time become irreversible, develop in the target organs and in the proximal neuron. Motor end-plates atrophy and disappear (Bowden & Gutmann 1944); the denervated muscles undergo fibrosis. Bowden and Gutmann (1944) recorded that after 3 months' denervation it became increasingly difficult to identify the end-plates. From 3 years on they found fragmentation of structures, and reckoned that this represented irreversible change. Luco and Eyzaguirre

(1955) found that the nearer the lesion was to the point of innervation the more rapidly did the changes in the end-plates appear. Cutaneous sensory end-organs atrophy more slowly (Figs 4.26 and 4.27). Dellon (1981) found that they degenerate and eventually atrophy. The reaction of muscle spindles to denervation has been studied extensively. Sherrington (1894) found the spindles "very obvious amid atrophied extrafusal muscle fibres five months after denervation". Batten (1897) found in a case of complete paralysis after a lesion of the brachial plexus that atrophy of spindles did occur, but took place much later than was the case in ordinary muscle fibres. Tower (1932) found that the nuclear bag fibres showed only a slight reduction in diameter after denervation, whereas the chain fibres atrophied almost as rapidly as did the extrafusal fibres. Tower noted in particular the thickening of the capsule. De Reuck (1974) reported rather similar findings. Swash and Fox (1974) noted capsular thickening

Figs 4.26 and 4.27 Atrophy of cutaneous sensory receptors.

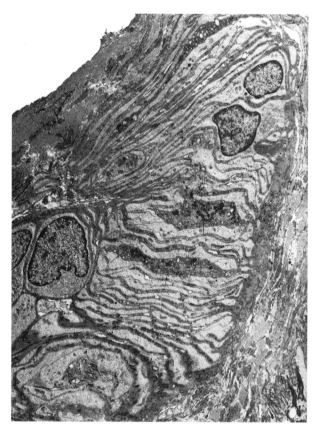

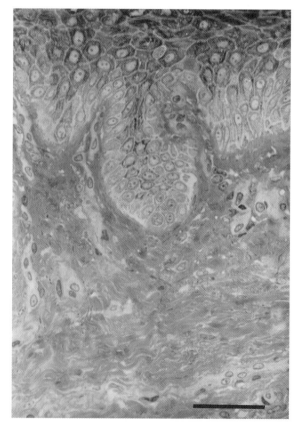

Fig. 4.26 A Meissner corpuscle in the skin of the index finger of a patient whose median nerve had been cut 3 weeks previously. × 3630.

Fig. 4.27 The skin of the index finger of a patient whose median nerve had been cut 1 year previously. No Meissner's corpuscles are recognisable. Scale bar: 50 μm.

Figs 4.28 and 4.29 Atrophy of the spinal cord after damage to the brachial plexus.

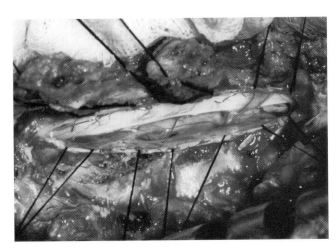

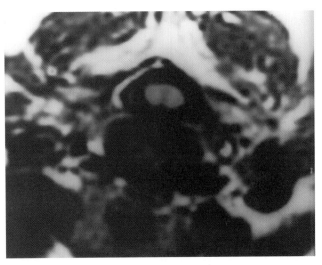

Fig. 4.28 Right side of the spinal cord at the level C5 to C8 seen at hemilaminectomy 6 months after intradural lesion of the plexus. Note the shrinking of the middle part of the cord at the level of the emergence of the seventh cervical roots, and the mouths of the pseudomeningoceles.

Fig. 4.29 Magnetic resonance image of the cord of a 12-year-old child who suffered an obstetric lesion of the brachial plexus. Note the loss of dorsal columns.

and atrophy of intrafusal fibres after sensorimotor denervation, and Myles and Glasby (1992) conclusively showed that atrophy of muscle spindles followed uncorrected denervation.

Loss of nervous control of the small peripheral blood vessels leads to defects of nutrition and subcutaneous tissues. There is atrophy of the proximal neuron. As long ago as 1913, Ramon y Cajal (1928d) noted that "as shown by the older observations of Dickinson (1868) and by the more modern ones of Gudden, Forel and Monakow (1882), there are cases where the neuron whose axon is mutilated or even functionally isolated shows morbid changes, and may even die". The changes in the nerve fibre and nerve cell proximal to the site of axonotomy have already been discussed. In the words of McComas et al

(1978), "the periphery is essential for the functional integrity of motor and sensory nerve axons".

Further evidence about the changes in proximal neural structures is available from studies of the spinal cord after intradural damage to the roots of the brachial plexus. At operation (hemilaminectomy) the ipsilateral cord is seen to be atrophic, doubtless from the damage to the motor and sensory pathways (Fig. 4.28). Further, magnetic resonance imaging plainly shows atrophy of the cord after birth injury of the brachial plexus (Fig. 4.29). It is a matter of interest that, despite the degeneration of the proximal process of the cells of the posterior root ganglion, these cells appear to retain for a long time their ability to sustain their distal processes, apparently without serious functional impairment (Bonney & Gilliatt 1958).

5. Regeneration

Regeneration: the cellular proliferation; importance of integrity of the basement membrane; neurotropins and neurotrophins; nerve growth factors; regeneration after intradural injury; predictors of recovery; regeneration of end-organs.

The cellular process of regeneration involves both proximal and distal stumps and any gap between them. Clearance of myelin debris by the action of macrophages prepares the distal stump for reception of the outgrowing fibres (Fig. 5.1). During this phase there is multiplication of Schwann cells (Figs 5.2 and 5.3). An increase in the collagen content of the distal stump may be related to the activity of Schwann cells or fibroblasts. The proximal stump is the site of intense activity and multiplication of Schwann cells, migrating from proximal and distal stumps, forming the "bands of Büngner" described by light microscopists. The axons of the proximal stump sprout, each sprout being tipped by a growth cone. *Collateral* sprouts arise from nodes of Ranvier at levels at which the axons are still intact; *terminal* sprouts arise from the tip of the surviving axon (Figs 5.4 to 5.6). With the entry of axonal sprouts into the distal stump there is a second wave of Schwann cell proliferation. Initially, there

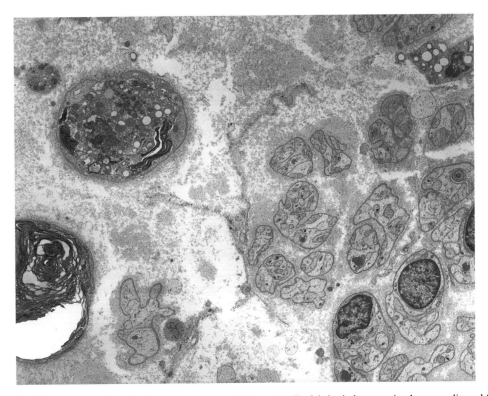

Fig. 5.1 The distal stump at 3 weeks. Macrophage (top left) clears myelin debris. A degenerating large myelinated fibre. Schwann cells. × 2880. (Electron microscopic study by Mr Stephen Gschmeissner.)

Figs 5.2 and 5.3 The distal stump at 3 weeks. (Electron microscopic studies by Mr Stephen Gschmeissner.)

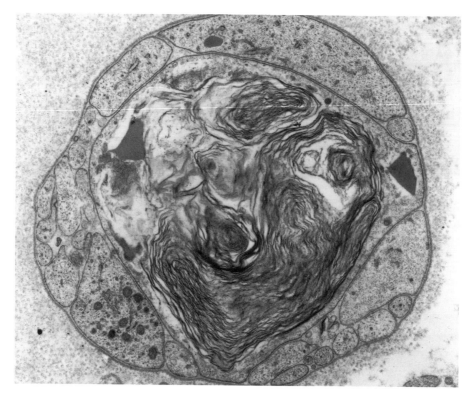

Fig. 5.2 Degenerating large myelinating nerve fibre, with proliferating Schwann cells. × 11 340.

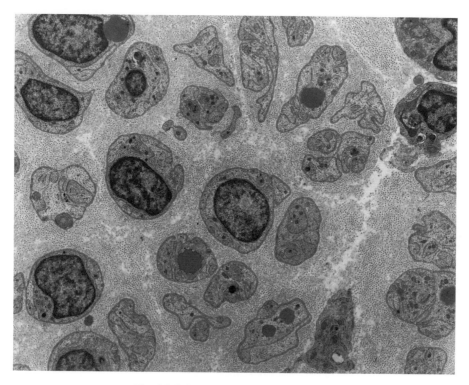

Fig. 5.3 Schwann cell proliferation. × 6840.

Figs 5.4 to 5.6 The proximal stump. (Electron microscopic studies by Mr Stephen Gschmeissner.)

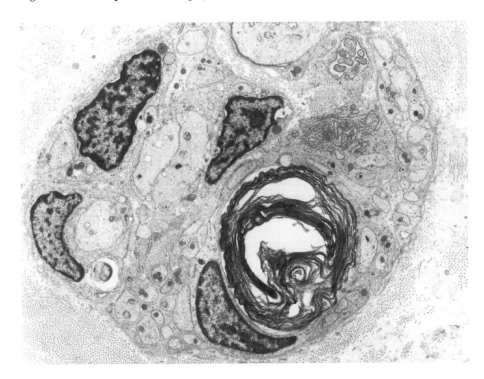

Fig. 5.4 At 3 weeks there is retrograde degeneration of one large myelinated nerve fibre. Sprouting axons. × 6960.

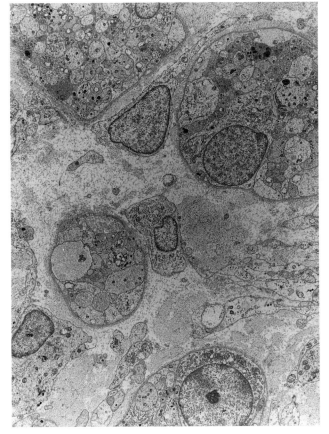

Fig. 5.5 Axonal sprouts and Schwann cells. × 3190.

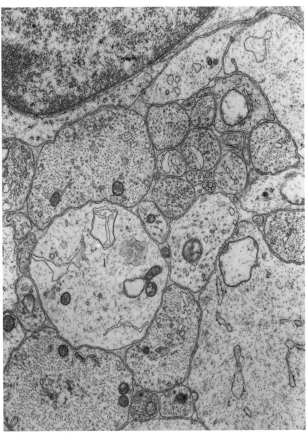

Fig. 5.6 Axonal sprouts adjacent to a Schwann cell nucleus. × 17 980.

are more axonal sprouts than there were axons in the intact nerve, but only those that establish connections with end-organs survive (Sanders and Young 1946).

Ramon y Cajal (1928a) described the process called "compartmentation" by Morris et al (1972), in which the proximal stump becomes divided into "minifascicles" that replace the original large bundles (Fig. 5.7). This arrangement is confined to the proximal stump and the gap; it gives way after some months to the more usual arrangement of fibres. Remyelination begins (Figs 5.8 and 5.9). As connections are established and the regenerating nerve matures, the original profusion of Schwann cells gives way to the more orderly arrangement characteristic of the healthy nerve. Vizoso and Young (1948) studied internodal length and fibre diameter in the developing and regenerating nerves of rabbits. They found that in regeneration the myelin was at first continuous over the surface of the nerve, and that segmentation followed later. In the adult the former relationship between fibre length and internodal length did not reappear: internodal lengths were always shorter in the regenerated than in the healthy nerve.

There is always a gap of some sort between the faces of the proximal and distal stumps. The gap is first filled with blood containing macrophages: a fibrin clot is then formed. Into this clot proceed capillaries and fibroblasts from the surrounding tissues and the nerve ends (Thomas 1966). The advancing axonal sprouts accompany Schwann cells. When the gap is bridged by a nerve graft, the latter acts as a source of Schwann cells for sustaining the axonal sprouts and for their conduction to the distal stump. Lundborg (1988c) studied the growth of axons across gaps in a mesothelial chamber and found that axons were able to traverse a 10-mm gap.

The success of axonal sprouts in surviving and developing in the new environment of the distal stump and in reaching their targets must depend on humoral factors. Lundborg (1991) helpfully defines the terms *neurotrophic* and *neurotropic* as applied to these factors. "A neurotrophic factor (νευρον (neuron) and τροφη (trophe): nutrition) is a substance influencing survival and growth of nerve cells. A neurotropic factor (νευρον (neuron) and τροπος (tropos): way, conduct) is a substance exerting an attraction, at a distance, on growing axons." That attraction is, presumably, specific as to tissue and as to topography. Thus, tissue-specific neurotropic factors lead sprouting axons into nerve tissue as opposed to muscle, skin or scar; topography-specific neurotropic factors lead sprouting axons of a particular nerve into the distal stump of that nerve. An even further degree of specificity may lead motor axons to motor endings, and sensory axons to sensory endings (Brushart & Seiler 1987, Brushart 1988). More recent work (Gu et al 1995) has clearly shown the neurotropic effect exercised on axons regenerating from the proximal stump of the transected sciatic nerve of the rat by the distal stump of the nerve. "In all cultures, neurites from the (excised neonatal dorsal root) ganglion extended directly towards the degenerated distal stump

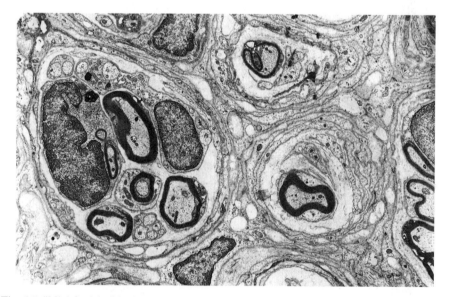

Fig. 5.7 "Mini-fascicles" in the proximal stump, with myelinated fibres and Schwann cells. × 2000.

Figs 5.8 and 5.9 The proximal stump. (Electron microscopic studies by Mr Stephen Gschmeissner.)

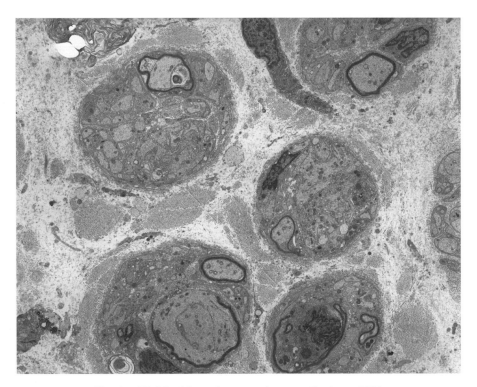

Fig. 5.8 Mini-fascicles and commencing remyelination. × 2784.

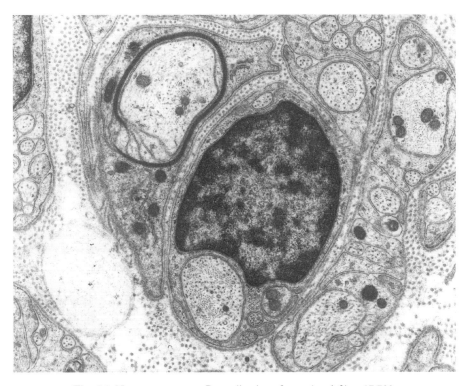

Fig. 5.9 Numerous sprouts. Remyelination of axon (top left). × 17 700.

and not towards the undegenerated nerve segment. Analysis of the supernatants of nerve homogenates ... demonstrated that 250 and 18 kDa proteins were upregulated in the degenerated distal stumps and that 89, 67 and 65 kDa proteins were expressed by these groups but not by normal nerve." Clearly, there are chemotropic (in this case neurotropic) substances in these bands; as Gu and colleagues indicate, the nature of these requires investigation.

The work of Brushart et al (1995) on the crossing of gaps by regenerating fibres indicated the limits of the ability of neurotropic factors to promote "correct" fascicular reinnervation. They found that, when the fascicular alignment of the stumps was reversed, axonal dispersion was determined by fascicular size rather than by fascicular identity. These results may stress the importance of correct fascicular alignment of stumps in suture and in grafting.

The production of nerve growth factors in the distal nerve by endoneurial fibroblasts and by Schwann cells, and of nerve growth factor and NEFR by the Schwann cells provides an environment friendly to regenerating axons. Indeed, Griffin and Hoffman (1993) remark: "given the environment of the dorsal stump, it is perhaps surprising that functional restoration is so seldom the consequence of nerve injury in humans". The perspective of most clinicians is perhaps rather different: they think that the results they obtain are not all that bad considering the natural difficulty encountered by regenerating nerve fibres in reaching their targets.

When there is a lesion "in continuity" or when healthy nerve end has been opposed to healthy nerve end, the elongating axon enters the environment most favourable to it: the denervated distal stump. Ramon y Cajal (1928b) plainly saw the system of guidance as being a combination of contact and chemotropism, and this view has in effect been confirmed by later work. If the "growth cone" encounters non-neural tissue, axonal elongation still occurs, and may even be followed by myelination. In some cases, doubtless, this process is sufficient to bridge a gap between the ends of the divided nerve. The growth cone contains growth-associated protein brought to the tip by fast axonal transport; this and other materials act with locally derived nerve growth factor to influence synthesis within the nerve cell. Cytoskeletal proteins are brought by slow centrifugal transport. As in the development of the nerve fibre, its regeneration is associated with further proliferation of Schwann cells. Enlargement of the diameter of the axon is the signal for myelination. The regenerating sprouts of unmyelinated fibres remain so. The rate of peripheral outgrowth of regenerating fibres is reckoned to be about 1 mm day in the human adult; that is, about the rate of slow transport of the neurofilament protein. The

rate is substantially faster in children, as indeed it is in young experimental animals. It is almost certainly faster after primary than after secondary repair, as was suggested by Birch and Raji (1991). It has been suggested (Lundborg 1988c), and the suggestion is supported by our experience, that the rate of regeneration is faster proximally than distally. We suggest a rate of 2 mm day after suture of clean wounds of nerves at clavicular level and in the proximal part of the lower limb. Why not? Such wounds are nearer to the nerve cell than are more distal injuries.

Regeneration after intradural injury

The intradural, preganglionic lesions of the brachial plexus, and to a lesser extent the similar lesions of the lumbosacral plexus, have to be discussed separately in the matter of regeneration. It has for some time been clear that repair of such lesions offered the best chance of restoration of function and avoidance of pain, but the formidable technical difficulties of this have for years deterred most aspirants. There was, in addition, the discouraging thought that, even if repair could be achieved, success required regeneration in the central nervous system. Although, as long ago as 1907 Kilvington (Glasby & Hems 1993) demonstrated the ability of the axons of the anterior horn cells to regenerate, and Tower (1943) showed the same, the matter was not systematically pursued. The latter indeed stated that the object of her work was "to prove unfounded the prevailing assumption that ventral nerve roots cannot regenerate if avulsed from the spinal cord". She did just that in experiments on cats. Freeman (1952) used plasma clot suture for intradural transplantation of anterior spinal nerve roots in immature male guinea baboons. He reported functional restoration of a spinal reflex pattern of activity, and drew the conclusion that regeneration had occurred. Ochs and Barnes (1969) showed regeneration of ventral root fibres into dorsal roots in the cat, as shown by axoplasmic flow of labelled leucine. Sanjuanbenito et al (1976) demonstrated axonal regeneration in the ventral roots of the cat.

The demonstration by Nathaniel and Nathaniel (1973) that in adult rats the dorsal root fibres could regenerate into the spinal cord after crushing, seemed to indicate that the proximal limb of the axon of the sensory cell could make its way into the substantia gelatinosa and posterior funiculi. Bonney and Jamieson (1979) achieved reattachment of posterior roots in the case of a man with a severe traction lesion of the brachial plexus, but that was not followed by recovery. Then Jamieson and Eames (1980) studied in adult dogs the regeneration of motor and sensory axons after avulsion and reimplantation. They found that, whereas there was significant regeneration of motor axons across the zone of repair, there was no regeneration of sensory axons. It appeared that, whereas the motor axons behaved as part of the peripheral nervous system, the central process of the axon of the sensory cell behaved as part of the central nervous system.

Interest was revived by the demonstration by Carlstedt et al (1986) that in the rat motor axons could grow out of the spinal cord into ventral roots reimplanted after avulsion, and that they could make functional connections. Cullheim et al (1989) confirmed the reinnervation of skeletal muscle after ventral root implantation into the spinal cord of the cat. It was not even necessary to reimplant the roots along the anterolateral sulcus; subpial implantation near the sulcus was all that was necessary. Carlstedt et al (1990) confirmed the regeneration of motor axons through the cord into implanted roots, and Smith and Kodoma (1991) confirmed that functional reconnection was possible. Carlstedt (1991) confirmed these results with experiments on primates. Hems and Glasby (1992a) and Hems et al (1994) followed with similarly rigorous studies in sheep, which put beyond doubt functional regeneration from motor cells into skeletal muscle. Carlstedt et al (1995) reported the results of repair in man, of one root by direct implantation and of another by an intervening graft. There was secure evidence of functional reinnervation. Thus it seems clear that, although the motor axon can pass through central nervous system tissue to its destination, the central process of the sensory axon is unable to do this in the adult. As work in this field expands, it will be necessary to examine the effect of a solely motor innervation of muscles on their function. Doubtless, the search for sensory reinnervation will have to continue.

Nerve growth factor

Ramon y Cajal (1928c) clearly established that there was no autogenous regeneration of the peripheral stump. His belief in the presence of some neurotrophic factor in the distal stump is expressed in the phrase: "The penetration into the peripheral stump implies a neurotrophic action, or the exercise of electrical influence by the latter." He named contact guidance "tactile adhesion". Young (1942), however, seemed to conclude that "successful nervous regeneration must depend mainly on the chances provided for adequate numbers of outgrowing fibres to establish connections resembling their original ones". A hint of belief in neurotrophins had however been given in his work with Holmes (Young & Holmes 1940).

Levi-Montalcini et al (1954), Cohen et al (1954) and Cohen and Levi-Montalcini (1956) described an agent found in mouse sarcomata which markedly promoted growth in the sympathetic and posterior root ganglia of chick embryos. They found that treatment with snake venom enhanced the activities of this agent, and that snake venom itself contained a potent growth-promoting agent. In 1956, Cohen and Levi Montalcini presented the results of partial purification and characterisation of this nerve growth factor (NGF). They suggested that the active material was a protein or bound to a protein. Levi-Montalcini and Angeletti (1968) indicated the specific action of NGF on sensory and sympathetic nerve cells: "the control exerted by the NGF on sensory and sympathetic nerve cells stands out by virtue of the magnitude of its effects, its target specificity, and the plurality of its actions". Politis and Spencer (1983) showed the neurotropic effects of diffusible factors in the distal stumps of cut nerves. The factor was further examined by Gunderson and Barrett (1979), Martini and Schachner (1986), Heumann et al (1987), Rich et al (1989) and Hurst and Badalmente (1991). Brushart and Seiler (1987), using horseradish peroxidase (HRP) to label motor neurons, found evidence of selective innervation of the motor stump. They rightly concluded that "augmentation of this phenomenon to produce specific reunion of individual motor axons could dramatically improve the results of nerve suture". So it could. Windebank (1993) defined growth factors as "soluble extracellular macromolecules that influence the proliferation, growth and differentiation of target cells by a cell surface–receptor mechanism". Nerve growth factor interacts with receptors in cells throughout the central nervous system. In the peripheral nervous system the cells of the ganglia of the posterior root and autonomic system are responsive to NGF. Those of the anterior horn appeared not to be, but the existence of a motor neuron growth factor with similar properties was inferred (Hollyday & Hamburger 1976).

The importance of NGFs in regeneration and in the quality of reinnervation can hardly be overestimated, but effective clinical application awaits the outcome of current work. It is perhaps in this field in particular that peripheral neurologists must look for advance in methods for improving results after repair. Levi-Montalcini (1987) herself reviewed the situation regarding NGF in her Nobel Prize lecture "The Nerve Growth factor 35 Years Later." She reviewed the extraordinary history of its discovery, and indicated the current state of affairs in the field. Later, Drago et al (1994) summarised the current situation in a rapidly changing field. They defined NGF as a trophic agent for developing sensory and autonomic neurons, and went on to narrate the identifications of its three homologues: brain derived neurotrophic factor (BDNF), neurotrophin-3 (NT-3) and neurotrophin-4 (NT-4).

Each of these was found "to exert distinct but overlapping activities within the developing peripheral and central nervous systems". Other growth factors were also found to exert significant effects in the developing nervous system. They included ciliary neurotrophic factor (CNTF), leukaemia inhibitory factor-cholinergic differentiation factor (LIF/CDF), acidic and basic fibroblast growth factors (FGF-1 and FGF-2), epidermal growth factor (EGF) and platelet derived growth factor (PDGF).

Clearly, the question arose of whether any of these many growth factors could be used with advantage in neurological disorders. Drago et al went on to examine the role of NGF in the treatment of diabetic neuropathy and adumbrated the need for study of the role of NGF, BDNF, CNTF and LIF/CDF in the treatment of injured nerves. Their later discussion concerned the possible role of neurotrophic factors in various diseases of the central nervous system. In this, the role of CNTF and LIF, in particular, in the survival of motor neurons is considered. Discussing the implications for Parkinson's disease in particular, Drago et al noted the work of Lin et al (1993) on the isolation of a neurotrophic factor derived from glial cell line (GDNF), which suggested that dopaminergic neuron-specific neurotrophic factors would be identified. Through the goodwill and courtesy of Dr Anand, Dr Terenghi and his colleagues we are able to reproduce microphotographs showing NGF, GDNF and GDNF receptor activity in the human peripheral nerve and dorsal root ganglion (Figs 5.10 to 5.13 and 5.24, 5.25; see also Plate section). Anand et al (1994d) investigated the role of NGF deprivation in the development of diabetic neuropathy; they also studied accumulation of NGF in the distal stump of injured nerves, and the consequent deprivation in the proximal stumps and cell bodies. The role of CNTF in regeneration of motor neurons was also examined. Anand et al also speculated on the role of NGF in the regulation of nociception. Their important work is continuing. A recent application of NGF is given by Whitworth et al (1996). They had earlier studied fibronectin (a matrix glycoprotein, relevant in wound repair) as a potential scaffold for regeneration of nerves. When fibronectin mats were impregnated with NGF, regeneration of Schwann cells and axons across defects in the rat sciatic nerve was enhanced.

Evidently, important questions regarding the role of neurotrophic factors in regeneration of peripheral nerves and in the causation of pain and cutaneous hyperaesthesia are raised by the continuing work in this field. Once those questions are answered, the therapeutic role of these factors will almost certainly be explored and developed.

Predictors of recovery

In clinical practice, most injuries of nerves short of transection inflict damage of all three grades of severity. The quality of reinnervation and hence of recovery depends first on the extent of damage causing degeneration and in particular loss of continuity of the basement membrane. A nerve fibre recovers completely after conduction block (neurapraxia), so long as the causative factor ceases to operate. Since this recovery does not have to be determined by axonal regrowth, it occurs over minutes, hours, days, weeks or, – rarely, – months. A nerve fibre will regenerate to its correct target after axonotomy so long as the basement membrane is preserved and the causative factor is removed. But recovery will take as long as it takes for the axon to reinnervate its target. Thus, recovery is the rule after "axonotmesis". A nerve fibre will only regenerate to its correct target after axonotomy with interruption of the basement membrane if it is correctly directed to its target field or is drawn there by the operation of growth factors.

Thus, in the case of individual nerves, when the promptitude and quality of primary treatment is equal the quality of recovery will depend on

- the nature of the lesion
- the incidence of axonotomy
- the incidence of interruption of the basement membrane
- the obstacles posed to correct targeting by the complexity of functional representation in the nerve and the consequent liability to axon/target confusion
- the distance of the lesion from the target organs.

We have already indicated that there are in effect no "purely motor" or "purely sensory" nerves, but the liability to axon/target confusion is plainly greater in a nerve such as the median, which has an extensive motor and cutaneous sensory distribution, than it is in the posterior interosseous nerve, which has no cutaneous sensory distribution. It is not doubted that full maturation of the regenerating nerve fibre depends on the establishment of the connection with its end-organ.

The quality of recovery after repair is far better in children than it is in adults. The reason for this difference has been sought in the better quality and quantity of reinnervation in the child and in the better adaptation of the child's central receptor and effector mechanisms to change in the pattern of innervation. Certainly, neurotrophic factors are more active and more effective in the growing child than they are in the adult.

Regeneration of end-organs. There is, evidently, a limit to the period during which an end-organ can be denervated and yet recover after reinnervation. All end-organs have been studied: the earliest were perhaps the motor end-plates (Bowden & Guttman 1944). The effect of reinnervation on muscle spindles was studied by Myles and Glasby (1992), Schröder et al (1979) and Barker et al (1986, 1990). The work of Barker et al (1986) on muscle

Figs 5.10 to 5.13 Neurotrophic factors visualised through immunoreactivity. (Micrographs courtesy of Dr Praveen Anand and colleagues.)

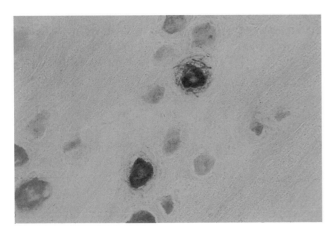

Fig. 5.10 Brain derived neurotrophic factor (BDNF) immunoreactivity in medium-sized neuronal cell bodies and associated axons in human dorsal root ganglion after avulsion of spinal root. × 150. (See also Plate section.)

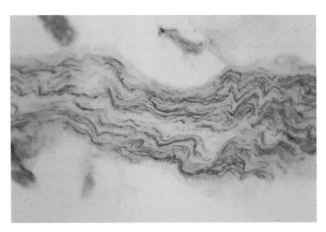

Fig. 5.11 Glial derived neurotrophic factor (GDNF) immunoreactivity in Schwann cell of healthy human sural nerve. × 150. (See also Plate section.)

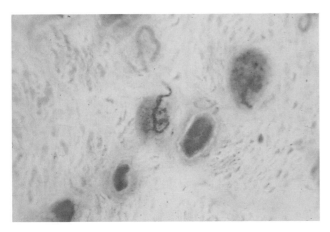

Fig. 5.12 GDNF immunoreactivity in neuronal cell bodies and adjacent axons in human dorsal root ganglion after avulsion of spinal root. × 150. (See also Plate section.)

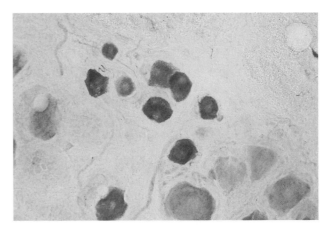

Fig. 5.13 GDNF receptor C ret immunoreactivity in neuronal cell bodies of human dorsal root ganglion after avulsion of spinal roots. × 150. (See also Plate section)

spindles denervated for long periods seemed to indicate that the quality of response after reinnervation would be impaired. However, later work (Barker et al 1990) indicated that delaying repair for up to 8 weeks "did not give rise to any significant detrimental effect on such reinnervation". Bowden and Gutmann (1944) did an extensive study of the response of the motor end-plates to denervation, finding that after 3 months it became increasingly difficult to identify the organs. Denervation for up to 3 years produced no degeneration or disruption of the muscle fibres themselves. However, "shrinkage and increase of connective tissue may be too advanced to allow recovery after reinnervation". After 3 years, disruptive changes occurred in the muscle fibres. Gutmann and Young (1944) investigated the reinnervation of muscle in rabbits, and found that when muscles were kept denervated for increasing periods the proportion of old end-plates that became reinnervated was progressively reduced. "Most of the nerve fibres escape and run along between the muscle fibres, ultimately making contact with the sarcoplasm and forming new plates." They had the opportunity of examining the extensor carpi radialis muscle of a patient whose radial nerve was repaired 5 years earlier after it had been interrupted. There was no recovery of motor power. Examination of a piece of this muscle showed that "although abundant nerve fibres were present they had failed to make connexions with the much-atrophied muscle fibres".

The changes are not confined to the end-organs of the motor apparatus: the cutaneous sensory receptors similarly undergo a slow degenerative change after denervation. After 3 years they may in fact disappear. Reinnervation tends to reverse these changes, though the longer the period of denervation has been, the less complete will be the regeneration.

The quality of recovery after neurotmesis and repair depends chiefly on the number of axons reaching their correct targets and on the later development and myelination of those axons. Factors influencing such reinnervation are:

- the promptitude of repair
- the quality and viability of the opposed nerve ends
- the quality and accuracy of fascicular matching
- the degree of damage to the nerve ends during suture
- the length of gap after resection
- the number of channels provided by the interposed graft for the regenerating columns
- the extent of fibroblastic infiltration of the stumps and of the interposed grafts.

As Birch (1989) remarks, "the evidence that nerve grafts of the calibre of the sural or medial cutaneous nerve of the forearm can survive in an unscarred bed is secure"

Figs 5.14 and 5.15 Regeneration through a graft in the rat.

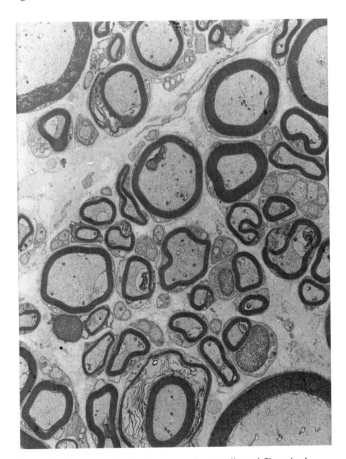

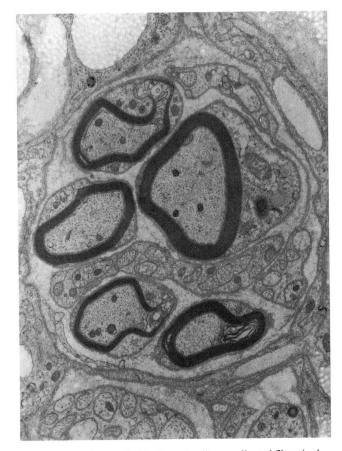

Fig. 5.14 Primary graft. Myelinated and unmyelinated fibres in the graft. × 3190.

Fig. 5.15 Secondary graft. Myelinated and unmyelinated fibres in the distal stump. × 10 440.

Figs 5.16 to 5.18 Failure of regeneration through a graft inserted 3 years previously to bridge a gap in a median nerve.

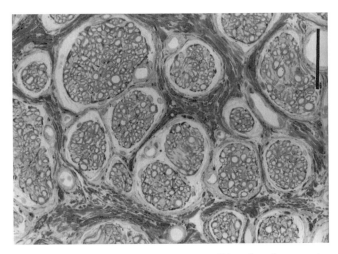

Fig. 5.16 The proximal suture line. Many small bundles of regenerating myelinated fibres. Scale bar: 100 μm.

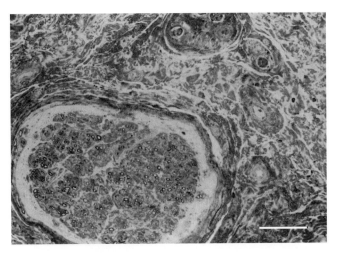

Fig. 5.17 The middle of the graft. Increasing fibrosis and loss of neural elements. Scale bar: 100 μm.

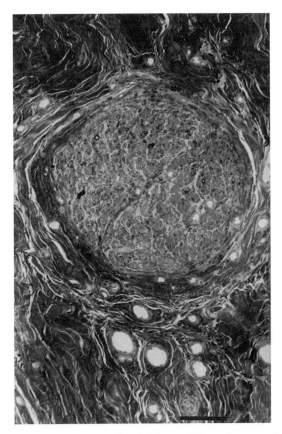

Fig. 5.18 Distal segment of graft. Obvious failure of regeneration. Scale bar: 100 μm.

(Figs 5.14 and 5.15). Even so, regeneration through such grafts may fail (Figs 5.16 to 5.18). More certain is the failure of main nerves when used as grafts (Holmes 1947, Birch 1989). The nerve pedicle graft (Barnes et al 1946, Strange 1947, 1950) was developed to permit use of a main nerve as a graft without risking central necrosis. With the later development of techniques of microvascular anastomosis, free vascularised trunk nerve grafts became practicable. Birch (1989) reproduces a section through such a graft showing numerous myelinated and unmyelinated fibres (Fig. 5.19). Perhaps disappointingly, he also reproduces sections through a failed vascularised sural nerve graft in which the vascular anastomosis remained patent and yet regeneration failed (Figs 5.20 to 5.23).

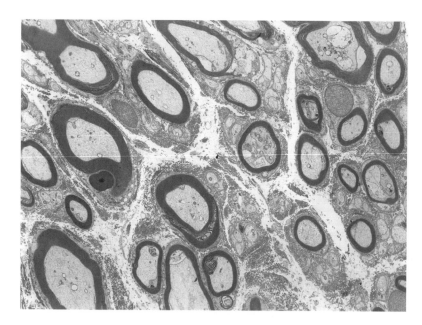

Fig. 5.19 Regeneration through a vascularised ulnar nerve graft (fifth cervical nerve to lateral cord). Although the biceps muscle recovered well, the appearance of the hand led the patient to demand amputation. Note the numerous myelinated and unmyelinated fibres, without excessive collagenisation. × 2142.

Figs 5.20 to 5.23 Failure of regeneration through a vascularised sural nerve graft used to repair a long defect in the median nerve. At re-exploration 2 years after operation the vascular anastomosis was found to be patent.

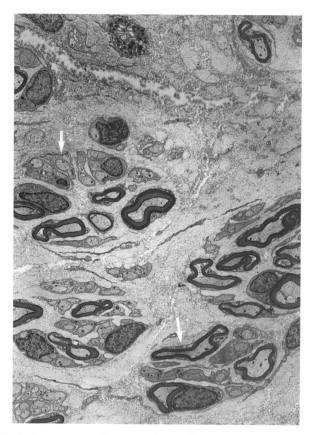

Fig. 5.20 Just distal to the proximal suture line. "Mini-fascicles" of myelinated (heavy arrows) and unmyelinated nerve fibres (thin arrows). × 2108.

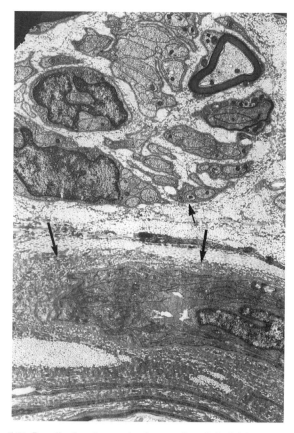

Fig. 5.21 Just distal to the proximal suture line. A "mini-fascicle" of myelinated (heavy arrows) and unmyelinated (thin arrows) nerve fibres lies just outside the perineurium of one of the vascularised strands (heavy arrows). × 6270.

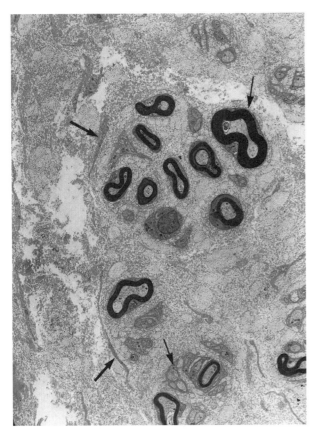

Fig. 5.22 The middle part of the graft. Much endoneurial fibrosis; myelinated and unmyelinated fibres (thin arrows); a suggestion of new perineurium formed from fibroblasts (heavy arrows). × 1770.

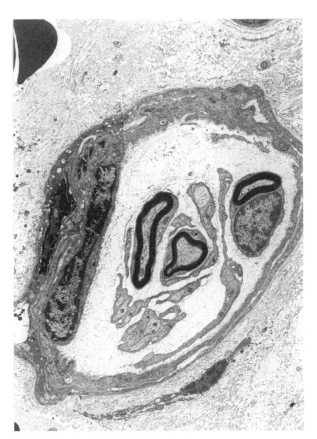

Fig. 5.23 The distal quarter of the graft. This shows one of the few surviving clusters of neural elements. Myelinated and unmyelinated nerve fibres in a lamellar cellular tube. Nucleus of new perineurial cell (left) abuts on interior of tube. × 4408.

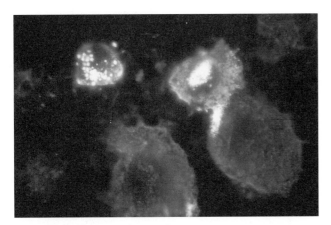

Fig. 5.24 NGF immuno-reactivity in primary sensory neurones in human dorsal root ganglion, which was avulsed from spinal cord six weeks earlier. Immuno-reactivity, identified by green fluorescent staining, is localised to cells of the small type. The yellow intracellular granules are lipofuchsin deposits which exhibit auto-fluorescence. Indirect immuno fluorescence method × 50 (see also Plate section).

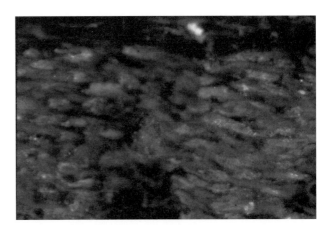

Fig. 5.25 NGF immuno-reactivity localised to most of the Schwann cells in the distal stump of a human common peripheral nerve. Indirect immuno fluorescence method × 50 (see also Plate section).

6. Clinical aspects of nerve injury

Clinical aspects: acute injury; symptoms and signs; importance of recognition of differential affection of fibres of different sizes; examination; recording; signs of regeneration; significance of Tinel sign; aids to diagnosis; causes of susceptibility to damage.

In the acute injury the object of the clinician must be to recognise the fact of injury as soon as possible after the event, and later to go on to determine the nerve or nerves affected, the level or levels of injury and the extent and depth of the lesion or lesions. That this is not always easy nor always appreciated is apparent to anyone who has been able to study the records of the medical defence organisations.

The history is important: high velocity injury, compound fracture and wounding, accidental, criminal, surgical, or all three, are likely to mean that there has been a serious lesion. The use of a knife, often enough in the hand of a surgeon, is an indication that a nerve is likely to have been partly or completely severed. In cases of gunshot injury, the distinction between shotgun on the one hand and handgun or rifle on the other can usually be made. The diffuse effect and relatively restricted penetration of shotgun pellets has to be compared with the more limited effect and greater penetration of a single missile. It is obvious that the immensely destructive effect of close-range shotgun injury is much more than that of

wounds from more distant discharge. It is, however, rarely possible to determine from the history whether a jacketed or soft-nosed bullet has been used (Fig. 6.1). Wounds from bomb fragments and shell splinters have some of the characteristics of shotgun injury, though on a larger scale and with a higher velocity (see Ch. 8).

Associated signs

The site and nature of the wound or wounds must be observed. In closed injuries the presence of swelling and bruising may give some indication of severity (Fig. 6.2). In all cases of limb injury the adequacy of perfusion, as judged by the state of the pulses, by color and by temperature, must be observed. Indications of associated fracture must be sought. In cases of serious injury, special attention

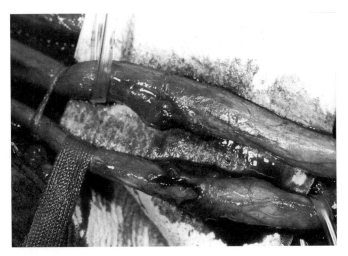

Fig. 6.1 Bullet wound of the left ulnar (bottom) and median (top) nerves just below the axilla. The bullet has tumbled or flattened, and the damage to the ulnar nerve is severe.

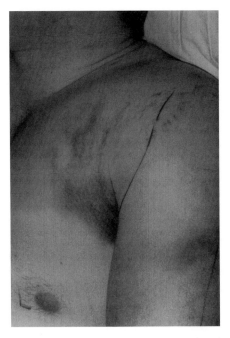

Fig. 6.2 Bruising and swelling of the left shoulder, neck and upper arm a few hours after a motor cycle injury causing avulsion of most of the roots of the brachial plexus.

has to be given to the patient's general condition, as shown by colour, pulse, blood pressure, respiration and other indicators.

The early symptoms of acute nerve injury are abnormal sensations, alteration or loss of sensibility, weakness, motor paralysis, impairment of function and sometimes pain. Rarely, the patient is aware of warming and dryness of all or part of an extremity. Abnormal sensations or paraesthesiae, most often pins and needles, are usually associated with continuing noxious process. They are of course commonly associated with recovery of a transient conduction block. Their mechanism in that process was ingeniously explored by Merrington and Nathan (1949). Alteration and loss of sensibility are not necessarily associated with continuing noxious process, nor are motor weakness and paralysis and impairment of function. The patient's failure to observe warming and anhidrosis is, regrettably, often shared by the examining clinician.

Pain, though not always present, is a most important symptom. It may be immediate or delayed; episodic or continuous; of all grades of severity. Its occurrence after injury often means that the noxious process is continuing; such as when a nerve is stretched over a bony projection or compressed by a hard object or constricted by, for instance, a suture. It is a regular feature of injury by heat and of lesions caused by critical ischaemia; it occasionally follows simple transection. Two rare and easily recognisable forms of severe pain quite often begin soon after injury. These are:

- the pain associated with intradural damage to nerve roots, particularly in traction lesions of the brachial plexus
- causalgia.

These and related matters are the subject of separate study in Chapter 16.

Examination should enable the clinician to extend the knowledge afforded by the history and the narrative of symptoms to permit accurate diagnosis to be made. All findings should be recorded in such a manner that the record will be intelligible later, not only to the examiner but also to others. Unfortunately, the signs of acute nerve injury have to be sought at a time when the patient may be the least able to co-operate in an examination: that is, soon after wounding, when there is likely to be distress and when the general condition may be affected by loss of blood and other injuries. The examination often has to be done in the often unfavourable surroundings of an accident department. The patient may be a distressed child, an older child, an adolescent or an adult; the last three may be affected by drink or drugs, or by both. When the lesion has been inflicted by a surgeon or anaesthetist, the patient's response is likely to be distorted by postoperative pain, by the effects of recent general anaesthesia or by sedative or analgesic drugs. The patient's ignorance of the medical process and even his or her trust in "the doctor" may lead him or her to think that pain and paralysis after operation is just something to be expected. That faith or even deference may inhibit him or her from voicing a complaint. These are no conditions for a quiet and comprehensive "neurological examination", yet this is the time when the fact of nerve injury must at least be recognised if the best result is to be obtained from treatment. *The examiner should at all times bear in mind that if there is a wound over the line of a main nerve and if there is any suggestion of loss of sensibility or impairment of motor function in the distribution of that nerve, it must be regarded as having been cut until and unless it is proved otherwise.*

Recognition of the depth of injury

Some of the most serious mistakes in the diagnosis and treatment of patients with injured nerves are made because the examiner fails accurately to assess the depth of injury; that is, to distinguish between degenerative and nondegenerative injury and to estimate the extent in the nerve of each type of lesion. Some atavistic urge seems to cause clinicians to play down the severity of nerve injury. Perhaps beneath this urge there is a feeling that, if there is a serious injury, much hard and possibly unrewarding work is going to be required. The tendency is of course particularly marked in cases of closed injury and of injury during operation. Too often the mantra "neuropraxia" is pronounced: too often the soothing words "just some bruising of the nerve" are uttered.

The diagnosis of the depth of the injury depends on history and signs and on the simplest electrical examination. Serious injuries are likely to cause serious lesions of nerves. Severance of a nerve with a cutaneous sensory component will lead to well-defined loss of sensibility and to complete motor, sudomotor and vasomotor paralysis in the distribution of the nerve. Simple conduction block is likely to produce a patchy loss of sensibility and a patchy motor loss. Further, it is likely to bear more heavily on the large axons than on the small ones: vibration sense and sensibility to light touch are likely to be impaired, whereas pain sensibility may be unaffected.

If the axons are damaged (degenerative lesion), stimulation of the nerve below the level of the lesion 6 days after injury will not elicit a motor response (Landau 1953). If the axons are intact (conduction block) stimulation will evoke a motor response. It will, equally, be possible to stimulate and record from the nerve below the level of the lesion. This simple, but rarely used, test can permit the early recognition of the depth of the lesion. *A firm diagnosis of neurapraxia should never be made unless 1 week after the injury stimulation of the nerve below the level of the lesion produces a motor response.*

SIGNS

The early signs of nerve injury are alteration or loss of sensibility, weakness or paralysis of muscles, vasomotor and sudomotor paralysis in the distribution of the affected nerve or nerves, and abnormal sensitivity over the nerve at the point of injury. For the reasons given above, testing of sensibility is often difficult soon after wounding, or when nerve injury is associated with fracture of a long bone. In addition, it may even be that for a few hours there is conduction across a clean transection without retraction of nerve ends (Smith & Mott 1986). The actions of some muscles can be simulated by the actions of others, so that the fact of paralysis can be missed in the early stages after nerve injury. However, one almost infallible sign is always present in the first 48 hours after deep injury of a nerve with a cutaneous sensory component: because of the affection of small as well as of large fibres, the skin in the distribution of the affected nerve is warm and dry (Fig. 6.3) (Bonney 1983, Birch 1986). In the small child, there may be an abnormal posture of the denervated digits (Fig. 6.4).

When there is no breach of the skin and the injury of the nerve is caused by pressure or distortion, there is usually differential affection of fibres. Szabo et al (1984), working with volunteer human subjects on the effects of an acute rise of pressure on the median nerve in the carpal tunnel, plainly showed that vibratory thresholds were the earliest measure of a decrease in nerve function. The largest fibres were in fact the most susceptible to pressure. The use of vibratory stimuli as a noninvasive diagnostic test may, as the authors suggest, have a significant role in clinical work and in research. The smaller ones are spared, so that there is rarely any sudomotor or vasomotor paralysis, and delayed pain sensibility is preserved. We have, however, seen at least one case in which pressure paralysis was deep enough to affect the autonomic fibres. That was in a young girl whose attempt at suicide with narcotic drugs led to prolonged pressure on the tibial and common peroneal nerves. In her case, there was prolonged vasomotor and sudomotor paralysis of the foot.

In the case of intraneural haemorrhage or injection, the situation is different: small fibres are early affected, sometimes, as with injection of local anaesthetic, before the large fibres. When the injected fluid is itself noxious, there is early affection of all sizes of fibre.

Peripheral ischaemia is usually signalled by pain, but in cases in which the vascular injury is associated with fracture, the significance of that pain may not be recognised. Ischaemia affects first the large fibres: discriminative sensibility and vibration sense are first affected (Mackinnon & Dellon 1988b). It is not easy to test these modalities when ischaemia is developing because of damage to a main vessel associated with a fracture of a long bone, but if action is not taken until superficial sensibility is lost, it will come too late.

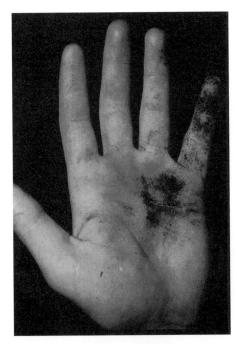

Fig. 6.3 An old photograph showing anhidrosis in the area of supply of the median nerve some months after injury. The sweating of the ulnar-innervated area is shown by the darkening of the quinizarin powder.

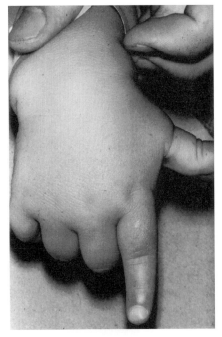

Fig. 6.4 Infant's hand 24 hours after section of the palmar nerves to the index finger and thumb. Note that the anaesthetic digits are held out from the others. There was no tendon injury.

So far as possible, sensation to light touch and pin prick, vibration sense and position sense should be tested, and the area of skin affected should be recorded (Figs 6.5 to 6.12). The timing of the response to pin prick should, if possible, be noted. Anhidrosis is easily perceptible; vasomotor paralysis is shown by warming of the skin and, in the finger tips, by capillary pulsation.

Testing motor function. It is usually simple enough to test the action of the large proximal muscles of the limbs. It is more difficult to test the muscles connecting the limbs to the trunk, and more difficult still to test the action of the flexors of the fingers and the intrinsic muscles of the hand and foot.

Figs 6.5 to 6.8 Cutaneous distribution of the median nerve.

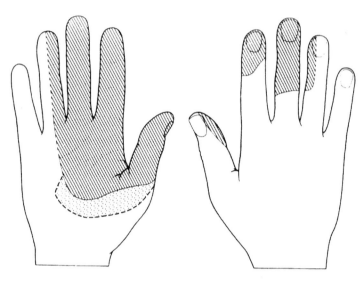

Fig. 6.5 Drawing showing the usual distribution.

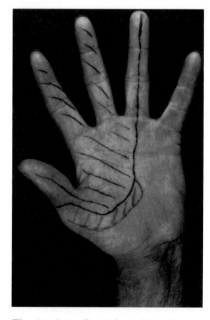

Fig. 6.6 Area of loss of sensibility after division of nerve in forearm.

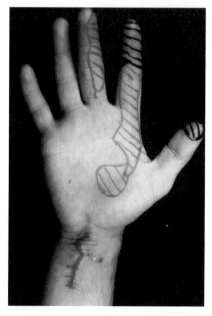

Fig. 6.7 An unusually restricted area of loss of sensibility after division of the nerve at the wrist.

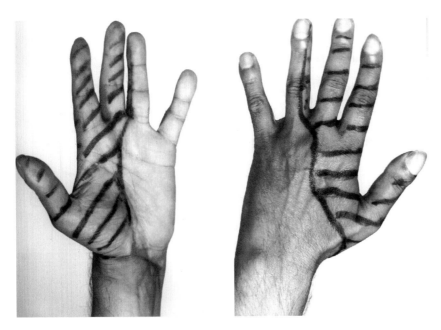

Fig. 6.8 An extended area of loss of sensibility after division of the median nerve.

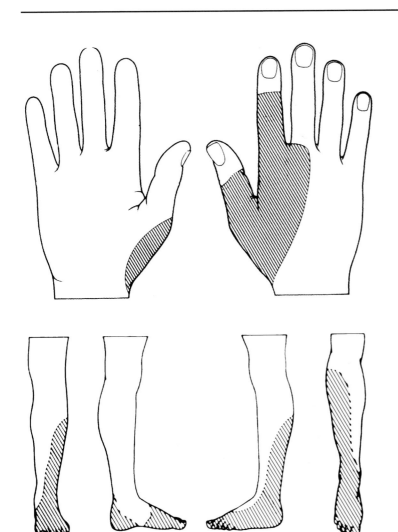

Fig. 6.9 Cutaneous distribution of radial nerve.

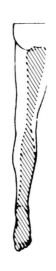

Fig. 6.10 Cutaneous distribution of sciatic nerve.

Figs 6.11 and 6.12 Cutaneous distribution of the sacral plexus.

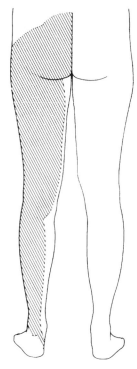

Fig. 6.11 Drawing of area of skin affected.

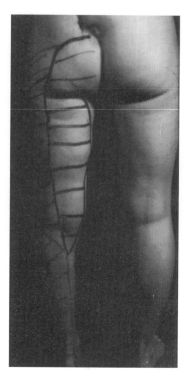

Fig. 6.12 Area of loss of sensibility in a case of damage to the sacral plexus associated with fracture–dislocation of the pelvis.

Thoracoscapular, thoracohumeral and scapulohumeral muscles

Much the best way of testing the serratus anterior muscle is to ask the patient to press against a wall with both hands. Weakness is shown by winging of the scapula on the affected side (Fig. 6.13). The method is, unfortunately, inapplicable just when it is most needed: in paralysis of the upper limb from a complete lesion of the brachial plexus. The examiner supports the paralysed upper limb with one arm; the index finger and thumb of the examiner's other hand grip the lower pole of the scapula; the patient is asked to push forward. Protraction of the scapula shows that serratus anterior is not paralysed.

The trapezius muscle is tested by asking the patient to elevate the limb or to press forward against resistance (Figs 6.14 and 6.15). The lower fibres can be tested by asking the patient to put a hand behind the back and press it against the trunk. The rhomboids are tested by pressing

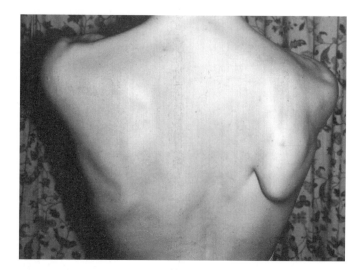

Fig. 6.13 Winging of the right scapula in paralysis of the serratus anterior. Note the border of the lower part of the trapezius medial to the scapula.

Figs 6.14 and 6.15 Paralysis of trapezius. Note the wasting of the upper fibres of the muscle.

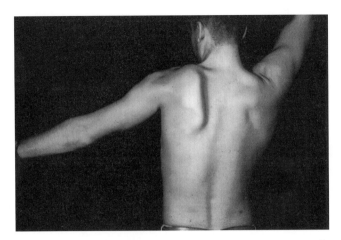

Fig. 6.14 Scapular winging without prominence of the lower fibres of the trapezius (compare with Fig. 6.13).

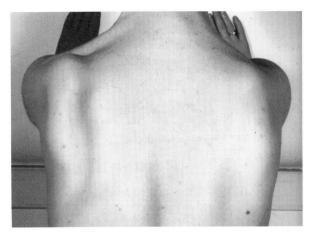

Fig. 6.15 "Winging" produced by pressure against wall.

in the opposite direction. The action of the levator scapulae muscle is best felt at the beginning of abduction of the shoulder from a resting position of 30° of abduction.

The infraspinatus and teres minor are lateral rotators of the scapulohumeral joint; the subscapularis and teres major are medial rotators. The latissimus dorsi is especially active in adduction of the scapulohumeral joint; the supraspinatus in abduction. The supraspinatus can in fact manage abduction in the absence of the deltoid; on the other hand, the deltoid cannot by itself initiate abduction (Figs 6.16 to 6.18). The subscapularis, teres major and the sternal part of the pectoralis major are medial rotators of the scapulohumeral joint. Testing the power of flexion and extension of the elbow is usually simple.

The power of supination and pronation of the forearm should be tested from the neutral position: it is important to remember that both biceps and supinator contribute to supination, and that the long flexor muscles of the forearm can often give useful pronation when the pronator teres muscle is paralysed or weak.

The long flexors of the fingers

The flexor superficialis, usually innervated by the median nerve, acts on the interphalangeal joints of the medial four digits. Its action on individual fingers is best tested by holding three of the digits almost straight and asking the patient to flex the free finger. Because the tendons of the superficialis are largely independent of each other and those of the profundus are not, the former muscle will act to flex the proximal interphalangeal joint.

The medial half of the flexor digitorum profundus is usually innervated by the ulnar nerve; the lateral part, by the median nerve. With the exception of that to the index finger, the tendons are closely associated with each other, and independent movement is in some cases hardly possible. The test for the integrity of the profundus requires the subject to flex the distal interphalangeal joint of one finger with the proximal joints of that finger and all joints of the other fingers stabilised (Fig. 6.19).

The division of the supply of the intrinsic muscles of the hand between the median and ulnar nerves varies from subject to subject (Rowntree 1949). The most common arrangement is for the ulnar nerve to supply all muscles, with the exception of the first lumbrical, the abductor brevis and opponens pollicis, and part of the flexor brevis pollicis. Most of the intrinsic muscles act on the meta-carpophalangeal joints to flex, adduct and abduct. The particular action of the thenar muscles is to *oppose* the thumb to the little finger, and the muscle particularly responsible for rotating the metacarpal bone during that movement is the opponens. When the median nerve has been cut the opposing action of the thenar muscles can be mimicked by the combined action of an ulnar-innervated flexor brevis and the abductor longus muscle. Comparison with the intact side will usually show that this combined action does not reproduce the rotational action of the opponens (Fig. 6.20). Similarly, the abducting action of the abductor brevis can, in the absence of the median nerve function, be imitated by the action of the abductor longus muscle. These points are important in the early stages when there is no wasting to guide the examiner.

Figs 6.16 to 6.18 Elevation of the upper limb by the supraspinatus in the absence of the deltoid.

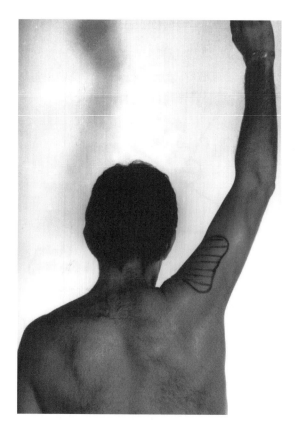

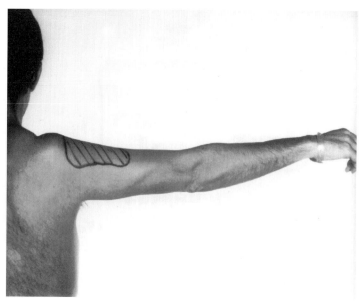

Fig. 6.16 (Left and right) Full elevation possible.

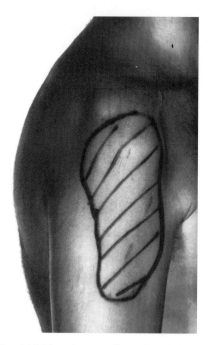

Fig. 6.17 Note the area of loss of sensibility.

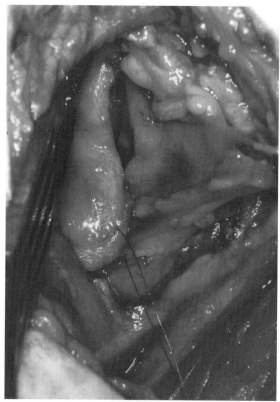

Fig. 6.18 The ruptured circumflex nerve seen at operation.

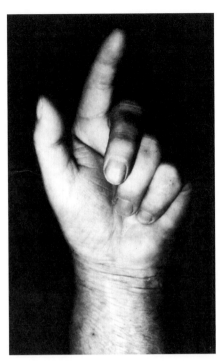

Fig. 6.19 Testing the flexor digitorum superficialis and profundus. High median nerve injury: no active flexion of the index finger.

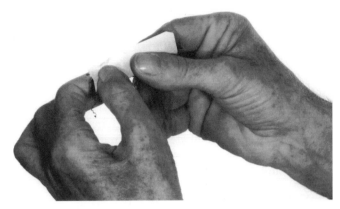

Fig. 6.20 Opposition of the thumb. There has been a lesion of the left median nerve, with failure of recovery. An "opposition transfer" has been done, but the failure of the left thumb to rotate in "opposition" is plainly seen in contrast with the right.

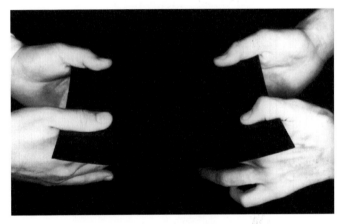

Fig. 6.21 Testing the thenar muscles. "Froment's sign" is positive in the patient's left hand (right).

The action of the thumb in pinching against the forefinger is modified by the loss of the stabilising action of the flexor brevis pollicis on the first metacarpophalangeal joint. Without that action, pinch has to be mediated by the action of the flexor longus pollicis on the interphalangeal joint (Fig. 6.21). The power of the ulnar-innervated muscles of the hand is best tested by examining the power of abduction and adduction of the fingers. The ease with which a sheet of paper may be pulled from the grasp of two fingers gives some indication of this power.

The lower limb

There is no great difficulty in testing the muscles connecting the pelvis to the femur in the healthy subject, but things are different when this has to be done soon after replacement arthroplasty. Our observations suggest that in this situation there is also quite often a certain reluctance to look. In one case, a "drop foot" was observed soon after arthroplasty, but it was not until a year later that another examiner found a paralysis of most of the muscles of the buttock. The integrity of the smaller glutei is tested with the patient standing, that of the rotators of the hip with the patient seated, and that of the gluteus maximus with the patient prone. The flexors of the knee are best examined with the patient prone: it is usually possible to distinguish the action of the biceps femoris from that of the medial hamstrings.

It is necessary, in testing the power of the flexors of the ankle, to make sure that the action is in fact effected by the soleus and gastrocnemius: the tibialis posterior and the flexors of the toes can produce ankle flexion, though they cannot sustain the patient's weight. Both tibialis muscles effect inversion of the foot; the anterior muscle is the principal extensor of the ankle.

We know of no really satisfactory way of testing the integrity of the intrinsic muscles of the foot. Some individuals can use these muscles independently of each other, most cannot.

Late signs of nerve injury

Two weeks after a complete degenerative lesion, the area of loss of sensibility is well defined; the beginning of wasting indicates the extent of the motor affection. Anhidrosis is still present, but with the degeneration of peripheral fibres the warm isothermia of the skin gives way to poikilo-thermia and later to cold isothermia.

As time goes by, the changes of disuse appear: thinning of the skin; even ulceration from accidental injury; loss of substance in the tips of the digits; loss of skin markings; constant coldness and cyanosis; stiffness of joints; contractures; and unmistakable wasting (Figs 6.22 to 6.24). At a late stage in partial denervation or with incomplete recovery after a deep lesion there may be muscle spasms and spontaneous fasciculation. Prolonged denervation of a growing limb leads to defective growth: this is of course well seen after birth injury of the brachial plexus. Lewis and Pickering (1936) thought that the changes in denervated limbs were simply the result of disuse rather than that of the loss of a "trophic" function of the nerves. However, it is a fact that in cases of greatly prolonged conduction block the changes are always far less than they are in degenerative lesions. In the case in which vasomotor and sudomotor paralysis was produced by prolonged pressure (see p. 77) the toes of the affected foot were dry and warm 3 months after injury. We have seen that in degenerative lesions profound changes take place in both motor and sensory end-organs. The distal axon normally maintains a dense population of end-organs in skin and sweat glands and in the muscular component of arterioles. It is hard to resist the conclusion that the changes of "disuse" are at least in part due to the loss of distal axons and of their end-organs, and to the effects of that loss on superficial tissues.

By the time the changes of degeneration are present, the patient is a better candidate for the examination halls than for restorative treatment. The object of the clinician must be to make the diagnosis before the signs of peripheral degeneration have appeared; that is, before the best time for intervention has passed. Unfortunately, the peripheral neurologist is still likely to be presented with cases in which delay in diagnosis has permitted the development of these signs. The last are at this stage well marked; their absence in association with persistent partial motor and sensory paralysis almost certainly means that the lesion was partly or wholly a conduction block.

Figs 6.22 to 6.24 Late changes after nerve injury.

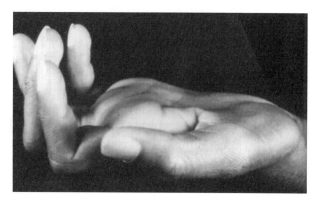

Fig. 6.22 Severe wasting of the hand with contractures a year after stab wound of the lower part of the plexus.

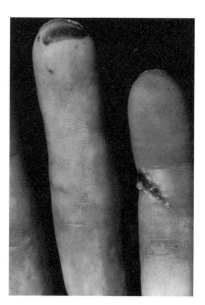

Fig. 6.24 Ulceration of the skin of middle finger and accidental injury to index finger after median nerve injury.

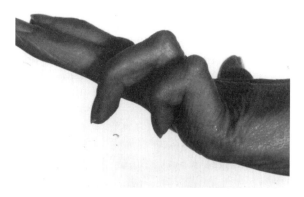

Fig. 6.23 Clawing after failure of recovery of a lesion of the ulnar nerve at wrist level.

Recording of motor power and sensory function

No system for recording of motor power has really super-seded that proposed in 1942 by Highet (1954) to the Nerve Injuries Committee of the Medical Research Council (MRC) (Table 6.1). The place of the system for recording sensory recovery (Table 6.2) is less certain, largely because of the later development of more refined methods of testing sensibility, and because the system in effect ignored input from receptors in muscles, tendons and ligaments. Narakas (1977) used the MRC system as a basis for his method of grading progress in lesions of the brachial plexus. Kline and Hudson (1995a) modified the MRC motor and sensory systems and combined these in their system for grading "whole nerve injury". Certainly, both systems give the examiner and his or her successors a better idea of the progress of function than did the original tables of the individual muscles and the grades. Trumble et al (1995) made objective measurements of muscle power by the use of force transducers; they used the results to "quantitate" the MRC grades. Thus, they reckoned that grade M3 represented 17–42% of the function of the healthy muscle, and that grade M4 represented 66–79%. The use of this technique is, unfortunately, too time-consuming for use in most clinical work, but it should be

considered very carefully in the construction of a research project.

All systems fail to a greater or lesser extent in

- failing adequately to record the stamina of muscles
- failing adequately to record function of the sensory end-organs in muscles, tendons and articular capsules and ligaments.

Special apparatus is indeed available for testing stamina of muscles, in particular those of the hand. The amount of time involved is, however, too great to permit the routine use of these methods. Evidently, tests such as Moberg's "pick-up" test to some extent examine deep as well as superficial sensibility, but there is no good measure of the extent of reinnervation of muscle spindles. The examination of tendon reflexes is, evidently, a coarse method of testing the function of the Golgi organs and muscle spindles, but more precise methods are lacking. We do not know how much the function of a muscle recovered after nerve repair is impaired by defect of input from it.

Our systems are discussed in Chapters 8–10.

Signs of reinnervation

The detection of initial and continuing reinnervation is often very important in aiding a decision about intervention. After such intervention, it is important as an indicator of success or failure, and consequently as a guide to a second intervention. In cases in which long spatial and temporal distances separate a lesion from the nerve's target, the "Tinel" sign (Tinel 1915, 1917b) is useful but can mislead. Tinel (1915, 1917b) was probably the first to draw attention to the indication of the "growing point" of the regenerating axons signalled by the production of paraesthesia by tapping over the course of the nerve. Buck-Gramcko and Lubahn (1993) remind us that Tinel made the observation at about the same time that Hoffman, working on the other side of the Western Front, made a similar discovery (Hoffman 1915a,b). Properly, the sign should be called the "Hoffman–Tinel sign". Tapping the skin over the course of a recovering nerve reveals the presence of regenerating axons by the production of paraesthesiae in the sensory distribution of the nerve. Pearce (1996) does well to remind us of Tinel's words and of the limitations of the sign. His translation of Tinel (1916) runs as follows: "The all important sign is formication. We find that sudden pressure or percussion of the nerve trunk, below the lesion, calls forth a tingling sensation in the cutaneous region of the nerve ... It appears about the third or fourth week ... Then it gradually becomes more pronounced and it is possible to follow, week by week, in the course of the nerve, the progress of this provoked formication, pari passu with the advance of the axis cylinders. The formication sign is thus of supreme

Table 6.1 Motor function

M0	No contraction
M1	Return of perceptible contraction in the proximal muscles
M2	Return of perceptible contraction in both proximal and distal muscles
M3	Return of function in both proximal and distal muscles of such degree that all *important* muscles are sufficiently powerful to act against resistance
M4	Return of function as in stage 3 with the addition that all *synergic* and independent movements are possible
M5	Complete recovery

Table 6.2 Sensory function

S0	Absence of sensibility in the autonomous area
S1	Recovery of deep cutaneous pain sensibility within the *autonomous area* of the nerve
S2	Return of some degree of superficial cutaneous pain and tactile sensibility within the autonomous area of the nerve
S3	Return of some degree of superficial cutaneous pain and tactile sensibility within the autonomous area with disappearance of any previous overreaction
S3+	Return of sensibility as in stage 3 with some recovery of two-point discrimination within the autonomous area
S4	Complete recovery

importance since it enables us to see whether the nerve is interrupted, or in the course of regeneration; whether a nerve suture has succeeded or failed, or whether regeneration is rapid and satisfactory, or reduced to a few insignificant fibres." In Pearce's published letter, "significant" has been printed for "insignificant". All authors will recognise this sign. The element of unreliability is introduced by the fact that some of those regenerating axons are not on their way to any target. However, these points can be stated:

- a strongly positive Tinel sign over a lesion soon after injury indicates rupture or severance
- after repair which is going to be successful, the centrifugally moving "Tinel sign" is persistently stronger than that at the suture line
- after repair which is going to fail, the "Tinel sign" at the suture line remains stronger than that at the growing point
- failure of distal progression of the "Tinel sign" in a closed lesion indicates rupture or other injury not susceptible of recovery by natural process.

After a degenerative lesion, recovery proceeds centrifugally, so that the first sign of reinnervation is voluntary contracture in the muscle most proximally innervated. Sensibility too recovers centrifugally. As Head et al (1905) observed, its quality improves over successive months, doubtless with remyelination of the larger axons (see Chs 2, 3 and 5). Recovery of sensibility may be preceded by recovery of sweating; indeed, sweating may be restored without any later recovery of sensibility.

In nondegenerative lesions, recovery is not necessarily nor even generally centrifugal: distal muscles may well recover before proximal ones; loss or alteration of sensibility may anyway be patchy; vasomotor and sudomotor paralysis is rare. Because the lesion depends so much on demyelination, and in particular on demyelination of large fibres, a dissociated loss of position sense and vibration sense may be a good indicator of its type.

Very often, in recovery after both degenerative and nondegenerative injuries, the patient experiences radiated pain and paraesthesiae and asks the clinician whether these feelings indicate progressive recovery. We have seen that Merrington and Nathan (1949) explored the nature and origin of paraesthesiae after conduction block: certainly, such feelings indicate recovery in that condition. They do not necessarily, nor even often, have that significance in the case of degenerative lesions.

Features of imperfect recovery. Imperfect recovery, common in the adult after repair of a degenerative lesion, is apparent to the patient through:

- weakness and sometimes wasting
- alteration of sensibility
- dysfunction
- pain (sometimes)

- sensitivity over the site of the lesion (sometimes)
- exaggerated reaction of the affected part to external cold
- stiffness and even deformity of the joints of the affected part.

The exaggerated reaction to cold requires some further comment; all other aspects are treated elsewhere. Cold affects healthy nerves: it affects even more severely those in which the number of functioning axons is reduced. So, conditions of cold that would not seriously affect healthy nerves are liable badly to affect damaged nerves in which regeneration has been imperfect. Both motor and sensory function are affected. The cold affects not only nerve function; it affects too the skin and deep tissues of the affected limb, which is quick to cool and slow to warm.

AIDS TO DIAGNOSIS

Electrophysiological examination

Electrophysiological examination (Wynn Parry 1953, Payan 1987, Peterson & Will 1988, Morgan 1989) is certainly the foremost aid to diagnosis, although in the acute stage the process is often hampered by pain and by local conditions. It must be done expertly and results must be interpreted expertly. It is no substitute for clinical observation; it must not be used as device for deferring decision and delaying action. It can help in diagnosis of the site and depth of a lesion and in the recognition and measurement of recovery. The extension of the process to the detection and measurement of potentials evoked from the cortex provides valuable evidence in the case of suspected avulsion of the roots of the brachial plexus. Perhaps the simplest, yet often neglected, technique of most electrophysiological examination is that of stimulating the nerve below the level of the lesion and observing the motor response. If, 3 days after injury, stimulation below the level of the lesion produces a normal response in the muscles supplied by the nerve, the odds are that the lesion is a conduction block. If there is no motor response or if the response is much subdued, then the lesion is degenerative.

The introduction of electrophysiological process during operation has brought massive advantages, in particular in:

- determining neural continuity across a lesion in continuity
- determining the site of a conduction block
- determining which part of a nerve has suffered axonal interruption
- determining whether an apparently intact component of the brachial plexus has intact central connections.

We are profoundly glad that the whole matter is considered at length in Chapter 14 by an expert in the field.

X-ray examination

Seddon (1975) was evidently sceptical about the value of neurography with contrast media, and experience has confirmed that view. Myelography was widely used in the diagnosis of intradural damage to the brachial plexus, and still finds a place in that field. Our preference has been for computed tomography with enhancement, which enables the intrathecal roots to be seen (Marshall & de Silva 1986). Unfortunately, it is difficult to apply this method to very young children.

Magnetic resonance imaging

The capacity of magnetic resonance imaging to show major nerve trunks (magnetic resonance neurography) is revealed by Fahr and Sauser (1988), Taylor et al (1993) and Filler et al (1993). By this means Pangeyres et al (1993) convincingly showed the site and extent of lesions in thoracic outlet syndrome. West et al (1994) showed changes of signal in denervated muscles (Fig. 6.25). Using fast spin-echo magnetic resonance imaging, Francel et al (1995) have been able to shorten the time of the procedure sufficiently to permit examination of infants with birth lesions of the brachial plexus.

Three very important papers from the western USA were published in 1995 and 1996. Britz et al (1995) used T1- and T2-weighted, proton density and short τ inversion recovery (STIR) sequences to study the median nerve in control subjects and in patients with carpal tunnel syndrome. Britz et al (1996) used STIR sequences to study the ulnar nerve in control subjects and in patients with entrapment of the nerve at the elbow. Dailey et al (1996) used a phased-array coil system to obtain high-resolution coronal T1-weighted spin echo, coronal and axial T2-weighted fast spin echo with fat saturation, and coronal and axial fast STIR weighted images of the cervical spine and spinal nerves in three patients with cervico-brachial pain and in one control subject aged 38 years.

The studies of the median nerve showed increased signal in 95% of cases, those of the ulnar nerve showed increased signal in 97% of cases, and those of the neck showed increased signal in the affected spinal nerve in all three cases. The abnormalities were shown in the median nerves in the carpal tunnel, in the ulnar nerve usually in the cubital tunnel, and in the cervical nerves distal to the site of compression. The pathological basis for these findings are, presumably, oedema and interference with axonal transport. Filler et al (1996) defined magnetic resonance neurography as "tissue-selective imaging directed at identifying and evaluating characteristics of nerve morphology: internal fascicular pattern, longitudinal patterns in signal intensity and caliber, and connections and relations to other nerves and plexuses." They outlined the imaging protocols necessary for these purposes, and showed the remarkable degree of contrast achieved between the fascicles and the endoneurial epineurium.

The portentous question is soon going to be raised, or perhaps has already been raised, of whether magnetic resonance neurography can be a substitute for exploration

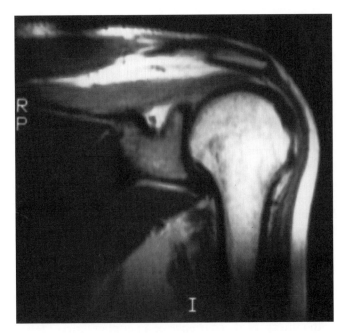

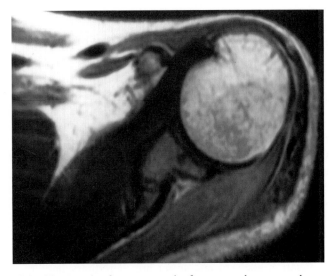

Fig. 6.25 Denervated muscles defined by magnetic resonance imaging. Image of shoulder 6 weeks after axonotmesis of suprascapular nerve and rupture of circumflex nerve. Note the contrast between the subscapularis muscle and the supraspinatus, infraspinatus and deltoid muscles.

aided by the microscope and the apparatus for stimulating and recording. Certainly, the demonstration of an intact fascicular pattern without local hyperintensity would negate the intention to operate as surely as demonstration of loss of continuity or obliteration of fascicular pattern would indicate operation. At present the bar to routine use of these methods in peripheral nerve work in England and Wales is expense. In the 1980s the development of centres for magnetic resonance imaging was left to individual enterprise and to the operation of the profit motive, and no attempt was made to create a national network of such centres, the capital cost of which was, and is, so high. The routine use of magnetic resonance imaging in traumatic lesions of nerves would hardly be acceptable, even though the hidden costs of other methods of diagnosis and of failure of diagnosis could well make that "cost–benefit analysis" unreliable.

At present, magnetic resonance neurography is uniquely informative in the diagnosis and accurate measurement of extent of tumours in and near nerves, in the more difficult entrapment syndromes and in some closed injuries of peripheral nerves. Considerable further study is needed to define the particular areas of usefulness of imaging and of exploration, but it is likely that the former will supersede the latter in many cases and that increasingly it will become a routine preliminary to operation.

Seddon (1975c) mentioned the sweating test only to dismiss it as a practical investigation. Interest was revived by Wilson's (1985) introduction of a simple device for measuring the moisture content of the skin and, by extrapolation, its degree of innervation. Unfortunately, the small sudomotor fibres may regenerate more effectively than the larger fibres, so that the accuracy of the test is vitiated. There is still a place for nerve biopsy and, in particular, for the examination of nerve roots under the electron microscope. Magnetic measurement of nerve action currents during operation (Hertz et al 1986) seemed to be a promising development, but it does not seem to have caught on.

CONDITIONS CAUSING ABNORMAL SUSCEPTIBILITY TO INJURY

Serious mistakes can arise from concentrating on local and peripheral manifestations to the neglect of enquiry into an underlying cause. There are many causes of generalised neuropathy; many general disorders which by their local manifestations cause local neuropathy. "Carpal tunnel syndrome" may be the first symptom of rheumatoid arthritis; a peripheral neuropathy may be the first symptom of carcinoma of the lung.

The conditions causing neuropathy which the operating clinician is likely to encounter are: hereditary liability to pressure paralysis, alcoholic neuropathy, diabetes mellitus, hypothyroidism, acromegaly, disorders of the immune system, carcinoma and the presence of a more proximal lesion of the nerve. In haemophilia, of course, the disorder of the blood – the universal fluid – predisposes all soft tissues, including nerves, to damage by induced or spontaneous bleeding.

Inherited susceptibility to pressure paralysis

Davies (1954) first reported inherited susceptibility to pressure paralysis. He was followed by Wahle and Tonnis (1958) and by Earl et al (1964). The last described the condition affecting members of four families, many of whom gave histories of recurrent and transient lesions of peripheral nerves, in addition to which there were a number of persistent paralyses. There were in some of these patients symptomless electrophysiological abnormalities of nerves at sites where "entrapment syndromes" occur, such as the ulnar at the elbow and the median at the wrist. Behse et al (1972) were able to examine the sural nerves of six patients from three families showing this abnormality. They found that the diameter of the axons of large fibres were smaller than normal and that there was a lowered ratio of axonal to external diameter, with multiple defects in the myelin sheath. Electrophysiological examination showed a slowing of conduction by 20–70%.

Having examined the sural nerves of four patients suffering from "neuropathy with focal thickening of the myelin sheath", Madrid and Bradley (1975) suggested the term "tomaculous neuropathy". They noted the axonal constriction, the sausage-shaped thickenings of the myelin sheath, the segmental demyelination and the early "onion bulb" formation. Yoshikawa and Dyck (1991) found a widespread asymptomatic abnormality, with lowering of conduction velocity and focal thickenings in the teased myelinated fibres of clinically unaffected nerves. Electron microscopy showed regions where the lamellae of myelin were uncompacted.

Our experience of this condition is limited to the case of one patient, a man in his forties, who did not in fact have a history of peripheral affection. He suffered a lesion of the left fifth lumbar and first sacral nerves after a left lower lumbar disc protrusion, which persisted for a long time after removal of the nucleus. Three years later there was a similar sequence of events on the right. Electrophysiological examination 6 months after the second episode (Dr N. Murray) showed widespread abnormalities affecting both median nerves as well as the nerves of the lower limbs.

Alcohol

It is impossible to know the incidence of symptomless alcoholic neuropathy, which is brought to light, perhaps, by the unexpected occurrence of a peripheral nerve lesion during the course of treatment, operative or otherwise. On the other hand, the clinician is familiar with the presenting features of established neuropathy with impairment of peripheral sensibility associated perhaps with encephalopathy and evidence of impairment of liver function. The features of alcoholic autonomic neuropathy are also well known. The alcoholic is often reticent, even deliberately evasive, about his or her drinking habits, though often enough the finding in the blood of a persistently high mean corpuscular volume gives the game away. It may well be that some of the nerve lesions ascribed to mistakes in operation represent the effect on susceptible neural tissue of trauma which would be tolerated by a healthy nerve. The work of Monforte et al (1995) appears to confirm the view that alcoholic neuropathy is produced by the direct, dose-related action of alcohol or its metabolites on the axon or the cell body, and that associated malnutrition is not a factor. These workers further found that one-third of their patients with high alcohol intake showed electrophysiological abnormalities of the peripheral nerves. Evidently, it is as well to be particularly cautious about the handling of nerves of patients who admit to an alcohol intake of more than 100 g/day or whose mean corpuscular volume is over 100 µl.[3]

Diabetes

Diabetic neuropathy usually comes to attention as an affection of sensibility beginning proximally and extending proximally. Early work (Jordan et al 1935, Jordan 1936) established the changes in the phospholipid content of the nerves of diabetics, and showed that the change was present even in the absence of clinical evidence of neuropathy. Discussing his classification of diabetic neuropathies, Jordan (1936) noted particularly that in a number of cases pressure was a precipitating cause. Gilliatt and Willison's (1962) study of neuropathy in diabetes indicated a predominant affection of large myelinated fibres, but in fact fibres of all dimensions and all functions may be affected. The lesion is predominantly axonal (Thomas & Lascelles 1966); the small unmyelinated fibres and the myelinated sensory fibres are the most commonly affected.

The property of nerves of diabetics that principally interests or ought to interest the operating surgeon is that of abnormal sensitivity to pressure. Mayer and Tomlinson (1983) studied the axonal transport of adrenergic enzymes in the nerves of rats. They found that experimentally produced diabetes caused at 3 weeks a reduction in orthograde transport of choline acetyltransferase, possibly preceded by a defect in retrograde transport of the enzyme at 1 week. Dahlin et al (1986a) similarly used streptozotocin to produce diabetes in rats. They found that compression caused a significantly greater accumulation of axonally transported proteins in the nerves of the diabetic animals than in the nerves of the controls. Their conclusion was that "diabetes may lead to an increased susceptibility of peripheral nerves to compression". The clinician can draw but slight encouragement from the earlier finding (Castaigne et al 1966) that sensory nerve action potentials are retained longer during ischaemia in diabetics than in healthy persons. The practical conclusion from all this is that the routine testing of the urine of all new patients and of all inpatients, now in many centres fallen into desuetude, remains mandatory.

Hypothyroidism

As Pollard (1993) remarks, "neurologic complications of hypothyroidism are well recognised". Most clinicians know that "carpal tunnel syndrome" may be the symptom that brings hypothyroidism to attention. However, reliable figures are lacking for the percentage of cases of carpal tunnel syndrome in which hypothyroidism is a determining factor. Murray and Simpson (1958) established the connection between "acroparaesthesiae" and myxoedema; Fincham and Cape (1968) found evidence of alteration of conductivity in the median and ulnar nerves of four patients with myxoedema. Nemni et al (1987) examined the clinical, electrophysiological and morphological changes in four patients with "secondary hypothyroidism" and polyneuropathy. They found not only changes in conductivity but also, in three cases, evidence of axonal degeneration in sural nerve biopsies. The neurophysiological changes were reversible with replacement therapy. Wise et al (1995) indicated the importance of the findings of slow relaxing reflexes in the diagnosis of this condition.

We think that, in all cases of "carpal tunnel syndrome" in women in which no local or systemic cause is apparent, tests of thyroid function (free and total thyroxine) should be done.

Acromegaly

"Carpal tunnel syndrome" may be the presenting symptom of acromegaly (Johnston 1960). O'Duffy et al (1973) found that 35 of 100 acromegalic patients suffered from carpal tunnel syndrome. Their analysis showed that the combination indicated "ongoing pituitary overactivity" ($P < 0.001$). Low et al (1974) studied the frequency of peripheral neuropathy in acromegaly, and studied the electrophysiological and pathological changes in the nerves of 11 patients with clinical and radiological evidence of the condition. A little unfortunately, perhaps, neither set of workers indicated the sex distribution in their series. Low et al (1974) found a high incidence (8 of 11 patients) of generalised peripheral neuropathy, with increase in endoneurial tissue and reduction in density of myelinated fibres. The fascicles were larger in the nerves of acromegalics than in healthy nerves. The changes were independent of the presence of diabetes mellitus. Doubtless, extraneural changes contribute to the compression of the median nerve in this condition (Kellgren et al 1952).

Evidently, the possibility of acromegaly ought to be considered in all cases of carpal tunnel syndrome in men without evidence of a local or other systemic cause.

Immune disorders

Orthopaedic surgeons in particular should be interested in the association of neuropathy with rheumatoid arthritis, but the vasculitis that, at any rate in part, is responsible in this condition is common to many disorders of the immune system. Hart and Golding (1960) discussed 42 cases of "rheumatoid neuropathy". It is interesting to find that examination of peripheral nerves in their five patients who died showed arteritis in only one and demyelination in one other. Certainly, extraneural changes are in part or wholly responsible for the nerve lesion in some cases of "rheumatoid mononeuropathy". In one of Hart and Golding's cases that was certainly so: division of a thickened arcuate ligament sufficed to give complete and lasting relief in a case of ulnar neuropathy. Pallis and Scott (1965) and Pallis (1966) later considered in detail the clinical features in pathology of "rheumatoid neuropathy", stressing the frequency of arterial lesions "like those of polyarteritis nodosa".

Hughes et al (1982) examined the common cause of neuropathy in immune disorders. They found necrotising vasculitis in biopsy specimens of the sural nerve in a case of systemic lupus erythematosus presenting with multiple mononeuropathy. Allan et al (1982) examined the clinical characteristics of vasculitic mononeuropathy; Dyck et al (1987) clarified the distinction between systemic vasculitic neuropathy affecting patients with polyarteritis, systemic lupus erythematosus, rheumatoid arthritis and other conditions, and nonsystemic vasculitic neuropathy, in which clinically only nerves are affected. The occurrence of neuropathy in Sjögren's syndrome was studied by Mellgren et al (1989) and by Griffin et al (1990); Hagen et al (1990) discussed association of trigeminal sensory neuropathy with immune disorder in a series of 81 patients.

Clearly, clinicians must be aware of the possibilities of immune disorder presenting as a mononeuropathy and of abnormal susceptibility of peripheral nerves to pressure and ischaemia in cases with an established diagnosis of rheumatoid disease. In this connection, it is as well to remind clinicians operating on patients with rheumatoid arthritis that nerves in wasted limbs have less protection against external pressure than do nerves in healthier limbs.

Carcinoma

This subject is considered in detail in Chapter 15. Henson et al (1954) described carcinomatous neuropathy and myopathy; in the same year, Heathfield et al (1954) described the association with bronchogenic cancer. In 1964, Grunberg et al, reviewing systemic manifestations associated with carcinoma, included a survey of various types of neuropathy. Croft et al (1965) went further into the immunological basis, a subject which was examined in more detail by Patey et al in 1974. Campbell and Patey (1974) further examined electrophysiological changes. Walsh et al (1976) reported sympathetic overaction in response to direct invasion, and Handforth et al (1984) reported an unusual case of polyneuropathy associated with breast cancer. Most cases of carcinomatous neuropathy arise in connection with lung cancer; here too it is important to recall that neuropathy may be the sole presenting symptom, and that the nerves of patients with lung cancer may be unduly susceptible. We hope that the question of abnormal susceptibility of nervous tissue in patients with breast cancer may be explored during the investigation of radiation injury of the brachial plexus.

Among other conditions that may come to the attention of surgeons dealing with peripheral nerves are motor neuron disease in its early stages, and the singular disturbances of motor conduction described by Krarup et al (1990) and Tahmoush et al (1991). The former described a syndrome of asymmetric limb weakness with motor conduction block; the latter described a "cramp–fasciculation" syndrome.

A more proximal lesion of the trunk nerve

The matter of the susceptibility of the distal part of a nerve because of a symptomless lesion in the more proximal part of the trunk (the "double-crush syndrome") is considered in Chapters 12 and 13.

7. Operating on peripheral nerves

Operating on nerves: indications for operation; conditions and requirements; general principles of operation; intraoperative diagnosis; methods of repair and possibilities of stimulating regeneration; possibilities of intradural repair; approaches to individual nerves.

INDICATIONS

The decision whether to intervene on a nerve after injury is rarely easy, except perhaps in the acute case of an open wound and in cases in which nerve injury is associated with damage to major bones and blood vessels. The indications for operation are probably as follows:

- deep paralysis after wounding over the course of a main nerve or injection close to the course of a main nerve
- deep paralysis after closed injury, especially high velocity injury, associated with severe damage to soft tissues, bone or joint
- deep paralysis after closed traction injury of the brachial plexus
- association of a nerve lesion with evidence of an associated arterial lesion
- association of a nerve lesion with fracture of a related bone requiring early internal fixation
- increase in depth of a nerve lesion under observation
- persistent symptoms and signs of affection of conducting tissue at any interval after exposure of the part to ionising radiation
- failure to show evidence of recovery at the expected time after a closed lesion initially thought to be an axonotmesis
- failure to show evidence of recovery in conduction block within 6 weeks of injury
- persistent pain at almost any interval after injury
- in entrapment neuropathy, persistence of symptoms and evidence of increasing depth of the lesion.

This list probably covers most contingencies except that of delay between injury and consultation. Evidently, there is a time limit for successful intervention, except perhaps in the case of persistent pain. Whereas it is reasonable to explore and repair the median nerve of an adult that was cut 3 months previously, it is hardly reasonable to explore an adult's sciatic nerve cut 3 years previously, with a similar object in view. On the other hand, such an exploration could be justified by persistent or increasing pain. No one should forget the lesson of case 3 in Birch and Strange's (1990) series. There, exploration and decompression of the sciatic nerve in the notch 3 years after injury was followed by recovery of a paralysis affecting the common peroneal component. That lesion was, of course, a conduction block prolonged by external causes.

It is, in general, fruitless to expect motor recovery in the adult if the operation is delayed for more than a year after a degenerative lesion. Operation to restore sensibility may fare better, though the quality of restored sensation is certain to be defective. The limits are much more elastic in children before the age of puberty: we have seen motor and sensory recovery after nerve transfer in an arm denervated for 3 years. Indeed, regenerative powers in children are so great that it is sometimes difficult to determine whether recovery is due to the intervention or to wholly independent natural process.

The clinician must always bear in mind that the sooner the distal segment is connected to the cell body and proximal segment the better the result will be. In the extreme case of replantation after traumatic amputation, O'Brien (1975) showed that primary suture of nerves gave the only hope of recovery. Merle et al (1986), Leclerq et al (1985), and Birch and Raji (1991) have all shown the ill effect of delay in the repair of the median and ulnar nerves.

CONDITIONS FOR OPERATION

The results of operating on peripheral nerves depend to an extent hardly matched in any other branch of surgery on the skill of the surgeon and the quality of the technique. The results obtained by surgeons regularly engaged in these procedures are regularly better than those obtained by occasional operators on nerves. It is therefore a matter for regret that these considerations, long known to clinicians, have not led in the UK to the establishment of regional centres for the investigation and treatment of surgical disorders of the peripheral nerves. We have already remarked on the great advances that flowed from the establishment, under the hammer of war, of such regional centres. It is, however, vain to repine: surgeons must do what they can. This is particularly so in departments receiving accident and emergency cases. Operation on most uncomplicated open injuries of nerves can safely be left for 24 hours in order to receive attention from an experienced surgeon. When the injury is associated with damage to a major vessel or with increasing pressure in a fascial compartment, and peripheral ischaemia is threatened, such deferment is not permissible: it is better for the surgeon who is available to act rather than to risk the consequences of ischaemia until it is too late by waiting for a surgeon with special experience.

Most operations on injured peripheral nerves are best done with general anaesthesia. If the anaesthetist uses a muscle relaxant, he or she must be prepared to reverse its effect when the nerve stimulator/recorder is being used. Most work on the nerves of the limbs is best done at first in a bloodless field; it is of course important to recall that nerves that have been ischaemic for 15 minutes or more will conduct either defectively or not at all.

Because these operations are usually time-consuming, it is especially important adequately to protect the pressure points at the knee, the elbow and elsewhere with suitable padding. In operations on the nerves of the neck in particular, special care must be taken to avoid air embolism, to recognise it if it does occur and to be prepared to deal effectively with any such occurrence. In the case of severe injuries to the brachial plexus, when there may be a sudden release of spinal fluid, it is necessary to be prepared quickly to alter the position of the patient to avoid "coning" of the medulla. If it seems likely that a nerve graft is going to be needed, the donor site should be prepared and the drapes should be placed accordingly.

APPARATUS AND INSTRUMENTS

Special apparatus required includes bipolar diathermy, stimulating and recording apparatus, and instruments for magnification. For simple stimulation and observation of motor response only the simplest uni-or bipolar stimulator is necessary. For stimulation and recording from muscle and nerve, more elaborate apparatus is required. We use a Medelec MS 91.

A bipolar stimulator with platinum electrodes is used. Recording is from a bipolar electrode on the surface of the nerve or fascicle or from a concentric needle electrode in the muscle. Further refinement of stimulating and recording electrodes is possible, and probably desirable. For stimulation and recording of sensory evoked potentials from the neck and scalp we use the Medelec MS 91 monitor. The settings are as follows: filter 20 Hz to 2 kHz; time base 1, 2, 3 or 5 ms; volts/division 20–50 µV; duration 0.2 single; stimulation intensity 1–50 V. The placement of the electrodes is shown in Figures 7.1 to 7.3.

For magnification we use loupes or the operating microscope. The microscopes are OPMI 6SD FC and OPMI 6 (both Carl Zeiss, Oberkochen); the stand is the universal S3B (Carl Zeiss, Oberkochen).

The instruments specially required are: fine skin hooks; plastic slings and light clips; malleable retractors; fine forceps and scissors for work under the microscope; Lahey swabs held in tonsil forceps; brain syringes or other irrigators and saline; 6/0, 8/0 and 11/0 nylon sutures with appropriate needles and needle holders; plasma "glue" Tisseel (TM) (Immuno Limited, Arctic House, Rye Lane, Dunton Green, Sevenoaks TN14 5HB, UK); light arterial clamps; and Fogarty catheters. A selection of instruments that we have found particularly useful is shown in Figure 7.4.

OBJECTS OF INTERVENTION

The objects of intervention are:

- to confirm or establish diagnosis
- to restore continuity to a severed or ruptured nerve
- to remove a noxious agent compressing or distorting or occupying a nerve.

"It has all been done before" (Holmes 1881). The *British Medical Journal* of May 15, 1915 – a dismal date for the British nation and its Army – carried a report of an address by Inspector General E. Delorme to the Académie de Médecine on the treatment of gunshot wounds of the nerves. In this address most of the procedures to be recommended here are canvassed, including the use of electrical stimulation during operation. Alas! The medical world then was evidently unprepared for Delorme's proposals, many of which were sharply criticised by the great and good of French neurology. Bland-Sutton (1930) relates that in the 1870s J.W. Hulke, then surgeon to the Middlesex Hospital in Mortimer Street London, repaired the cut median and ulnar nerves of a woman. Bland-Sutton continues: "The operation was successful and this was the first instance of a successful secondary suture of a divided nerve in London. Surgeons had been afraid to suture cut nerves in this way for fear of tetanus." Interestingly enough, the possibilities of nerve grafting are here adumbrated.

In cases of injury, diagnosis is always easier the earlier the exploration is done. Not only is the field free from scar tissue, but the axons of the distal stump continue to conduct and neuromuscular junctions continue to function for a few days. Stimulation of the distal stump produces a motor response, which permits the operator to identify bundles with a predominantly motor function. This is nowhere better shown than in the case of the brachial plexus; it is easy to diagnose rupture up to 3 days after injury (Fig. 7.5), but it is progressively more difficult after that time (Figs 7.6 to 7.8). With early operation it is

Figs 7.1 to 7.3 Placement of electrodes for recording sensory evoked potentials.

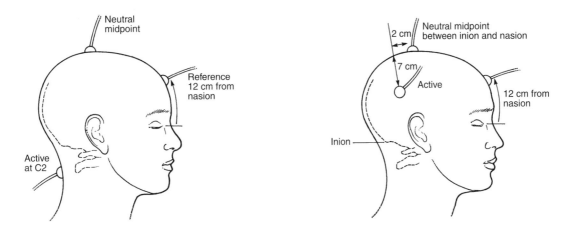

Fig. 7.1 Placement for cervical (cord) and cortical recording.

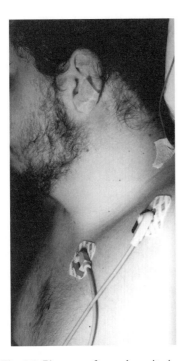

Fig. 7.2 Placement for cord monitoring.

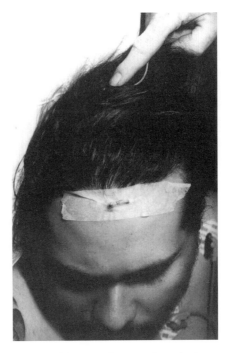

Fig. 7.3 Placement for cortical monitoring.

possible to match fascicular arrangements of the stumps; as time goes by, the matching becomes progressively more difficult. This is not all; with delay there is progressive intraneural collagenisation.

Possibly the most difficult decision for the peripheral neurosurgeon is that of whether to leave alone a lesion in continuity or to resect and bridge the gap. That decision is made particularly difficult when there is clinical evidence of some recovery through the neuroma and the neuroma involves the whole thickness of the nerve. Things are much easier when it is clear that there are some intact fascicles in one or more sites in the substance of the neuroma. There are no other completely satisfactory guides. The operator can derive from the consistency of the neuroma some idea of its connective tissue content: a hard neuroma is likely to contain much connective and little conducting tissue. The

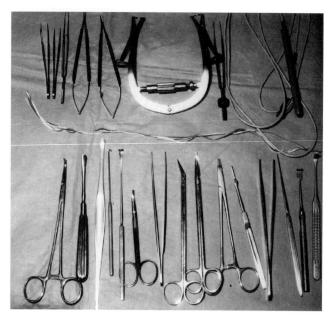

Fig. 7.4 Some of the instruments that we have found useful.

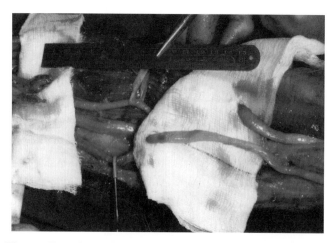

Fig. 7.5 Ease of diagnosis at operation done soon after injury. There has been an infraclavicular traction injury of the left brachial plexus. At operation 24 hours after injury, the rupture of the nerves of the arm is clearly seen.

surgeon can make a trial incision and view the interior of the neuroma through the loupe or microscope; the finding of nerve bundles traversing the neuroma indicates the chance of spontaneous recovery. The operator can stimulate the nerve above the neuroma and look for distal motor response. He or she should not omit to stimulate too below the neuroma, for it is possible that part or all of the lesion may be a conduction block and that there may be functioning axons below the lesion.

Most informative of all is to stimulate above the lesion and to record from the nerve or from individual fascicles below it: a response of good amplitude may well indicate a

good prognosis. Or, a response in individual fascicles may allow differentiation of an intact part of the nerve from the damaged portion. The tendency, in cases in which there is no recovery at the time of operation, must surely be towards resection and repair. We have rarely regretted taking such action; we have often regretted failure so to act. So bold a line is probably justified in most cases in which at the time of operation there is imperfect recovery, but such patients must clearly be warned before operation that after it there may be a temporary falling-off of function.

GENERAL PRINCIPLES OF OPERATION

All tissues must be treated gently. They are, after all, alive, and on their continued viability depend the healing of the wound without infection and the recovery of the nerve lesion. Indeed, avoidance of infection probably has more to do with tender handling of the tissues and accurate haemostasis than has the administration of antibiotics. The line of the proposed incision should be marked and cross-hatched with Bonney's Blue (Berkeley & Bonney 1920). In operations on the neck in particular, a dilute haemostatic solution (POR 8 Wirkstoff, Ornipressin, Sandoz AG, Nürnberg) can be injected subcutaneously along the line of the incision. Incisions should, whenever possible, follow the lines of relaxed skin tension indicated by Copeland (1995a). They should be planned with cutaneous innervation in mind: lasting trouble can follow wounding of an apparently trivial cutaneous nerve; it is an ill matter for a surgeon purporting to assist healing of lesions of peripheral nerves to damage one set of nerves on the way to repairing another. The more important cutaneous nerves are shown in Figures 7.9 to 7.17.

In the neck, the skin flaps should include the platysma; elsewhere, they should be cut to full thickness. Skin flaps should be held with fine skin hooks; if the procedure is going to take a long time, the flaps should be sutured back to the surrounding skin. So far as possible, dissection should be done with the knife or with sharp blunt-ended scissors. Although in the limbs the pneumatic tourniquet can be used during dissection and exposure, it must be released for stimulation, repair, and closure. The best possible haemostasis must be secured after the cuff has been deflated, by diathermy, ligation and haemostatic sponge. Cut bone surfaces should be sealed with wax or similar preparation.

Once the flaps are raised, the field should be kept as free of blood as possible, but it must be kept moist by regular irrigation. Even well-shielded operation lamps generate enough heat to accelerate desiccation of the tissues. When muscles have to be divided, their ends should be marked with sutures and, if necessary, labelled, so that when the procedure is completed they can accurately be reunited. Nerves should be handled with extreme care; they should be retracted with very fine skin hooks in

Figs 7.6 to 7.8 Difficulties with late operation.

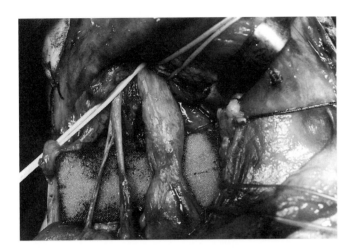

Fig. 7.6 Upper trunk of left brachial plexus seen at operation 8 weeks after injury. It is possible to deduce that there has probably been a rupture.

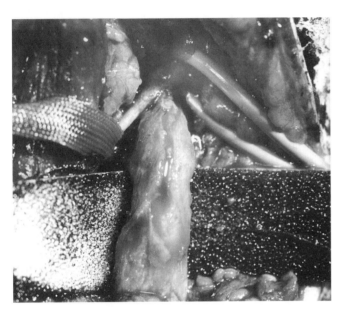

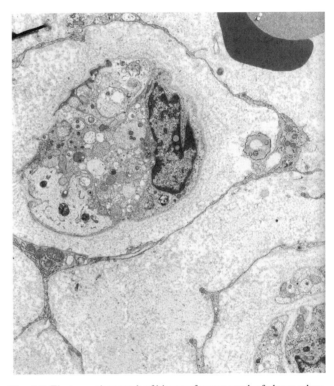

Fig. 7.7 A more difficult case. The upper trunk again, 3 months after injury. It is very hard to determine from inspection alone the nature of the injury.

Fig. 7.8 Electron micrograph of biopsy of upper trunk of plexus taken 8 months after injury. There is dense collagenisation. × 5270. (Electron microscope study by Mr Stephen Gschmeissner.)

the epineurium or with plastic slings. They should not be mobilised over such a length as to impair their blood supply.

When the decision has been made to resect and repair, the proximal section should be done first. A new large blade mounted on a handle should be used, and the nerve should rest on a firm surface during this procedure. It is important to cut rather than compress, and to make the section as near as possible to a right angle with the line of the nerve. If before resection it is plain that there are intact fascicles or an intact fascicle crossing the zone of the lesion, those fascicles or that fascicle should be separated from the

nerve before resection begins. Sometimes there is sufficient bleeding from the cut surface of the proximal stump to require checking by bipolar diathermy. The amount of resection should be enough to expose pouting bundles in each stump, and, if possible, to reach mobile epineurium.

The wound should not be closed before bleeding points have been checked; even with good haemostasis it is wise to use a suction drain in most wounds. However, the business end of the drain should not be placed near the site of repair, for fear of damage to the anastomosis by the suction or by later withdrawal of the drain. Divided

Figs 7.9 to 7.17 Some of the more important cutaneous nerves.

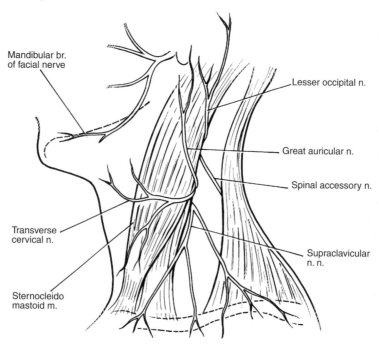

Mandibular br. of facial nerve

Lesser occipital n.

Great auricular n.

Spinal accessory n.

Transverse cervical n.

Supraclavicular n. n.

Sternocleido mastoid m.

Fig. 7.9 The neck. Note that the mandibular branch of the facial nerve comes at one point below the lower margin of the mandible. The cervical branch has been omitted.

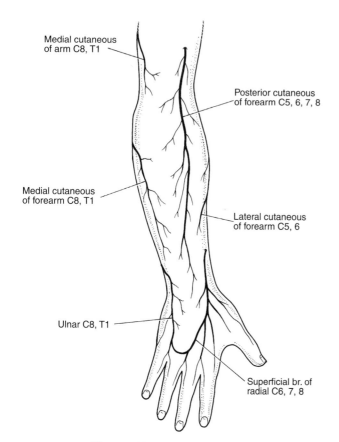

Medial cutaneous of arm C8, T1

Posterior cutaneous of forearm C5, 6, 7, 8

Medial cutaneous of forearm C8, T1

Lateral cutaneous of forearm C5, 6

Ulnar C8, T1

Superficial br. of radial C6, 7, 8

Fig. 7.10 The back of the forearm.

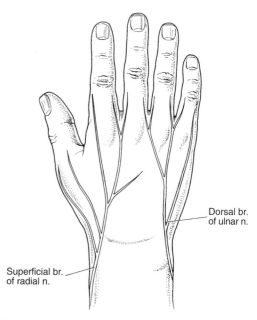

Dorsal br. of ulnar n.

Superficial br. of radial n.

Fig. 7.11 The back of the hand. Note in particular the site of the radial nerve.

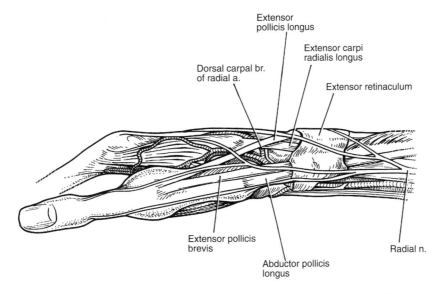

Fig. 7.12 The radial side of the hand, with further warning about the terminal branches of the radial nerve.

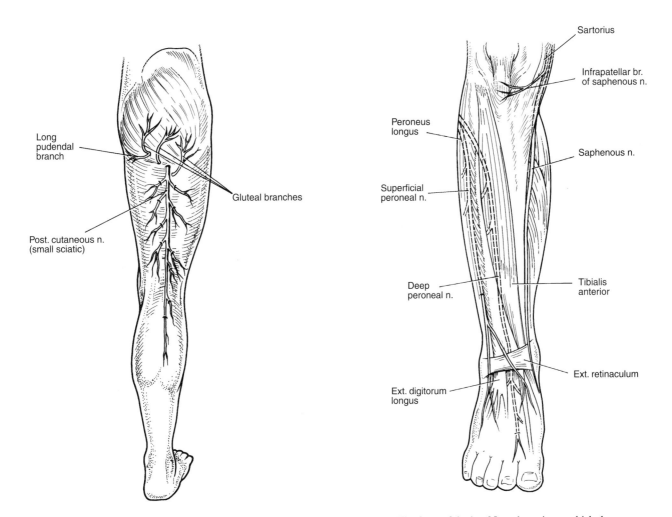

Fig. 7.13 The back of the thigh and leg, showing the posterior cutaneous nerve of the thigh, rather larger than life.

Fig. 7.14 The front of the leg. Note the point at which the cutaneous component of the superficial peroneal nerve pierces the deep fascia.

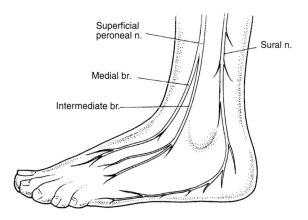

Fig. 7.15 The lateral side of the foot.

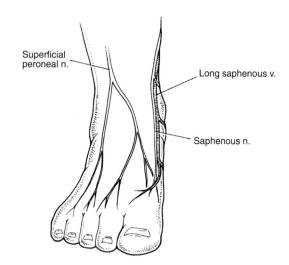

Fig. 7.16 The dorsum of the foot.

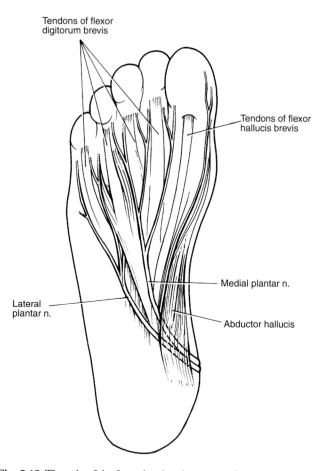

Fig. 7.17 The sole of the foot, showing the course of the plantar nerves.

muscle layers should be repaired accurately and securely. In the neck the platysma should carefully be closed with interrupted sutures; in the limbs, a subcutaneous suture should generally be used.

Although with careful handling of tissues wound infection is rare, the exposure is often so much prolonged that prophylactic use of antibiotics is advisable. Such cover should always be used if there is any liability to ischaemia or if there is an associated fracture. We use antibiotic cover (cefuroxime 750 mg intravenously three times in 24 hours starting just before operation and continued for 72 hours) in all cases of major intervention on the brachial plexus, in all compound nerve injuries, in interventions on the proximal part of the sciatic nerve, and in most second operations on main nerves.

The record should carefully be maintained: it is best to follow a standard form (Fig. 7.18) and to supplement this with a diagram and photographs. Under no circumstances must descriptions of the lesion, of the state of the stumps after resection or of the gap after resection be omitted. The operation record should be written or dictated by the operating surgeon as soon as possible after completion of the procedure.

METHODS OF REPAIR

Once the decision has been made for or by the surgeon, the nerve ends are cut back progressively until healthy pouting bundles show in the cut surfaces (Figs 7.19 and 7.20). Then the ends must be united, preferably by end to

RNOH STANMORE: PNI OPERATION RECORD

Name:

Date of birth:

Address:

Hospital number:

Ward:

Operation:

Code:

Surgeon:

Assistant:

Anaesthetist:

Duration of GA:

Tourniquet time:

Blood loss/replacement:

Operation date:

Preoperatively:

Position:

Incision:

Procedure/findings:

Repair:

Closure:

Records/specimen:

Comment:

Signature:

Distribution:

Fig. 7.18 An example of a standard form for an operation record (not to scale).

end suture so long as the gap after resection is small, little mobilisation of the nerve is needed to close it, and the repaired nerve lies without tension, without excessive flexion of adjacent joints. The experimental work of Clark et al (1992) clearly showed the ill effect of tension on the repaired nerve. We take as guides these principles:

1. End to end suture of the nerves of the brachial plexus above the clavicle or of the accessory nerve is never practicable.
2. It is impracticable to bridge with grafts gaps in lesions of the whole sciatic nerve. Sufficient graft material is not available. The gap has to be closed by flexion of the knee and extension of the hip and later maintenance of that position for the appropriate time.
3. Anterior transposition of ulnar or radial nerves gives at most 3 cm.
4. No gaps in the median nerve in the forearm can be closed by end to end suture.

It will be seen that in many circumstances it is better to bridge a gap with a graft than to force direct suture; it is better to resect to healthy bundles and create a wide gap than to resect too little in order to facilitate direct suture.

The advantages of the autogenous cable graft (Sanders 1942, Seddon 1947, Sunderland & Ray 1947, Sedel & Nizard 1993) are now so well known that we tend to forget that earlier this century surgeons obtained what we would now consider remarkably good results with grafts which would now not be used. Thus, Mayo-Robson (1917) reported a good result after repair of a lesion of the median nerve with an allograft of median nerve, and another good result after repair of another lesion of the median nerve with a length of the spinal cord of a rabbit. Cable grafts remain the favoured method of bridging gaps. The advantages of vascularised grafts of various sorts and of freeze-dried muscle will be canvassed elsewhere.

Ideally, it is best to match bundle to bundle, sensory fibres to sensory fibres, and motor fibres to motor fibres. It is often easy to match bundle to bundle simply by looking at the nerve end under the microscope or with the loupe, though the changing architecture of the nerve along its length makes this difficult when a long gap has to be bridged. When operation is done soon after injury, it is easy, as Vandeput et al (1969) suggested, to determine the sites of motor fascicles in the distal stump and to effect an "electrophysiological orientation" however, the late distinction between motor and sensory fibres requires more advanced methods. Gruber and Zenker (1973) attempted this distinction with a test depending on histochemical assessment of acetylcholinesterase activity. Gruber and Zenker (1973) had shown that by this technique motor and sensory funiculi could be stained differentially. An interval of 2–3 days between differentiation and repair was necessary, and the method was applicable only in acute cases. Riley and Lang (1984) studied the cytochemical

Figs 7.19 and 7.20 Good and bad stumps after resection in traction injury of the brachial plexus.

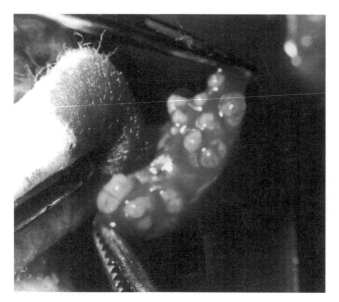

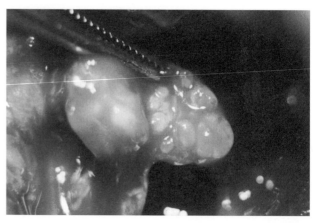

Fig. 7.20 The proximal stumps of the right fifth (left) and sixth (right) cervical nerves. There is evidently much intraneural collagenisation in the fifth nerve; the bundles are very poorly defined. The condition in the stump of the sixth nerve is clearly better.

Fig. 7.19 The distal stump of the lateral cord of the plexus. There are clearly separated "pouting" bundles.

localisation of carbonic anhydrase activity in rat peripheral sensory and motor nerves, dorsal root ganglia and dorsal column nuclei. Riley et al (1984) used carbonic anhydrase histochemistry to distinguish motor from sensory fibres. Axoplasmic staining characterised sensory fibres: myelin staining was characteristic of somatic motor fibres. It was left to Yunshuo and Shizen (1988) to establish a clinically feasible method of improving the accuracy of nerve repair. They described a method for acetylcholinesterase histochemical identification of motor and sensory fibres, which was in theory applicable to clinical practice. Perhaps the most practical contribution is that of Gschmeissner et al (1991), who offered a 2-minute assessment of the quality of the stumps by examination of frozen sections. Since failure so often depends on inadequate resection of nerve ends, this method could be important in avoiding this error. Considerable further steps in the organisation and management of nerve injuries will be needed, in the UK at any rate, before such methods enter common practice.

Methods of suture

The relative advantages of perineurial (fascicular) and epineurial suture have been canvassed by Edshage (1964), Terzis and Strauch (1978), Donoso et al (1978), Lilla et al (1979), Brunelli (1980a), Millesi (1973, 1981), Jàbaley (1981), Snyder (1981), Sunderland (1981) and Tupper et al (1988). The last workers confirmed the general experience that over the general field there was no difference between the results of epineurial and fascicular suture. Orgel (1987) described a modified fascicular suture: "group fascicular suture". Millesi (1981) proposed that the epineurium was the main source of the infiltration of the suture line by fibroblasts. In his technique of fascicular suture he practised resection of epineurium from the proximal and the distal nerve stumps and subdivided the trunks into clusters of bundles. Millesi further shielded the suture lines by grafts of healthy muscle or fat. Orgel (1987) concluded that, since there was little difference between the results of epineurial and perineurial suture, epineurial suture was "the technique of choice for most acute nerve lacerations". He pointed out that it was easier and faster and entailed less manipulation of the internal structure of the nerve than did fascicular suture. Kline and Hudson (1995b) indicate a restriction of fascicular suture to "some oligofascicular nerves". We reserve bundle suture for primary repair of clean transections of most trunk nerves.

In both types of suture, the areolar adventitial tissue is pushed back from each stump to expose the true epineurium. In fascicular suture, matched bundles, identified by size and by position in the nerve, are united by perineurial sutures of 11/0 nylon (Fig. 7.21). Once these "key" bundles have been united, the union is completed by passing a few sutures of 10/0 nylon through perineurium and epineurium (Fig. 7.22). Birch (1991b) rotates

Figs 7.33 and 7.34 Protection after repair.

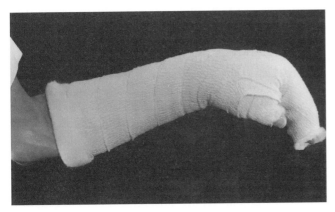

Fig. 7.33 Plaster after repair of both nerves and flexor tendons at the wrist.

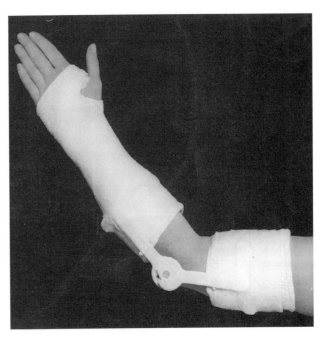

Fig. 7.34 Hinged plaster with adjustable check.

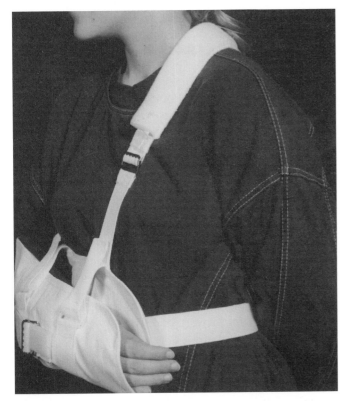

Fig. 7.35 Evelyn Hunter's sling for control of the forequarter after repair of the brachial plexus. Note the check on lateral rotation at the glenohumeral joint.

movement of related joints, and to rely on the patient steadily to restore movement of those joints. There is particular difficulty in controlling movement of the forequarter on the axial skeleton after repair of the brachial plexus. This difficulty may be even more of a problem when it becomes necessary to protect roots reunited to the spinal cord. At present we rely on a sling for the upper limb of the adult: the best, in our experience, is that designed by Evelyn Hunter RGN (Fig. 7.35).

It is, of course, very important during the period of recovery to maintain the mobility of the joints, some or all of the governing muscles of which are paralysed, and to warn the patients of the danger, especially in cold weather, of accidental damage to the anaesthetic skin. Most of the work on passive movements of the joints can be done by the patient or by his or her carers, but weekly supervision by a physiotherapist is useful in keeping the mind concentrated on the work during the long march towards recovery. In the case of the metacarpophalangeal joints of the fingers and the carpometacarpal joint of the thumb, "lively" splints are useful, but the problem of the stiff metacarpophalangeal joint in the paralysed hand persists.

Acceleration of regeneration

A number of attempts have been made to accelerate regeneration. Thus, Cockett and Kiernan (1973) showed acceleration of regeneration of nerves in the rat by exogenous triiodothyronine, and Melsaac and Kiernan (1975) repeated this success, measuring the effect of triiodothyronine on neuromuscular reinnervation. On the other hand, Verghese et al (1982) were unable to find any difference between the rate of regeneration in the treated and untreated groups when they examined the effects of adrenocorticotrophic and cerebral gangliosides on nerve regeneration in the rat. Danielsen et al (1986) reverted to the hormonal concept, and showed some acceleration of axonal growth in response to experimental hyperthyroidism. Raji and Bowden (1983) tried a new approach, and managed to show an acceleration of the processes of degeneration and regeneration by exposure to a high-peak electromagnetic field. Pomeranz et al (1984) showed that sprouting of axons of the saphenous nerves of rabbits was enhanced by application of electric fields at the growth tips.

Evidently, there is at present no wholly reliable nor practical method of accelerating the regeneration of axons in man. Developments in the field of nerve growth factors must surely bring nearer the time when such methods are available (Becker et al 1989).

APPROACHES TO INDIVIDUAL NERVES

THE NECK

The nerves associated with the neck are:

- the cervical and brachial plexus
- the spinal accessory nerve
- the suprascapular nerve
- the sympathetic chain.

For exposure of the supraclavicular part of the brachial plexus we have generally used the anterior (or anterolateral) approach described in Chapters 9, 10 and 12. The disadvantage of this approach is that the vertebral artery stands between the operator and the most proximal parts of the nerves. The demonstration by Cullheim et al (1989) and later by Hems et al (1994), and the clinical evidence provided by Carlstedt et al (1995) that axons from anterior horn cells would reinnervate anterior roots which had been detached and later reattached through grafts, opened at last the prospect of true repair of intradural lesions of the brachial plexus. Our thoughts have been directed to the evolution of the best route for this or a similar procedure, and we have accordingly canvassed the possibility of using the anterior transvertebral approach described by Cloward (1964) for gaining access to the anterior aspect of the spinal cord. Cloward, who successfully performed anterolateral cordotomy through this approach, indicated the ease of access to the anterior and lateral aspects of the cord. He stemmed the flow of spinal fluid by drainage through a flexible spinal needle

inserted before operation into the lumbar theca. We have thought that it would be possible to approach the anterior aspect of the cervical spine between the visceral tubes and the carotid sheath, and through the same incision to expose the detached plexus lateral to the sternocleido-mastoid muscle. The spinal canal would be opened by excision of the lateral part of the appropriate vertebral bodies to expose the dural lesion and, eventually, the anterior aspect of the cord. Either the roots would be drawn back into the spinal canal to permit reattachment of the anterior roots to the anterolateral sulcus, or the detached posterior rootlets would be used as a free graft to bridge the gap between the anterolateral sulcus and the proximal ends of the anterior roots. Such an approach would avoid the difficulty experienced by Bonney and Jamieson (1979) in obtaining access to the anterolateral aspect of the cord. They used a dual approach, by hemi-laminectomy and anterior exposure, and felt obliged, due to the danger of the prolonged rotation of the cord needed for reattachment of the anterior roots, to limit their reattachment to selected posterior roots.

Hoffman et al (1993b) found that the anterior transvertebral approach was practicable in cats for the reattachment of anterior roots, though the mortality was high. The chief risk to be apprehended from such a procedure in man soon after intradural injury of the plexus would, we think, be that of bleeding from epidural veins in a spinal canal robbed of pressure exerted on the walls by an intact theca. Indeed, the major surgical problem, "contributing to death in some cases", encountered by Hoffman et al was loss of blood. They found, however, that with increasing skill in operating and with the use of plasma expanding fluid, hypovolaemic complications could greatly be reduced. In man, it would almost certainly be necessary to stabilise the operated segments by graft after completion of reattachment. Another possible route for approaching the anterior aspect of the spinal cord is opened by the recent experience of one of us working with Dr Thomas Carlstedt. A 10-year-old boy with complete lesion of the brachial plexus was operated at 2 weeks from injury. The seventh and eighth cervical and the first thoracic nerves were avulsed. A small arthroscope introduced through the foramen of C8 gave a surprisingly good view of the cord, and of the stump of the ventral root of C8. The presence of useful stumps at C5 and C6, and the state of the avulsed nerves persuaded us against replantation, but the possibility of doing this through the enlarged foramina, with proper care for the vertebral artery, is attractive.

The posterolateral route

Kline and Hudson (1995c) and Dubuisson et al (1993) expand on the experience of Kline et al (1978) with the "posterior subscapular" route. We have only rarely used a posterolateral approach and, when we did, we used one more resembling that of Adson and Brown (1929) than that of Kline et al. We recognise that it offers very good access to the most proximal parts of the nerves and, in particular, to the nerves in the intervertebral foramina. Carlstedt et al (1995) has used an approach like that of Kline et al for the reconnection of anterior roots to the cord.

Kline et al (1978) describe a position in which the patient is almost supine, with the limb on the affected side resting on a separate table. The incision is convex medially, truly parascapular. The scapula is freed by the division of the trapezius and rhomboid muscles and, if necessary, the levator scapulae. It is retracted laterally and the upper ribs are exposed. The first rib is defined and extraperiosteally removed, if necessary after the second rib has been removed subperiosteally to facilitate exposure. The scalenus medius muscle is partly liberated during the removal of the first rib, and further liberation permits its upward retraction to display the brachial plexus. Kline et al (1978) warn that it is necessary to avoid damage to the nerve to serratus anterior during this process. By medial retraction of the posterior paravertebral muscles the foramina can be opened by facetectomy and partial laminectomy. Closure after completion of the procedure is by reuniting the muscles carefully over a drain or drains.

Dubuisson et al (1993) frankly draw attention to the fact that the posterior approach is more extensive than the anterior approach, and that it can "occasionally result in winging of the scapula". They append a very good list of indications for the use of this approach which includes the three *potential* complications: winging of the scapula, instability of the cervical spine if more than two facet joints are removed, and damage to various related structures. We certainly accept as firm indications:

1. In thoracic outlet syndrome: prior operation by transaxillary or supraclavicular route for removal of first thoracic or seventh cervical rib, when the posterior third of the rib remains.
2. In tumours of the plexus: tumours with intraforaminal and extraforaminal lateral components.
3. In radiation neuropathy: when there is extensive change in the skin and deep tissues of the neck and chest wall.
4. In traumatic lesions: when the evidence is that a reparable lesion is in or near the foramen.

It may be that we have been too hesitant in using this method. Certainly, the paper by Dubuisson et al (1993) is required reading for all who work in this field.

Our posterolateral approach owes more to Adson and Brown (1929) than to Kline et al. It affords a less extensive view than does Kline's to the more distal (lateral) part of the supraclavicular plexus. The patient is put in the lateral position, the affected side uppermost, and the limb is included in the field. The incision, convex laterally, is centred over the seventh cervical vertebral spine (Fig. 7.36). The flaps are raised. The trapezius is divided close to the midline and the muscle is retracted laterally (Fig. 7.37). The next layer then comes into view: the upper part of the rhomboids, and the lower part of the splenius capitis

---

Figs 7.36 to 7.40 Posterior approach to the left brachial plexus.

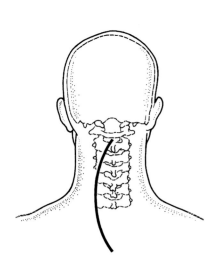

Fig. 7.36 The incision.

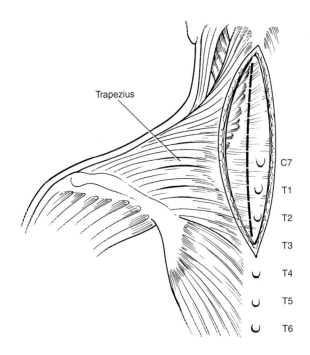

Fig. 7.37 The division of the trapezius.

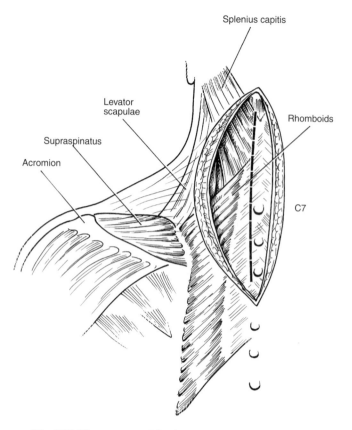

Fig. 7.38 The exposure of the rhomboids and splenius capitis.

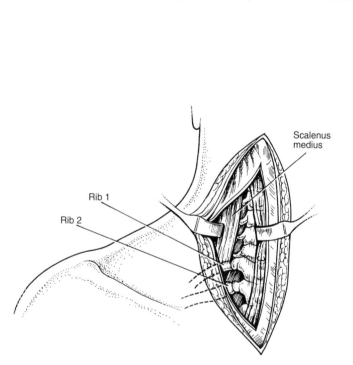

Fig. 7.39 Exposure of the posterior elements after division of the second muscular layer.

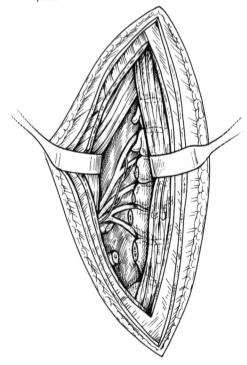

Fig. 7.40 Removal of posterior elements and detachment of scalenus medius to expose the proximal part of the plexus. Note that the nerve to serratus anterior is shown. In many cases of proximal injury to the plexus, it will have been damaged with the main nerves.

(Fig. 7.38). The levator scapulae, running from the scapula to the upper cervical transverse processes, and the splenius cervicis, running from the third to the sixth thoracic vertebral spines to the upper cervical transverse processes, are rather lateral. The upper part of the rhomboids and the lower part of the splenius capitis are divided near the midline and the erector spinae group is exposed. Lateral to this the transverse processes of the first thoracic and lowest four cervical vertebrae can be felt. The transverse processes and lateral masses are exposed by blunt dissection, with medial retraction of the erector spinae group (Fig. 7.39). The back of the first rib is exposed at the lower end of the field, and the scalenus medius is cleared from its upper surface. That muscle is detached from its origin on the posterior tubercles of the lowest three of four cervical transverse processes. The nerves are then shown distal to the transverse processes, the proximal branches of the fifth, sixth and seventh vertebrae going into the scalenus medius to form the nerve to the serratus anterior. Now the posterior tubercles of the fifth and sixth vertebrae and part of the transverse process of the seventh are nibbled away to show the most proximal parts of the nerves. If necessary, the first thoracic transverse process and the first rib can be removed to increase the exposure of the lowest part of the plexus (Fig. 7.40). Later, if necessary, one or two interfacetal joints can be removed to show the nerves in their dural sheaths in the foramina.

As in "anterolateral decompression", it is necessary to proceed carefully and methodically in this exposure, securing good haemostasis at each stage. It is not an easy exposure, but it is the preferred route when there is a very proximal lesion and access by the anterior route is barred by the sclerosis of a previous intervention. Two muscular layers and one subcutaneous layer are closed over a suction drain.

The infraclavicular part of the brachial plexus; the axillary artery

The infraclavicular part of the plexus is most commonly displayed in association with exposure of the supraclavicular part, by an extension of the collar incision traversing the clavicle and running along the line of the deltopectoral groove. The skin flaps are raised. The middle part of the clavicle is cleared above and below, with opening up of the deltopectoral groove by a small detachment of the deltoid and pectoralis major muscles from the clavicle. It is sometimes necessary to divide the clavicle in cases of vascular injury, in dealing with tumours and when there is damage to the retroclavicular part of the plexus. Before the bone is cut a plate should be shaped and fitted and holes drilled for its later fixation. In other circumstances, the view of the plexus is developed above and below the bone and completed by division of the subclavius muscle. The cephalic vein is usually retracted laterally.

With the full opening of the deltopectoral interval the pectoralis minor muscle is exposed crossing the field to its attachment on the coracoid process. Below and above it is the neurovascular bundle, covered by a layer of fascia and, in the lower part of the field, by the flat reflected tendon of the sternal part of the pectoralis major. The pectoralis minor is divided through its tendon and the lower part of the muscle is drawn downwards, care being taken of the medial pectoral nerve piercing it and going on to the pectoralis major. Now the fascia over the plexus is divided above and below the former site of the pectoralis minor. If it is absolutely necessary, the flat reflected tendon of the pectoralis major too can be divided. Thus the whole neurovascular bundle is displayed. The lateral cord is the most prominent component, the axillary artery is behind it and the axillary vein medial to it. In the lower part of the field the median nerve is formed from the contributions from the medial and lateral cords. Just at the formation of the lateral cord the lateral pectoral nerve arises to pierce the clavipectoral fascia and enter the pectoralis major. The posterior cord lies deep to the lateral cord and axillary artery; the medial cord is deep to the axillary vein. Some mobilisation of both great vessels is necessary for the full display of the cords.

The musculocutaneous nerve arises from the lateral cord above the level of the coracoid process and runs laterally into the coracobrachialis muscle. It may be a single branch; it may consist of several branches arising at different levels from the cord.

The posterior cord and its lateral and terminal branches are exposed between the lateral cord and the axillary artery. The three subscapular nerves are seen, and in the lower part of the field the separation of the trunk into radial and circumflex, nerves is visible. Birch (1995a) comments that "reflection of coracobrachialis from the tip of the coracoid process improves exposure of the anterior 'door' of the quadrilateral space", to permit exposure of the distal stump of a ruptured circumflex nerve.

When there is need rapidly and urgently to expose the axillary artery, the exposure described by Fiolle and Delmas (1921) and recommended by Birch (1991a) is the best. Henry (1957) added some helpful touches to the description of this procedure. We use a transclavicular incision extending from a supraclavicular limb, following the deltopectoral interval to the anterior axillary fold (Fig. 7.41). The tendinous insertions of the pectoralis major muscle are defined and divided. The muscle is reflected medially to expose the plane of the clavicle, clavipectoral fascia and pectoralis minor. The pectoralis minor is divided through its tendon, and the clavicle is defined and divided at about the junction of the middle and medial thirds. The subclavius muscle is divided. This approach offers access to the neurovascular bundle from the first rib to the lower part of the axilla.

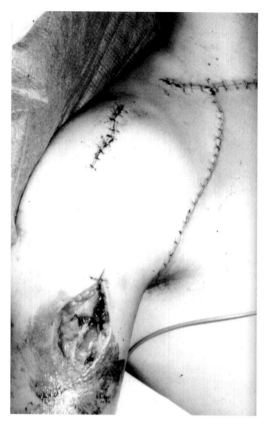

Fig. 7.41 Incision for the Fiolle–Delmas exposure. The two incisions over the humerus were made for the purpose of inserting a medullary nail. More information about this approach is given in Chapter 9.

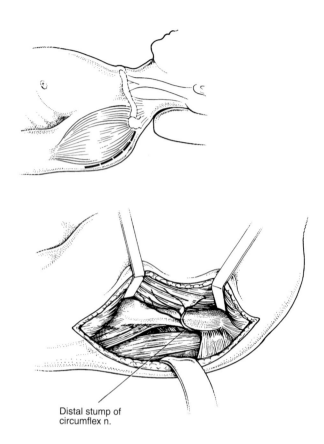

Distal stump of circumflex n.

Fig. 7.42 Approach for the exposure of the distal end of a ruptured circumflex nerve. (Top) The skin incision, (bottom) the exposure.

When the procedure is finished the fragments of the clavicle are united with a plate and screws. It is often tiresome and unnecessary, and even unwise, to reunite the divided pectoralis minor, but the pectoralis major muscle should be reattached. One or two suction drains should be placed before closure.

The circumflex nerve

The circumflex nerve may be damaged on its own in association with dislocation of the shoulder and humeral fracture or in association with wider supra- or infraclavicular damage to the brachial plexus. The preferred anterior exposure is made through the incision in the deltopectoral groove. Birch (1991b) reckons that in cases of rupture the anterior (proximal) stump is always found just below the coracoid process and that repair sometimes requires exposure of the posterior (distal) stump through a separate posterior incision (Fig. 7.42). It is sometimes difficult to repair a ruptured circumflex nerve through a single axillary incision, even when the distal stump can be brought into view by lateral rotation of the humerus. As Birch (1991b) remarks, open wounds of the circumflex nerve are uncommon: it is almost always a matter of rupture with

separation of the stumps or of a lesion in continuity, which may or may not require resection. Repair has to be effected by graft, and it is certainly easier to secure good placement and attachment through two incisions than through one giving limited access.

The suprascapular nerve

Access to the suprascapular nerve for relief of compression in the suprascapular notch has to be obtained by a posterior incision, though the preforaminal part of the nerve can be exposed through the anterior incision for exposure of the brachial plexus. Copeland (1995c) prefers a lateral position and a vertical incision; Kline and Hudson (1995a) prefer the prone position and a transverse incision. We prefer the lateral position and a transverse incision. The flaps are raised, and the supraspinous part of the trapezius muscle is detached from its origin and raised to show the supraspinatus muscle (Fig. 7.43). Alternatively, the fibres of trapezius can be split to show the underlying supraspinatus, which is lifted from its scapular origin to show the suprascapular nerve traversing the notch. The accompanying artery is usually superficial to the transverse ligament or bony bridge.

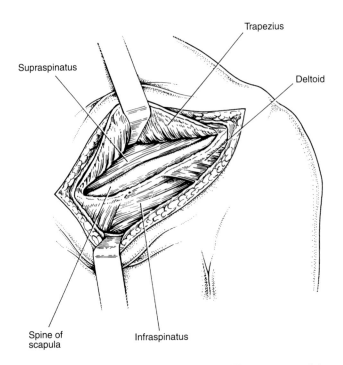

Fig. 7.43 Approach to the suprascapular nerve. The upper part of the trapezius has been lifted from the spine of the scapula to expose the spine and the supraspinatus muscle.

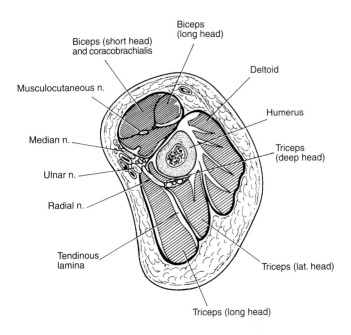

Fig. 7.44 Transverse section through the arm above the level of the insertion of the deltoid muscle, just below the level of the posterior movement of the radial nerve.

The spinal accessory nerve

As Birch (1995a) remarks, the siting of the incision is often dictated by the placing of that through which the nerve was originally damaged. Often enough, the original incision can be extended either as a "Z" or in the direction of the lines of skin tension. The usual site of injury is in the posterior triangle between the sternocleidomastoid muscle and trapezius muscles, though occasionally the nerve is wounded in its course through the former muscle or proximal to it. The exposure of the nerve should begin in unscarred tissue, and the lesion should preferably be exposed after both proximal and distal sections have been defined. The distal part is usually found beneath the anterior part of the upper fibres of trapezius. There is no point in attempting end to end suture after resection: the gap is usually too great, and in any case the mobility of the forequarter on the axial skeleton forbids the use of such a method because of the hazard of disruption.

MEDIAN AND ULNAR NERVES IN THE ARM AND THE AXILLA

The incision crosses the anterior axillary fold and the axilla, and descends the medial side of the arm. The flaps are raised and the axillary fat displaced downwards. The neurovascular bundle is found in its sheath in the lower part of the axilla: most medial is the axillary/brachial vein; the nerves are grouped around the lower part of the axillary and the brachial artery. The axillary artery is embraced by the two roots of the median nerve, which starts on its lateral side and crosses it in the arm. The musculocutaneous nerve most commonly arises as a single branch from the lateral cord at or below the level of the coracoid process, but it may consist of several branches arising at intervals along the line of the lateral root of the median nerve. It passes laterally into the coracobrachialis muscle and the flexors of the elbow. The ulnar nerve and the medial cutaneous nerve of the forearm are on the medial side of the artery. The former passes posteriorly about half way down the arm to pierce the medial inter-muscular septum and to lie between it and the medial part of the triceps muscle, to which it usually gives a branch. Deepest of all is the radial nerve, which soon passes posteriorly between the long and medial heads of triceps, to cross the back of the humerus deep to the lateral head of the triceps and to gain the lateral aspect of the lower part of the arm by piercing the lateral inter-muscular septum (Fig. 7.44).

The neurovascular bundle can be traced up into the axilla to expose the cords and the origin of the circumflex and radial nerves. If this exploration is undertaken for the repair of an extensive infraclavicular lesion of the median and ulnar nerves, the incision can be continued distally behind the medial epicondyle and the whole skin flap can be raised to show the median and ulnar nerves at and below the elbow. This incision avoids a scar in front of the elbow, but it is important to take the full thickness of the skin and to make sure that the base of the flap is sufficiently long.

THE RADIAL NERVE

The proximal part of the radial nerve is quite easily displayed in the upper part of the axillobrachial incision; the distal part is easily found through an anterolateral incision in the lower part of the arm and by entering the interval between the biceps and brachialis medially and the brachioradialis and extensor carpi radialis longus laterally. Finding the middle part – the part most likely to be in trouble – is rather more difficult. It is to be found through a sinuous posterior incision, and by separation of the superficial part of the triceps (the long and lateral heads) from its deep part (the medial head). The flaps are raised and the lower part of the deltoid muscle and the superficial part of the triceps muscle are exposed (Fig. 7.45). The V-shaped interval between the upper parts of the long and lateral heads is now defined, by defining the

upper part of the long head and following its lateral border distally. The "seam of the half sleeve" (Henry 1957) – that is, the junction of the long and lateral heads of the triceps – is now opened from the top towards the olecranon (Fig. 7.46). This shows the radial nerve and the profunda brachii artery crossing the deep head and the bone and piercing the lateral intermuscular septum (Fig. 7.47). The further exposure of the radial nerve has to be lateral to the lateral head of the triceps muscle, by entering the interval between the biceps/brachialis and the brachioradialis/ extensor carpi radialis longus. If there is difficulty in bridging a gap after resection, some length can be obtained by rerouting the distal stump towards the upper medial aspect of the arm deep to the biceps and brachialis muscles. For exposure of the more distal part of the nerve the incision may be extended round the side of the arm to the medial side of the brachioradialis. Thence it runs across the anterolateral aspect of the elbow into the forearm. With this anterior approach the radial nerve and its terminal branches are found in the interval between, on the one hand, the biceps/brachialis and, on the other, the brachioradialis/extensor carpi radialis longus.

Figs 7.45 to 7.47 The exposure of the radial nerve in the arm. (After Henry (1957).)

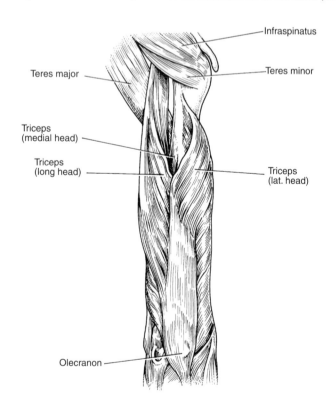

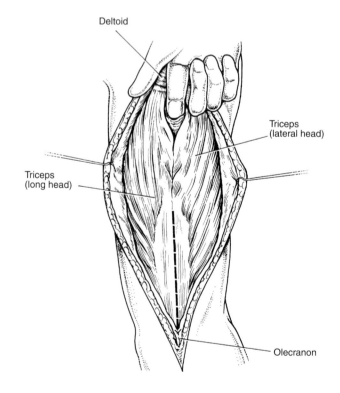

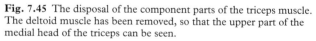

Fig. 7.45 The disposal of the component parts of the triceps muscle. The deltoid muscle has been removed, so that the upper part of the medial head of the triceps can be seen.

Fig. 7.46 The "seam of triceps" (A.K. Henry). The finger is introduced between the long and lateral heads, and the latter two are separated.

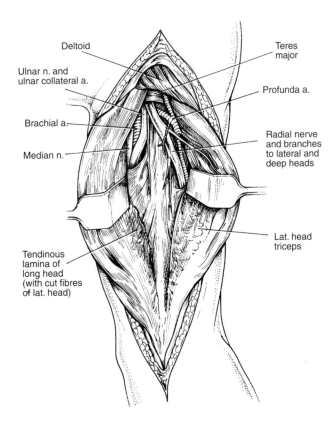

Fig. 7.47 The opening of the "seam" reveals the radial nerve from the start of its course on the back of the humerus to the piercing of the lateral intermuscular septum.

THE POSTERIOR INTEROSSEOUS NERVE

In the Henry (1957) approach, the incision is made on the posterolateral aspect of the upper forearm between, on one hand, the mobile mass of the brachioradialis and the radial extensors of the wrist, and, on the other, the extensor communis digitorum. The interval between the extensor carpi radialis brevis and the extensor communis digitorum is then opened and the supinator muscle is exposed. The posterior interosseous nerve passes between the superficial and deep parts of the muscle, to emerge at the lower margin of the superficial part and to run for about 4–5 cm before breaking up into its terminal (motor) branches. Henry indicated exposure of the nerve by a short incision in the supinator muscle. However, the point of emergence can quite easily be found, and the nerve can be followed proximally by division of the superficial part of the muscle along its line (Figs 7.48 and 7.49).

The lower part of the radial nerve and its terminal branches are very well exposed by a more extensive procedure. The incision runs down the line of the lateral supracondylar ridge, turning posteriorly at the epicondyle. The whole mass of the brachioradialis and extensor origin is then lifted from the supracondylar ridge and lateral epicondyle to expose the lateral and posterior aspects of the capsule of the elbow, the anconeus, and the supinator muscle. With this mobilisation, the lower part of the radial nerve, its superficial branch and the posterior interosseous nerve are well shown. The motor branches to the brachioradialis and radial extensors are protected, and a good view of the whole course of the posterior interosseous nerve is obtained.

THE LOWER PART OF THE MEDIAN NERVE

The median nerve is easily displayed at and just below the elbow and in the lower part of the forearm through a sinuous incision winding down from the elbow. At elbow level it is found medial to the brachial artery. It then descends between the superficial and deep heads of the pronator teres where it gives off its deep muscular branch the anterior interosseous nerve. The median nerve can be traced down into this tunnel, and can to some extent be mobilised by division of the deep (ulnar) head of the pronator teres. Having negotiated the pronator teres, the

Figs 7.48 and 7.49 Exposure of the posterior interosseous nerve. (After Henry (1957).)

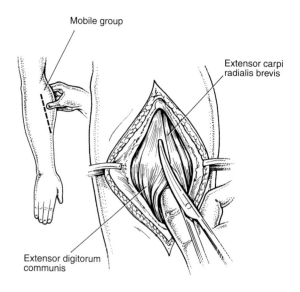

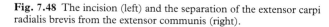

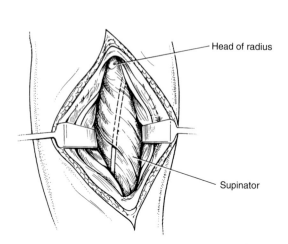

Fig. 7.48 The incision (left) and the separation of the extensor carpi radialis brevis from the extensor communis (right).

Fig. 7.49 The posterior interosseous nerve and supinator exposed.

nerve runs down the forearm between the deep and superficial flexor muscles, loosely attached by areolar tissue to the deep surface of the flexor digitorum superficialis. It can be exposed in this part of its course by separating the flexor superficialis from its radial origin and retracting the muscle. The nerve enters the hand just deep to and between the tendons of the palmaris longus and flexor carpi radialis. Its course and exposure in the hand are considered in Chapter 12.

THE ULNAR NERVE AT THE WRIST AND IN THE HAND

The ulnar nerve divides into its superficial (sensory) and deep (motor) components at about wrist level. Both components run into Guyon's space (the pisoretinacular space of Denman (1978)). The superficial branch passes superficially to supply the palmaris brevis and the skin of the medial two digits; the deep branch runs between the abductor and the flexor of the little finger to pierce the opponens and run across the deep palmar space with the deep palmar arch, ending by supplying the adductor and flexor brevis of the thumb and the first palmar interosseous muscle. Deep as it is, the deep branch is vulnerable to wounds from glass or knife. It is best followed by an incision beginning above the wrist, entering the ulnar side of the palm and curving across the distal palm

in a crease. The nerve is isolated in the upper part of the incision lateral to the tendon of flexor carpi ulnaris and medial to the ulnar artery. It is followed to its bifurcation. Then the deep branch is followed between the hypothenar muscles. Its deep course has to be revealed by mobilisation of the deep and superficial flexor tendons. The multitude of the motor branches of this nerve, to most of the intrinsic muscles of the hand, has to be borne in mind during this exposure, though it is impossible to avoid some of these in a scarred field. Lassa and Shrewsbury (1975) warn of dangers posed by the occasionally anomalous course of this nerve.

NERVES IN THE ABDOMEN AND PELVIS

The lumbar and sacral plexus are accessible through the lower quadrant of the abdomen, by the same transverse muscle cutting incision and extraperitoneal approach that is used for lumbar sympathectomy. This approach gives good access to the lumbar plexus in the psoas muscle and to the femoral and obturator nerves on each side of the lower part of the psoas. Access to the lumbosacral plexus is rather restricted through this extraperitoneal approach; a transperitoneal approach makes access easier, but the viscera have to be mobilised, and there are consequently risks of ileus after operation and of late complication from adhesions.

The femoral nerve can be traced down to the level of the inguinal ligament from above through an abdominal incision and exposed again in the thigh through a separate anterior crural incision. Alternatively, as Kline and Hudson (1995) suggest, the crural incision can be extended laterally above the inguinal ligament, and the lower abdominal muscles can be split to give an extraperitoneal approach.

THE SCIATIC NERVE

A limited view of the sciatic nerve at the hip and in the great sciatic notch can be obtained by splitting the gluteus maximus muscle as in the posterior approach to the hip. For a more extensive view, the approach described by Henry (1957) should be used. Henry compares the "gluteal lid" with a parallelogram the shorter sides of which are almost longitudinal and the longer (upper and lower) sides of which are oblique. The caudal edge is virtually unattached.

The prone position is used. The incision can follow the "question-mark" shape advised by Henry, or can run from the iliac crest at the junction of the gluteus maximus and the iliotibial tract to run obliquely down the back and lateral side of the buttock to reach the great trochanter and then turn medially to descend in the midline of the thigh (Figs 7.50 and 7.51). It is necessary to look out for the posterior cutaneous nerve of the thigh, piercing the deep fascia in the upper part of the thigh and descending in the midline. It should be identified under the fascia below the lower border of gluteus maximus. Now the gluteus maximus is detached from its insertion to the femur: the cephalic side of the muscle is detached from the iliotibial tract, and both tendinous and muscular insertions to the femur are divided (Fig. 7.52). Then, with continued care for the posterior cutaneous nerve of the thigh, the gluteal lid is hinged back on its pelvic origin. The structures displayed are the gluteus medius and the short lateral rotators of the hip, the superior and inferior gluteal vessels and nerves, the pudendal nerve and vessels and the sciatic nerve (Fig. 7.53). The sciatic nerve can be followed into and through the great sciatic notch by division of the tendon of the piriformis and retraction of the muscle. Downward extension of the vertical limb of this incision permits display of the whole of the sciatic nerve (Fig. 7.54).

Careful closure of this wound is essential: in particular, the gluteus maximus must be reattached laterally and cephalad. One or two suction drains should be used; subcutaneous tissues should be closed.

Figs 7.50 to 7.54 Exposure of the sciatic nerve. (After Henry (1957).)

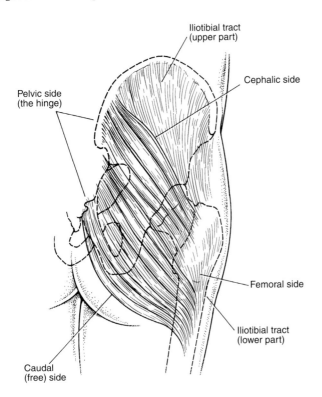

Iliotibial tract (upper part)

Cephalic side

Pelvic side (the hinge)

Femoral side

Iliotibial tract (lower part)

Caudal (free) side

Fig. 7.50 Surface markings.

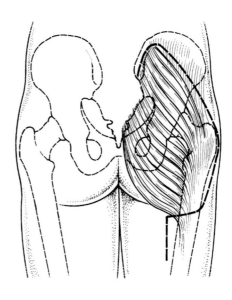

Fig. 7.51 The incision.

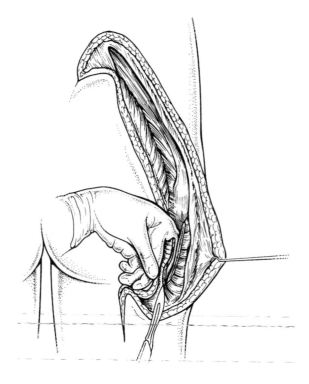

Fig. 7.52 The division of the upper and lateral sides of the gluteal "lid", to facilitate its lifting.

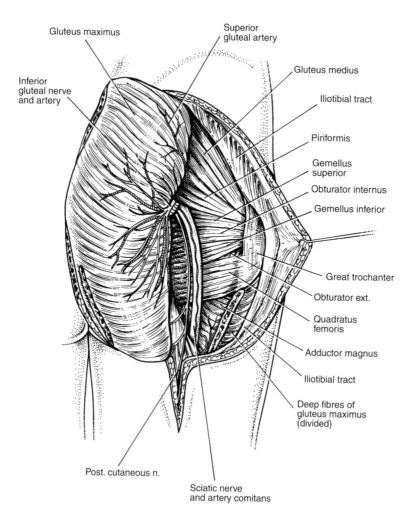

Gluteus maximus

Superior gluteal artery

Inferior gluteal nerve and artery

Gluteus medius

Iliotibial tract

Piriformis

Gemellus superior

Obturator internus

Gemellus inferior

Great trochanter

Obturator ext.

Quadratus femoris

Adductor magnus

Iliotibial tract

Deep fibres of gluteus maximus (divided)

Post. cutaneous n.

Sciatic nerve and artery comitans

Fig. 7.53 The gluteus maximus reflected, to show the sciatic and inferior gluteal nerves and the lateral rotator muscles of the hip.

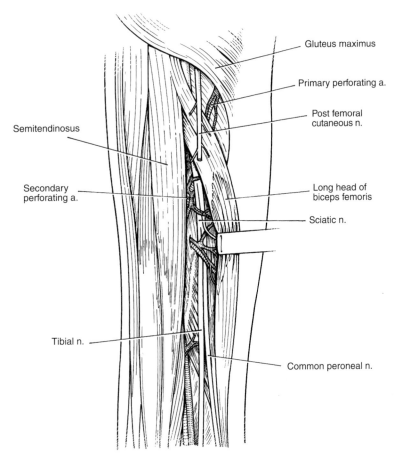

Gluteus maximus

Primary perforating a.

Post femoral
cutaneous n.

Semitendinosus

Long head of
biceps femoris

Secondary
perforating a.

Sciatic n.

Tibial n.

Common peroneal n.

Fig. 7.54 Showing the exposure of the sciatic nerve below the buttock.

THE TIBIAL AND COMMON PERONEAL NERVES IN THE POPLITEAL FOSSA AND BELOW

The incision starts above the back of the knee and skirts the crease to return to the midline below the knee and to descend in the midline for about 10 cm. The flaps are raised. Care must be taken of the sural nerve arising from the tibial nerve and descending in the midline, at first just under the deep fascia and piercing that in the proximal part of the leg (Fig. 7.55). The tibial nerve and popliteal artery and vein are found above in the midline; the common peroneal nerve has at this level deviated laterally to lie close to the tendon of the biceps femoris (Fig. 7.55). The gastrocnemius is split in the midline to expose the underlying soleus muscle, which also is split to show the nerve and vessels below the knee (Fig. 7.56).

The tibial nerve in the leg and behind the ankle is exposed through a straight or sinuous incision over the medial head of the gastrocnemius and medial to the tendocalcaneus. The medial head of the gastrocnemius is exposed and freed and retracted laterally, to expose the medial part of the soleus. Then the medial part of the

soleus is mobilised by division of the medial "pier" of its tendinous arch and of its medial origin. The soleus is then retracted laterally, to expose the deep compartment of the leg with the tibial nerve and vessels (Figs 7.57 and 7.58).

Exposure of the common peroneal nerve necessarily takes the popliteal incision laterally, to descend on the lateral side of the leg and permit exposure of the deep and superficial peroneal (musculocutaneous) branches in which the nerve terminates just below the neck of the fibula. The operator must remember that the common peroneal nerve is very close to the surface behind the fibular head and lateral to the fibular neck. We have seen it partly divided by the initial skin incision.

THE LOWER TIBIAL NERVE AND THE PLANTAR NERVES

The lower part of the tibial nerve is easily found on the medial side of the ankle, under the flexor retinaculum, between the flexor tendons of the hallucis and the flexor digitorum. The terminal plantar branches are traced into the foot by division of the retinaculum and then by bringing back the abductor hallucis muscle after defining its superior edge and detaching it from its origin on the distal part of the retinaculum. The plantar nerves are found between the deep and superficial layers of the plantar muscles – the plane between, on the one hand, the two abductors and the flexor brevis digitorum and on the other, the flexor accessorius and the tendons of the long flexors (Figs 7.59 and 7.60).

SYMPATHETIC GANGLIONECTOMY

Cervicothoracic sympathectomy

The long controversy about the best approach for cervico-thoracic sympathectomy began to move towards its conclusion with Atkins' (1949) description of a transthoracic approach, which he attributed to R.H. Goetz. Atkins enlarged on this account in 1954, and in 1956 Palumbo described an anterior transthoracic route. For some time transaxillary sympathectomy through the bed of the third rib was the favoured procedure for uncontrollable hyperhidrosis of the axilla and hand in young girls. It was left to Kux (1978) and his successors Weale (1980), Göthberg et al (1990), Salob et al (1991), Mussad et al (1991), Edmondson et al (1992), Rosin (1993) and Robertson et al (1993) to develop and perfect the technique of endoscopic transthoracic sympathectomy by electrocoagulation or excision. The best accounts of the procedure are those by Nicholson and Hopkinson (1993) and Nicholson et al (1994). If the apical part of the pleural sac is more or less clear, a very adequate sympathectomy can be done by this method, without serious disturbance to the patient, so long as the operator is thoroughly familiar with the practice of endoscopic surgery. Graham et al (1993) dealt with problems in anaesthesia associated with bilateral operation. Wilkinson (1984) indicates a method in which coagulation of the ganglia is affected by radiofrequency probes introduced by a paravertebral approach.

In our view, formed in the days when we did cervicothoracic sympathectomy by the supraclavicular route or through the axilla, the resection should extend below the fourth ganglion and should stop below the junction of the

---

Figs 7.55 to 7.58 Exposure of the tibial nerve in the upper, middle, and lower parts of the leg. (After Henry (1957).)

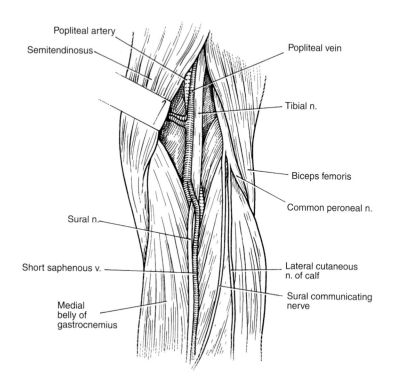

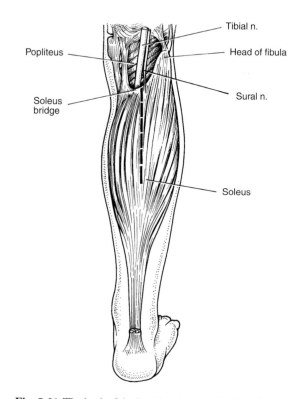

Fig. 7.55 The tibial and common peroneal nerves above and at the level of the popliteal fossa. Note the origin of the sural nerve and its connection with the common peroneal nerve.

Fig. 7.56 The back of the leg, showing the line for splitting the soleus.

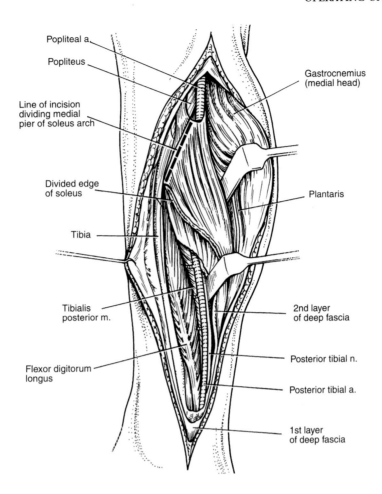

Popliteal a.

Popliteus

Line of incision
dividing medial
pier of soleus arch

Divided edge
of soleus

Tibia

Tibialis
posterior m.

Flexor digitorum
longus

Gastrocnemius
(medial head)

Plantaris

2nd layer
of deep fascia

Posterior tibial n.

Posterior tibial a.

1st layer
of deep fascia

Fig. 7.57 The soleus
exposed, and the line for
its detachment shown.

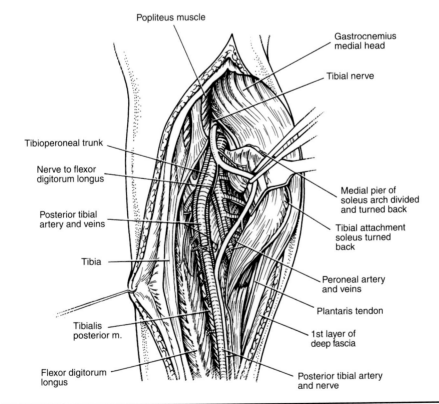

Popliteus muscle

Tibioperoneal trunk

Nerve to flexor
digitorum longus

Posterior tibial
artery and veins

Tibia

Tibialis
posterior m.

Flexor digitorum
longus

Gastrocnemius
medial head

Tibial nerve

Medial pier of
soleus arch divided
and turned back

Tibial attachment
soleus turned
back

Peroneal artery
and veins

Plantaris tendon

1st layer of
deep fascia

Posterior tibial artery
and nerve

Fig. 7.58 The tibial nerve
and vessels revealed by the
retraction of the soleus.

Figs 7.59 and 7.60 Exposure of the plantar nerves through a medial incision. (After Henry (1957).)

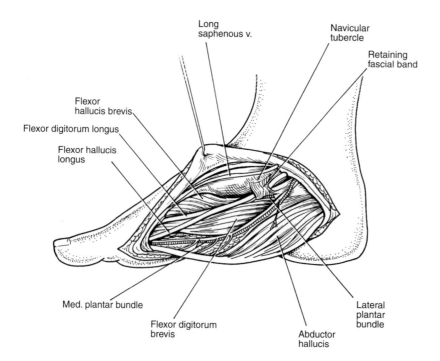

Fig. 7.59 Retraction of abductor hallucis reveals the medial plantar nerve.

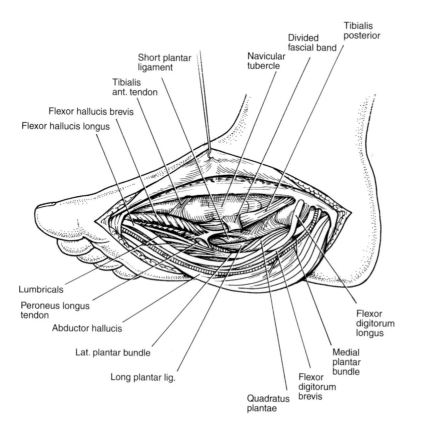

Fig. 7.60 Release of the tendon of the flexor longus hallucis gives access to the whole of the deep compartment of the sole.

first thoracic white ramus with the lower part of the stellate ganglion. That resection produces an effective sympathectomy, with minimal risk of causing a Bernard–Horner syndrome. The question of asking the patient to pay the price of a permanent Bernard–Horner syndrome for a complete sympathectomy to gain relief of pain is less often raised now than formerly: the introduction of guanethidine "blockade" (Hannington-Kiff 1974, 1977, 1979) has very greatly reduced the need for making this hard decision.

When the routes across the pleural cavity and extrapleural space are blocked it is necessary to revert to the supraclavicular and even posterior routes. In the former the apical pleura is exposed by mobilisation of the subclavian artery and identification of the lower trunk and first thoracic nerve after division of scalenus anterior. After division of the suprapleural membrane, the pleura is eased away from the inner side of the heads and necks of the upper ribs and the sympathetic chain is defined. The last is then resected from below up: usually from below the fourth ganglion to below the entry of the first thoracic white ramus into the stellate ganglion.

If the supraclavicular route is hopelessly blocked by scarring from injury, previous operation, or both, the posterior route (Adson & Brown 1929) is used. The approach has been described. Resection of the posterior end of the second rib and the related transverse process permits entry to the extrapleural space for resection of the ganglia.

If with any of these methods there is uncertainty about the identity of the first thoracic white ramus, it is no great matter to stimulate the suspected ramus and observe the ipsilateral pupil for dilation.

Lumbar sympathectomy

Occasion for this operation has declined, perhaps rather more than is really necessary. In our field it finds its chief use in the treatment of causalgia. The transverse unilateral or bilateral incision is made between the rib cage and the iliac crest. The external oblique muscle is split and the deeper muscles cut, with opening of the lateral part of the rectus sheath. The underlying fascia is delicately opened and the peritoneum is swept away from the abdominal wall and vertebral column. On the right the chain is found behind the lateral part of the inferior vena cava; on the left it is found just in line with the edge of the aorta. It is firmly bound to the vertebral column and the medial margin of the psoas by its rami. It should be transected below the fourth ganglion, usually found behind the iliac vessels, and lifted up and traced through the medial arcuate ligament so that the first ganglion can be removed. It is unwise to remove both first lumbar ganglia in men. Division of segmental arteries should, in general, be avoided, in case of interference with blood supply of the cord or cauda equina; however, sometimes this is inevitable. One or more segmental veins may require ligation and division. After haemostasis, the peritoneal sac is allowed to fall back into place, and the abdominal wall is carefully closed in separate layers.

8. Compound nerve injury

Compound nerve injury: definition; the wound; the vascular lesion in general and particular; the skin lesion; the penetrating missile injury; the nerve lesion; nerves and bone and joint injuries; particular problems in the upper limb; lesions of the lumbosacral plexus and compound nerve lesions in the lower limb; burns; experience and recommendations across the field.

We define "compound nerve injuries" as those in which damage to a nerve or nerves is associated with major damage to other tissues or organs such as skin, muscle, the skeleton, viscera and major vessels at the *same site*. There are some obvious categories:

- penetrating missile injuries
- severe open wounds, partial or complete amputation
- nerves injured by fracture or dislocation, open or closed, notably at the shoulder, elbow, pelvis, hip and the knee
- burns.

The timing of nerve repair in compound injuries remains controversial. Horn (1959) practised primary suture of median and ulnar nerves at the Accident Hospital in Birmingham. From 1956 onwards primary suture of severed nerves was practised at St Mary's Hospital whenever it was possible. There, in 1965, Michael Laurence achieved an outstanding result from primary repair of all flexor tendons, radial and ulnar arteries and median and ulnar nerves sectioned at the wrist. O'Brien (1975), one of the founders of modern microsurgical work, proved that primary repair of nerves was better, even in the most severe injuries, in reattached limbs amputated by crush or traction. We think that the general contraindications to primary repair include:

- the poor condition of the patient
- inexperience of the surgeon and defect in the facilities available to him or her
- most, but not all, penetrating missile injuries
- burns
- cases of severely contaminated wounds from machinery, road accidents or agricultural injuries, in which the prevention of sepsis must be the priority.

There are three general factors that determine the final outcome of nerve injury and repair and which strongly influence the timing of that repair. They are: the nature of wound and the risk of sepsis; vascular injury; and loss of skin.

THE WOUND

One of the achievements of Robert Jones was to secure agreement amongst the surgeons on the Allied side on the Western Front in 1917 to a common policy of treatment of missile wounds. The elements of this included the debridement, in its true sense of unbridling or decompression, wound excision and delay in primary closure. Ruscoe Clarke's (1959) discussion of the treatment of wounds in the Libyan Campaign is worth reading. He considers that debridement is properly extending the wound and argues against needless excision: "the scalpel cannot and need not excise all microorganisms", acknowledging in this Almroth Wright's (1942) work on the resistance of wounds to infection, an essential contribution by this St Mary's bacteriologist. Omer (1991) pointed out that the incidence of gas gangrene, 7% in World War One, dropped to 0.7% in World War Two and to 0.08% in the Korean War, and thought this was a reflection of the contribution of antibiotics because the principles of the primary treatment of war wounds had not changed in this time. It might equally be recognition of the importance of adequate tetanus prophylaxis and rapid evacuation.

It seems that these principles of the early treatment of wounds must be relearned at every conflict. Cooper and Ryan (1990), in commenting on the trend in civilian practice to minimal surgical intervention and primary closure of wounds with increasing reliance on antibiotics, say: "it is timely to remind our civilian colleagues that this approach, transferred to the battle field will result in catastrophe for many of the wounded". One might add for many of those wounded in civilian practice too, as shown by Dudley (before his translation to the Chair of Surgery at St Mary's Hospital) et al in 1968, and by Odling-Smee (1970). We have had to treat four cases of gas gangrene in which fundamental principles had not been followed. For these patients only urgent amputation or radical excision of the limb compartments availed.

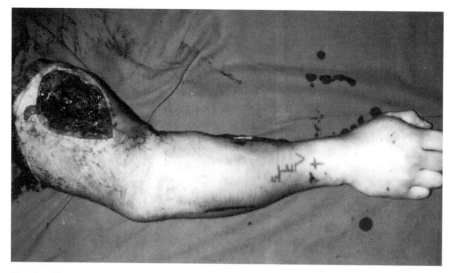

Fig. 8.1 Gas gangrene.

Case report. An 18-year-old man suffered a closed traction lesion of the brachial plexus with rupture of the axillary artery, and closed fractures of humerus and both forearm bones. Circulation was restored through a prosthesis. At his arrival to St Mary's Hospital, 18 hours after this operation, the diagnosis was immediately obvious. He had a heliotrope complexion, an extraordinary sang froid and a racing pulse. Gas was palpable under the skin of the arm. Emergency amputation was performed through the upper humerus, the skin flaps were closed 72 hours later. The errors which led to this outcome include: failure to stabilise the skeleton; failure to decompress the limb; and, to a lesser extent, use of a prosthesis rather than a vein graft (Fig. 8.1).

Case report. A 28-year-old man suffered fracture of the femur, complicated by a sciatic nerve palsy in a road traffic accident. The fracture was open, and the skin wound, which was 3 cm in diameter, was sutured before the patient was transferred to us. He arrived with gas in the muscles of the thigh. Excision of all of the flexor muscles of the thigh was necessary. One of us is reminded of the demonstration by Peter London, at the Accident Hospital in Birmingham: on being presented with a thigh after the fracture had been reduced and the skin closed, London immediately manipulated the limb so that the ends of the fracture were forced through the wound. Road tar and a cigarette stub were impaled onto a spike of the femur.

For those not already familiar with this work we think that Coupland's (1993) writing on war wounds of limbs, which sets out the International Red Cross Wound Classification, is valuable to those surgeons interested in accident work. Tables 8.1 and 8.2 set out elements of this classification. We have not regretted our policy of delaying closure of skin wounds in all cases sent to us with open fractures complicated by nerve or arterial damage.

Table 8.1 The Red Cross Wound Classification (from Coupland (1993))

1. The field wound score

E	Entry		Diameter of entry wound (cm)
X	Exit		Diameter of exit wound (cm)
C	Cavity	0	Wound cavity too small to take two fingers
		1	Wound cavity admits two or more fingers
F	Fracture	0	No fracture
		1	Simple fracture
		2	Comminuted fracture
V	Vital structure	0	No injury to brain, vessels or viscera
		1	Injury to the above
M	Metallic body	0	No metal fragment seen on radiograph
		1	One fragment
		2	More than one fragment

2. Subsequent analysis

(a) Extent of tissue damage

Grade 1	E + X < 10:	F0 or F1	Low energy transfer
Grade 2	E + X > 10:	C1 or F2	High energy transfer
Grade 3	E + X > 10:	C1 or F2	High energy transfer

(b) Type of wound according to structure injured

ST	F0. V0.	Soft tissue only
F	F1 or F2	V0
V	F0	V1
VF	F1 or F2 and V1	

Table 8.2 Categories of wound (from Coupland (1993))

	Grade I	Grade II	Grade III
ST	Small simple wounds	2ST	3ST
F	1F	2F	3F
V	1V	2V	3V
VF	1VF	2VF	3VF

THE VASCULAR LESION

Advances in arterial and venous surgery, with the introduction of antibiotics, blood transfusions and improvements in anaesthesia are the basis of modern surgical practice, particularly in the treatment of severe wounds. It is a source of dismay that trends in training make it less likely that orthopaedic surgeons of the future will be as capable of dealing with the injured artery, or for that matter coping with the problem of skin loss, as were those who contributed to these advances. Bonney (1963) and Kirkup (1963) successfully dealt with femoral arterial injury caused by fractures of the femur (Fig. 8.2). We think that the first successful replant of the hand was performed by

Mr David Harris, an orthopaedic surgeon, and that one of us was perhaps the first to successfully replant an amputated thumb in the UK. We think that Bonney (1963), "Surgeons treating fractures of long bones must be prepared to treat associated vascular injury", London (1967), "there is nothing so difficult about sewing up an artery as to make it the strict preserve of the vascular specialist", and Birnstingl (1982), "the ability to repair blood vessels should now be part of the repertory of every accident surgeon", are right. Of course, as De Mello and Khan (1990) emphasise, severe vascular injury can follow a blunt crushing injury; such injuries are by no means benign.

Hunter (1793) noted the effect of transection of major arteries in the limbs of the boar and the dog. The vessels constricted "before the animal weakened" (Figs 8.3 and 8.4). Hallowell (1761) wrote to John Hunter telling him of repair of a brachial artery by means of a Farriers stitch. Murphy (1897) was probably the first successfully to repair a severed femoral artery. The foundations of modern surgical technique were laid by Carrel (1902), who was awarded the Nobel Prize, and by Guthrie (1912), whose contributions were no less significant. Pringle (1913) used vein grafts to repair two cases of aneurysm. Sherrill (1913) described successful suture of a brachial artery "by the method of Carrell employed by Crile", and there are occasional reports from these years from German surgeons such as Lexer (1913). The First World War saw very important work from surgeons whose contributions are little known, perhaps because they were on the losing side. The Serbian surgeon Subbotich (1913, 1914) described his experience in the Balkan Wars, in which he reported repairs of 135 arterial injuries and of 32 arteriovenous fistulae. The

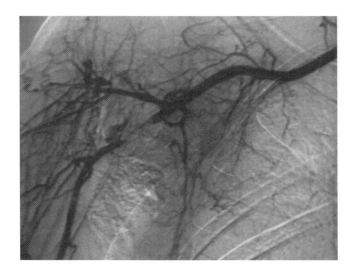

Fig. 8.2 Thrombosis of the femoral artery from fracture of the shaft of the femur.

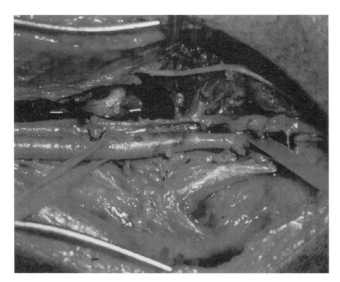

Fig. 8.3 A glass wound to the axilla transected the axillary artery. Spasm of the stumps prevented catastrophic bleeding.

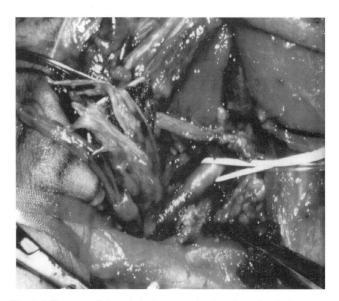

Fig. 8.4 Rupture of the subclavian artery in closed traction lesion. There was little haemorrhage.

Russian surgeon Weglowski (1925) (see also Shumacher 1990) described 51 vein grafts for arterial repair in the wounded of the Eastern Front. Markins (1919) advised suture of arteries in selected cases, but most such injuries were treated by ligation.

The Second World War inevitably saw advances. The work of the Vascular Injuries Committee of the Medical Research Council, chaired by Sir Thomas Lewis, was summarised in the Medical Research Council War Memorandum No. 13 (1944). We think it should be re-issued, slightly modified, to all accident and orthopaedic surgeons. "The memorandum is intended for guidance of those who have had only limited previous experience of the early treatment of arterial wounds". It described pathological changes and principles of diagnosis, and strongly recommended axial anastomosis for stab wounds of vessels and the use of artificial tubes where tension was too great for end to end suture. "In the war of 1914–1918 Tuffier's cannula usually failed in its purpose, because thrombosis occurred within a few hours; the use of heparin, however should prevent this." This technique was designed to maintain blood flow for 3–4 days before necessary removal of the tube and ligation of the artery. During this time collateral circulation increased. The memorandum referred to early work with free vein grafts, commenting that heparin was necessary, and adding "they are considered unsafe for use in heavily contaminated wounds and are likely to be applicable only in special vascular injury centres". However, ligation was widely practised, and the results of this are shown by DeBakey and Simeone (1946, 1955) in a series of nearly 2500 arterial injuries. A total of 346 of 502 limbs were amputated after ligation of the popliteal artery. Overall, nearly 50% of limbs came to amputation after ligation of an axial vessel. The results following arterial repair in 120 cases were a good deal better even in those difficult times when the average interval between wounding and operation was 10 hours. Arterial repair was regularly practised during the Korean War, a conflict in which the incidence of arterial injuries in those surviving wounding increased, and in which the interval from injury to operation dropped to 6 hours. An amputation rate of 13% was recorded by Hughes (1958) and Jancke (1958). Significant publications describing experiences in civilian practice came from Porter (1967), who described 100 cases of arterial injury seen at the Accident Hospital in Birmingham between 1956 and 1965. Eighteen of 19 major vessels were successfully repaired. In 48 cases the condition of the limb was such that amputation was elected. Morris et al (1960) reported 220 cases. Arterial repair was successful in 86%. Early in the series, 14 major vessels were ligated, which led to five amputations, hemiplegia in two of three carotid arterial lesions so treated and two deaths.

The conflicts in Vietnam and Ulster saw the most recent stage in the evolution of arterial repair in emergencies, so that failure is now the exception. In 1966, the Vietnam Vascular Registry was established at the Walter Reed Hospital, carrying on a tradition of centralisation of information, so permitting analysis and improvement, a tradition established in this country and now, sadly, abandoned with the same alacrity as the bandwagon of audit and outcome studies rolls inexorably forwards. Rich et al (1970) reviewed 1000 arterial injuries: in 42% there were associated peripheral nerve injuries; there were fractures in 28.5%. Arteriovenous fistulae were treated by Hewitt et al (1973) and by Rich et al (1975) who discussed 558 false aneurysms and arteriovenous fistulae. The popliteal artery remained a problem; an amputation rate of 30% was recorded by Rich et al (1974). The results of Barros d'Sa and his colleagues in Belfast are impressive (Elliot et al 1984, Barros d'Sa 1989, Barros d'Sa & Moorhead 1989). The technical principles for urgent arterial repair are set out in Barros d'Sa's chapter in Eastcott's work (1992). In describing intraluminal shunts for the early restoration to the leg after kneecapping injury, in which a close-range shotgun blasts the contents of the popliteal fossa and fragments the femur and tibia, he comments that shunts have revolutionised the treatment of vascular injuries complicating fractures of the lower limbs. In his Hunterian Lecture (Barros d'Sa 1982) the principles of treatment in 188 major vascular injuries in the lower limbs of 118 patients were set out: revascularisation within 4 hours; fasciotomy of all four compartments; vein grafting for the artery; and repair of at least one major vein. This has led to an amputation rate of 5% for cases of popliteal artery arterial injury, the lowest of any civilian or military series yet published. Most patients were admitted within 30 minutes, indeed one-half were admitted within 15 minutes of injury. The use of shunts permits early perfusion, so that fasciotomy was not regularly done when these were used. Shunts also permit adequate fixation of a fracture before definitive repair of a vessel.

We make no apology for repeating the comments of Hughes and Bowers (1961), who write of the incidence of gangrene after ligation of a major artery: "It is realised that these percentages, derived from battlefield wounded may be slightly higher than may be encountered in many injuries in civilian life; these should serve as a grim reminder of the dangers of ligation of major arteries and may deter some individuals so inclined. We have been amazed at the lack of interest and knowledge of many surgeons who have no idea as to which vessels may be safely ligated." Harsh words! Sadly, we have found them applicable today. Perhaps now is as good a time as any to comment on arterial spasm. We have never seen a case of spasm alone producing obstruction in an adult; we have seen it in children. As to sympathetic block, or sympathectomy, Seddon (1964), when writing of acute ischaemia, said: "let us hope that the completely futile sympathetic block will not have been done". Birnstingl (1982), vascular

Table 8.3 Arterial injuries in association with nerve lesions, 1975–1996

	Closed		Open	
	Total	Repaired	Total	Repaired
Vertebral	1	0	4	1
Subclavian	82	40	9	9
Axillary	63	54	31	27
Brachial	7	6	35	31
Radial and ulnar	5	2	211	198
Common femoral	0	0	3	3
Superficial femoral	2	2	4	4
Profunda femoris	2	1	2	1
Inferior gluteal	2	0	1	0
Popliteal	14	9	12	9
Posterior tibial	3	1	7	4
Anterior tibial	9	2	3	1

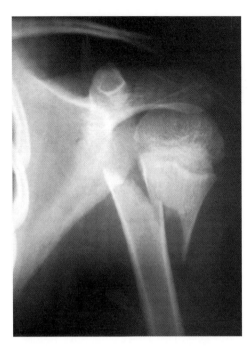

Fig. 8.5 Displaced fracture in an 11-year-old boy which occluded the axillary artery and caused multiple nerve palsies.

surgeon to the Royal National Orthopaedic Hospital for some years, said: "sympathetic block is useless"; "sympathectomy has no place in the treatment of acute ischaemia; spasm should never be diagnosed unless the artery has been exposed at operation and either distended with saline or opened to exclude an intimal tear". There is, lastly, the view of Eastcott and colleagues in his monumental work *Arterial Surgery* (1992): "sympathetic block or denervation are practically useless in the treatment of acute limb ischaemia".

Our own experience in the treatment of arterial injuries complicated by nerve lesions of one sort or another is set out in Table 8.3, and methods of exposure and repair for the subclavian–axillary arterial lesion associated with injuries of the brachial plexus is described in Chapter 9. We now acknowledge the consistent and generous advice and support given to us by colleagues at St Mary's Hospital: Mr Felix Eastcott, Mr Iain Kenyon, Professors Averil Mansfield and Andrew Nicolaides, and Mr John Wolfe from the Department of Vascular Surgery, and Dr David Sutton and Dr Al Kutoubi from the Department of Radiology.

Arterial lesions are sufficiently common a complication of injuries to three joints – the shoulder, the knee and the elbow – as to require separate consideration.

Dislocation of the shoulder

The dangers of late closed reduction were shown by Flaubert (1827), who described attempted late dislocation by traction applied by six (!) medical students which led to rupture of the axillary artery, avulsion of the brachial plexus, injury to the spinal cord and death (perhaps this experience stimulated his son to describe the fate of the wretched Hippolyte in *Madame Bovary*); and by Calvet et al (1942) who collected 90 cases of arterial injury from dislocation, in 68 of whom late reduction had been attempted. There was a 50% mortality. Watson-Jones (1936) reported a fatal outcome from rupture of the axillary

artery in a man with recurrent anterior dislocation of the shoulder. Although Baratta et al (1983) described a case of a 13-year-old boy with rupture of axillary artery from dislocation of shoulder attendant on arm wrestling, these are on the whole injuries of the elderly (Fig. 8.5). Stableforth (1984) found four arterial injuries in his series of 81 cases of four part fractures of the proximal humerus. Bigliani et al (1991) say that ruptures of the axillary artery, secondary to shoulder fractures or dislocation, account for 7% of all arterial injuries. Cases were reported by, amongst others, Henson (1956), Smyth (1969), Theodorides and De Keyzer (1977), Drury and Scullion (1980), Laverick et al (1990) and Nicholson (1991). Puri et al (1985) made this significant observation: "the intima had fractured cleanly and circumferentially".

Vascular injury in the older patient

There is a group of older patients who suffer damage to the axillary artery from fractures of the proximal humerus from low energy injuries. The nerves are injured indirectly, as a consequence of ischaemia or of compression by an expanding haematoma or aneurysm. We have seen eight such cases. Particular lessons can be drawn from two of them.

Case report. An 83-year-old woman suffered a closed fracture of the proximal humerus in a fall in the street. There was no neurovascular deficit. She was treated in a collar and cuff. At 18 weeks there was no radiological evidence of union. Two weeks later she re-presented with massive swelling in the shoulder. A computed tomography scan suggested haematoma, and an intra-arterial digital

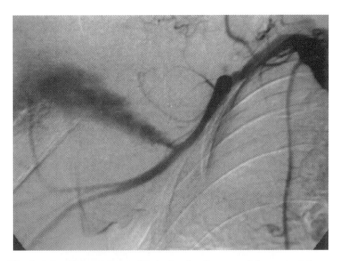

Fig. 8.6 Leaking aneurysm, 20 weeks after fracture of the neck of the humerus in an 83-year-old woman.

subtraction angiogram confirmed active bleeding from the third part of the axillary artery (Fig. 8.6). Before operation the patient was noted to have massive swelling in the shoulder and axilla, a palpable but weak radial pulse, a complete musculocutaneous and radial nerve palsy, and partial palsy of the median and ulnar nerves. The artery was exposed, 3 l of fresh haematoma were evacuated, and rupture of false aneurysm at the junction of the axillary artery with the subscapular artery was found. Direct suture of the deep defect in the axillary artery was possible. A full radial pulse was restored. No attempt was made to reconstruct the proximal humerus. At 2 months there was virtually full neurological recovery, with radiological evidence of reconstitution of the humerus.

Case report. A 66-year-old man fell 6 feet from a ladder on to his right shoulder, sustaining a four-part fracture of the proximal humerus. On presentation there was no radial pulse, with complete radial palsy. A digital subtraction angiogram confirmed a block in the third part of the vessel. Immediately before operation there was complete loss of power and sensation in the forearm and hand, and the patient was in very severe pain. In this case the artery had been directly damaged by the fracture. There was a segmental fracture of the atheromatous intima. The vessel was repaired with a 5-cm reversed vein graft. Conduction was still present in the musculocutaneous, radial and ulnar nerves, but not in the median nerve. This was found matted to the artery in dense oedematous tissue. A full radial pulse returned after release of clamps; the radial, musculocutaneous and ulnar nerves recovered rapidly to near-normal levels of function by 3 months, but recovery of the median nerve was only partial at 18 months. There was early relief of pain, within days of the operation. The median nerve was directly damaged by bleeding and the lesion was deeper than in the other trunks, which exemplify ischaemic conduction block.

The elbow

The brachial artery is the lifeline of the forearm and hand. The consequences of neglect in treatment of injuries to this vessel can be as severe as those flowing from a failure to repair the popliteal artery. An excellent review of injuries to the brachial artery is set out by Gross and Yao (1982) in Thomas Wadsworth's work "The Elbow". In commenting on spasm they write: "of all peripheral arteries in the body, the brachial is the most prone to spasm. Arterial spasm is usually self limiting and disappears within a few minutes following relief of the external local stimulus. In the treatment of trauma, any persistent ischaemia should be considered arterial injury and not caused by spasm; if distal ischaemia persists after reduction of a fracture or dislocation, it should be assumed that arterial occlusion is the result of vessel damage or thrombosis rather than spasm". Barros d'Sa (1992) describes causes of injury and he refers to risks of accidental injury, intra-arterial injection of thiopentone, diazepam and other drugs. He comments that "these arterial occlusions should not be regarded as innocuous and should not be left to the novice, as opportunities to obtain a good result diminish with each repeated attempt. Experience of meticulous technique are essential and repair should be performed under magnification using fine instruments". We think that repair of the brachial artery is technically easier than it is in other more deeply seated vessels and it must be a matter of very grave concern to all engaged in the treatment of patients with musculoskeletal injury or in training surgeons entering into this field that there are still so many examples of neglect in diagnosis and in repair of this vessel which is, after all, the first artery to have been successfully repaired in the human. A complacent approach to the pulseless forearm ought to be inconceivable. The evidence set out in Chapter XVII (Reconstruction) suggests that such a complacent approach still exists in certain quarters as is shown by the following case report.

Case report. A 23-year-old woman fell downstairs, suffering fractures of the distal humerus. On arrival at hospital the arm was noted to be pulseless. The fracture was fixed through a posterior approach. The artery was not explored and the forearm was not decompressed. Twelve hours later an operation was performed attempting to restore circulation, which failed. The patient was advised to undergo cervical sympathectomy, advice which she declined. She was then referred to St Mary's Hospital where prompt decompression of the extensor muscles saved them. The flexor muscles of the forearm were necrotic; indeed, they were liquified and were totally excised.

The knee

The arrangement of the popliteal artery, of its branches and of collateral vessels makes it particularly vulnerable to

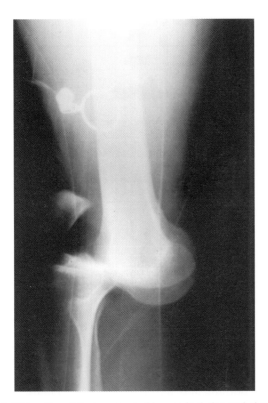

Fig. 8.7 Dislocation of the knee treated by manipulation and plaster of Paris splint.

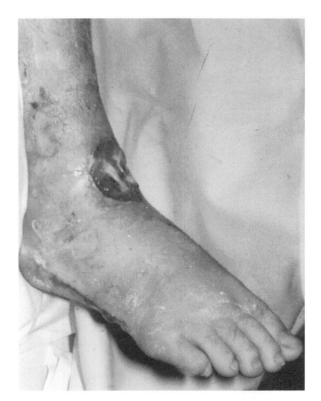

Fig. 8.8 The appearance of the foot on removal of the splint some days later.

injury, adds greatly to the difficulties of repair, and leads to the most severe consequences in the event of failure. We think these are among the most technically difficult of peripheral arterial injuries. Eastcott's phrase "the lifeline of the leg" is clearly shown by the amputation rate in such civilian series as the one reported on by Orcutt et al (1983), who found survival of the leg after repair of the popliteal artery in 95% of the penetrating wounds, but in only 70% of those from blunt injury, and by a recorded amputation rate following popliteal artery injury from dislocation of the knee of from 30% to 80% (Lefrac 1976, Green & Allen 1977, Alberty et al 1981).

Four fractures are notably associated with arterial injury. Arterial rupture occurs in 3% of supracondylar fractures of the femur, in 30% of dislocations of the knee (Figs 8.7 and 8.8), and in 10% of fractures of the proximal tibia, and fractures of the proximal part of the fibula are associated with damage to the anterior tibial artery (Fig. 8.9). Technical difficulties of repair increase with the more distal injuries as they approach the trifurcation of the popliteal artery, and in these cases there is more likely to be gross injury to the skin, muscle and nerve.

Case report. A 58-year-old man was knocked down by a car and suffered open fractures of femur and tibia, with rupture of the popliteal artery. The limb was critically ischaemic and had been so for 3 hours by the time the

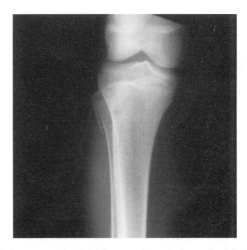

Fig. 8.9 An apparently trivial fracture through the neck of the fibula ruptured the anterior tibial artery. Necrosis of the anterior muscles.

patient reached theatre. The skeleton was stabilised by a Küntscher nail passed from the hip to the ankle, a procedure which took 15 minutes. Then, with the patient prone, the femoropopliteal trunk was exposed. The vessels were atheromatous, and the gap between the prepared stumps was 15 cm. A reversed vein graft from the distal femoral to the posterior tibial and to the anterior tibial (by means of a

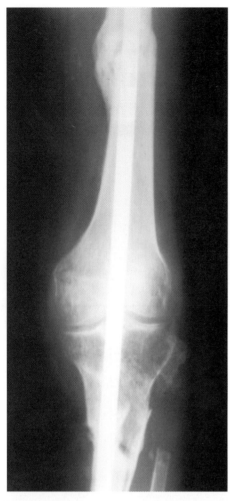

Fig. 8.10 Open fractures of the femur and tibia, with rupture of the tibial artery. Internal fixation and reversed vein graft to the vessel.

Table 8.4 Traumatic false aneurysms and arteriovenous fistulae with associated nerve lesions

Region	Aneurysms	Arteriovenous fistulae
Artery		
Posterior triangle of neck	3	2
Axillary	14	3
Brachial	4	1
Femoral	3	1
Profundus femoris	2	0
Inferior gluteal	1	0
Popliteal	5	2
Posterior tibial	2	0
Anterior tibial	1	0

preserved (Dunkerton & Boome 1988). In some of our cases diagnosis was delayed, and in four cases of false aneurysm preoperative diagnosis was neurotmesis (see Ch. 9). Larger areriovenous fistulae produce local and systemic responses, as described by Sumner et al (1992): "the drop in total peripheral resistance is the essential pathophysiological aberration". This fall leads to a drop in diastolic pressure, an increase in pulse rate, an increase in cardiac output, and ultimately to heart failure. There is hyperventilation. The local effects are a reflection of deprivation of blood, which may lead to venous insufficiency. The part is swollen, dry, and discoloured. Clinical diagnosis is made by listening to the murmur, which is continuous but louder in systole (Table 8.4).

Case report. A 28-year-old soldier was wounded in the posterior triangle of the neck by a fragment from an exploding tank. He presented with complete loss of function of C5, C6 and C7. A rumbling bruit in the neck with palpable thrill diagnosed an arteriovenous fistula. The diagnosis was confirmed by Dr Al Kutoubi, who embolised the lesion. The subsequent repair of the plexus itself was straightforward (Fig. 8.11).

Case report. A 28-year-old man suffered gunshot injury to the right axilla and presented to us at 6 weeks with median, ulnar and musculocutaneous palsy. He was in great pain. The hand was dry, the limb engorged and purplish, and there was dilation of the skin veins. His pulse rate was high and the jugular venous pressure elevated. There was a loud, continuous rumbling murmur from the axillary vessels. Digital subtraction angiogram (Dr Al Kutoubi) demonstrated a complex fistula not suitable for embolisation. At operation the fistula was displayed; there were several communications between the artery and the veins, which were enormously dilated. The arterial lesion was successfully excised and grafted, and two veins were sutured. The musculocutaneous and the ulnar nerves were stretched by the vascular lesion, but not embedded within the false sac. The median nerve was so enveloped and one-third of it had been sectioned by a bullet (Fig. 8.12). Circulation was restored, there was considerable relief of

branch) successfully restored circulation. The fractures healed; persisting discharge from the tibial fracture ceased at 9 months after removal of the nail. The patient had no pain, normal function of the leg and foot, and a range of flexion of the knee of 0–80° (Fig. 8.10).

The false aneurysm and arteriovenous fistulae
(Figs 8.11–8.16)

The effects of aneurysms and fistulae on nerves are interesting. Both lead to a general decline of function, which is all the more rapid with expansion of the vascular lesion. Nerves embedded within the sac of a false aneurysm or fistula are badly damaged; recovery is always imperfect, and may not occur at all. Those more remotely affected will recover after prompt treatment. Pain indicates that nerves are closely related to the false sac; in these, complete loss of autonomic function is the rule, even when deep pressure sense and other modalities are still partially

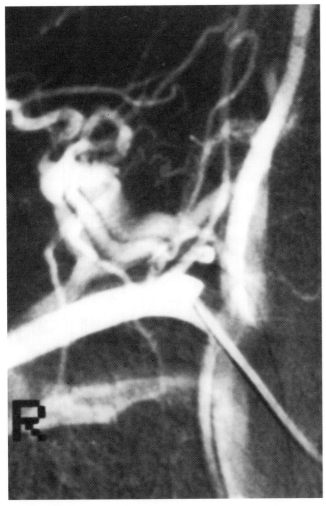

Fig. 8.11 Arteriovenous fistula between the subclavian artery and vein, successfully embolised by Dr Al Kutoubi.

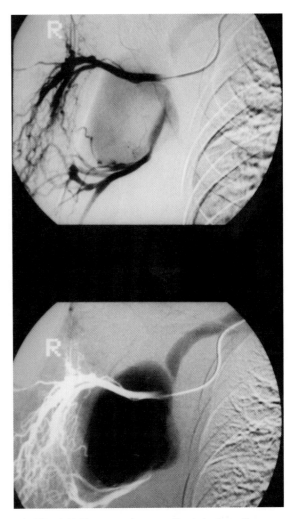

Fig. 8.12 Large arteriovenous fistula in the axilla.

pain, although still an element of post-traumatic neuralgia from the median nerve. There was rapid recovery of both musculocutaneous and ulnar nerves.

We have seen a number of iatropathic cases. Some are described in Chapter 13. One patient, the narration of whose case is salutary, was treated by Professor Averil Mansfield. The patient presented in severe pain after an ill-advised and badly performed osteotomy of the tibia. There was a complete lesion of the tibial nerve, with sympathetic paralysis in the foot. Repair of the false aneurysm of the posterior tibial artery was followed by rapid and complete relief of pain.

Case report. Lateral meniscectomy through the arthroscope was performed in a 31-year-old man. He experienced intense pain on awakening, which was not controlled by morphine. The leg became swollen, blue and cold. He was given anticoagulants on the suspicion of deep vein thrombosis. The true diagnosis, of false expanding aneurysm of

the lateral genicular artery, was not made until it was too late to prevent massive ischaemic fibrosis of all muscles in the leg (Fig. 8.13). One remarkable feature in this case, amongst others, was the sharp condemnation by lawyers and doctors of one of us who had had the temerity to suggest that 5 years without any form of active treatment was a touch unreasonable!

Case report. A 36-year-old woman developed intense pain, true causalgia, after excision of an axillary lipoma. Arteriography confirmed occlusion of the brachial artery. At operation we found false aneurysm of the vessel, and the median nerve was splayed out over the sac; the epineurium was disrupted, so that individual bundles were separated, and enveloped in inflammatory tissue. The artery was repaired with reversed vein graft, and an indwelling catheter used to infuse local anaesthetic for 5 days postoperatively. There was early relief of pain, but little recovery of the nerve (Fig. 8.14).

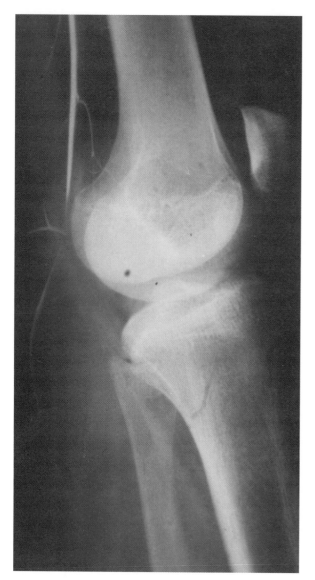

Fig. 8.13 Massive false aneurysm from the lateral genicular artery.

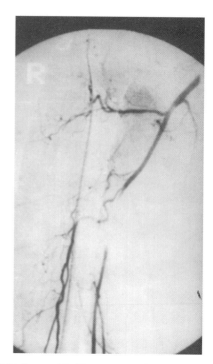

Fig. 8.14 Iatropathic false aneurysm in the brachial artery.

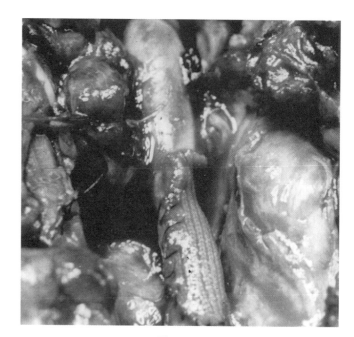

Fig. 8.16

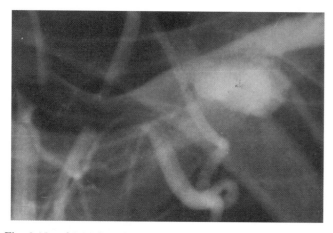

Figs 8.15 and 8.16 Saccular aneurysm from a bullet wound to the subclavian artery. Fig. 8.15 Arteriograph shows the aneurysm. Fig. 8.16 shows repair by dacron patch.

SOME TECHNICAL COMMENTS

The first principle of exposure is to secure proximal control of the axial artery as quickly as possible. Approaches are discussed in Chapters 7 and 9. It is perhaps worth emphasising that we have found the exposure of Fiolle and Delmas most effective in providing access to and control of the subclavian and axillary arteries.

We have used reversed vein grafts in nearly all cases where direct suture was not possible and prefer interrupted sutures of 5/0 to 8/0 prolene. These are muscular vessels and a continuous suture causes stenosis. End to side suture is valuable when there is mismatch in the calibre of the vein graft and artery. We agree with the comments of Narakas (1987) on synthetic grafts: "in cases where vascular repair has been undertaken immediately and nerve repair carried out later immense technical difficulties arise because it is almost impossible to expose the plexus without damaging the vascular graft or even prosthesis if one has been used ... Vascular prostheses should not be used in young patients with brachial plexus injuries. Prostheses cannot adapt to changes in the calibre of anastamotic site and may leak causing minor or massive haemorrhage which afterwards embeds the nerve trunks in a fibrotic mass." Heparin may be injected into the distal arterial tree, but systemic anticoagulants are not used. We do not use Fogarty's catheters, having seen cases where repeated passage of these so damaged the intima that later repair of the artery was well nigh impossible. Papaverine and procaine are useful in reducing spasm of the vein graft. It is essential to keep the patient warm and to replace lost blood. Exposure of the vein graft must be kept to as short a time as possible: if nerves must be repaired, grafts should be elevated by one surgeon, whilst others continue the arterial repair, and then inserted with as little delay as possible. Decompression of the axillary sheath and of the brachial bundle is always necessary. In cases of arterial repair at 24–48 hours after injury we have noted considerable constriction of the distal artery by oedema within those sheaths. Fasciotomy is not performed if flow is restored within 4 hours in clean sections or ruptures without distal injury. It is done in all other circumstances. The skin is incised when there is swelling from distal contusion or fractures of the forearm or leg.

Ischaemia and the nerve

It is difficult, in the clinical situation, to separate the effects on the nerve of pure ischaemia from those of ischaemia associated with compression, traction, and distortion. Certainly we see:

1. Ischaemia of the nerve trunk itself. Seddon (1975) described several cases. In one case of severe Volkmann's ischaemic contracture, amputation was performed: the branches of the median nerve within the palm of the hand, where they were not compressed, were completely infarcted. Lamerton et al's (1983) case is interesting as an example of painful ischaemia of the sciatic nerve relieved by the reconstruction of the internal iliac artery.
2. Ischaemia associated with compression or stretching of the nerve by haematoma or aneurysm, which is worse when the nerve is embedded in the sac.

3. Ischaemia of nerves compressed distally by swollen muscle. Parkes (1945) recognised the effect of compression by swollen muscles and noted venous obstruction rather like strangulation of hernia leading to irreversible changes in the nerve at between 12 and 24 hours. Barros d'Sa (1992b) emphasises that the increased permeability of vessels from hypoxia leads to increase of pressure within compartments by exudation.

The blood supply of nerves and the effects of ischaemia are described in Chapter 4. It is relevant to cite the role of arteries proper to the median and sciatic nerves as examples of the importance of the extrinsic circulation. In one case in which the entire flexor compartment of the forearm was excised for ischaemia the median nerve was nourished by the longitudinal supply over a length of 24 cm. The nerve recovered. In another case, in which the posterior muscles of the thigh were excised for gas gangrene the sciatic nerve was maintained by its longitudinal supply over a length of 38 cm. There was useful recovery. In one of our early replants we noticed that the median artery was so large as to provide sufficient circulation to the hand while more elaborate reconstruction went on.

Effects on the tissue – compartment syndrome

When an artery is occluded there is death of tissue. It is wrong to apply the term "compartment syndrome" to the events which follow ligation of a popliteal or anterior tibial arteries, to the gangrene of peripheral vascular disease or the gangrene of arterial embolus. However, muscles confined within semi-rigid spaces bounded by bone and inelastic fascia are vulnerable to perfusion block, which may occur as a result of arterial injury and in the event of delayed restoration of circulation, but it may also occur because of swelling within the compartment, as in bleeding from a fracture or haemophilia or infusion of fluids. The swelling following unaccustomed exercise or after the prolonged compression sustained in coma is more akin to the effect of delayed restoration of circulation. All these effects may be exacerbated by tight external bandages or splints. The term "compartment syndrome" was introduced by Matsen (1975, 1980). This is useful, for it draws attention to the "final common pathway" of ischaemia. The subject is extensively reviewed by Pellegrini and McCollister Evarts (1991).

The first event is the closure or obstruction of perfusing arterioles when tissue or extravascular pressure exceeds the critical closing pressure of those vessels (Burton 1951). Of course, abnormal events occur before this. There is collapse and block of flow through low pressure systems, first the lymphatic and then the venous. There is now tissue hypoxia and derangement of fluid and electrolyte exchange across cell membranes, so that fluid passes from vessels to the extravascular compartment. The vicious cycle is complete (Eaton & Green 1972). Fluid entering the compartment cannot get out; it continues to leak into the compartment until the pressure within that compartment is so high that inflow is blocked. The tissues will now die.

Our material is described in Chapter 17. It is always worth remembering that in Volkmann's original description he clearly recognised that late muscle contracture was a consequence of muscle death, which was in turn a consequence of block to arterial inflow. Thomas (1909) described 107 cases, some from contusion and others in which no external bandages had been used, and Jones (1928) recognised that the contractures could follow from "pressure within, pressure without or both". Brooks (1922), in experimental work, commented on the importance of obstruction to venous return. Jepson (1926), whose experiments with animals induced contracture, was probably the first to recommend decompression, although as we have seen this concept was regularly applied by military surgeons. Tavernier et al (1936) recognised that muscles became infarcted. Griffiths (1940) emphasised that muscle death followed hypoxia, and believed that spasm was important, an idea later dispelled by Kinmonth et al (1952), who were unable to induce spasm in large arteries by stimulation of the sympathetic system or dispel it by sympathectomy.

There have been a large number of publications on the consequences of ischaemia within limbs or compartments. We pick just a few. That from Ashbell and Lipscombe (1967), describing a series from the Mayo Clinic, points to different types of injury to the brachial artery – contusion, tear or perforation. Perry et al (1971) made the important observation that 25% of limbs with major arterial injuries still had peripheral pulses. Natali and Benhamar (1979) described 125 cases of iatropathic vascular injuries. Two amputations followed plating of forearm fractures: 20 cases of ischaemic contracture were caused by plaster of Paris splints. Mubarack and Carrol (1979) described 58 limbs in 55 children seen over the course of 20 years at the Sick Children's Hospital in Toronto. In 23 cases the lower limb was affected; Bryant's traction was particularly dangerous. They commented that the incidence of postischaemic contracture had not changed. Regrettably, we think that the situation is no better now. Holden's review (1979) is particularly good. In speaking of sympathetic block in impending ischaemic contracture he says: "this futile time wasting manoeuvre should finally be abandoned". One cannot add to his criteria for clinical diagnosis and action, which are, first and foremost, pain persisting after reduction of fracture and refractory to moderate analgesia, and, second, tense swelling of the afflicted compartment.

Monitoring of intraoperative compartmental pressure was introduced by Whiteside et al in 1975, and there has been extensive and, at times, really very tedious debate about its role ever since. There is no doubt that monitoring is useful in patients unable to speak for themselves because they are unconscious or too young or too old. It may also have a role in those with multiple injuries or in those with nerve injuries preventing experience of pain. The findings of compartmental monitoring should never replace or overrule clinical judgement. The debate about the role of monitoring in the leg has been closed by two welcome papers from Edinburgh. McQueen et al (1996) studied 25 cases of compartment syndrome from fracture of the leg. In 13 of these patients pressure was monitored, and the mean time to decompression was 16 hours. In 12 patients monitoring was not done, and the mean time to decompression was 36 hours. Ten of those in the latter group had persisting contractures and muscle weakness and there was significant delay to union in this group. None of the patients who had fasciotomy and whose pressures were monitored developed contractures or weakness. In the second paper, McQueen and Court-Brown (1996) defined the pressure threshold for decompression in a study of 116 with fractures of the leg. This is the difference between diastolic pressure and the compartment pressure. Fasciotomy is indicated when this falls below 30 mm (which is less than the critical closing pressure of muscle arterioles). Fasciotomy was necessary in three of the patients studied. None of the other patients developed contractures, even though compartmental pressures were high; 34 patients had recorded pressures of more than 40 mm.

Compartment syndromes are a very real problem. Ellis (1958) found 4.3% of ischaemic contractures in his series of tibial shaft fractures, and Owen and Tsimboukis (1967) found clawing of toes from contracture of the deep flexor compartment in no less than 10% of such fractures. In the upper limb the compartments most at risk are the flexor compartment of forearm, then the extensors of the forearm, the small muscles of the hand, especially the interosseous muscles and adductor pollicis, and the pronator quadratus. We have seen cases involving the deltoid and pectoralis major. In the lower limb the deep flexor compartment of the leg leads the way, followed closely by the anterolateral compartment. Then, the other compartments of the leg, and the small muscles of the foot; the syndrome is not rare in the gluteal muscles, and on occasion it also involves the muscles of the thigh. We have already outlined the indications for decompression after arterial injury. We agree with Holden that clinical suspicion is the most important indication for intervention, and that this is preferably noted and acted upon before neural deficit. We think that the papers from Edinburgh have resolved the debate about monitoring in the leg, and have accurately defined its place.

Absence of a pulse in the presence of a fracture is an indication for exploration: pain and tense and tender swelling is an indication for decompression of a compartment even in the presence of a distal pulse. Sensible monitoring of intracompartmental pressure in the leg is useful.

SKIN

The safe and regular closure of major defects in the skin is the third and most recent of technical advances in the surgery of wounds. It rests upon anatomical studies of blood supply to skin and the recognition that large areas of skin can be elevated on a pedicle of one artery and its vena comitans (as in the groin flap); that blood supply may pass to skin through perforating vessels from underlying muscle (the major myocutaneous flaps); or through deep fascia (the lateral forearm flap). Hallock (1992) presents detailed discussion of fasciocutaneous flaps. Although for many years orthopaedic surgeons used latissimus dorsi in functional reconstruction of the upper limb, the implications of this were not grasped until McGregor and Jackson described the groin flap in 1972. This represented a real revolution for those brought up with the difficulties of split skin grafts or the cumbersome random or tubed flaps. This, the first axial pattern flap, remains exceptionally valuable in the emergency treatment of the hand and the distal forearm. In these years microsurgical techniques advanced so that there are now a large number of flaps which are in regular use for free tissue transfer. Godina (1986) was among the first to use these in urgent cases or in complex injury to the extremities, and his work is graciously acknowledged in the review by Lister (1988) of emergency flaps.

It is a considerable mistake for the fracture or orthopaedic surgeon to decline knowledge of these advances. With vascular repairs, they must remain part of the repertoire of any accident surgeon. Surgical details, indications and complications are reviewed by Gilbert et al (1990), who described flaps for the upper limb, and by Oberlin et al (1994) who described flaps for both upper and lower limbs. These last authors used a charming grading of between 1 and 4 for technical difficulty, akin to mountaineering terminology (or, for the more sedentary reader, the Michelin star system). Grades 1 and 2 encompass those flaps which have served us well, and such flaps do not need elaborate equipment or extensive experience in microvascular work. Indeed, the review of anatomical and technical details of pedicle flaps prepared in masterly fashion by Mathes and Mahai (1979) demands no knowledge of those things.

Flaps that we use regularly in the emergency treatment of wounds of the extremity include: the latissimus dorsi flap for the shoulder and arm, which, being a free flap, can be used virtually anywhere; the groin flap for the distal forearm and hand; the gluteal flap for the sacrum; and the tensor fasciae latae flap for the trochanteric region. The medial or lateral gastrocnemius flaps are useful for cover about the knee and upper leg, and the soleus flap for the upper one-third of the tibia. The latissimus dorsi is the largest, and it remains the most reliable and versatile of all flaps. It was first used in reconstruction of the breast by

Tansini (1906), for defects in the upper limb by Silverton et al (1978) and as a free flap by Baudet et al (1976). Bostwick et al (1979) described their results in 60 cases, and the development of applications of the flap is reviewed by Lassen et al (1985). These flaps are invaluable in situations where urgent cover of bone or joint, vascular repair or nerve repair is necessary. Their use in difficult cases for provision of cover for the irradiated plexus (in collaboration with Professor Roy Sanders) is set out in Chapter 13 and for the damaged or amputated forearm and hand (in collaboration with Mr David Evans) in Chapter 17.

With these lessons in mind we turn to the first group of "compound nerve injuries".

PENETRATING MISSILE INJURIES

Delorme (1915), then Inspector General of the Medical Services of the Armies of France, outlined a method of treatment for shell and bullet wounds based on three principles: resection of scar until a healthy bed is secured; excision of damaged nerve until healthy stumps are reached; and tension-free suture by adequate mobilisation and flexion of adjacent joints or grafting. His paper was heavily criticised by the great and good of the French Academy, but the verdict of history goes to Delorme and against his detractors. Tinel (1917b) supported the proposals of Delorme, adding: "when the distance between the segments of the nerve trunk is too great to permit direct suture *the only legitimate operation is nerve grafting* as recommended by J. and A. Déjerine and Mouzon". He further added: "there is nothing but nerve tissue can serve as a conductor for regenerating axis cylinder," and roundly castigated "mischievous" operations such as lateral implantation, transplantation of a motor nerve into a sensory one and isolation of nerve by foreign body. Only the interposition of a "muscular – or better still, a fatty – layer" between a nerve and callus or bony projection is permitted. It seems difficult to add to this.

Owen Smith (1981) and Omer (1991) wrote extensively of high velocity bullet wounds, pointing out that the effects of such injuries were well known in the 19th century. Horsley (1894) showed that the wound was caused by transmission of energy from the bullet to the tissues, and Woodruff (1898) introduced the term "cavitation" for the damaged caused at a distance from the bullet track.

The Red Cross Wound Classification focuses the mind on the wound, not the weapon; Lindsey (1980) pithily condemns "the idolatry of velocity, or lies, damn lies and ballistics". A number of writers have described the dangerous nature of the close-range shotgun wound. Raju (1979) reported 39 shotgun wounds and 72 gunshot vascular injuries over 13 years, finding the shotgun injuries much the most severe. Shephard (1980) emphasised the significance of the mass of shotgun pellets in his series of 42 cases; so did Luce and Griffen (1978), who reported 77 cases of penetrating missile injuries of the upper limb collected over 7 years. Forty-five of these patients had nerve lesions; the shotgun wounds fared particularly badly. Of the nine patients with combined injury to the brachial plexus and major vessels, only one had a useful result and three came to amputation. We should not forget the lesson given us by McCready et al (1986) who found good recovery of the nerves after prompt decompression of haematomas compromising the brachial plexus in their series of 34 cases of open wounds of the subclavian and axillary vessels. The devastating effect of close-range shotgun wounds was shown by Stewart and Kinnimonth (1993) from the Royal Infirmary in Glasgow, who treated 23 patients with 28 shotgun wounds to limbs over the course of 4 years. Their valuable paper uses the Red Cross Wound Classification. No limbs were amputated for vascular injury alone, but three amputations in the lower limb were considered necessary because of the associated injury to the sciatic or tibial nerve. The functional outcome was disappointing in three more cases of shotgun injury to the forearm in which median and ulnar nerves had been torn. These were treated by early grafting; skin cover was achieved by free flap transfer. The authors comment that: "nerve repair was unsuccessful and left the patients with significant pain and disability two years after injury". It is possible that the pedicled ulnar nerve graft developed by St Clair Strange is applicable in such injuries.

As Nicholls and Lillehei (1988) point out, success in vascular repair leaves us with the problem of the nerve injury, which they found in 60–70% of upper limb wounds and in 25% of the lower limb wounds. Evidently, a proportion of these people recover spontaneously. Omer (1980a) made a prospective study of 500 cases, and saw some spontaneous recovery in 67% in both high and low velocity injuries. Sunderland (1978) recorded a similar outcome in untreated cases. A distinctly contrary view comes from Seddon (1975), who described the varying injury to a nerve following "through and through" missile injuries: "the shock wave has caused more or less disturbance of function and structure in the nerve, ranging from fleeting paralysis (many combatants remark that the injured limb 'went completely dead' for a few minutes) to neurapraxia and axonotmesis, and to internal disruption sufficient to cause moderate or severe intraneural fibrosis; all this short of actual severance of the nerve. The longitudinal extent of the fibrosis is a reflection of the distortion that the nerve has suffered and in this there is probably an element akin to traction" (Fig. 8.17). Seddon emphasised that secondary repair is obligatory because the extent of intraneural fibrosis could be recognised only after a few weeks. In his series of 379 median and ulnar nerves damaged by missiles, no less than 70% had been divided or partially divided, and in commenting on nerves injured by missiles he said "patients who present with complete paralysis require exploration anyway, because there is no

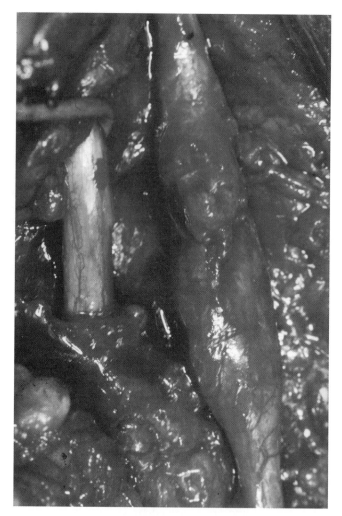

Fig. 8.17 Bullet wound of divisions of the sciatic nerve in the thigh. The common peroneal nerve was transected and repaired (neurotmesis). The tibial nerve (sling) recovered spontaneously (axonotmesis).

other means of knowing whether the nerve has been completely severed. Discovering it to be in continuity is fortuitous. The debate then centres on finding reason why resection and suture should *not* be performed."

Seddon's experience was enormous. In addition to the 379 cases mentioned above he also followed and described outcome in over 240 cases of missile injury to the sciatic nerve or its major divisions. It is clear that he felt exploration was indicated in those cases with no clear evidence of clinical recovery as soon as the patient's condition permitted. But Seddon used grafts for nerve repair at a time when this was not fashionable. Even so, this quite decisive view is a little at odds with the less positive approach adopted by Seddon and the Medical Research Council towards the treatment of injuries to the brachial plexus. There was, perhaps, a feeling that useful recovery could not follow repair of such proximal lesions. It must be admitted that results were not particularly encouraging

Table 8.10 Upper limb nerve injuries complicated by arterial injury in adults, 1977–1995 (excluding penetrating missile injuries and amputations)

Level of lesion and artery	Number of patients		Number of nerves	
	Open	Closed	Open	Closed
Infraclavicular (axillary artery)	21	55	48	108
Arm, elbow (brachial artery)	27	5	31	9
Forearm, wrist (radial and ulnar arteries)	188	5	279	3
Total	236	65	358	120

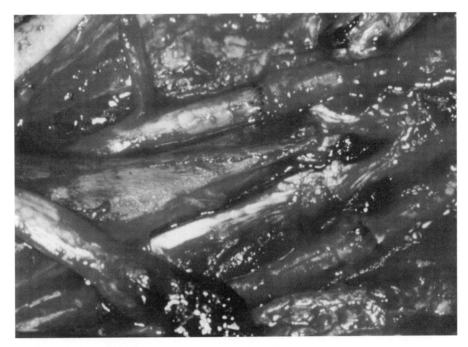

Fig. 8.22 Stab wound of the axilla; suture of the artery and median and ulnar nerves. The radial nerve (top) was grafted. Recovery for the radial and median nerves, and useful recovery for the ulnar, with intrinsic muscles regaining power (Medical Research Council grade 3+).

to use the tourniquet when the wound is in the forearm or wrist, permitting display and identification and repair of the radial and ulnar arteries within 90 minutes before proceeding, in more leisurely fashion, to repair of muscles and tendons. Birch and Raji (1991) emphasised that the synovium be repaired over each tendon at the wrist, which diminishes adhesions between the tendons and between the tendons and the nerve trunks.

The closed infraclavicular lesion

We think that this is among the worst of all true peripheral nerve injuries. It is characterised by the violence of the causal lesion, by the high incidence of rupture of the axillary artery (about 25% in our cases), and by the complexity of the nerve lesion (Figs 8.23 and 8.24). It is common to find nerve trunks ruptured at different levels up and down the limb, and it is not rare to find them avulsed from muscle bellies. Alnot (1988) described a large series of severe infraclavicular lesions, finding injuries of the cords or terminal branches in 105 of 420 patients with a closed traction injury to the brachial plexus. In 15 of these the nerves were damaged at two levels, with both preganglionic and more distal lesions. The axillary, suprascapular and musculo-cutaneous nerves were most vulnerable, and Alnot emphasised the technical difficulty of nerve repair when there had been widespread longitudinal nerve injury.

Some of our material is set out in Table 8.11. We think that the advantages of urgent repair of the vessel and of the nerves are overwhelming. They include: ease of identification of ruptured structures; the use of the nerve stimulator to detect more distal nerve injuries; and the ability to diminish the gap between nerve stumps, which retract widely after ruptures. The exposure of Fiolle and Delmas, which is described in Chapter 9, is ideally suited to these cases.

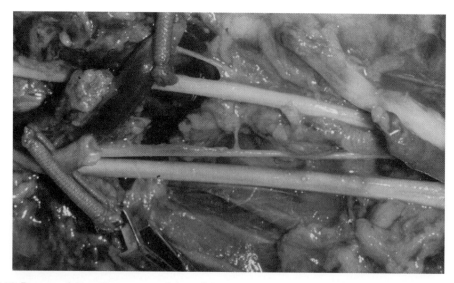

Fig. 8.23 Rupture of the axillary artery and the radial nerve associated with closed fracture of the upper humerus.

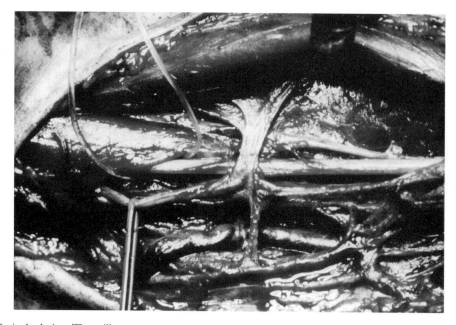

Fig. 8.24 Closed infraclavicular lesion. The axillary artery was ruptured at the level of the coracoid. Musculocutaneous and ulnar nerves were ruptured, and the distal stumps retracted into the arm.

Table 8.11 Infraclavicular lesions

Lesion type	Total	Open	Vascular
Involving suprascapular and circumflex nerves	126	6	6
Caused by shoulder dislocation; no nerve rupture	26	0	2
Caused by shoulder dislocation; with vascular injury but no nerve rupture, in older patients	8	0	8
Multiple ruptures of nerves (the true infraclavicular lesion)	282	54	62
Total	442	60	78

Cavanagh (1987) presented the results of the repair of 91 nerves ruptured in closed infraclavicular lesion. In some later cases, nerve repair was abandoned because of technical difficulty or because the state of the tissues in the arm was so bad. As might be expected, the results were a good deal better for the suprascapular, the circumflex, the radial, and the musculocutaneous nerves than they were for the median and the ulnar nerves. What was particularly striking was the effect of delay. Results were very much better when the nerves were repaired within 14 days of injury than in those repaired later (average time in this group being 12 weeks), and this was particularly true for the median and ulnar nerves. These and other findings are discussed in Chapter 11.

NERVES AND BONE AND JOINT INJURIES

Nerves are injured by damage to the adjacent skeleton by: traction from displacement, which commonly ends in rupture; laceration by a fragment of bone; entrapment within the dislocated joint or in a fracture; and late entrapment and compression from callus. On the whole, dislocations are more damaging. It seems to be widely assumed that the prognosis for nerves injured in this way is good, but this is not generally the case. Our own indications for exploring the nerve are governed by: the violence of the injury, which indicates the extent of displacement of bones and their fragments; the depth of lesion; and pain. A surgeon who considers that the fracture requires open reduction and internal fixation will rarely regret exposing the afflicted nerve at the same time, and we think that a nerve palsy is added indication for open reduction.

Seddon (1975) had the following comment to make in speaking about nerves injured in the arm and at the elbow. He thought that recovery could be awaited if two conditions were met: "The first is reasonable apposition of the bony fragments and the other *complete certainty that there is no threat of ischaemia of the forearm muscles.*" In referring to sciatic palsy in fracture of the femoral shaft, Seddon said "it is wise always to explore the nerve". One of the earliest series on nerve injuries from fractures and dislocations comes from Watson Jones (1930), and it remains one of the best. More than 100 nerve lesions were analysed from 5000 consecutive patients seen in the Liverpool Fracture Service over the course of 2 years. The nature of the injury to the ulnar nerve from fracture of the medial epicondyle, and to the common peroneal nerve from fracture of the fibula, was clearly described. In noting the vulnerability of the median nerve distal to the pronator quadratus, Watson Jones made this tart comment about excision of the lunate bone: "The writer's opinion is that it would be as reasonable to suggest excision of a four week old dislocation of the hip."

Both Watson Jones and Platt (1928) were strongly in favour of the exploration of nerves injured by fractures.

Siegel and Gelberman (1991) reviewed the subject thoroughly, finding 85% of nerve palsies recovering from closed fractures and 65–70% after open fractures. Of those nerves which went on to recovery, 90% had done so by 4 months. These cannot have been wholly degenerative lesions. Siegel and Gelberman's indications for intervention include:

- the fracture needs internal fixation
- there is associated vascular injury
- wound exploration of an open fracture is necessary
- a fracture or dislocation is irreducible.

We might add to this two more:

- the lesion deepens while it is under observation (Fig. 8.25)
- the lesion occurred during operation for internal fixation.

The association between displaced fragments of bone and serious nerve lesions is relevant too. Goldie and Powell (1991) described a case where the median nerve was transfixed by a fragment of the distal radius. They intervened urgently, on the basis of a near-complete nerve lesion and radiological evidence of a skeletal cause. Recovery was good. We have seen several cases where displaced fragments from the clavicle impaled or compressed the retroclavicular brachial plexus. In Omer's (1974) prospective study, 83% of nerve palsies from closed upper limb fractures recovered and 90% of these had done so by 3 months. If there was no recovery by 7 months then there would be none. Seddon's own figures are interesting: 146 from 212 of cases of nerves injured in fractures or dislocations of the upper limb spontaneously recovered to near normal levels, but less than one-half of his 57 cases of nerve palsies after

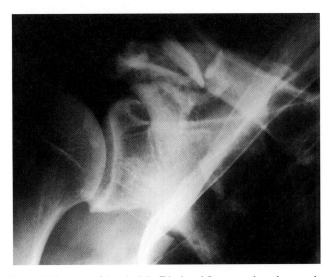

Fig. 8.25 Fracture of the clavicle. Displaced fragments have lacerated the subclavian artery and the brachial plexus.

skeletal injury in the lower limb did so. One-third of his own series of radial nerves so injured did not recover, but of course these were referred cases. Seddon described the information given to him by Böhler on the fracture services of Salzburg and Vienna. There were 57 cases of radial palsy in 765 closed fractures of the humeral shaft, an incidence of 7.4%. Spontaneous recovery occurred in 47, so the incidence of unfavourable radial lesions in this series was less than 2%.

We shall consider in more detail five regions: the shoulder girdle and the glenohumeral joint; the elbow (and radial palsy in humeral fracture), the pelvis, the hip and the knee.

The shoulder girdle and glenohumeral joints

Bonnel (1989) estimated that one-quarter of the nerves of the brachial plexus pass to this complex of joints, which permits an extraordinarily wide range of movement for the upper limb. One cranial and three peripheral nerves are of particular significance: the spinal accessory (eleventh cranial) nerve, the nerve to the serratus, and the supra-scapular and circumflex nerves. Understanding of their role, and of the consequences following lesions, has been increased by such studies as those reported by Comtet et al (1993a), Narakas (1993c) and Coene and Narakas (1992). Some lessons learnt from renewed interest in re-innervation of the shoulder after adult plexus lesions are described in Chapter 9, and from the complex problem of the shoulder in birth palsies in Chapter 10. The forma-tion, course, distribution and function of these nerves are outlined in earlier chapters. Pain is usual after injuries to these nerves, particularly to the accessory and the nerve to the serratus anterior, and now is as good a time as any to dispel a commonly held misconception that the three nerves without a cutaneous sensory component are purely "motor" nerves. This is quite wrong. All three contain large numbers of Aδ and C fibres. Biopsies of the supra-scapular nerve weeks after proven preganglionic injury to the fifth and sixth cervical nerves showed that over 30% of the larger myelinated fibres survived, these presumably being those responsible for proprioception with cells in the dorsal root ganglion. Williams et al (1995) showed that one-half of the fibres within the accessory nerve were Aδ or C fibres (Fig. 8.26). Williams et al reported their clini-cal findings in 64 cases as set out in Tables 8.12 and 8.13.

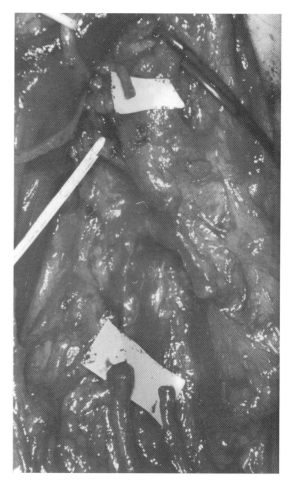

Fig. 8.26 Iatropathic section of the spinal accessory nerve and of two supraclavicular nerves in the posterior triangle of neck.

Table 8.12 Lesions of the spinal accessory nerve

Cause	Operation	
	Neurolysis	Repair
Stab wound	2	10
Penetrating missile wound	1	2
Traction	1	3
Iatropathic	12	31
Irradiation	2	0
Total	18	46

(Reproduced by permission of the Editor of Annals of the Royal College of Surgeons of England.)

Table 8.13 Classification of recovery

	Outcome	Grade	No.	Treatment
A	No change	Poor	7	4 graft; 3 neurolysis
B	Pain improved	Fair	10	6 graft; 4 neurolysis
	Movement improved			
C	Almost normal (difficulty with overhead work)	Good	15	13 graft; 2 neurolysis
D	Normal (from patient's point of view)	Excellent	4	1 graft; 3 neurolysis

From Williams et al (1996). (Reproduced by permission of the Editor of Annals of the Royal College of Surgeons of England.)

Ruptures of the suprascapular and circumflex nerves account for about 1% of the larger series of peripheral nerve injuries (Sunderland 1978). We think that they are a good deal more common than this; amounting to nearly 10% of our own repairs of all peripheral nerves (excluding brachial plexus lesions), and we suspect that they have suffered a degree of neglect in the past. It is remarkable that Seddon wrote only briefly about the suprascapular nerve. It is a lamentable fact that we are seeing increasing numbers of injuries to all four of these nerves incurred during the course of treatment. The subject of iatropathic nerve lesions is discussed in Chapter 13.

The suprascapular and circumflex nerves

Combined injury of these two nerves is not uncommon, and it therefore seems reasonable to consider them together.

The suprascapular nerve passes away from the upper trunk about 3 cm above the clavicle. It is not unusual to find it arising entirely from the fifth cervical nerve. It passes laterally and posteriorly deep to the omohyoid to the scapular notch, entering the supraspinatus fossa deep to the superior transverse ligament; it traverses the fossa deep to the supraspinatus muscle to wind around the lateral border of the spine of the scapula to enter the infraspinus fossa. The nerve contains 3000–4000 myelinated nerve fibres. Its course renders it particularly vulnerable to traction lesions, and we have seen it so injured where it branches from the upper trunk, in the posterior triangle, at the supraspinus notch and within the supra- and infraspinus fossae. The nerve is essential for abduction and lateral rotation at the glenohumeral joint; indeed, patients with isolated paralysis of the deltoid with an intact

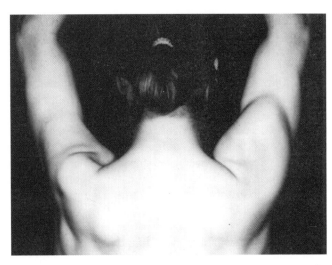

Fig. 8.27 Shoulder elevation in complete paralysis of deltoid. Note the activity in the clavicular head of pectoralis major.

suprascapular nerve of rotator cuff are usually able fully to abduct and laterally rotate the shoulder (Fig. 8.27).

The circumflex nerve is the terminal branch of the posterior cord and it contains 6000–7000 myelinated nerve fibres which pass through the fifth and sixth cervical nerves. The nerve divides into two branches within the quadrilateral tunnel: the anterior division continues around the neck of the humerus to innervate the anterior deltoid, and the larger posterior branch innervates the teres minor and the posterior deltoid. One cutaneous branch, the upper lateral cutaneous nerve of the arm, is a useful landmark where it pierces the deep fascia over the posterior border of the deltoid (Fig. 8.28). Spilsbury and Birch's

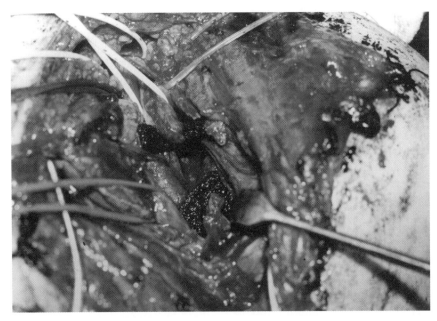

Fig. 8.28 Circumflex nerve rupture. The stumps prepared. The distal trunk displayed after reflection of coracobrachialis.

(1996) investigations suggest that the deltoid is responsible for over 50% of the power of abduction, about 30% of forward flexion power and 80% of extension power at the shoulder.

It is our experience that British orthopaedic surgeons tend to adopt an expectant approach to circumflex palsy, unlike their more energetic approach to other injuries of peripheral nerves, notably to the brachial plexus. Leffert and Seddon (1965) and Seddon (1975) found that many closed injuries to the circumflex nerve went on to recover spontaneously, and it is true that the nerve is only partially injured in many cases. Blom and Dahlback (1970) described 24 cases of isolated circumflex nerve lesions; all of these went on to full recovery, even though electromyographic abnormalities were found in nearly all. In an electrophysiological study, Liveson (1984) showed that the lesion extended beyond the circumflex nerve. Rockwood et al (1991) found an incidence of circumflex palsies in 30% of shoulder dislocations, and this was higher in older patients. de Laat et al (1994) made a detailed study of 101 patients with nerve lesions after shoulder dislocation. The circumflex nerve headed the field, followed by the suprascapular and musculocutaneous nerves. Electromyographic abnormality was detected in 45%, and this was more evident in the elderly and in those with obvious haematomas. There was no spontaneous recovery of the nerve lesion in eight cases; not an insignificant number in these cases of low energy injury.

In a significant paper describing the treatment of combined injuries of the circumflex and suprascapular nerves, Ochiai et al (1988) showed that the suprascapular nerve might be serially damaged at several places. They recommended that the nerve should be exposed along its entire course as far as the infraspinatus. Petrucci et al (1982) described 21 cases treated by nerve graft and neurolysis. Millesi (1980) and Narakas (1989) published series of repairs of the nerve, and of the total of 45 repairs reported in these three papers, 80% gave good or excellent results. Nunley and Gabel (1991) say that: "if no evidence of clinical or electromyographic recovery is seen at two to three months after injury, exploration should be performed … Recovery is unlikely after twelve months of denervation, and surgical treatment is of negligible benefit in this setting." We think that Nunley and Gabel are right. Narakas (1991) described a large series of operated cases, with isolated lesions of the circumflex nerve in 62 cases and combined injuries of the circumflex and suprascapular nerves in 27. In 16 patients rupture of the rotator cuff was associated with a lesion of a circumflex nerve or the suprascapular nerves.

Spilsbury and Birch (1996) reported findings in 129 nerve injuries in 98 of our patients. There were 62 ruptures of the circumflex and 22 of the suprascapular nerve. Lesions in continuity were seen in 26 circumflex and 19 suprascapular nerves. In 31 patients both nerves were damaged, and in at least eight more there was an associated rupture of the rotator cuff. Open wounds from stabbings, missiles or surgeons accounted for 25 nerves in 16 patients. Results were described using the MRC Medical Research Council of power and the scoring system of Narakas, and in 28 patients myometric measurements of strength and stamina were done. Spilsbury thought that results were good in 27 of 56 grafts of the circumflex nerve and fair in 23 more. Results were rather better for the 20 grafts of the suprascapular nerve. Only six of the 23 lesions in continuity of the circumflex nerve, treated by neurolysis, went on to good recovery. Eight of the 16 lesions in continuity of the suprascapular nerve did so. Myometric measurements of strength and stamina revealed a rather more unfavourable picture. The stamina of the shoulder with paralysis of the deltoid was no more than about 30% of the normal side, and ranged between 40% and 45% in those cases where there had been some recovery through lesions in continuity. Stamina of the shoulder after successful repair of the suprascapular nerve, with an intact circumflex nerve, reached 70% of normal. Where the circumflex nerve had been grafted the shoulder achieved only 50% of normal stamina. In many patients with paralysis of the deltoid, extension behind the plane of the body was impossible with the shoulder abducted. With the arm adducted the latissimus dorsi muscle compensated.

Some recognised causes of failure are described in Chapter 11 (Fig. 8.29). The most important is rupture of the rotator cuff, and we have been guilty of not recognising this associated injury until after recovery of the nerves. However, in three cases, not included in the above series, where we have repaired both the circumflex nerve and the rotator cuff, the results were poor and this injury is indeed a bad one.

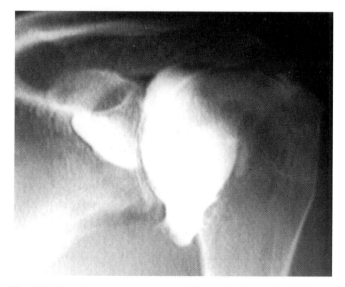

Fig. 8.29 Capsular contracture marred the result after repair of the circumflex nerve.

It would appear that a more vigorous approach towards palsies of the suprascapular and circumflex nerves is justified. If a patient with a clinical diagnosis of circumflex nerve lesion is unable to abduct the shoulder, then either the suprascapular nerve is damaged or the rotator cuff is torn. Probably the best single investigation to disentangle these elements is magnetic resonance imaging, which not only demonstrates damage to the rotator cuff but also indicates denervation of deltoid and supraspinatus muscles. The suprascapular and circumflex nerves can be seen at the notch and in the quadrilateral space, respectively. The single most important factor in advising operation is the history of injury, an indication of the extent of violence expended upon the shoulder. Urgent exploration is justified in open wounds and, obviously, where there is associated vascular lesion, as there was in eight of Spilsbury's cases. We think that urgent steps should be taken when there are apparently combined suprascapular and circumflex nerve palsies, and that exploration is justifiable if there is no clinical evidence of recovery in isolated palsy of the circumflex nerve by 3 months. "The difficulties attending diagnosis and treatment of the combined lesion, to circumflex and suprascapular nerves, are considerably eased by two important contributions from Tokyo. Ochiai et al (1997) describe a method of exposure: Mikami et al (1977) report encouraging results after repair".

We have already referred to large published series which suggested that the prognosis for radial nerve palsy in closed fracture of the proximal or midshaft of humerus was good. We are not sure about this. It may be that our experience is coloured by the referral of patients who have suffered high energy injuries and by a trend to favouring internal fixation of the bone. In any event these injuries are by no means benign. The surgeon embarking on an operation of open reduction and internal fixation in a patient with radial nerve palsy should expose that nerve during the operation. The presence of such a nerve palsy adds weight to the argument for open intervention (Fig. 8.30).

The elbow

The elbow is a notorious area of difficulty in treating nerve injuries, especially in children. The close proximity of all trunks to bone makes them vulnerable; there is, of course, the constant risk of damage to the brachial artery and of compartment syndrome in the flexor muscles of the forearm. There are a large number of reports of nerve injuries in relation to this joint, all of which contribute, and we refer here to some of them.

Duthie (1957) described a radial nerve entrapped within a tunnel after supracondylar fracture. Post and Hashell (1974) repaired a median nerve which had been damaged by supracondylar fracture. Recovery, after suture, was good. Symeonides et al (1975) and Lalnandham and Lawrence (1984) described radial and ulnar nerves entrapped in callus. Jessing (1975) recognised the vulnerability of the radial nerve and the posterior interosseous nerve in Monteggia fracture dislocation, especially if the head of the radius was displaced anteriorly. Beverly and Fearn (1984) reported a case of anterior interosseous nerve palsy after dislocation of the elbow, and Hallett (1981) described a series of median nerves entrapped within dislocations of the elbow in a valuable paper which provoked St Clair Strange to open the debate on indications

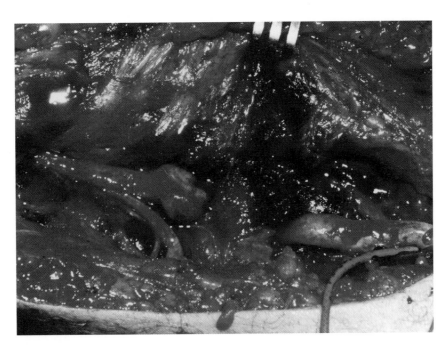

Fig. 8.30 Rupture of the radial nerve in a closed fracture of the humerus. The stumps are embedded within the fracture.

for resection and repair. Other series were reported by Sorrel and Sorrel Déjerine (1938), who described 252 children's fractures of the distal humerus in which 21 nerves were injured. Some of these were explored. Linscheid and Wheeler (1965) found ulnar palsies in 14% of elbow dislocations. Kurer and Reagan (1990) reviewed 1708 completely displaced supracondylar fractures in children. Wilkins (1991), in discussing fractures and dislocations of the elbow region in children, found and incidence of nerve palsy of 11% in 285 patients, but a failure to recover in only one nerve. Ottolenghi (1971) described 830 cases of supracondylar fractures in children: 39 of these required treatment for vascular complication, an incidence of 5%. He emphasised that the earlier this was done the better. Ottolenghi recognised three types of median and arterial damage:

- both were tented over the spike of the proximal fracture when the proximal fracture intervened between the artery
- nerve which was entrapped within the fracture
- both were entrapped within the fracture.

We have seen all three.

Dutkowsky and Kasser (1991) wrote a comprehensive review of nerve injuries associated with fractures in children, and they recommend exploration of the nerve if the fracture itself warrants operation. They comment: "an irreducible supracondylar fracture with associated nerve damage represents an indication for open reduction and exploration", and noted the risks of using the percutaneous approach for insertion of the medial pin in fixation, preferring a short incision to expose the medial epicondyle. Their reference to Panas (1878) who first recognised this tardy ulnar palsy takes us to the late complication for the ulnar nerve. Miller (1924) found that half his cases of ulnar neuropathy were associated with fracture of the lateral condylar physis in childhood, with an average range of age at onset of symptoms of 30–40 years. Gay and Love (1947) described 100 cases with an average age of onset of 22 years. Wadsworth (1972, 1982) has written definitively on this subject, and said "this is the most important complication of injuries to the capitular epiphysis ... even in the well treated case there is no absolute certainty that tardy ulnar palsy may not follow in adult life; however this probability is minimised by proper case."

Our own experience is set out in Table 8.14. Of the 190 nerve lesions repairs were necessary in 45. Operation was performed when the lesion was complete and degenerate, when there was pain, when there was any hint of vascular impairment, when further operation on the fracture was necessary, and when the nerve lesion became evident only after primary operation. Of the 106 lesions in children, one radial, five ulnar and two median nerves were damaged during operations for internal fixation of fracture. Seventeen of the nerves damaged in supracondylar fractures were found entrapped within the fracture, or impaled on a bone spike. The remainder were compressed by swelling or fibrosis at or distal to the fracture, and recovery after decompression was uniformly good. Entrapment of the ulnar nerve after "reduction" of a fracture of the medial condyle is a particular pitfall. We have seen seven cases – the outline of one should suffice. A 10-year-old boy

Table 8.14 Nerve lesions associated with fractures and/or dislocations at the elbow, and displayed at operation

Skeletal injury	Nerve	No.	
Children			
Supracondylar fracture	Median	38	
	Ulnar	35	
	Radial	9	
Medial condyle fracture	Ulnar	7	
	Median	1	
Dislocation	Median	9	
	Radial	2	
	Ulnar	1	
Monteggia fracture dislocation	Radial–posterior interosseous	4	
Total		106	
Adults			
Fracture dislocations about the elbow	Radial	16	3 entrapped 8 ruptured 5 iatropathic
	Median	17	6 entrapped 7 ruptured 4 iatropathic
	Ulnar	18	7 entrapped 8 ruptured 3 iatropathic

was seen 72 hours after closed manipulation of this injury. He had a complete ulnar nerve palsy. Inspection of the radiographs showed imperfect reduction. The ulnar nerve was trapped within the fracture, and liberated. Recovery was complete.

Surgeons faced with children in whom the nerve trunks are entrapped in the joint after dislocation, or are embedded, are faced with a difficult decision. In two cases we decided against resection and grafting. We were wrong. That the interval between injury and intervention is an important factor is shown by the following two cases:

1. A 9-year-old girl presented with complete median nerve palsy 10 days after closed reduction of dislocation of the elbow. Mr Jamie McLean (Perth) extricated the nerve from the joint. Recovery was complete at about 1 year (Figs 8.31 to 8.33).
2. An 8-year-old girl presented with complete median nerve palsy 11 months after closed reduction of dislocation of the elbow. Mr Boyd Goldie (London) found the nerve irretrievably lodged within the joint, and elected to reset the damaged segment and graft it. Recovery was good.

We think that both surgeons acted correctly – in the early case, retrieval of the nerve was possible; in the later case, it was not.

The 84 lesions in the adult cases were much less favourable, and severe pain was a common complication (Figs 8.34 and 8.35).

The risk of arterial injury must always be remembered. The following case is the exception which does not disprove the rule.

Case report. A 7-year-old boy presented 4 months after closed supracondylar fracture. The reduction had been imperfect. There were no distal pulses; the median nerve lesion was complete and that of the ulnar nerve only partial. At operation both nerve and artery were found jammed in the fracture site. The median nerve was liberated: it had not been lacerated and was left alone. The brachial artery was reduced to a pulseless cord over a length of 3 cm, and preparations were made to take a vein graft from the dorsum of the foot to repair it. Fortunately, we reinspected the artery before incising the skin of the

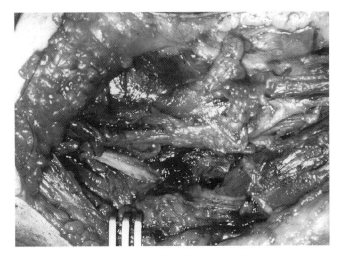

Fig. 8.32 The nerve entering the joint. (Courtesy of Mr Jamie McLean.)

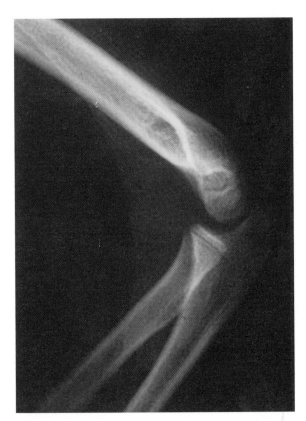

Fig. 8.31 Post reduction radiographs of dislocation of elbow in a child, complicated by median palsy. (Courtesy of Mr Jamie McLean.)

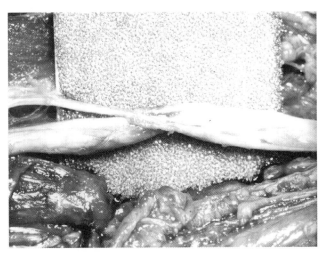

Fig. 8.33 The extricated nerve. (Courtesy of Mr Jamie McLean.)

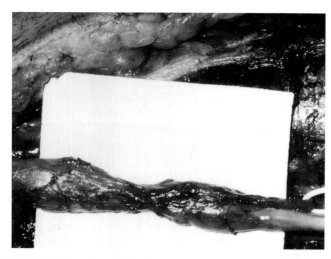

Fig. 8.34 Dislocation of elbow in a 28-year-old man. The appearance of the median nerve after extrication from the elbow. Recovery after graft was poor.

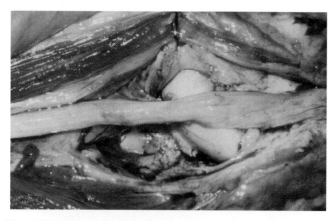

Fig. 8.35 A 43-year-old man. The appearance of the ulnar nerve after removal from within the elbow joint. Recovery was poor and complicated by severe pain.

foot, and saw that it had expanded and become pulsatile and that the radial pulse had returned.

Such an unusual event does not permit ignoring the clear advice given by Gross and Yau in Wadsworth's book *The Elbow* (1982) (see page 134).

Conclusion

Complete nerve lesions should be explored after fractures or dislocations about the elbow, when the palsy occurs after reduction or operation, when the palsy progresses, or if radiographs are unsatisfactory. Severe pain is a strong indication for operation. If the nerve is lacerated, resection and repair is justified, particularly in a child. Above all, impairment of circulation which begins after good reduction of the fracture by closed manipulation is an *absolute* indication for exploration.

THE LOWER LIMB: THE LUMBOSACRAL PLEXUS

The brachial plexus is vulnerable because of the mobility of the forequarter on the trunk such that the attachment of its constituent spinal nerves to the spinal cord is the weakest link in the chain. By contrast, the lumbosacral plexus is protected by the stability of the pelvic girdle. The ilium is bonded to the lumbosacral spine by massive ligaments, and there is no joint between ilium and pubis. These features are one reason for the relatively scant literature on and only occasional report of repair of injuries to the lumbosacral plexus. Such injuries can only occur from massive injury of a life-threatening nature. There is also the matter of technical difficulty. Some clear descriptions of the injury come close on 100 years after equivalent descriptions of the pathological lesions in the upper limb. Finney and Wulfman (1960) wrote of the case of avulsion of lumbar spinal nerves confirmed by myelography. Barnett and Connolly (1975) described what they thought was the fourteenth published case – a patient sent to them after below knee amputation who continued in intractable pain. The stump had been explored, and sympathectomy performed. The diagnosis was made at 6 years after injury when myelography revealed the true cause. Pain was eased by transcutaneous nerve stimulation. Radiographs confirmed that the original injury had caused displacement of the hemipelvis (Figs 8.36 to 8.38).

The anatomical disposition of the lumbosacral plexus is set out by Horwitz (1939), who performed 228 dissections and described 13 variations from the standard pattern, noting that these variations were related to the formation of the lumbar spine. The shorter (sacralised) spine is associated with a prefixed plexus; the longer spine with the extra vertebral body is associated with postfixed plexus formation. Webber (1961) dissected 50 cadavers, and found variations in the formation of the lumbosacral trunk, in the origin of the cutaneous nerves, and in the presence or absence of accessory obturator and femoral nerves.

Lam (1936) and Bonnin (1945) described nerve injuries from fractures of the pelvis and sacrum, and London (1961) emphasised that the nervi erigentes were particularly vulnerable within severe pelvic fractures "judging from the fact that about one man in twenty is more or less impotent (but not sterile) after major fractures". He also described cases of sciatic paralysis from narrowing of the sciatic notch, and a case of "an unimportant looking fracture that was shown to have the sciatic nerve trapped in it". The displacement of the fracture was far greater than the radiographs suggested. Räf (1966) described the displaced fracture of pelvis, the double vertical fracture, as an injury with a particularly high incidence of nerve injuries. Huittinen and Slätis (1972) described a series of 31 patients with nerve injuries, from a total of 68 patients with unstable fractures, which included fractures of the pelvic ring and of the sacroiliac joint. L5 and S1 were most

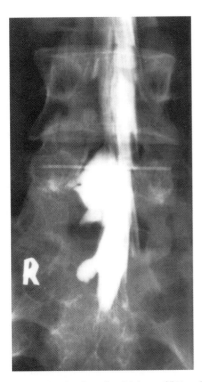

Fig. 8.36 Myelogram showing intradural injury of L5 and S1, associated with fracture dislocation of the pelvis.

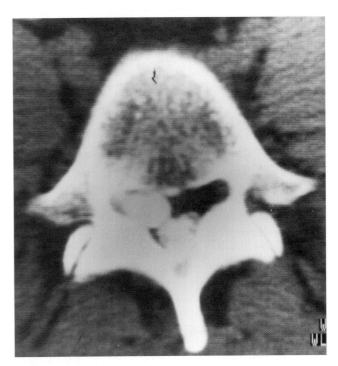

Fig. 8.37 Computed tomography scan – myelogram of lumbosacral junction.

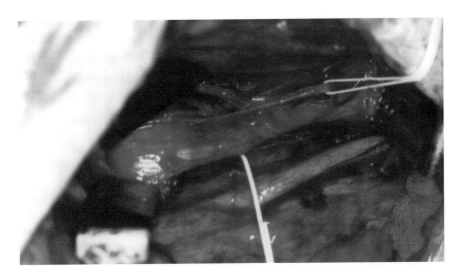

Fig. 8.38 Lesion of the lumbosacral plexus; grafted. (Courtesy of Mr Thomas Carlstedt.)

commonly affected, and six patients were incontinent. These authors estimated that the incidence of significant nerve injuries from all pelvic fractures was about 10–12% and the natural history for spontaneous recovery in their cases was poor.

Huittenen (1972) went on to postmortem studies of 42 cases of pelvic fracture. There had been unstable vertical fractures in 38 of these, and nerve injuries were demonstrated at 20 necropsies, involving four nerves. Traction

lesions accounted for 21 of these, 15 more nerve trunks had been ruptured. The roots were damaged in six cases, the anterior rami in seven, and the trunk nerves in 27. The lumbosacral and superior gluteal nerves were the most vulnerable (23 cases). Injuries to these two nerves was associated with hemipelvic dislocation with outward rotation and upward displacement. Comminution of the lateral sacral mass caused compression of the sacral nerves and the intradural injuries were caused by comminution and displacement of the sacroiliac joints. Huittenen described the lumbosacral trunk as "three to four centimetres long and oval in cross section about 10 mm wide and 4 mm thick. It contained about 40 funiculi and many vasa nervorum. It lies under the psoas major muscle from which it descends obliquely in front of the lateral sacral mass, traverses the front of the sacro-iliac joint behind the common iliac vessels and enters the sacral plexus at the upper border of the piriformis muscle. The lumbo-sacral trunk participates in the nerve supply of the 4th and 5th lumbar myotomes and dermatomes and when it has been damaged these are the segments where motor, sensory and vaso motor disturbances are to be expected."

Stoehr (1978) described no less than 53 cases, 31 of which were from injury (usually a fracture of the sacrum) and 22 of which were postoperative (17 of these following arthroplasty of the hip). In his series the lumbar plexus was most often involved, and two-thirds showed useful spontaneous recovery by about 18 months. Operations were not performed in this series. Moossy et al (1987) made an important contribution in their description of six cases of avulsion of spinal nerves from the conus presenting with intractable pain. These patients had suffered violent injuries. There had been three amputations, two of which were hemipelvectomy; two patients were paraplegic. The pain was characteristic of deafferentation, being constant and burning in nature, but there was also paroxysmal pain. Five of these six patients were cured or eased of their pain by coagulation of the dorsal root entry zone (DREZ lesion). Narakas edited and summarised discussions from a joint symposium of the French and Spanish Hand Societies and the Groupe pour l'Avancement de la Microchirurgie, held at Sitges, where a particularly valuable collection of papers was presented. Aramburo (1986) described exposure of the lumbosacral plexus by the retro- and intraperitoneal approaches; Linarte and Gilbert (1986) described the transsacral approach to the sacral plexus, in which the patient lies prone and the sacrum is lifted up like a lid, permitting bypass grafting to the sciatic and gluteal nerves in the buttock. Brunelli and Vigasio (1986) described 12 cases, outlining indications for extra- and intraperitoneal approach with repair.

Other reports come from Wood (1991) and Millesi (1987) who described useful recovery after repairs of open wounds. Our experience is limited to attempted repair of four intrapelvic injuries: two from penetrating wounds and two from iatropathic causes. In one case, the lumbosacral trunk was repaired, but there was no recovery. Repair was not possible in any of the other three. Thomas Carlstedt has kindly given us information about his experience of four cases in whom operation was performed for diagnosis. Repair was performed in three.

Case report. A 28-year-old soldier suffered severe pelvic fracture from crush injury. Complete loss of power and sensation followed in the right lower limb 7 months after injury. The lumbosacral trunk and first sacral nerves were displayed by intraperitoneal approach and found to be ruptured. The 8 cm gap was bridged by 10 grafts. By 3 years there was useful recovery into the muscles at the hip, the flexors of knee, and of ankle, with trophic sensation throughout the foot (Fig. 8.39).

In a second case there was intradural extramedullary rupture (preganglionic injury) of S1, S2, and S3. Eight months after injury the damaged roots were repaired by graft. There was recovery into the gluteal and thigh muscles. In a third case, an emergency repair of ruptures of S1 and S2 performed during reduction and fixation of sacroiliac dissociation was followed by functional recovery into the tibial division of the sciatic nerve.

Meyer (1982) repaired the third and fourth lumbar nerves, severed by glass, at 3 months after injury in a young woman. Five years after repair function, was close to normal throughout the lower limb.

These are difficult injuries to diagnose and to treat. The technical problems are forbidding, but results such as those obtained by Carlstedt and Meyer suggest that a more vigorous approach is justified in patients suffering from severe neural deficit or in severe pain.

We have seen other examples of lumbosacral plexus lesion caused by haematoma (similar to the two cases of Rajashekhar and Herbison (1974)), irradiation and intraperitoneal sepsis. Allieu et al (1977, 1986) studied the effects of haematoma on nerve function, particularly in the femoral and sciatic trunks. Their advice is salutary: "conservative treatment of a haematoma is to be condemned". Ultrasound is useful in diagnosis. Decompression is a matter of urgency.

Lumbosacral plexus lesions in infancy

Mills (1949) was probably the first to describe lumbosacral plexus lesions as a complication of birth. He suggested that the cause was thrombosis of the inferior gluteal artery. However, Meyer (1931) had described a case in which necropsy revealed haematomyelia within the sciatic nerves, and Fahrni (1950) described 11 cases implicating umbilical arterial injection as a possible cause. Teot (1986) and his colleagues from Montpelier described six cases in the Children's Service which had been explored and followed. The cause was obscure; no direct injury to the sciatic nerve was displayed. Recovery was very limited, and a more proximal cause was proposed. Canale (1991) discussed pelvic fractures in childhood, finding a 1.6% incidence of neurological lesions. Most recovered spontaneously, but causalgia persisted in one child.

The hip

The sciatic nerve is at risk in fracture dislocations of the hip, and the incidence is highest in posterior column fractures.

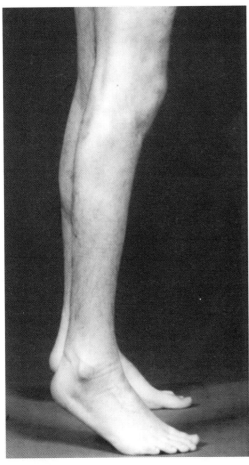

Fig. 8.39 Functional recovery into the flexor muscles of the knee and ankle at 3 years. (Courtesy of Mr Thomas Carlstedt.)

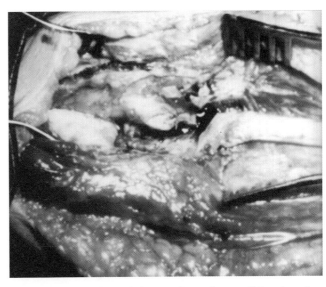

Fig. 8.40 Rupture of the sciatic nerve from a fracture dislocation of the hip.

Epstein (1980), in his personal series of 830 cases, found 68 nerve injuries, an incidence of 8%. There was good recovery in 43%, but the outcome was poor in 32%. Siegel and Gelberman (1991) found a range of 6–20% in published series, and commented that injuries to the sciatic nerve were a good deal more common in types 2, 3 and 4 of the Thompson–Epstein classification (1951), in which dislocation is associated with fractures of the rim or floor of the acetabulum, than in uncomplicated dislocation (Thompson–Epstein type 1). Letournel and Judet (1981) recorded 57 nerve injuries in 469 of their patients treated by open reduction and internal fixation, a preoperative incidence of 12%, which rose to 17.4% in the posterior column group. Their recommendations about diminishing the risks to the nerve during operations for fracture dislocation repays study. Sciatic palsy occurred in 30 of their patients after operation, and recovery was poor in 13 of these. They found that meticulous handling of nerve, and combining femoral traction with flexion at the knee during operation, reduced the incidence of intraoperative injury from 18% to 9%.

Badger (1959) said: "sciatic nerve damage is an indication for early manipulation followed immediately by open reduction of the fracture and repair of the sciatic nerve if practicable", advice which is given by others with substantial experience. London (1967) thought that moderate or increasing sciatic palsy, especially when the dislocation was complicated by a fracture, was an indication for urgent operation. Siegel and Gelberman thought that exploration of the nerve was not indicated in one circumstance – when a computed tomography scan confirmed that reduction was congruent and there were no bone fragments lying posterior to the hip. They noted "a specific fracture pattern that requires early exploration is one with displaced acetabular bone fragments, where there is an associated primary sciatic nerve injury. At exploration, these fragments have been found commonly compressing or impaling the nerve". Further, they recommend exploration of the nerve for sciatic palsy of delayed onset. Heterotopic bone formation is one explanation for this event.

Our experience comprises 19 operations for exploration of the sciatic nerve damaged in fracture dislocations of the hip. Operations were performed in complete lesions, partial lesions with severe pain, lesions occurring after open reduction, and lesions of increasing depth. This approach was justified in those cases where the nerve was entangled around a bone fragment or entrapped within the joint or compressed by callus. In four cases the nerve was found transected and was repaired, but useful recovery followed in only one of these (see Fig. 8.40). As far as we can see, exploration of the nerve did not improve the outcome in cases where the nerve had been violently stretched but had not ruptured. Injury to the lumbosacral plexus is likely in such cases.

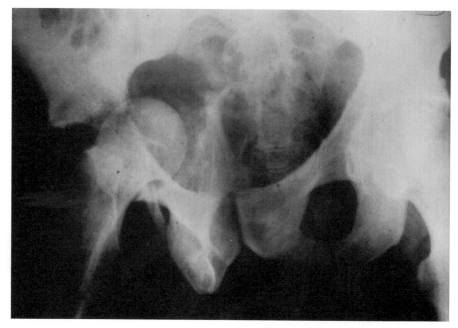

Fig. 8.41 Neglected fracture dislocation of the hip complicated by lumbosacral lesion.

Case report. A 43-year-old pathologist suffered posterior fracture dislocation of the hip complicated by complete sciatic palsy. The fracture was never reduced, and when we came to expose the nerve at 10 months from injury we found it intact, although stretched over the posterior aspect of the displaced acetabulum (Fig. 8.41).

The outlook is less dismal following repair of the sciatic nerve ruptured in the thigh by fracture of shaft of femur. Urgent exploration of the nerve is warranted, unless there is evidence of recovery or the general condition of the patient forbids operation.

The knee

The common peroneal nerve is commonly damaged in severe varus injuries of the knee. The lesion is caused by traction and the nerve may be damaged over a segment of 20 cm or more (Fig. 8.42). Platt (1928) and Watson Jones (1931) described the mechanism of injury, and Sunderland (1972) noted certain features of the nerve which make it vulnerable: the nerve is superficial; it is tethered to the sciatic trunk above and at the neck of the fibula below; and it has less supporting connective tissue and fewer autonomic fibres than the tibial nerve, so that the larger motor and sensory fibres bear the brunt of any injury. We think that the segment of nerve between the midthigh and the fibula is relatively ischaemic, because it is remote from major arteries and contributions to the epineurial circulation are few.

The traction rupture has a bad reputation. However, Sedel and Nizsard (1993) described the results of repair of

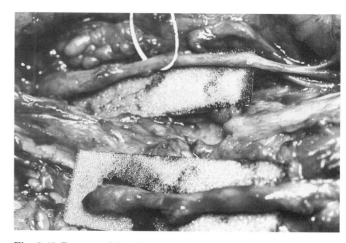

Fig. 8.42 Rupture of the left common peroneal nerve in a girl of 17 following severe adduction of the knee; appearances 5 days after injury.

17 cases. The gap ranged from 7 to 20 cm. Good function was regained in six cases, and a fair result was achieved in six more. A later posterior tibial transfer improved five patients. Sedel and Nissar emphasised that an abnormal and scarred nerve should be resected before grafting, and they did not find that the length of the gap was critical. Wilkinson and Birch (1995) described results in 27 of our patients operated on over a 10-year period. These were a mixed group, pure traction accounting for 11 injuries. The results are close to those of Sedel and Nissard. However, patients with arterial injury were excluded from our study: results of repair in such cases are undoubtedly poor. Delay between injury and repair is important. In all, we have

seen 38 cases of traction rupture of the common peroneal nerve. In nine cases repair was not performed, either because of delay or because the condition of the leg was too poor. Of the 25 cases adequately followed, the result was good in 11. These included the four cases where the opportunity was taken to graft the nerve at the primary operation for ligament repair.

Mr D. Roussow (London) performed urgent repair, by graft, of a closed rupture of the common peroneal nerve, at the same time as he repaired the lateral ligament complex of the knee. We saw his patient at 22 months – there was excellent function. This is a remarkable result – the defect in the nerve was over 15 cm long.

BURNS

It would be impertinent for us to draw conclusions from our limited experience in the treatment of burns of peripheral nerves. Tubiana (1988) made rather sombre observations on the evolution of the treatment of these injuries during a long and illustrous career, noting little significant improvement. Kline and Hudson (1993) were not impressed by the outcome in their seven cases of electrical burns to nerves.

The physical effects of different types of thermal injury are described by Thomas and Holdorff (1993) and by Hobby and Laing (1988). Hobby and Laing recognised four groups of electrical injury in 169 cases from a total of 3300: true electrical injury, from current passing from the conductor through the skin to the tissues; "arc" burn, where current passes external to the body to the ground; secondary flame burn, from ignited clothing; and direct burn, from a hot electrical element. Nerves were injured in 10% of their cases. Reasonable spontaneous recovery occurred in those cases where the blood supply to the adjacent tissues was not destroyed. Di Vincenti et al (1969) reported 69 cases of electrical burns, mostly from high tension injury. The median and ulnar nerves were the most frequently damaged, this damage was often severe and irreparable – because nerves are good conductors, the neurovascular bundles may be destroyed. Gruber (1990) recommended delayed, palliative, reconstruction in such cases. Salisbury and Dingeldein (1988) and Salzberg and Salisbury (1991) provide extensive reviews, emphasising the necessity for early incision of the encircling eschar. A clear description of the technique, with emphasis on avoiding damage to underlying nerves, is given. Wilkinson and Clarke (1992) reported two cases of burns to the brachial plexus in patients who fell asleep with their arms draped over the back of heated towel rails. Later decompression was performed in one case, revealing extensive fibrosis of the nerves and adjacent tissues. Recovery was poor in both these cases. Rousso and Wexler (1988) discuss the problem of pain relief, noting that thermal injuries to nerves "are often associated with sympathetic dystrophy".

9. Traumatic lesions of the brachial plexus

The brachial plexus: anatomy, including blood supply; incidence and mechanism of injury; patterns of injury; types of intradural lesion; diagnosis; indications for operation; the arterial lesion; approaches; techniques of nerve repair; neurotisation; special problems with the infraclavicular lesion; the advent of reimplantation.

There must be a beginning of any good matter, but the continuing to the end, until it be thoroughly finished yields the true glory.

(Drake to Walsingham)

SPECIAL ANATOMICAL CONSIDERATIONS

Leffert (1985) has discussed the topographical anatomy of the brachial plexus in detail, referring particularly to the work of Ker (1918) and Walsh (1877). These last two performed over 400 dissections, finding abnormalities in the formation of the plexus in some 2% of cases. Other important works include those of Harris (1904) and Hovelaque (1927). We shall discuss here some anatomical features that have particular significance for the surgeon embarking on repair.

The roots of the brachial plexus are formed from dorsal and ventral rootlets which join the spinal cord at, respectively, the posterolateral and the anterolateral sulcus. Berthold et al (1993) described the junction between the roots and the spinal cord, identifying a central–peripheral transition zone lying outside the spinal cord at varying levels along the roots. The peripheral component is characterised by a high extracellular element, the endoneurium, which is rich in collagen and contains Schwann cell–axon complexes. The central component has very little extracellular space; collagen is sparse and axons are embedded in oligendrocyte and astrocyte processes. The transitional zone is relevant to the level of intradural injury: it has been assumed that the lesion is commonly one of *avulsion* from the spinal cord. Jamieson's observations (Bonney & Jamieson 1979) suggested that, in this one case at least, there was actual rupture of roots – possibly at the level of the transitional zone. Gschmeissner (personal communication) has examined by electronmicroscopy a number of avulsed rootlets from our cases: he has found that most ruptures occurred in the peripheral nervous segments. We now recognise two types of intradural injury – intradural rupture and avulsion – of which the former may be the more common. We also think that lesion confined either to the ventral or the dorsal rootlets, and the extent of displacement of the dorsal root ganglion should be recognised in a classification set out in Table 9.1 and Figures 9.1 to 9.11.

Herzberg et al (1989) emphasised certain anatomical features of the spinal nerve within the foramen of considerable clinical significance, for they found that the fifth, sixth, and seventh nerves were so arranged that they were less vulnerable to traction force than are the eighth cervical and first thoracic. The transverse radicular ligaments are well formed in C5, C6 and C7. They are absent in C8 and D1. There are proximal branches from the ventral primary rami to the phrenic nerve (C5) to the nerve to serratus anterior (C5, C6, C7) and to the scalene muscles (C5, C6). Again C8 and D1 do not have these proximal branches.

The vertebral artery lies anterior to the brachial plexus and is in particularly close relation to C5 and C6. It supplies radicular vessels to the spinal nerves, which are particularly abundant about C7. These communicate with the anterior spinal arteries. A Brown–Séquard syndrome of varying severity is found in about 5% of complete avulsion injuries, and it is tempting to speculate that this indicates impairment of the blood supply of the spinal cord. Bleeding following rupture of the radicular vessels may be profuse: we have seen, in one case of avulsion, compression of the trachea from bleeding of the vessels about C7 so severe as to demand urgent tracheostomy.

Table 9.1 Preganglionic injury

Type	
A	Roots torn central to transitional zone. True avulsion
B	Roots torn distal to transitional zone
Type 1	Dura torn within spinal canal, DRG displaced into neck
Type 2	Dura torn at mouth of foramen: DRG more or less displaced
Type 3	Dura not torn. DRG not displaced
Type 4	Dura not torn. DRG not displaced, either ventral or dorsal roots intact

DRG, dorsal root ganglion.

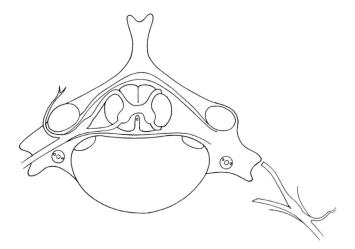

Fig. 9.1 Type A: avulsion distal to the transitional zone, the dura torn within the canal.

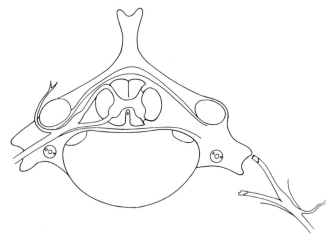

Fig. 9.2 Type B1: avulsion central to the transitional zone.

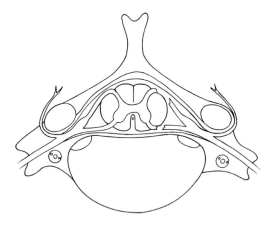

Fig. 9.3 Type B2: rupture of roots within the spinal canal without displacement of the dorsal root ganglion or rupture of the dura.

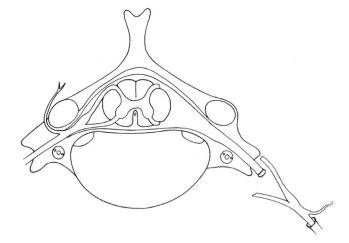

Fig. 9.4 Type B3: the dural sleeve is intact as far as the mouth of the foramen.

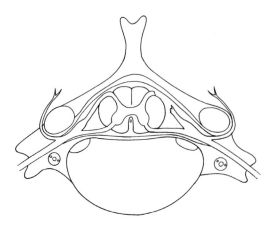

Fig. 9.5 Type B4: avulsion confined to dorsal (as shown) or ventral root.

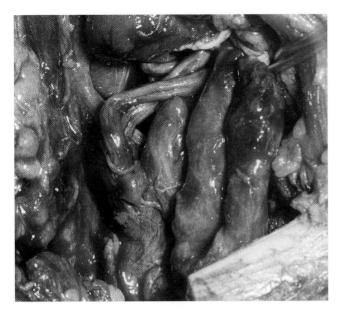

Fig. 9.6 Total avulsion. Note the variation in level of rupture of the dura and extent of displacement of dorsal root ganglia.

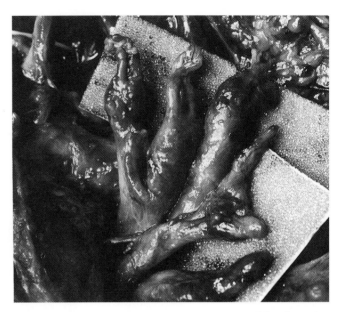

Fig. 9.7 Total avulsion. The dorsal and ventral roots of T1, C8, and C7 are seen. The ruptures of the roots of C6 and C5 are more distal.

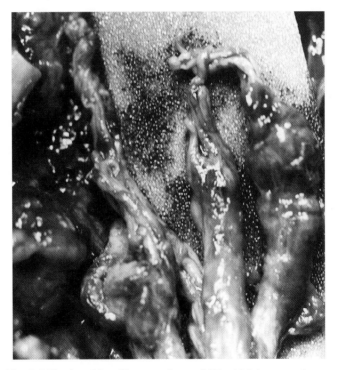

Fig. 9.8 Total avulsion. The ventral root of C6, which is stouter, is ruptured more peripherally than the dorsal root. Note the varying levels of rupture of the rootlets of the other avulsed spinal nerves.

Figs 9.9 to 9.11 Intradural rupture seen at hemilaminectomy.

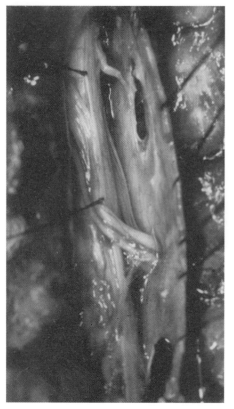

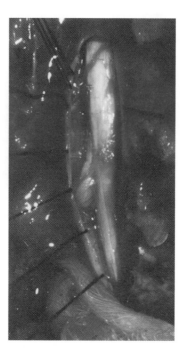

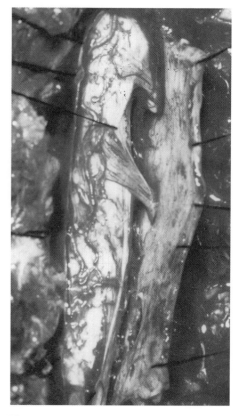

Fig. 9.9 Avulsion of C5 and C7. Intact C6. Note the peripheral rupture of the dorsal root of C5.

Fig. 9.10 The ventral root of C8 is intact, the dorsal root has been avulsed central to the peripheral zone.

Fig. 9.11 Intact C5 and C6; central avulsion of C7 and C8.

Course in the neck

The anterior primary rami enter the posterior triangle of the neck as the *roots* of the brachial plexus between scalenus anterior and scalenus medius. The first thoracic nerve passes upward round the neck of the first rib, behind the pleura, and behind the vertebral artery and the first part of the subclavian artery. This course renders the nerve vulnerable in fractures or dislocations of the first rib. The formation of the *trunks* of the brachial plexus is fairly consistent. C5 and C6 form the upper trunk, the middle trunk is a continuation of C7, the lower trunk is from C8 and T1. These lie in front of one another rather than side by side, with the subclavian artery passing anteromedially. The relations with the cervical plexus and phrenic nerve are useful in identifying C5, and hence the rest of the plexus, in difficult dissections. The phrenic nerve crosses C5 to pass anteromedially on the surface of scalenus anterior. The transverse cervical and greater auricular

nerves wind round the posterior border of the sterno-mastoid no more than 1 cm cephalad; the spinal accessory nerve emerges from deep to the sternocleidomastoid about 5 mm further cephalad. Although much has been written about pre- and postfixation of the brachial plexus, in fact contributions from C4 are uncommon and contributions from T2 are extremely rare. A significant branch from C4 to C5 or to the upper trunk is encountered in 2–3% of operated cases. We have seen the suprascapular nerve arising directly from C4 in one case, the musculo-cutaneous nerve so arose in two instances. A branch from C4 to C5 gives further protection from avulsion to that root, a feature which we have found in six adult cases and in one case of obstetric palsy in which only the fifth nerve had suffered postganglionic rupture, all others having been avulsed. We have never encountered T2 innervating skeletal muscle in the upper limb, and have seen just one case where T1 did not contribute to the plexus (Fig. 9.12).

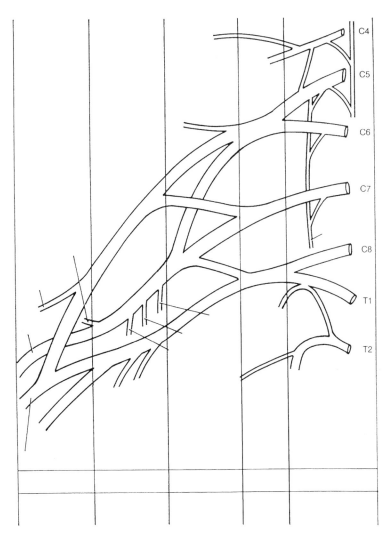

Fig. 9.12 Scheme of the brachial plexus.

Three significant nerves pass from the brachial plexus within the posterior triangle:

1. The nerve to serratus anterior is formed by rami from C5 and C6, which pass deep to scalenus medius: they may be compressed by a fibrous arcade. C4 contributes to this nerve in one-third of cases, and C7 in about one-half.
2. The nerve to the rhomboids (C5) may be conjoined with the ramus to the nerve to the serratus. It leaves C5 within the foramen lying posterior to the main trunk.
3. The suprascapular nerve passes away from C5, or from the proximal part of the upper trunk a finger's breadth above the clavicle, passing laterally and then posteriorly through the suprascapular notch.

The *divisions* of the brachial plexus lie deep to the clavicle and their display in a scarred field can be particularly tedious. The posterior division of the upper trunk is consistently larger than the anterior; this is true also for the middle trunk. In some 10% of cases there is no posterior division of the lower trunk. The formation and relations of the three *cords* are variable, and indeed their designations are somewhat misleading. Immediately inferior to the clavicle the posterior cord lies *lateral* to the axillary artery, the medial cord *behind*, and the lateral cord *in front*. The cords assume their appropriate relations about the axillary artery deep to pectoralis minor. Miller (1939) found considerable variation in 9% of 480 dissections of the neurovascular axis. Most commonly the axillary artery lies anterior to the three cords and median nerve.

The branches of the posterior cord, the largest of the three trunks, are consistent: in sequence they are the sub-scapular, the thoracodorsal and the circumflex (axillary) nerves. The branches of the medial cord too are usually predictable: the medial pectoral nerve, the medial cutaneous nerve of the forearm, and then the division into the medial root of the median nerve and the ulnar nerve. Not infrequently, the ulnar nerve arises as two or three branches. The greatest variation in formation of trunk nerves is found within the lateral cord. In about 10% of cases the musculocutaneous nerve arises more distally than usual, springing directly from the lateral cord as two or three branches, or even from the median nerve itself. Sometimes the highest of these branches enters the coracobrachialis muscle no more than 2–3 cm below the coracoid process, and in this site it is at risk during operations for habitual dislocation of the shoulder. The lateral root of the median nerve may arise as two or three branches, and in some cases it appears as a branch of the musculocutaneous nerve. It is useful to be aware of these variations of the formation of the plexus and of its relation to the great vessels, because they can cause difficulties during urgent exploration.

Blood supply

Abdulla and Bowden (1960) showed that the blood supply of the brachial plexus arose through vessels from the subclavian and vertebral arteries. Important branches pass from the vertebral artery to the roots of C6, C5 and the more proximal cervical nerves. Branches from the costocervical trunk provide a rich supply to T1 and C8. Two major arteries arise from the thyrocervical trunk: the suprascapular, which runs behind the clavicle, in front of the brachial plexus and the subclavian vein, and into the supraspinous fossa; and the superficial cervical artery, which crosses anterior to the phrenic nerve and the scalenus anterior, becoming bound down to the upper trunk of the brachial plexus by the prevertebral fascia. Here the artery is 2–3 mm in diameter and it is very useful in vascularising a free ulnar nerve graft. The dorsal scapular artery may arise from the third part of the subclavian artery to pass between the upper and middle trunks. It is a cause of substantial bleeding in a scarred field. In at least one-third of cases the superficial cervical artery and the dorsal scapular vessel arise as the transverse cervical artery, a branch of the thyrocervical trunk. The great vessels and their branches are particularly at risk in severe closed traction lesions and in open wounds. Obliteration of the transverse cervical vessels is a frequent finding in irradiation neuropathy: thrombosis of the subclavian–axillary artery being a recognised late complication of irradiation (Butler et al 1980, Barros d'Sa 1992a).

Functional distribution

The cutaneous distribution of the fifth cervical nerve does not extend below the elbow; the sixth cervical nerve consistently innervates the thumb and index finger; the first thoracic nerve does not innervate the skin of the hand. There are, however, frequent and important variations.

The variations of supply amongst the spinal nerves within the brachial plexus are far more important than pre- or postfixation, and this is particularly true for the 7th and 8th cervical and first thoracic nerves.

The fifth cervical nerve regularly controls extension, abduction, and lateral rotation of the shoulder. The sixth cervical usually innervates biceps, brachialis, brachioradialis, pronator teres, supinator and extensor carpi radialis longus. The seventh cervical nerve gives widespread innervation throughout the limb: in those unusual instances where it alone is damaged, the patient will note a rather diffuse loss of function throughout the upper limb, without complete anaesthesia or paralysis of any significant muscle group. It consistently supplies latissimus dorsi. The eighth cervical nerve innervates the extensors of the digits and of the thumb in at least one-third of cases, and the first thoracic nerve does this and also innervates the triceps in at least 10%. It is useful to bear these variations in mind in clinical examination of the injured plexus and in interpreting neurophysiological evidence (Figs 9.13 to 9.15).

Microanatomy

The arrangement of nerve fibres within their bundles has been extensively analysed by, among others, Sunderland (1978), Narakas (1978), Slingluff et al (1987) and Bonnel (1989). Their work was stimulated by interest in repair of traction lesion and, although no really accurate map of the changing arrangement of the bundles throughout the brachial plexus exists, this is an essential basis in operations for repair. There is agreement that the total number of myelinated fibres in the brachial plexus in the adult is between 120 000 and 150 000, and that fully 25% of these innervate the shoulder girdle and glenohumeral joint. The fifth cervical and first thoracic nerves contain the least number of myelinated fibres, between 15 000 and 20 000; the eighth nerve is usually the largest, containing about 30 000 myelinated fibres. Harris (1904) suggested that the proportion of motor fibres was highest in C5 and then C8 and was least in C7 and D1. He thought that the sensory contribution was greatest in C7, then C6 and then C8. The segregation of nerve fibres is established well proximally, so that the suprascapular nerve can be traced to an anterior bundle within C5 at the level of the anterior tubercle. One bundle, controlling the radial extensors of the wrist, can be consistently displayed within the posterior division of the upper trunk when exploration is performed within 36–48 hours after injury. This, of itself, is a strong argument in favour of urgent exploration in appropriate cases. This anatomical evidence has further been supported by microneurography. Schady et al (1983) stimulated within fascicles of the proximal median nerve in volunteers, and showed segregation of muscle and sensory fibres.

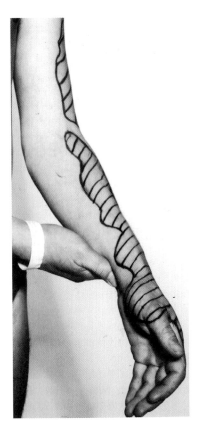

Fig. 9.13 Rupture of C5 and C6. Sensory loss does not extend to the thumb and index finger.

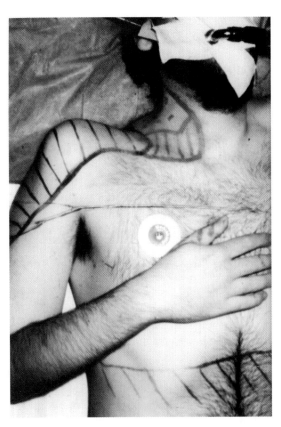

Fig. 9.14 In this patient with T6 spinal cord lesion and on clinical examination, C5 and C6 lesion, operation showed avulsion of C5, C6 and C7.

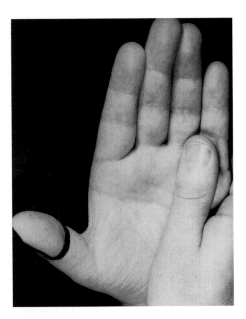

Fig. 9.15 This patient had full power in intrinsic muscles and in the digital flexor and extensors. There was sweating throughout the hand. Loss of sensation was confined to the tip of the thumb. At operation, C5, C6, C7 and C8 were found avulsed; only the first thoracic nerve was intact.

HISTORY OF TREATMENT OF LESIONS OF THE BRACHIAL PLEXUS

Injuries of the brachial plexus are the worst of all peripheral nerve lesions. In many cases the damage lies between the posterior root ganglion and the spinal cord. To these injuries Bonney (1954) applied the term "preganglionic", and this designation will be used here interchangeably with "intradural" to signify rupture or avulsion of roots within the spinal canal. There are two types of this injury. Intradural rupture implies tearing of the rootlets at or peripheral to the transitional zone; avulsion means that rootlets are torn from the spinal cord itself, and the injury is central to the transitional zone. We think that cord damage, in the form of the Brown–Séquard syndrome, found in 2–5% of complete lesions, is caused by these central avulsion injuries. Most of these lesions are caused by great violence, and the subclavian or axillary artery is frequently ruptured. Life-threatening associated injuries to the head, the chest and the viscera are common, and associated fractures of long bones are the rule. There is a long history of surgical endeavour in repair of the brachial plexus, and review of the literature shows alternation between optimism and pessimism. Our own approach can be summarised in quite bald terms: accurate diagnosis is essential in determining prognosis; all reasonable attempts should be made to improve that prognosis. From this flows a policy of early exploration and repair, of urgent attention to the vascular injury and of treatment designed to neutralise associated fractures.

Probably the first suture of a closed traction lesion of the brachial plexus was performed by Thoburn of Manchester in 1896 (Thoburn 1900). The patient, a mill girl, was aged 16 years, and 7 months previously had been injured at work. The limb was completely paralysed. At operation he excised a massive neuroma of the upper trunk and approximated the ends with fine silk sutures. Some recovery was noted at 7 months. Ultimately his patient regained partial flexion of the elbow and of the wrist. *Kennedy*, of Glasgow, described three cases of repair in 1903. One of these was an infant with birth lesion, and Kennedy noted a good return of shoulder and elbow function after suture of the upper trunk. Clark et al (1905) amassed a series of cases of repair, numbering over 70 by 1920, and Sharpe (1916) reported on 56 cases of operative treatment of birth palsy. This early endeavour fell away because of difficulty of intraoperative diagnosis and difficulty in accurately assessing outcome of the nerve repair, and also because there were postanaesthetic deaths. The work of these pioneers, and of those who followed them, is admirably set out by Leffert (1985) and Narakas (1991). One early contribution particularly worthy of note is that of Frazier and Skillerne (1911), who performed cervical laminectomy with the aim of posterior rhizotomy for the relief of pain in a patient with closed traction lesion of the brachial plexus.

They showed that the left "anterior and posterior roots of the 6th, 7th and 8th cervical nerves were absent. The roots evidently had been torn completely from the cord."

The Medical Research Council's (1954) report on peripheral nerve injuries is an example of detailed and systematic study which has not been surpassed. Brooks (1954) reviewed the outcome from 170 cases of open wound of the brachial plexus. He concluded that "with the possible exception of lesions of the upper trunk, operative repair is valueless". In fact, few of these patients had operations for repair. Seddon (1963) took a similar view about repair in the closed traction lesion, indicating that, with the possible exception of upper trunk lesions, this too was worthless. The pessimistic approach gained further support from Nulsen and Slade (1956), who contributed to the monumental work edited by Woodhall and Beebe which described peripheral nerve injuries treated in the Veterans Administration Hospitals in the USA during the Second World War. They reported on 117 cases, and concluded that the prognosis for stretch injuries of the brachial plexus could not be improved by operation. It is not a little surprising that this verdict was returned at a time when the diagnostic and technical basis of virtually all modern work had already been established, mainly in the UK. Bonney (1954) made plain the distinction between pre- and postganglionic injury, and devised physiological tests to discriminate between the two. Davis et al (1966) and Yeoman (1968) confirmed the value and the limitations of myelography. Seddon (1947 and 1963) referring to much of Brooks' work had given nerve grafting respectability, and Seddon (1963) recorded the first clearly documented success from intercostal transfer to restore active flexion of the elbow, the operation performed with Yeoman. Strange (1947) developed the technique of the pedicled ulnar nerve graft, the forerunner of the free vascularised nerve graft. Young and Medawar (1940) introduced fibrin clot glue as an alternative to suturing.

In the 1960s and early 1970s, many patients in the UK with complete lesions of the brachial plexus were treated by early amputation, glenohumeral arthrodesis, and fitting with a prosthesis. Ransford and Hughes (1977) showed that only a small minority of patients actually used their prosthesis. Although Bonney persisted with operations to establish diagnosis and, where reasonable, to effect a repair, renewed interest was stimulated by the work of Millesi, Narakas, and others in Europe and, a little later, by surgeons in Japan. Millesi's first publication appeared in German in 1968, that from Narakas and Verdan in 1969. In 1977 they presented their preliminary results, Millesi of 56 patients with a 5-year follow-up, Narakas with 107 patients of whom 60 had been followed for more than 2 years. They analysed the findings at operation and showed that useful results could be obtained using microsurgical techniques for nerve repairs. Allieu (1975) described 34 of his own cases, and referred to the work of

Alnot, Mansat and Sedel. Jamieson and Bonney (1979) analysed findings at operation in 76 patients, and Jamieson and Hughes (1980) studied the results in 31 of these patients who underwent repair. They found that "the surgical repair of the plexus does produce reasonable results, while late repair is unrewarding". Alnot et al (1981) reported on 100 cases operated on between 1974 and 1979. Sedel described the natural history in over 100 cases in 1977, and in 1988 described the results of repair in supraclavicular lesions. Much of this work is set out in the volumes edited by Alnot and Narakas (1989 and 1986) which are essential reading. Millesi reviewed his experience in 1991, in the same volume as that in which Narakas wrote a masterly account of nerve transfer.

Epidemiology: natural history

Three publications describe the natural history of severe traction lesion where no nerve repair had been performed. Bonney (1959) followed 25 patients for a minimum of 2 years and found that pain was worse in those with no recovery. Yeoman, whose work is extensively referred to by Seddon (1975), studied 180 patients; of the 99 patients with complete lesions, only 13 showed useful recovery. He noted that in two-thirds of patients presenting with an injury of the 5th and 6th cervical nerves useful flexion of the elbow recovered spontaneously, and this occurred in 40% of the patients presenting with injuries to the 5th, 6th and 7th nerves. Yeoman noted that severe pain persisted in 32 of his 46 cases of complete paralysis; of the 40 with paralysis but later recovery of elbow flexion, 22 noted severe pain. Wynn Parry et al (1987) took the opportunity to follow over 500 cases, first at RAF Chessington, later at the Royal National Orthopaedic Hospital. They found increasing severity of the injury, and collected a total of 181 patients with complete lesions. Although he found that about two-thirds of patients with C5 and C6 lesions regained elbow flexion, this occurred in only one-third of those with C5, C6 and C7 lesions, and very few of his complete lesions regained any worthwhile function at all.

Epidemiology: incidence

Although individual units have accumulated much experience and large series, accurate information about the incidence, causation, social background and social consequences of a brachial plexus injury is hard to find. In 1987, Goldie and Coates (1992) asked Fellows of the British Orthopaedic Association for information about patients with closed traction lesions. They received replies to 55% of requests, 402 in all, and uncovered 254 patients admitted with complete or partial lesions. From this it seems reasonable to assume that between 450 and 500 patients suffer severe and permanent damage from closed supraclavicular lesion every year in the UK. Wilbourn

(1993) reviewed published work from the military series from World War One and World War Two, finding that the injury to the brachial plexus accounted for 4–9% of all peripheral nervous lesions and 6–12% of injuries within the upper limb. Rosson (1988) made two studies of motor cyclists transferred to our unit (1987–1988). He found that 91 of 106 patients injured in motor cycle accidents were aged less than 25 years, and of these 43 held only a provisional licence. One-third of their machines had an engine capacity of 125 cc or less. In his 1987 study of 102 motor cyclists treated in the years 1985 and 1986, he discovered a mean age of 21 years, injury to the dominant upper limb in 65, and severe injury to the head, the chest, the viscera or other limbs in 51. Over one-third of his patients followed for more than 1 year remained unemployed. Two-thirds of his patients remained in severe pain at over 1 year from injury.

Epidemiology: mechanism of injury

The earliest description of traction lesion is that by Flaubert (1827), who described the late reduction of dislocation of shoulder by manual traction. Six students pulled upon the limb, the result was catastrophic and the patient later died. Flaubert noted a Bernard–Horner sign long before this was formally described, and also described an affection of the cord. At necropsy a rupture of C5 was found, with avulsion of C6, C7, C8 and D1, and rupture of the subclavian artery. The radicular vessels had also been ruptured, leading to a haematoma within the spinal canal. In order to study the mechanism of damage, Horsley (1899) dropped cadavers on their heads; Duval and Guillain (1898 and 1901) studied the effects of direct traction upon the nerve roots. Barnes (1949) recognised the importance of the posture of the arm, pointing out that with the limb adducted the brunt of injury was borne by the upper roots of the brachial plexus, whereas with the arm abducted and extended the lower roots were more vulnerable. His analysis gives some understanding of the infraclavicular injury, which in fact is caused by violent extension of the upper limb with the arm abducted.

Leffert (1985) draws on Steven's model (1934). With the arm at 90° of abduction the axis of force passes through C7. With the arm adducted, the first rib concentrates the force on the lower roots. If a weight falls on the shoulder, however, the upper roots suffer most. If the arm is abducted, then the coracoid acts as a pulley and force is transmitted along the line of the cords, falling chiefly on the lower roots of the plexus. Brunelli and Brunelli (1991) described four cases of an intermediate type of plexus injury, part of the injury being borne by C6, C7 and the middle trunks.

In fact there is one common element underlying closed traction lesion, and that is the violent distraction of the forequarter from the head, neck and chest. The angle

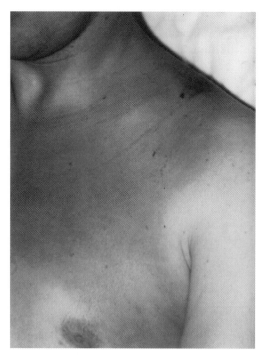

Fig. 9.16 This motor cyclist struck his shoulder against a traffic bollard. There was total avulsion.

between the head and shoulder is open, and one of the most important physical signs supporting this proposal is the presence of linear abrasions on the chin and on the face, with corresponding abrasions and bruising at the tip of the shoulder. We have seen complete avulsion of the brachial plexus from weights falling on the shoulder. In other cases the patient was able to give a clear history of the shoulder colliding with an immovable object. In these cases there was avulsion or high rupture of C5, C6 and C7. Although it is often said that these are injuries of high speed accidents, we have also seen complete avulsion in pedal cyclists and in motor cyclists whose speed at the time of accident was 25 mph or less (Fig. 9.16).

Wilbourn (1993) proposes causation by: traction; contusion, as from a gunshot wound; compression, as from exuberant callus after fracture of the clavicle; laceration; and ischaemia. His last group is particularly relevant in understanding the cause of lesion in radiation neuropathy and in neurovascular injury.

Epidemiology: major types of lesion

It is convenient to separate supraclavicular from retro- and infraclavicular lesions. The supraclavicular lesion is the most common: it is caused by distraction of the head from the upper limb; it is characterised by a high incidence of rupture or of pre-ganglionic injury to the spinal nerves forming the plexus. Rupture of the subclavian artery

occurs in about 15% of these cases, damage to the spinal cord is found in 5% of complete lesions. The retroclavicular lesion is surprisingly infrequent: it involves the divisions of the brachial plexus, and there is a high incidence of associated vascular lesions. In the infraclavicular injury there is rupture of the axillary artery in nearly 30% of cases; the neural injury is complex and variable, with ruptures of cords or of the terminal branches, the proximal stump usually being at the level of the coracoid deep to the pectoralis minor. In about 20% of cases there is associated preganglionic injury of the lowermost roots of the brachial plexus. In general, the mildest form of infraclavicular lesion is that associated with anterior dislocation of the shoulder, although even here there may be rupture of nerves, in particular of the circumflex.

The distinction according to level is to some extent artificial: there is overlap between these categories, with double lesions of supraclavicular lesion combined with more distal rupture occurring in about 10% of cases. Alnot (1988) and Narakas (1984a) found this double lesion in 8.5–15% of their cases. Nonetheless, we agree with Leffert in recognising the infraclavicular lesion as a distinct entity, taking the true retroclavicular lesion as being rather rare. It is caused by violent hyperextension at the shoulder; there is almost always a fracture of shaft of humerus or injury to the glenohumeral joint; the incidence of vascular injury is much higher; the level of proximal rupture is deep to pectoralis minor, which acts as a guillotine on the neurovascular bundle (Fig. 9.17).

It is useful to separate the more common and more difficult lesion above the clavicle, with its high incidence of injury to the roots and of intradural injury, from those predominantly below the clavicle. The cause, the pattern of injury, and the surgical approach are quite distinct.

DIAGNOSIS

Clinical features

Careful clinical examination allows a fairly accurate diagnosis, not only of the extent but also the level of injury, in the majority of cases. Particularly important features from the history include the violence of the injury and the mode of application of force to the damaged limb.

Case report. A 19-year-old rugby player went in for a low tackle, his shoulder struck the opponent's shin and he noted a severe lightning shoot of pain extending from the shoulder to the tip of the thumb. After this the whole arm was paralysed, but he rapidly regained function of the forearm and hand. He continued to experience burning pain along the radial aspect of the forearm, with occasional shooting bursts of pain. On examination paralysis was confined to those muscles supplied by the 5th and 6th cervical nerves. There was no Tinel sign. At operation preganglionic injury of C5 and C6 was confirmed.

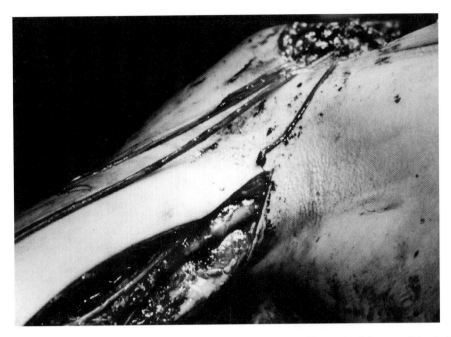

Fig. 9.17 A 21-year-old motor cyclist whose extended arm was struck by an oncoming lorry. He sustained fracture of the shaft of the humerus, rupture of the axillary artery deep to the pectoralis minor, and rupture of all trunk nerves at different levels in the upper limb. The ulnar and musculocutaneous nerves were ruptured in the arm; the radial and median nerves (above) were avulsed from the forearm.

In five other patients, injured in tobogganing or climbing accidents, who were able to give a clear account of a violent impact on the shoulder, the findings at operation were similar. A more extreme example of the value of knowing how the injury occurred is given by a 48-year-old seamstress who was walking along the road and was struck on her right side by a collapsing wall. She remembers the wall striking her shoulder; she suffered severe contusion of the chest and multiple fractures of ribs. In her case, C4 to T1 were avulsed. The description of pain in a proximal injury to the brachial plexus is characteristic, and in at least one-half of patients it begins at the moment of injury. In those who are rendered unconscious, pain is noticeable on recovery from the head injury. The description of pain is so precise that in many cases diagnosis of preganglionic lesion can be made from the history alone. There is a constant crushing or burning pain, sometimes described as intense pins and needles experienced chiefly in the forearm and hand in the area of anaesthesia. The superimposition of lightning shoots of pain coursing down the whole of the limb with extreme severity is diagnostic of preganglionic injury to the spinal nerve innervating that part of the limb. We might contrast this with the case of multiple cranial nerve palsies described by Smith (1995). His patient, a motor cyclist, was knocked off his machine, sustaining a head injury, fracture of left clavicle and crush fracture of the eighth thoracic vertebral body. The left side of the neck was bruised and swollen, and there was a friction burn from the strap of the helmet which had been wrenched from his head. He presented at 2 months with left-sided palsies of the spinal accessory (anterior to sternomastoid), hypoglossal superior laryngeal and cervical sympathetic nerves. The level of lesion was clearly established by the site of the burn: the prediction of good prognosis, for this was crush injury, not a traction lesion, was confirmed by later progress to full recovery.

The distribution of abrasions or bruises about the neck and shoulder girdle is important. Occasionally deep linear cuts passing from the face towards the tip of the shoulder indicate the violence of distraction of the limb from the head; a fractured or battered motor cycle helmet is useful in confirming this. Deep bruising in the posterior triangle is a most important sign, indicating rupture of the prevertebral muscles and, possibly, rupture of the subclavian artery (Fig. 9.18). Linear bruising along the limb suggests rupture of a distal nerve trunk. The extent of anaesthesia is worth careful examination, for when this extends above the clavicle, involving the branches of the cervical plexus, proximal injury of C5 and of C6 is certain (Figs 9.19 and 9.20). Measurement of muscular power is difficult in the early hours after injury in a patient who is in great pain or, at least, confused, but weakness of the trapezius and paralysis of the serratus anterior are important evidence of intradural injury of the upper roots of the plexus. Swelling in the posterior triangle indicates one of two things: collection of spinal fluid from avulsed roots, or an expanding haematoma from rupture of vessels. The Bernard–Horner sign is an important indication of the fate of the lower

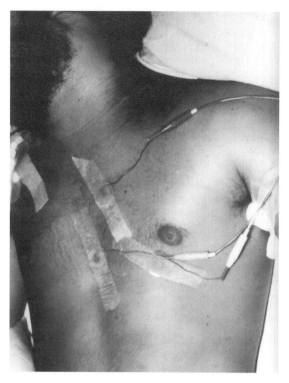

Fig. 9.18 Rupture of subclavian artery with total avulsion.

roots (Fig. 9.21). It is not an absolute indication of avulsion of C8 and T1. Narakas and Hentz (1988) found this sign in 10% of their patients who later went on to recover function through the lower trunk, and they also found the sign was not present in a further 10% of cases in which avulsion of C8 and D1 was confirmed. Furthermore, it may not be evident for the first 48 hours after injury. Nonetheless, it remains a strong indicator of the level of lesion (Fig. 9.22). One physical sign is of particular significance in the detection of a postganglionic rupture, and it should be sought with care. Tinel described this in 1917: "when compression or percussion is lightly applied to the injured nerve trunk, we often find, in the cutaneous region of the nerve, a creeping sensation usually compared by the patient to that caused by electricity. Formication in the nerve is a very important sign, for it indicates the presence of young axis cylinders in process of regeneration."

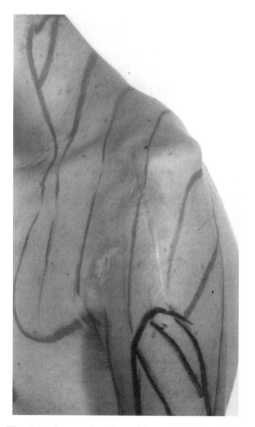

Fig. 9.19 Sensory loss in avulsion of C4, C5 and C6.

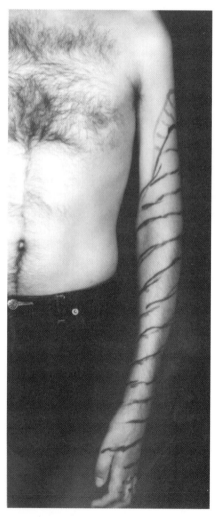

Fig. 9.20 Sensory loss in avulsion of C5 to T1. C4 innervates the skin of the outer aspect of the shoulder; T2 innervates the skin of the inner aspect of the arm.

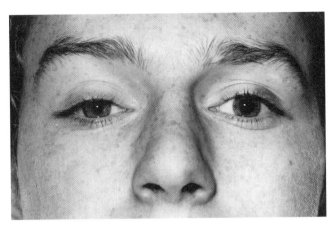

Fig. 9.21 Bernard–Horner sign in avulsion of C7, C8 and T1.

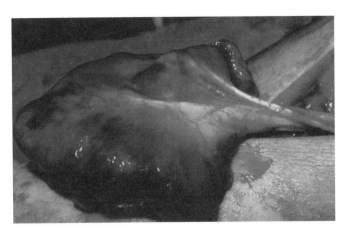

Fig. 9.22 Complete avulsion. At the elbow we found the pronator teres avulsed from its origin, there was rupture of the median nerve and of the radial artery.

Although Tinel thought that this sign appeared at about the fourth to sixth week after the wound, we regularly find it within days of closed traction lesion. Percussion deep to the sternomastoid may elicit really quite painful paraesthesiae in the relevant dermatome. We have found this to be an extremely reliable indication of rupture of C5 (radiation as far as the elbow), C6 (to the thumb and index) and C7 (to the dorsum of the hand). When the Tinel sign is weak or where the area of paraesthesia is confined to the skin over the deltoid, then avulsion is more likely, and the sign indicates injury to C4. Copeland and Landi discussed the usefulness of this sign in 1979.

SPECIAL INVESTIGATIONS

These can be summarised as physiological and imaging.

Physiological

Bonney (1954) developed the concept of pre- and postganglionic injury, distinguishing between injuries to the spinal cord and those to peripheral nerves. He described persistence of the axon reflex after injection of histamine, and in 1958 he and Gilliatt recorded sensory action potentials for the median and ulnar nerves of a patient with a complete preganglionic injury of the brachial plexus. Damage to the proximal limb of the axon of the posterior root ganglion cell appeared not to affect the distal axon or its myelin sheath. These two investigations confirmed that afferent axons remain myelinated if they are still in continuity with the dorsal root ganglion, and they are the foundation of all the current neurophysiological investigation work. Recognising that the histamine test is difficult to apply in the hand, Bonney then introduced the cold vasodilation response (1954). If normal fingers are immersed in water at 5°C they cool, rapidly; 5–20 minutes later there is vasodilation and a considerable rise

in skin temperature. This does not occur in denervated fingers, but it does in preganglionic injury.

The histamine response is difficult to use in the hand and in pigmented skin, but it remains very useful in diagnosis for the C5, C6 and D1 dermatomes. Recording of sensory action potentials (SAPs) is also a simple investigation, and it is reliable. If on stimulation of the skin of the thumb (C6), the middle and ring fingers (C7), and the little finger (C8) SAPs can be recorded for median and ulnar nerves, then the injury must be preganglionic. These tests can be applied no sooner than 2 weeks after injury; before this time Wallerian degeneration is incomplete and results may be confusing. Interpretation is modified by variations in distribution within the plexus, by the presence of separate, distal ruptures of nerve trunks, and by the death of nerve cells within the ganglia subjected to such violence that they are pulled into the posterior triangle of the neck or even beyond.

Useful evidence of the level of lesion is acquired by examining those muscles innervated by the dorsal primary ramus. Bufalini and Pescatori introduced this technique in 1969 and showed a reasonable correlation between denervation of the erector spinae muscles and intradural injury of C5 and C6, but the overlap of segmental supply of these muscles does cause difficulties in interpreting the precise root injury. Celli and Rovesta (1987) developed refined and sensitive techniques of electrophysiological examination to determine the level of lesion and to distinguish between avulsion of the ventral and dorsal rootlets. Dissatisfaction with their results in 234 patients operated on between 1971 and 1982 caused them to supplement examination of the stump of the spinal nerve with the operating microscope with neurophysiological investigation. They combined electromyographic examination of paravertebral muscles with pre- and intraoperative sensory evoked sensory recordings from 1980. They found a difference in 8 of 47 roots, indicating selective avulsion of a ventral or dorsal rootlet. This confirms the findings of Bonney (1977), Alnot et al (1981), and Privat et al (1982), who noted that the ventral rootlets are more vulnerable when displayed at hemilaminectomy.

Case report. Mr Simon Kay kindly asked one of us to review a patient in whom the clinical evidence of pre-ganglionic injury to all dorsal rootlets, but preservation of the ventral rootlets of T1, was persuasive. At no time was there any clinical evidence of spinal cord lesion, or of upper motor neuron lesion. He noted the return of finger movement at 3 months; by 18 months there was good power in the intrinsic, long flexor, and extensor muscles. Pain began at the same time as finger movement. It was typical deafferentation pain: constant, in the forearm and hand, and crushing and burning in nature. There was no paroxysmal pain.

We examined the patient at 3 years and found no evidence of cutaneous sensibility – indeed there were scars from unnoticed injury. Sweating was profuse. There was, however, some limited preservation of joint position sense, and a reflex extension jerk of the index finger from tapping the flexed thumb. Intradermal histamine induced flares in the dermatomes of C5, C6, and T1 (medial aspect of the forearm). Dr Nicholas Murray recorded SAPs from the median nerve, but *not* from the ulnar nerve. A magnetic resonance imaging scan performed by Dr Saifuddin showed that the cervical spinal cord was displaced; there was a clearly intact ventral root for T1. The other ventral roots, and all the dorsal roots of the brachial plexus, had been interrupted.

While the absence of ulnar SAPs is inconsistent with this clinical diagnosis, we do think it possible that the afferent fibres responsible for joint position sense passed through the intact ventral root of T1 (see Ch. 2).

Landi et al (1980) recorded cortical evoked potentials through scalp electrodes from nerve stumps stimulated at operation. They compared preoperative with intra-operative somatosensory evoked potentials with surgical findings in 15 patients, finding the investigation most useful in determining the level of injury to the 5th cervical nerve. Jones (1987), Sugioka (1984), and Sugioka and Nagano (1989) report on detailed analyses of pre- and intraoperative neurophysiological records with the findings at operation. Hetreed et al (1992) demonstrated the sensitivity of recording sensory evoked potentials through epidural electrodes inserted into the upper part of the cervical canal. There are limitations to this mode of investigation. It is not quantitative. Our colleague Liang Chen has kindly released his, as yet unpublished, findings in 100 of our consecutive cases, followed for a minimum of 2 years. He found that repair of postganglionic ruptures of spinal nerves failed when sensory evoked potentials were abnormal or absent. Intraoperative recording is sensitive to scarring about the exposed spinal nerve, and sensory recording will not detect cases in which there is isolated intradural injury of the ventral rootlets alone. Absence of potentials in preoperative work indicates that afferent nerve fibres have degenerated, but this will not distinguish between degeneration caused by postganglionic rupture and that following death of the neuron within an injured dorsal root ganglion. We have used intraoperative evoked potential studies since 1977, and find these particularly important in early cases. As Tinel (1917) said: "Naturally we must not neglect the objective examination and physiological exploration of the nerve exposed by intervention; of all the processes suggested for this examination we shall find that there is only one that is logical and capable of being utilised: the electrical exploration of the exposed nerve as propounded and carried out by P. Marie and Meige."

In explorations performed within days of injury there is still the potential hazard of missing avulsion of the ventral rootlets, because the proximal branches of the spinal nerves will still conduct to their relevant muscles. Gilliatt and Hjorth (1972) found that, after section of a motor nerve, after 2 or 3 days there was cessation of conduction at the neuromuscular junction. Our observations suggest that after avulsion or rupture a motor response to stimulation of the distal stump persists for at least 2 or 3 days: we have seen this as late as 10 days from injury.

Imaging

Plain radiographs are a source of useful evidence. Fracture or dislocation of the first rib with avulsion of the tip of the transverse process of C7 indicates proximal injury of C7, C8 and D1. Elevation of the ipsilateral diaphragm confirms a phrenic nerve palsy, and is an indication of the level of injury of C5 and C6. Roaf (1963) noted the significance of the tilting of the spine away from the level of injury, and the opening of the intervertebral spaces, a feature of the most violent traction lesions and usually associated with avulsion of the whole of the plexus (Fig. 9.23). In one group of patients the radiological features are quite characteristic, showing depression of the shoulder girdle and lateral displacement of the scapula. This is the worst of all injuries to the brachial plexus. Avulsion of C4 to T1 is usually found; rupture of the subclavian artery is almost inevitable. Ebraheim et al (1988) identified 13 such patients: three died from haemorrhage, and seven of those who survived had complete plexus palsy (Fig. 9.24).

Yeoman (1968) compared myelography with findings at operation, and confirmed that the investigation was a useful one. He described the different radiological findings in preganglionic injury, and pointed out that meningoceles are more common for the 8th cervical and first thoracic nerves. He also emphasised the importance of the tilting of the cervical spine as an indication of severity of injury. Davis et al (1966) also compared radiological and

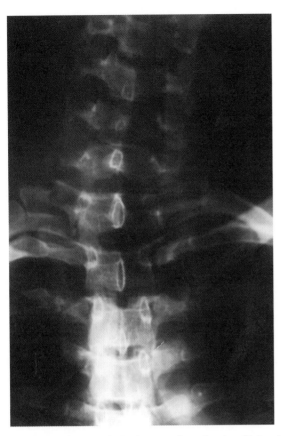

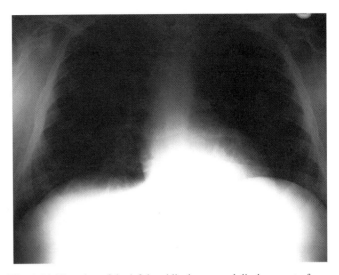

Fig. 9.24 Elevation of the left hemidiaphragm and displacement of the left shoulder girdle in C4 and T1 lesion, with rupture of the subclavian artery.

Fig. 9.23 Tilting of the cervical spine away from the site of injury in avulsion of C5, C6 and C7.

operative evidence. However, myelography particularly by oil-soluble media was found to underestimate the severity of injury, notably in the case of the 5th and 6th nerves. In early days we used myodil extensively, introducing the medium under general anaesthesia, screening it through the cervical region, and withdrawing it before proceeding to operation (Fig. 9.25). Nagano et al (1989c) reviewed 90 cases where metrizamide was used in patients whose plexus was later explored, and confirmed that the water-soluble medium does allow more precise delineation of the spinal nerves within the spinal canal (Fig. 9.26). David Sutton introduced computed tomography (CT) scanning with contrast enhancement at St Mary's Hospital, London, in 1983 and Marshall and De Silva (1986) compared the CT scan with the myelograph and the findings at operation in 16 cases. They confirmed that CT scans with contrast enhancement were a good deal more accurate, particularly for C5 and C6, than the standard myelographs, and that in some of their cases the dorsal and ventral roots could plainly be seen (Fig. 9.27). This most useful technique has now been widely adopted. Magnetic resonance imaging is of great value in displaying lesions of the spinal cord, but as yet it has been disappointing in demonstrating the intradural rootlets (Figs 9.28 and 9.29).

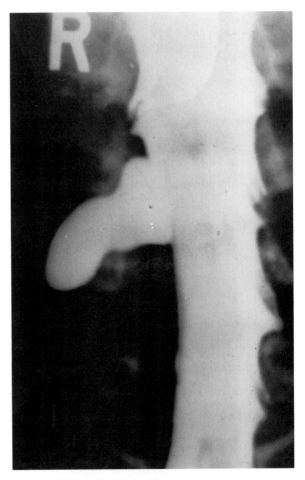

Fig. 9.25 Myelogram showing avulsion of C6, C7, C8 and T1. Note the deviation of the theca.

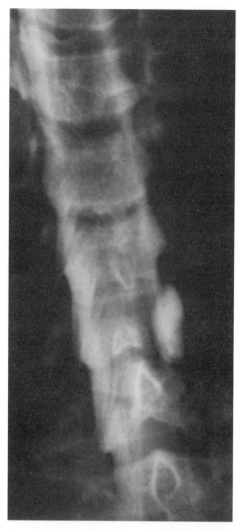

What then are the indications for urgent imaging techniques? Early myelography is most unpleasant for the patient, it is potentially hazardous in those who have suffered a head injury, and, because of the leak of contrast medium through the torn dura, interpretation may be impossible. We no longer use myelography in the acute phase. Magnetic resonance imaging is an excellent indicator of bleeding within the spinal canal with displacement of the spinal cord, and this method of investigation should surely be undertaken in a patient presenting with evidence of cord lesion. We hope that refinements in magnetic resonance imaging will permit the display of the ventral and dorsal roots, and the level of their lesion. The role of angiography will be discussed separately with the vascular lesion.

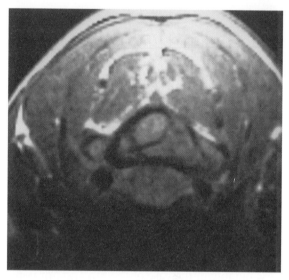

Fig. 9.28 Magnetic resonance scan in a 9-year-old boy with complete lesion. Note the displacement of the cord.

Fig. 9.26 Myelogram with water-soluble medium. The root shadows of C5 and C6 are blunted, there is a pouch at C7, and a defect in the contrast column at C8. All four nerves were avulsed.

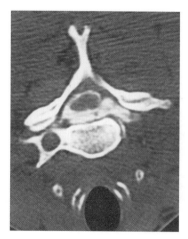

Fig. 9.27 CT myelogram showing avulsion of C6.

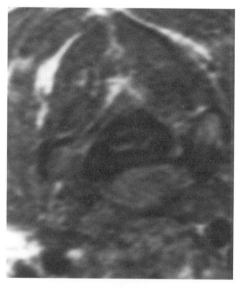

Fig. 9.29 Post-traumatic syrinx 8 years after complete lesion.

BRACHIAL PLEXUS: INDICATIONS AND TECHNIQUES OF OPERATION

Operation is indicated when there is evidence of section or rupture of the brachial plexus. We believe that in closed traction lesion operation should be performed on reasonable suspicion of rupture or avulsion as soon as the patient's general condition permits. Fractures of long bones are no contraindication; severe injuries to the head, chest or abdomen are. Vascular injury strengthens the case for urgent operation. While diagnosis is straightforward in the open wound, gunshot and missile injuries present added difficulty from contamination. Retained missiles embedded in the plexus are a notable cause of severe pain; in particular of causalgia. The gunshot injury to the neck and root of the limb is often fatal, but there are other cases in which limbs are salvageable. The extent of soft tissue damage and of contamination is severe and not always apparent on first examination. The associated vascular injury in these "untidy" wounds poses the very difficult problem of sepsis within ischaemic tissue. Because of the urgent necessity of treatment of many of the associated vascular lesions, we shall consider them first: those from gunshot wounds are considered separately in Chapter 8. The clinical material is set out in Table 9.2.

THE VASCULAR LESION

In the 1960s, one of us (G.B.) introduced a policy of urgent repair of nerve and vessels in the combined neurovascular injury, a policy which has been followed ever since.

Repair of nerves and of vessels was performed within 48 hours in 74 cases, and later than this in 44 more cases. Of 32 cases where repair of the artery was performed in the referring hospital, we found it necessary to revise this. Diagnosis of aneurysm or arteriovenous fistula was made between 10 days and 4 years from the causal injury. It seems to be incontrovertible that proper repair of the vascular lesion is the single most important factor in governing prognosis in all those within the surgeon's control. Furthermore, delay in the repair of nerves after arterial repair presents technical difficulty that is sometimes insuperable, and invariably diminishes the level of functional return.

Open

The level of arterial injury is not necessarily related to the entry wound. One false aneurysm was caused by a gunshot wound in the opposite arm, 4 years previously: a fragment in this arm migrated around the chest wall and embedded itself in the wall of the axillary artery of the opposite limb. In another case of high velocity missile injury the entry point was the anterior axillary line, and the exit wound lay at the spine of the scapula. Arteriovenous fistula between the subclavian artery and vein developed where these traversed the first rib.

Complete section of the artery does not inevitably lead to exsanguination, as the vessel may constrict in spasm, an observation first made by John Hunter. The partial wound is more likely to cause catastrophic bleeding, but may also lead to the formation of a false aneurysm from a breach of

Table 9.2 Operations for injuries of the brachial plexus, showing the incidence of open and vascular injuries, 1976–1996

Injury	Total	Vascular
Supraclavicular		
Complete avulsion (C4) C5 to T1; no repair	148	48
Incomplete or recovering lesions; no repair	262	20
Repairs in complete or partial lesions	687	42
Repairs by vascularised ulnar nerve graft	65	5
Total	1162	115
Infraclavicular		
Involving suprascapular and circumflex nerves	126	6
Caused by shoulder dislocation; no nerve rupture	26	2
Caused by shoulder dislocation, with vascular injury but no nerve rupture, in older persons	8	8
Multiple ruptures of nerves (the true infraclavicular lesion)	282	62
Total	442	78
Penetrating missile injury	51	

Note:
1. The first repair of a supraclavicular lesion at St Mary's Hospital was done in 1962.
2. From 1956 to 1974 there were 32 explored cases and three repairs.
3. From 1974 to 1978 there were 60 explored cases and 38 repairs.

the arterial wall. The sac contains thrombus, its wall being formed from perivascular soft tissues that may include nerve trunks. Aneurysms may also occur in closed traction lesion following the avulsion of such an offset as the supra-scapular, circumflex, humeral or subscapular arteries. We have encountered five such cases.

The slowly expanding false aneurysm causes profound loss of conduction in adjacent nerve trunks, and a deep-seated aneurysm may not be clinically diagnosed unless the potential significance of an earlier wound is noted.

Case report. A 37-year-old man suffered a perforating injury in the deltopectoral groove from fine steel wire. There was immediate loss of sensation in the hand. There was no local swelling. The patient was seen by us 3 months after the injury, with loss of elbow flexion, complete median palsy, a tender swelling in the axilla, and a positive Tinel sign radiating into the territory of the nerve. There was a good radial pulse. At operation a false aneurysm of the axillary artery was found. The musculocutaneous nerve had been severed, and the median nerve was wrapped around the wall of the sac. The sac was excised, the artery repaired by reversed vein graft, the musculocutaneous nerve was grafted, and a median neurolysis was done. Good circulation was maintained. At 9 months the biceps muscle regained power to Medical Research Council (MRC) grade 5. There was a Tinel sign for the median nerve in the middle part of the forearm, with recovery in the superficial forearm flexors.

Regrettably, iatropathic aneurysms are becoming more common. We have treated five that occurred following operations in the axilla. Their course was characterised by severe pain, progressive loss of nerve function, and, a notably early sign, sympathetic paralysis.

Case report. A 55-year-old woman developed intense pain after removal of a lipoma in the axilla. We saw her at 2 weeks because of suspected damage to the median nerve. The hand was red and dry, but not insensible; there was weakness of the flexor muscles of the forearm and the intrinsic muscles of the hand. The radial pulse was diminished. The arteriogram showed a block in the distal part of the axillary artery. At operation, a false aneurysm was displayed; its wall was formed from the brachial sheath and the median nerve, which was splayed out; the ulnar nerve was displaced and compressed. Eastcott (1992) has emphasised that arteriography can be misleading in the peripheral aneurysm and that ultrasonography may be the more valuable investigation. First, of course, one must think of the diagnosis.

Closed traction

The first injury is fracture of the intima, which in more violent injury progresses to rupture of all coats of the vessel (Fig. 9.30). The intimal injury can be seen easily as a pale crescent-shaped line, the damaged segment of the artery

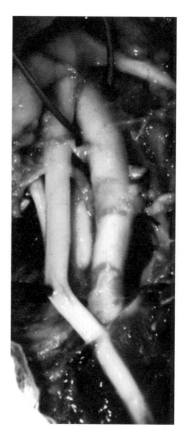

Fig. 9.30 Double circumferential rupture of the intima of the axillary artery with intervening thrombosis: in effect a floating segment of the vessel.

being filled with thrombus. Attempts to restore flow using embolectomy catheters are invariably futile in such cases and cause such extensive longitudinal damage to the intima that later repair is impossible. Torrential bleeding after rupture of the whole vessel is unusual in the closed traction lesion. The tips of the artery generally contract down but in one case the proximal stump of the vessel was plugged by an adjacent ruptured nerve trunk. There was torrential haemorrhage when this plug was removed. The length of damage ranged from 3 to 28 cm. The brittle atheromatous vessels of older patients are vulnerable even in low energy injuries.

The level of arterial rupture is remarkably consistent in the closed traction injury. In supraclavicular lesion the artery is occluded in its second part at the posterior margin of scalenus anterior. In the infraclavicular lesion it is occluded deep to the pectoralis minor (Fig. 9.31). There are exceptions; on occasion we have found the vessels lacerated by fractures of the clavicle or proximal humerus.

Potentially life-threatening injuries to head, chest or viscera are frequent in the high energy or missile lesion. Their treatment takes priority over that of the injured limb. In a number of cases avulsion of the right subclavian artery at its origin or rupture of the thoracic aorta was

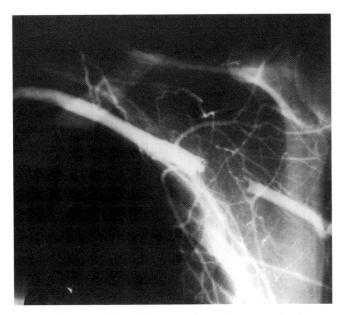

Fig. 9.31 Rupture of the axillary artery deep to the pectoralis minor.

successfully treated in the referring hospital. Extensive repair of the neurovascular injury in the upper limb is time consuming and, on occasion, amputation is necessary to save life. We have had to do this on six occasions: in two cases of gas gangrene occurring within 24 hours of successful arterial repair by prosthesis; for cases of upper limbs so badly damaged at several levels that there was no possibility of functional recovery; and in cases of limbs amputated through the glenohumeral joint where operation for replantation was abandoned because of uncontrollable bleeding from adjacent damaged soft tissues. Recognition of the vascular injury is usually straightforward in the open case. The diagnosis of aneurysm or of arteriovenous fistula may be delayed. Auscultation reveals the latter. Pain, with progressive loss of function, and sympathetic paralysis indicate an expanding haematoma or aneurysm compressing adjacent nerve trunks. In the closed lesion an expanding swelling with or without a bruit is certain evidence of arterial injury. A plain radiograph may be useful; fracture dislocation of the first rib is commonly associated with damage to the second part of the sub-clavian artery. A plain radiograph of the chest showing lateral downward displacement of the shoulder girdle with paralysis of the hemidiaphragm is characteristic of the worst form of supraclavicular lesion – one in which rupture of the subclavian artery can be expected.

Arteriography, whilst always valuable, should not unduly delay operation. A reasonable circulation to the skin is not the issue: what is important is whether muscle is perfused. Failure to restore flow through damaged axillary or common brachial artery within 6 hours of injury is almost always followed by, at least, severe ischaemic fibrosis. In most of our cases of closed infraclavicular lesion we did

not proceed to arteriography because the clinical evidence of arterial injury was strong. In these cases the posterior triangle was neither swollen nor deeply bruised; the sub-clavian pulse was palpable, whereas in the infraclavicular fossa there was swelling with bruising of the skin and the brachial pulse was absent. The axillary artery was ruptured deep to the pectoralis minor at the level of the coracoid process.

ACCESS AND CONTROL OF THE VESSELS

This is achieved by extension of a standard transverse supraclavicular approach. Eastcott (1973b) recommended excision of the clavicle, which gave excellent access to the subclavian and axillary arteries, but which presented later problems for the shoulder girdle and support of the limb. Fiolle and Delmas (1921) developed an approach that remains extremely useful; indeed, it is the method of choice for an exposure of the main artery from the second part of the subclavian to the terminal part of the axillary artery. Duval (attributed by Fiolle and Delmas) gave thought to access to the first part of the subclavian artery, considering the sternoclavicular joint as the barrier and advising that it be turned downwards. Bonney's (1977) transclavicular approach (Birch et al 1990) gives excellent access to the first part of subclavian artery, the first part of the vertebral artery, and the whole of the brachial plexus, but it is not easy to perform rapidly. It has been used in two emergency cases and on four more leisurely occasions for display of neurovascular injury at the root of the limb.

The exposure of Fiolle and Delmas grants access which is at least equal to that following excision of the clavicle; it is less destructive and is far superior to the exposure from the incision curving across pectoralis major to the inferior medial clavicle.

SUPRACLAVICULAR EXPOSURE

The incision is made one-finger's breadth above the clavicle and the platysma raised with the skin flaps (Fig. 9.32). The supraclavicular nerves are preserved. Flaps are elevated to the apex of the posterior triangle above, taking care for the accessory nerve above and showing the inferior margin of the clavicle below. The plane between the sternocleido-mastoid and external jugular vein is developed, displaying the omohyoid muscle which is divided between stay sutures and reflected (Fig. 9.33). The fat pad is divided and the transverse cervical vessels that lie deep to it are ligated. The phrenic nerve will be seen coursing obliquely across the scalenus anterior; it is mobilised and held in a nerve sling. Following the phrenic nerve cranially brings the surgeon to the 5th cervical nerve. Incision of the deep cervical fascia allows display of the 5th and 6th cervical nerves emerging from under the lateral margin of scalenus anterior (Fig. 9.34). The upper trunk and the

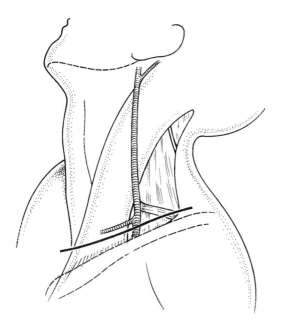

Fig. 9.32 Supraclavicular exposure: the incisions.

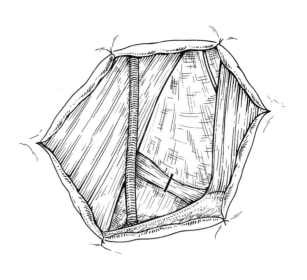

Fig. 9.33 Supraclavicular exposure: the flaps raised and the division of the omohyoid.

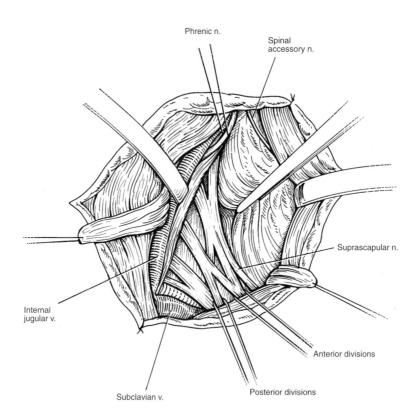

Fig. 9.34 Supraclavicular exposure: the plexus displayed.

suprascapular nerve are followed. The 7th cervical nerve is displayed between the scalenus anterior and the upper trunk. The nerve to the serratus anterior lies lateral and deep to the upper trunk. The lower trunk is displayed after division of the scalenus anterior; the plane between the muscle and the subclavian artery requires careful definition. The 8th cervical and first thoracic nerves are traced by following the plane between the artery and the lower trunk. This exposure allows access to the second and the third parts of the subclavian artery.

Full display of the supra-, retro-, and infraclavicular plexus of the second part of the subclavian to the terminal axillary artery and of the axillary and subclavian vein deep to the clavicle is achieved by the operation of Fiolle and Delmas. The operation secures rapid access and control of major vessels from scalenus anterior to the lowest part of the axilla. Exposure of the proximal subclavian vein is not so good as that of the artery. The plexus can be exposed from the spinal nerves above to the terminal branches below. It is a most valuable exposure in fresh cases of laceration or rupture of the great vessels deep to or below the clavicle, and in later cases of false aneurysm or for repair of the nerves after primary vascular repair. It is the exposure of choice in the closed traction lesion in infraclavicular rupture of vessels and nerves. The incision is T-shaped, the vertical limb running in the deltopectoral groove preserving the cephalic vein and then curving into the apex of the axilla underneath the fold of pectoralis major (Fig. 9.35). The platysma is reflected with skin flaps, and a Gigli saw is passed subperiosteally about the clavicle at the lateral edge of insertion of the sternomastoid. The fascia at the root of the axilla is divided, and the finger develops a plane between pectoralis major and

minor above and the underlying axillary bundle deeper. Pectoralis major is detached from the humerus, the plane between the inferior margin of the pectoralis minor and coracobrachialis is established, and the pectoralis minor is reflected taking care for the musculocutaneous nerve. The clavicle is divided obliquely, and the subclavius muscle and suprascapular vessels are divided between clamps. The limb is rolled into lateral rotation so that the trunks, divisions and cords of the brachial plexus are displayed with their accompanying great vessels. Reflection of omohyoid and division of the fat pad extends the exposure to the roots of the brachial plexus. Division of scalenus anterior extends exposure of the subclavian artery as far medial as the origin of the vertebral artery. The clavicle is repaired with a plate and screws. We have known of three cases of non-union, but have seen no deep infections in over 200 cases (Figs 9.36 and 9.37).

TRANSCLAVICULAR EXPOSURE

Bonney developed this operation in 1976 as an approach to the anterior aspect of the cervicodorsal spine for excision of a malignant cartilaginous tumour that had eroded the bodies of C7 and D1 and compressed the spinal cord. The approach was designed to give adequate exposure and control of the venous trifurcation, the first part of subclavian artery, the vertebral artery, and the recurrent laryngeal nerve. Duval attributed by Fiolle and Delmas (1921), faced with the problems of deep wounds in the neck, outlined a similar approach, describing it as "this major and hazardous intervention which should be undertaken only by the most consummate surgeon". Antibiotics, blood transfusion and advances in anaesthetics have greatly diminished some of these hazards, but the intervention remains an extensive and difficult one, calling for a high degree of anatomical knowledge and practical versatility. The exposure rests on the elevation of the osseomuscular flap, which comprises the medial portion of clavicle with the sternoclavicular joint and the sternomastoid. The whole of the brachial plexus can be displayed after some lateral work; the cervicodorsal spine can be seen from C3 to T4 by work between the carotid sheath and the visceral axis.

The transverse limb of the incision runs from the fold of the trapezius on the side of operation to the midpoint of the opposite posterior triangle. This limb can be extended to increase exposure. The vertical limb runs to the sternal angle. Flaps are widely elevated to include platysma (Fig. 9.38). The sternocleidomastoid muscle is defined anteriorly and posteriorly from its insertion below to the uppermost limit of the wound above. Care is needed for the accessory nerve. The clavicle is displayed subperiosteally at its midpoint. The pectoralis major is detached from the inferior portion of the medial clavicle, taking care for the subclavian vein. Strap muscles are released from the notch of the manubrium, and the plane

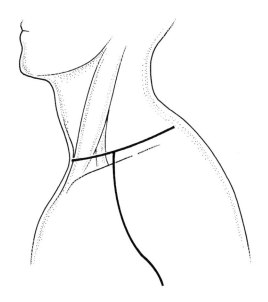

Fig. 9.35 The exposure of Fiolle and Delmas: the incision.

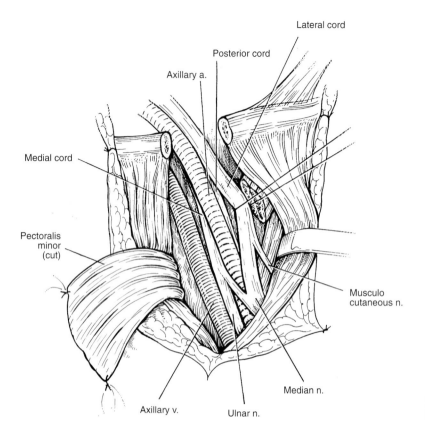

Fig. 9.36 Exposure of the infraclavicular brachial plexus.

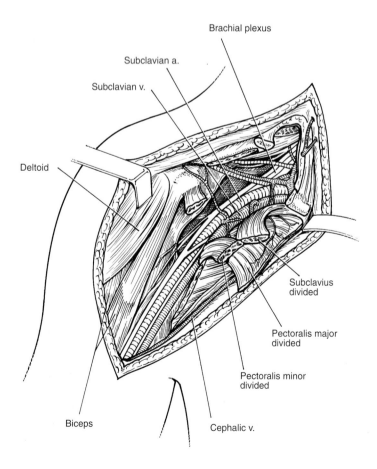

Fig. 9.37 Drawing showing the extent of exposure.

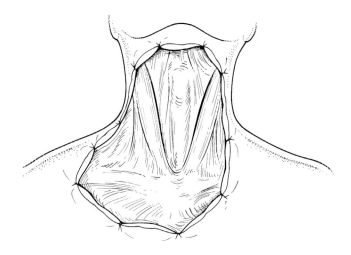

Fig. 9.38 Transclavicular approach: the skin incision.

deep to this developed carefully using a dental Howarth elevator and a curved Adson's dissector. The plane is enlarged with the finger, and a malleable retractor is passed. The first costochondral junction is defined after detaching the pectoralis major from the adjacent manubrium, and the interval between the first and second sternocostal junction is developed deep to the sternum by the means outlined above. A malleable retractor is passed to meet its fellow from above. The first costal cartilage is cut with a scalpel; a fine osteotome is used to divide the manubrium with an L-shaped cut (Fig. 9.39). The clavicle is now divided, and the medial clavicle, sternoclavicular joint and upper corner of the manubrium are elevated

on the sternomastoid muscle (Fig. 9.40). Residual strap muscles are released. The subclavius muscle and supra-scapular vessels are divided. The omohyoid muscle is divided and reflected. The internal jugular vein is now seen and traced to its junction with the subclavian vein. The innominate vein is traced and lightly held in a vascu-lar sling. The phrenic nerve is elevated from the scalenus anterior and the muscle is divided (Fig. 9.41). The first part of the subclavian artery, the vertebral artery, and the recurrent laryngeal and vagus nerves are seen (Fig. 9.42). To display the whole of the plexus, the pectoralis major is detached from the humerus, and pectoralis minor from the coracoid. When it comes to closure, the manubrio-clavicular fragment is reattached to the manubrium with wires, and to the clavicle with a plate and screws. The soft tissue layers are carefully closed. This exposure has been used in over 50 patients, chiefly for tumours of the brachial plexus. Osteomyelitis of the clavicle occurred in one case, and non-union in three more.

SOME TECHNICAL DETAILS

Having secured proximal and distal control of the injured vessel, any associated fracture of humerus is neutralised as rapidly as possible by insertion of an intramedullary rod or plate before arterial repair. Direct suture is occasionally possible in a fresh stab wound; a vein patch is better than lateral suture at the mouth of an aneurysmal sac. Reversed vein grafts were almost always necessary, and we agree with Narakas' comments on synthetic grafts (1987): "in those cases where vascular repair has been undertaken immediately and nerve repair carried out later, immense technical difficulties arise because it is almost impossible to expose the plexus without damaging the vascular graft even a prosthesis if one has been used … vascular prostheses should not be used in young patients with brachial plexus injuries. Prostheses do not adapt to changes in the calibre of the anastomosis site and may leak causing minor or massive haemorrhage which afterwards embeds the nerve trunk in a fibrotic mass."

Earlier work in the repair of small vessels by microsurgi-cal technique taught us the value of interrupted sutures, and these are better than continuous suture in the repair of a subclavian or axillary artery; they reduce the risk of stenosis at the suture line, they permit easier coaptation of vessels of different diameter, and they facilitate end to side suture. The apparent causes of failure of arterial repair in the 32 cases sent to us, and revised, were as follows:

1. Embolectomy catheters are contraindicated in the treatment of intimal fractures or tears. Flow may be restored temporarily, but the thrombosis inevitably recurs: overvigorous use of the balloon damages intima distally, so much that later repair is impossible (four cases).

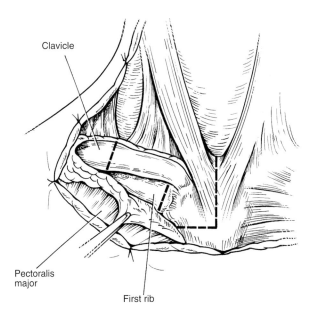

Clavicle

Pectoralis major

First rib

Fig. 9.39 Transclavicular approach: the bone flaps.

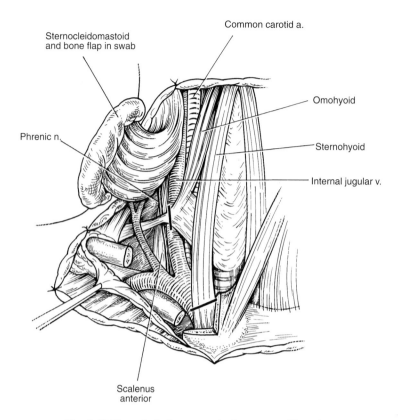

Fig. 9.40 Transclavicular approach: the venous trifurcation.

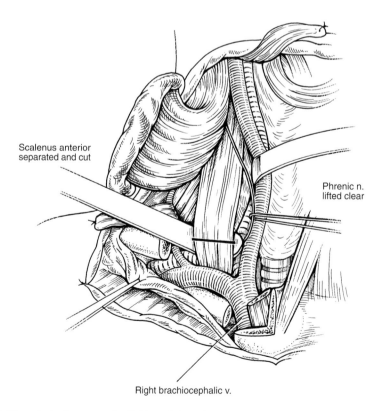

Fig. 9.41 Transclavicular approach: division of the scalenus anterior after elevation of the phrenic nerve.

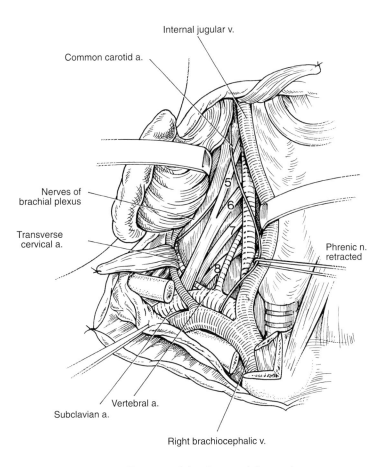

Internal jugular v.

Common carotid a.

Nerves of
brachial plexus

Transverse
cervical a.

Phrenic n.
retracted

Vertebral a.

Subclavian a.

Right brachiocephalic v.

Fig. 9.42 Exposure of the plexus and the arteries.

2. Continuous suture – running suture of a muscular vessel which is in spasm inevitably leads to stenosis and later thrombosis (20 cases).
3. Inadequate resection of the damaged vessel in closed traction lesion – longitudinal splits of the intima and media are common after missile or traction lesion, and vessel stumps must be resected back to where the intima is smooth and unblemished (eight cases).

In a number of other cases initial triumph in restoring arterial circulation was overturned by failure to decompress the limb. Division of the axillary and brachial sheath and of the deep fascia of the forearm is essential in all cases except those where a simple wound is successfully sutured within 3 hours of injury. "Closed" fasciotomy of the forearm is adequate if there is no distal injury of the elbow and forearm. In more severe cases a fasciotomy should include the skin: this is usually susceptible to delayed primary closure at about 48 hours. Anticoagulants are not used.

We have found constriction of the distal arterial stump and of the distal nerve trunks within the brachial sheath in cases explored several days after injury. Adequate perfusion was not restored until the brachial sheath had been released and the brachial artery traced as far as the elbow. Rupture of the axillary or subclavian vein is uncommon in closed lesion (six cases), but more frequent in open wounds (18 cases). Ischaemic fibrosis and joint stiffness are particularly severe in cases with such venous injury.

THE NERVE INJURY

OPEN WOUNDS

These fall into two groups. "Untidy" wounds from gunshot or other missiles are considered in Chapter 8. The tidy wounds from a knife, glass or a scalpel are among the most rewarding of all nerve injuries to repair. When the opportunity for repair within hours or days of injury is grasped, the results for C5, C6 and C7 wounds are excellent: better, by far, than equivalent results even for early repair of more distal nerve trunks ruptured by traction injuries. They are worthwhile for C8 and T1 too. We emphasise that in virtually no other nerve laceration is the harmfulness of procrastination so clearly shown as in the supraclavicular stab wound. On the other hand, the nature of the wound is such that other and more pressing problems frequently arise. Setting aside the cases of damage by scalpel there are three distinct patterns. When a blade or bottle is thrust from above down (as it was in Hector's case), the lower trunk, subclavian vessels and lung are damaged. Such wounds may be as rapidly fatal as they were for the Prince of Ilium. When the blade is thrust towards the face or neck, the 5th, 6th and 7th cervical and the phrenic nerves are damaged; in addition to the jugular and carotid vessels, the trachea and the oesophagus are at risk. However, in the cases coming to us, the vertebral body had shielded the viscera, and the knife point had glided laterally, severing the spinal nerves close to their exit from the intervertebral foramina. Lastly the lateral thrust had divided the upper and middle trunks, the nerve to the serratus anterior, and the accessory nerve (Table 9.3).

Table 9.3 Lesions due to stab wounds (knife or glass)

Lesion type	Total No.	Significant vascular involvement
Supraclavicular:		
Upper	8	2
Lateral	9	2
Lower trunk	5	2
Infraclavicular	23	7

The total number of lesions due to stab wounds is considerably exceeded by iatropathic lesions (see Ch. 8).

The temptation to suture the severed nerves directly should be resisted. Grafts are better, even if they are only 0.5 cm long.

Some examples are given below.

Case report. A 26-year-old man was stabbed in the neck. The internal jugular vein was ligated by the receiving surgeon, who gave us the opportunity to repair the neural lesion within 36 hours. The 5th, 6th and 7th cervical nerves had been severed close to their foramina; the phrenic nerve had also been severed. Twenty-four grafts were used to repair the 2-cm defect. By 3 years the only defect at the shoulder was in lateral rotation, which was restricted to 40° by capsular contraction. The sensation in the thumb and index and middle fingers was close to normal, without hypersensitivity. The power of deltoid, biceps, triceps, and wrist extension was 80% of the uninjured side. The phrenic nerve recovered, there was accurate localisation of touch, with two-point discrimination of less than 8 mm in the thumb and index and middle fingers (Fig. 9.43).

Case report. A 21-year-old nurse was assaulted and stabbed on her way home from duty in her accident and emergency unit. Mr Maelor Thomas (Kings College Hospital) transferred her to us so that repair was performed within 24 hours of injury. The knife had severed the upper and middle trunks and the nerve to the serratus anterior (Fig. 9.44). Nineteen grafts were used to bridge the 1-cm defect. At 4 years this patient considered function

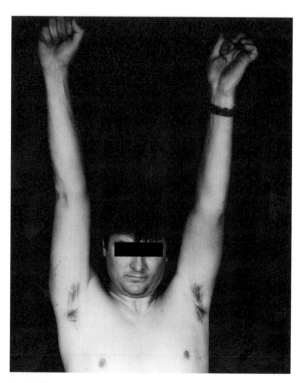

Fig. 9.43 The outcome at 3 years after repair of a stab wound of C5, C6 and C7 and the phrenic nerve.

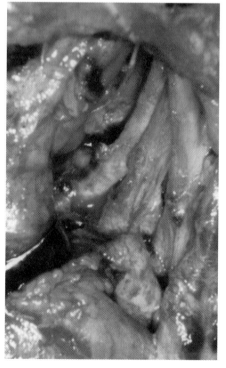

Fig. 9.44 Stab wound to the upper and middle trunks and nerve to the serratus anterior.

in her upper limb to be normal. The measured power of the serratus anterior, and of the muscles of the shoulder, arm, and forearm were MRC grade 5; power grip in the afflicted (dominant) hand was 90% of the uninjured hand. The two-point discrimination sense was 6–8 mm in the median territory of the hand. Early recovery of sympathetic function was the most striking feature in this case, as in the one described above.

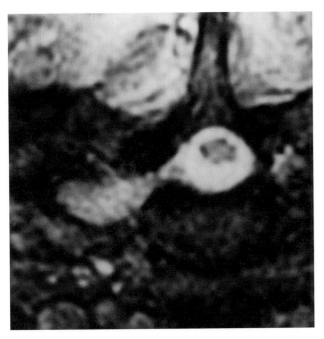

Fig. 9.45 Magnetic resonance scan showing the track of a knife which damaged C8 and T1.

Case report. A 22-year-old man was stabbed in the neck with a broken bottle and clearly remembered the downward thrust of the weapon, which entered the neck just above the medial one-third of clavicle. At emergency exploration copious bleeding from the offsets of subclavian vessels was controlled. The 8th cervical nerve was severed, together with about 50% of the 7th cervical nerve. The glass had scored the first rib, lacerating the pleura. Twelve grafts were used in the repair. At 2 years the one significant defect, function of thumb opposition, was mitigated by muscle transfer. Power grip for the whole hand was 85% of normal; the pinch grip between the thumb and index finger was 75% of the uninjured (dominant) side. There was no pain and no serious sensory deficit.

A striking feature of these and other cases of the urgent repair of stab wounds is the speed of recovery, the absence of pain, and a level of recovery superior to repair of more distal wounds of trunk nerves (Fig. 9.45).

THE SUPRACLAVICULAR CLOSED TRACTION LESION

We recognise distinct groups within this large population. The most important distinction lies between those cases where some roots are intact or recovering, from those where all roots are damaged. The prognosis for overall function is very different. Table 9.4 sets out the groups seen in 300 consecutive explorations done over 4 years, Table 9.5 shows the patterns of avulsion, and Table 9.6 details the lesions of the nerves.

Table 9.5 Common patterns of intradural injury seen in 300 consecutive operated cases, 1989–1993

Injured nerve	No.
C5–T1	52
C6–T1	39
C7–T1	54
C8–T1	10
C6	10
C7	13
C5–C6	21
C5–C6–C7	21
C6–C7–C8	10

Table 9.4 Patterns of injury in 300 consecutive operated supraclavicular lesions, 1989–1993

Lesion type	No.
Complete lesions: pre- and postganglionic injury	
Rupture of upper nerves C5 (C6, C7) Intradural lower nerves (C6, C7, C8) T1	83
Rupture of middle nerves (C6) C7 (C8) Intradural above and below	5
Rupture of lower nerves C8, T1 Intradural upper nerves C5, C6, C7	1
Rupture of C5, T1 Intradural C6, C7, C8	7
Total intradural C5–T1	52
	148
Incomplete lesions: some roots intact	
Damage C5, C6 (C7) Recovering or intact (C7) C8, T1	117
Damage C6, C7, T1 Recovering or intact C5, T1	23
Damage C7, C8, T1 Recovering or intact C5, C6	13
Total	153

Table 9.6 Injuries to individual spinal nerves in 300 consecutive operated cases, 1989–1993

Nerve	Intact or lesion in continuity	Rupture	Intradural
C5	41	154	105
C6	39	90	171
C7	76	24	200
C8	105	15	180
T1	133	7	170
Total	394	290	826

A. *The upper lesion: rupture or avulsion of C5 and C6 (C7) with intact (C7) C8 and T1.* This is the most favourable lesion because there is useful hand function, and it is in this group that all the endeavours of the last 25 years have borne the greatest fruit. Early repair, within a few days of injury, either by graft, by transfer, or both, can achieve such useful results that it is possible to argue that the problem of treatment in this group is now solved. This is a bold claim, and there are of course many failures and disappointments, but there are reasons for these which can be avoided, chief among them being delay. The aims of surgical treatment include restoration of: control of the thoracoscapular and glenohumeral joints; elbow flexion; and, if necessary, extension of the wrist and of sensation within the median territory of the hand. Table 9.7 outlines the injuries to C5, C6 and C7 in 51 patients with upper lesion seen in 108 consecutive operated cases the 2 years.

B. *The lower lesion: intact C5 and C6 (C7), with rupture or avulsion of C8 and T1.* The shoulder girdle, the shoulder and the elbow are intact, pronosupination is preserved, and there is extension of the wrist, with normal sensation for the thumb and middle and index fingers. There are opportunities for useful palliation, which is fortunate because recovery following repair of the lower roots of the plexus, while more promising than 20 years ago, remains uncertain and, on the whole, poor, except when the repair is performed within days of injury.

C. *The middle lesion: recovery of C5 (C6) and T1 (C8), with rupture or avulsion of (C6) C7 (C8).* This pattern is less common in adults than in the obstetric brachial plexus palsy. We have noted that avulsion of C7 induces a generalised loss of power throughout the limb without complete paralysis of any particular muscle groups, and is often attended by severe pain. There are other odd patterns: isolated avulsion or rupture of one or more roots, which, broadly speaking, fall into one or other of the above categories.

Table 9.7 Lesions of C5, C6, and C7 in 108 consecutive cases, 1993–1994

Total of repair of brachial plexus (graft or transfer or both)	108
Repairs of C5 and C6 (graft or transfer or both)	28
Repairs C5, C6, and C7 (graft or transfer or both)	23

The nerve injury in the 51 cases of C5 and C6, and C5, C6, and C7 lesion

Injured nerve	Intact or lesion in continuity	Rupture	Intradural injury
C5	0	38	13
C6	0	29	22
C7	26	16	9

D. *The complete lesion.* This can be divided into those in which some nerves are ruptured, in which case modest function can be expected from grafts, and those in which all nerves are avulsed. In the latter nerve transfer offers paltry mitigation, and for these the only real prospect of regaining useful function lies in replantation. We shall discuss that later. However, prompt repair of ruptures can achieve striking recovery.

Case report. A 27-year-old man suffered complete lesion of the brachial plexus on his dominant side in motor cycle accident. Operation within 72 hours confirmed rupture of all five spinal nerves. Repair by accessory to suprascapular transfer and graft of all five nerves was done. A leak of cerebrospinal fluid from the foramen of C5 was noted. Thirty-two grafts were used. At 18 months function at the shoulder and elbow was good; at 30 months there was functional return of the wrist extensors and the digital flexors, with early return of the intrinsic function. Temperature sensation was present and he could localise stimulae to the thumb, index, middle and ring fingers. At that time the gain on Narakas' system (see below) was 13 points for the shoulder, 8 points for the elbow, and 9 points for the forearm and hand, a total of 30. Recovery continues. This result was possible because of the alertness of Mr J Robertson (Southampton) who recognised the potential for early exploration.

THE CLOSED INFRACLAVICULAR LESION

The distinction between infraclavicular and supraclavicular lesions is of course to some extent artificial. A knife or a missile does not respect anatomical boundaries; even in closed traction injuries, there are in 15% of cases two-level lesions. The most common pattern of such lesions is preganglionic injury of the eighth cervical and first thoracic nerves with rupture of the lateral and posterior cords. Occasionally, a single peripheral nerve is ruptured in association with a lesion of the upper part of the plexus (Fig. 9.46). There is indeed some basis for the identification of a third type of closed lesion, the retroclavicular lesion, in which the plexus is, as it were, crushed between the clavicle and the first rib. Narakas (personal communication) used to think of this as damage to the plexus by the "costoclavicular scissors".

Cavanagh et al (1987) reviewed the results of repair of nerves in 89 cases operated over a 10-year period. They reckoned that infraclavicular lesions accounted for 20% of all brachial plexus lesions referred. In 46% there was damage to the axillary artery; in 52%, there was bony injury. They took as indications for operation signs of arterial injury, and evidence of severe local trauma with a deep neural lesion. A good case for primary repair was made out. Our later work has confirmed the last proposition.

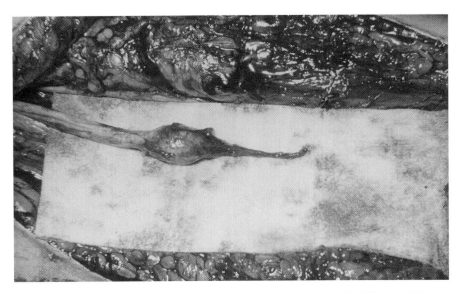

Fig. 9.46 The proximal stump of the left median nerve seen at operation 3 months after a closed injury which caused rupture of the fifth and sixth cervical nerves in the neck and of the median nerve in the arm. The top of the distal stump is just visible on the right.

Birch (1996), in a review of injuries of the brachial plexus, identified four types of infraclavicular lesion: lesions of the suprascapular and circumflex nerves (126 cases); traction lesions associated with anterior dislocation of the shoulder (26 cases); similar lesions associated with arterial injury (8 cases); and multiple ruptures of nerves (282 cases) (Table 9.7). He termed the last, the "true infraclavicular lesion". The first, third and fourth classes have been considered in Chapter 8; some more will be said here about the second class.

The injury to the infraclavicular plexus associated with anterior dislocation of the shoulder is produced by the intrusion of the head of the humerus into the axilla, beneath the cords and terminal branches of the plexus. The medial and posterior cords are predominantly affected; the lesion deepens and becomes more extensive while the humeral head is permitted to stretch the plexus. It seems that the large cords and main nerves are less susceptible to rupture than are the smaller suprascapular and circumflex nerves. In a few cases the lesion or part of it is permitted to deepen from recoverable axonotmesis to irrecoverable neurotmesis through failure to recognise the dislocation and the intrusion of the humeral head. The lessons are clear: recognise the anterior dislocation and reduce it before there is neural affection; if closed reduction is impossible, be prepared to reduce by open operation; recognise neural affection and act instantly to remove its cause; intervene without delay in cases in which unrecognised dislocation has produced a deep and extensive lesion of the infraclavicular part of the plexus. The common course of such lesions, properly treated, is to progressive recovery.

STRATEGIES OF REPAIR

There are summarised in Table 9.8. We rehearse again the arguments for urgent repair. Early exploration, by which we mean exposure within hours or days of injury, except when associated life-threatening injuries must take priority, permits accurate diagnosis and greatly eases the task of repair. The dissection is easier, the retraction of ruptured nerve trunks can be overcome, and regular use of intra-operative evoked potentials uncovers many instances of hidden intradural lesion. Nerve stimulation permits the recognition of bundles within the distal stumps passing to such critical muscle groups as those for wrist extension. Such stimulation work, within 48 hours of injury, gives evidence of distal ruptures – the so-called second level of lesion. In one case of a complete lesion, fractures of the humerus and dislocation of the elbow pointed to the possibility of distal lesion. Stimulation of the avulsed sixth, seventh and eighth cervical nerves failed to elicit elbow flexion or response in median innervated muscles. Distal exposure confirmed a rupture of the musculocutaneous nerve at the midarm level and rupture of the median nerve at the elbow.

A further advantage is the ease with which the ventral roots of an avulsed spinal nerve may be reinnervated by transfer of the accessory nerve or by suture to a ruptured spinal nerve. We have been able to do this in a number of cases since 1992.

Case report. A 27-year-old woman suffered complete lesion of the brachial plexus in a motor cycle accident. At exploration 4 days later, we found ruptures of C5 and C6 and avulsions of C7, C8 and T1. C5 and C6 were grafted

Table 9.8 Strategies of repair

Partial lesions

Ruptures of C5 and C6 (C7); intact (C7) C8 and T1
Accessory to suprascapular transfer
Standard graft for ruptures

Preganglionic C5 and C6; intact C7, C8 and T1
Reinnervation of nerve to serratus anterior necessary in 30% of cases
Accessory to suprascapular transfer
Intercostals T4 and T5 to circumflex transfer
Ulnar to biceps transfer (Oberlin)

Depending on sensory loss, and the presence of C7 fibres in the lateral cord, transfer the medial cutaneous nerve of forearm and/or superficial division of T3 and T6 to the lateral root of the median

Preganglionic C5, C6 and C7; intact C8 and T1
Reinnervation of nerve to serratus anterior usual
Accessory to suprascapular transfer
Ulnar to biceps transfer (Oberlin), or T3 and T4 to musculocutaneous
Superficial divisions T5 and T6, and/or medial cutaneous nerve to forearm to lateral root median nerve

If ulnar to biceps is used, T3 and T4 are available for the lateral pectoral and thoracodorsal nerves.

Early flexor to extensor tendon transfer (using flexor digitorum superficialis and palmaris longus) required in about 50% of cases

Mixed ruptures and preganglionic C5, C6, C7 and C8; intact T1
Combine grafts and transfers to reinnervate the limb

The aim in this group is to restore all major joint functions

Complete lesions

Ruptures C5 (C6, C7, C8); preganglionic (C6, C7, C8) T1
Accessory to suprascapular transfer:
  If three healthy nerve roots available: repair whole plexus
  If two healthy nerve roots available: repair upper and middle trunks, and T3, T4, T5 and T6 for ulnar nerve
  If one healthy nerve root available: repair lateral cord, and T3, T4, T5 and T6 for medial cord

Alternatively, transfer accessory and/or dorsal scapular nerve to ventral roots of avulsed spinal nerves *and* supraclavicular nerves to the nerve just distal to the dorsal root ganglion (see text)

Total preganglionic: phrenic nerve working
Nerve transfers for serratus anterior; suprascapular nerve; elbow flexion; median nerve sensation

Total preganglionic: phrenic palsy
Reinnervate serratus anterior (part of dorsal scapular nerve)
Accessory to musculocutaneous nerve
Intercostals, superficial divisions only, to median nerve

The aims of treatment in the complete avulsion group are much narrower: stability of shoulder girdle, elbow flexion and relief of pain

to the upper trunk: three grafts from C6 were passed to the 7th cervical nerve just distal to the dorsal root ganglion, which was excised. The dorsal scapular nerve was transferred to the ventral root of C7, and the accessory was transferred to the ventral root of C8. At 20 months the patient was free of pain. There was limited recovery

through the repaired C5 and C6 roots. The shoulder was stable, and the biceps reached MRC grade 3. Recovery through the repaired ventral rootlets was more impressive: triceps and latissimus dorsi, MRC grade 4; wrist flexors, MRC grade 3; and long finger flexors, MRC grade 2. There was light touch sensation in the palm of the hand and in the index and middle fingers. It seems that most of the patient's recovery was due to the transfer to C7 and C8.

It is now possible and reasonable to repair the whole of the plexus in those partial lesions where two or three nerves are intact. When the nerves damaged are the fifth sixth and seventh cervical nerves, useful functional improvement is usual. The outlook is very different in the complete lesion, particularly when all nerves have been avulsed. Nerve transfer offers only trivial mitigation in these cases. The benefit of free functioning muscle transfer is discussed in Chapter 17. The introduction by Professor Gu and his colleagues in Shanghai, of using the contralateral seventh cervical nerve to reinnervate the paralysed limb is described later. We believe that the only real prospect for restoration of useful function throughout the upper limb lies in replantation of the avulsed nerves into the spinal cord, and we shall return to this.

Standard graft

The available donor nerves, in order of choice, include the medial cutaneous nerve of the forearm, the superficial radial nerve and the cutaneous division of the musculocutaneous nerve, in addition to both sural nerves. Up to 160 cm of graft is available, but in favourable cases with many ruptures this is scarcely sufficient. We think that a minimum of five grafts is necessary to satisfy C5, and between six and eight grafts for the other spinal nerves. Ruptures of C5 and C6 and C7 will absorb about 18 grafts; 22 or more are necessary for repairs of four stumps. After preparation of the stumps, grafts are cut, allowing 15% of excess length with the head extended and the arm by the side. The ends are prepared by, using the operating microscope, cutting away epineurium and adventitia for the last 1–2 mm. Sutures are used for grafts passed to a specific nerve such as the phrenic nerve, the nerve to the serratus anterior and the suprascapular nerves. Haemostasis is tedious but essential. We use small pieces of absorbable sponge, and sometimes flood the bed of the graft with fibrin clot glue. It seems important to reattach the fat pad and repair the omohyoid over the graft in order to secure them and to aid revascularisation.

Vascularised ulnar nerve graft

In the early 1970s, the pedicled vascularised ulnar graft was used in suitable cases of the brachial plexus in which a hopeless prognosis for C8 and T1 had been established.

The operation was tedious, and it fell to Jamieson to propose the idea of taking the ulnar nerve from the forearm with the ulnar artery and veins, and transferring this as a free vascularised tissue transfer, an operation which he performed in 1977. We were concerned about taking a more major forearm artery, and in three cases repaired the ulnar artery with a vein graft, a procedure adding 2 hours to the time of operation in those days. Later, Jamieson suggested the superior ulnar collateral vessel as a pedicle, a suggestion which fell on stony ground until one of us, in 1981, during the second stage of St Clair Strange's operation, cut through the already prepared suture line. The remedy lay to hand, in the superior ulnar collateral vessel proposed by Jamieson. So was born a second type of vascularised ulnar nerve graft. The advantages were considerable. The operation was undoubtedly easier, the nerve trunk was unbranched, and the vessels were usually of adequate size (2 mm) but not essential for the perfusion of the limb. The ulnar nerve could be elevated on this pedicle from its origin to the wrist; preparation of two vascularised strands was quite straightforward, and with care three could be so prepared. As we shall see, the promise of the vascularised ulnar nerve graft was only rarely fulfilled, and we now think that the indications for it are narrow: for the severely scarred bed with a long gap, or as a means of bringing healthy nerves from the contralateral brachial plexus to reinnervate the upper limb or to innervate free muscle transfers (see Contralateral C7 transfer, p. 188).

NERVE TRANSFER

The idea of transferring an uninjured nerve to the distal stump of an injured nerve is not new. Narakas (1991) describes early work, pointing out that the principles for operations now performed were recognised decades ago. Harris and Low (1903) performed intraplexus nerve crossings on three patients, implanting the distal stump of a ruptured C5 or C6 spinal nerve end to side into a healthy neighbour. Tuttle, in 1912, transferred the deep cervical plexus nerves into a ruptured upper trunk. Chiasserini (1934) transferred sensory nerves in paraplegics, using the intercostal nerves.

Probably the first recorded success from nerve transfers in the brachial plexus was that by Seddon, who, with Yeoman, transferred intercostal nerves into the musculocutaneous nerve via interposed ulnar nerve (Seddon 1963). In 1965, Tsuyama adopted intercostal nerve transfer for patients with complete avulsion injury, and described the results in 179 patients (Nagano et al 1989b). The intercostal nerves were directly sutured to the musculocutaneous nerve, and over 80% of their patients regained functional flexion of the elbow. These extremely impressive results emphasised that delay is harmful; for patients presenting more than 10 months after injury, free muscle transfer is preferred. Dolenc (1987) described the outcome in 150 patients operated upon between 1972 and 1983, and emphasised the need for "better use of the scarce axons of the intercostal nerve." He recommended that repair should be performed within days of injury before Wallerian degeneration had occurred, for this allows recognition of the predominantly motor bundles of the major peripheral nerves.

Kotani et al (1972) and Allieu (1989) described the use of the distal part of the spinal accessory nerve in reinnervation of the upper limb, preserving rami to the upper fibres of trapezius. We are particularly grateful to Professors Laurent Sedel and Yves Allieu for describing their work to us at a time when they had not published it. Brunelli (1980) used the cervical plexus to reinnervate the upper limb. Brunelli and Brunelli (1987) reviewed results in 29 patients, achieving important improvement in many of these. They emphasised that nerve transfer should be limited to a few well-chosen muscles. Brunelli and Brunelli (1995) reported further studies of the anterior nerves of the third cervical ansa, estimating that some 2000 sensory and 4100 motor fibres are available for transfer. Bonnel et al (1979) estimate the number of myelinated nerve fibres in the spinal accessory nerve at about 1700; Alnot and Oberlin (1995) review the course and internal arrangement of the nerve. Williams Unwin and Smith (1995) estimated that 50% of the fibres within the nerve were Aδ or C fibres. Holle and Freilinger (1995) showed that the number of myelinated nerve fibres in intercostal nerves is 5500–8500 at the paravertebral region and that about 30% of fibres in T4 stained positive for acetylcholinesterase. The number of myelinated nerve fibres in the lateral cutaneous branch of this nerve was found to be 1000–1500. Oberlin et al (1994) estimate that the nerve to the biceps contains about 10% of the number of myelinated nerve fibres in the ulnar nerve in the arm at the same level.

The use of other healthy nerves

Use of the hypoglossal nerve (Slooff & Blaauw 1995) is mentioned in Chapter 10. Gu and his colleagues in Shanghai have great experience with ipsilateral phrenic nerve transfer, reporting a series of 164 cases in 1989. The nerve was transferred to the musculocutaneous nerve either by the interposed graft (9 cases) or by direct suture (40 cases) in 49 patients who were followed for a minimum of 2 years. Thirty-four patients achieved elbow flexion power to MRC grade 4 or better, 17 more achieved elbow flexion power of grade 3 or better. The obvious concern about respiratory capacity is to some extent relieved by their findings that only 5 of 40 patients had impaired diaphragmatic excursion at 5 years after operation. Ventilatory function was studied in 19 patients after operation: vital capacity dropped for the first year after operation, but had recovered to normal levels by 2 years. Gu and coworkers emphasise that the operation *should not* be performed in children. Gu and Ma (1996) showed, in an experimental study in rats, that the phrenic nerve is a better donor nerve than the accessory or intercostal nerves, and no significant impairment of ventilation was seen.

Contralateral C7 transfer

A more daring idea from the Shanghai school is the use of the contralateral 7th cervical nerve to reinnervate the limb after complete lesion of the brachial plexus. A vascularised ulnar nerve is used as an interposed graft in patients whose prognosis for C8 and T1 has been confirmed as hopeless. Gu et al (1992) describe promising results in 10 patients, with adequate follow-up, the first operations being performed in 1986. This innovation is supported by a considerable amount of experimental work. Chen and Gu (1994) found no detectable deficit of function in the donor limb in their rat experimental model. Chen (1996) showed quite decisively that the contralateral 7th cervical nerve was a more effective donor than the phrenic nerve, and also that the vascularised ulnar nerve graft was superior to the nonvascularised graft in reinnervation of biceps. A number of interesting clinical observations have been made. Gu and Shen (1994) examined their first 27 cases by electromyography and nerve conduction studies, finding "that severance of C7 caused no permanent functional damage to the upper limb". Gu and Shen (1994) recorded findings about sensory impairment after section of part or all of C7 in 50 patients. The most commonly afflicted digit was the index finger (34%), followed by the middle finger (58%) and the thumb (38%). Gu emphasised that sensory disturbance after cutting the posterior division of C7 (posterior division of the middle trunk) was considerably less, and in 7 of his 26 patients there was no loss at all. We understand that the Shanghai team now regularly use the posterior division of C7 as a donor in preference to taking the whole nerve. Xu (1996) studied 12 patients during operation, staining biopsies for acetylcholinesterase. He found that C7 contained about 27 000 myelinated fibres, and that the proportion of motor fibres in the posterior division was significantly higher than in the anterior division (30% versus 15%).

One of us was able to review some of Professor Gu's patients in Shanghai, and one of these (described below) is an outstanding example of what is possible.

Case report. A 27-year-old man sustained a complete brachial plexus lesion on June 18 1993. At 3 months, accessory to suprascapular and phrenic to muculocutaneous transfers were performed. At 4½ months intercostal nerves were transferred to the thoracodorsal nerve, and the contralateral C7 was sutured to the ulnar nerve from the damaged limb. At 8 months the graft was sutured to the median nerve. I saw this patient 18 months after reinnervation of the median nerve. Power in the long digital and wrist flexors was MRC grade 4. There was some activity in the abductor pollicis brevis and the patient was able accurately to localise touch, to the thumb and to the index and middle fingers. This patient had regained true hand function, which could have come only through the graft. Those of us examining him were unable to find any significant deficit of power or sensation in the donor limb.

Professor Gu's unit has shown that use of the posterior division of the contralateral seventh cervical nerve is potentially capable of restoring useful function to the hand in cases of complete avulsion. They have shown that delay is harmful and that the interposed graft should be vascularised. We do have reservations about applying this bold technique. Our experience with damage isolated to the seventh cervical nerve is that severe pain is common, and it does seem to be the case that severe pain, which is the rule in European patients, is much less common after closed traction lesion in Chinese and Japanese people. It does seem hard, too, to subject a patient to the risk, albeit slight, of significant loss of function in their one remaining arm. These comments in no way detract from the very real respect that we feel for this well-founded and openly presented work.

Technical considerations

It seems sensible to outline some of the pitfalls we have encountered in nerve transfer operations before describing the results.

Accessory to suprascapular nerve

It is essential that innervation of the upper fibres of the trapezius muscle is preserved. The operation fails if there has been any associated injury to the accessory nerve, if there is a second lesion of the suprascapular nerve, or if the rotator cuff has been torn. Function is poor if the serratus anterior remains paralysed and if there is no adductor function at the shoulder. With these provisions, the operation is useful, especially in partial lesions (Figs 9.47 and 9.48).

Reinnervation of the serratus anterior

This is essential in avulsion of C5, C6 and C7, or in cases of irreparable damage to the nerve in the posterior triangle of the neck or the upper axilla. However, we have encountered cases where C4 contributed to the muscle; in other cases there has been no contribution from C7. In six cases a branch of the dorsal scapular nerve was transferred to a ramus of the nerve to the serratus anterior arising from C5 or C6. In 22 cases we have used the deep division of T4 or T5 to reinnervate the nerve.

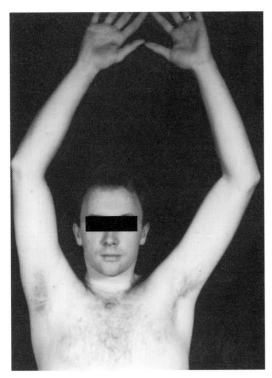

Fig. 9.47 A 22-year-old man: rupture to C5, avulsion to C6. Repair at 4 days: accessory to suprascapular transfer, and graft of the upper trunk. The result at 2 years.

Intercostal transfer

This operation cannot be performed when there have been multiple rib fractures. In cases of phrenic nerve palsy we use only the lateral cutaneous division. We try to preserve the fourth intercostal nerve in young women. Results in patients with Brown–Séquard syndrome are extremely poor.

The incision runs from the upper arm, across the axilla and along the chest wall behind the pectoralis major to the level of the nipple. The wound is deepened to expose nerve trunks within the axillary sheath, and the chest wound is then deepened to expose the artery to serratus anterior. The plane of dissection is anterior to the nerve to the serratus and follows the digitations of that muscle. Now the lateral cutaneous branches of intercostal nerves are identified. These are traced proximally, where they disappear into a tunnel in the serratus. The serratus anterior is sectioned anterior to this perforation and turned back as a flap to reveal the entry of the lateral branch into the intercostal tunnel. In this way T3, T4, T5 and T6 are found. The external intercostal muscle is incised, anterior to the lateral branch and the deep branch identified. The temptation to pull this out with a hook is resisted; rather it is traced with slight strokes of the scalpel as far as the anterior angle of the ribs. Now the external and middle intercostal muscles posterior to the perforating branch are incised and the two branches traced until they become common. Elevation of the nerve is now easy, as far as the posterior angle of the rib, taking care not to lacerate the pleura. A Jackson–Burrows retractor is very useful for spreading the ribs (Fig. 9.49).

Ulnar to biceps transfer (Oberlin's operation)

The ulnar nerve is identified, usually in the middle of the arm running parallel to a vascular pedicle. The ulnar nerve is exposed and its epineurium incised. The nerve contains 6–12 bundles here, and nerve stimulation of low intensity is used to distinguish between those bundles passing chiefly to the intrinsic muscles and those passing to the long flexors and flexor carpi ulnaris. One of the latter bundles is selected (Fig. 9.50).

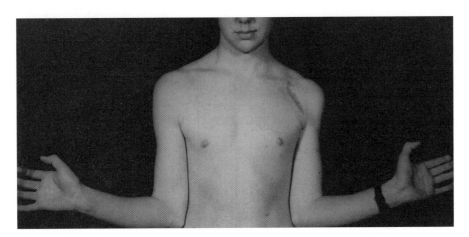

Fig. 9.48 A 17-year-old man: rupture to C5, avulsion to C6. Operation on the day of injury: accessory to suprascapular transfer, and graft of the upper trunk. The range of lateral rotation at 16 months; he had full abduction.

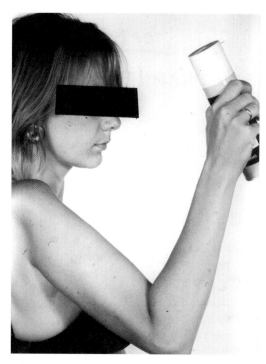

Fig. 9.49 A 28-year-old woman: avulsion at C5 and C6. Operation at 8 weeks: accessory to suprascapular transfer, and intercostal T3 and T5 with deep branch of T4 to musculocutaneous nerve. Function at 22 months; she could abduct to 120°.

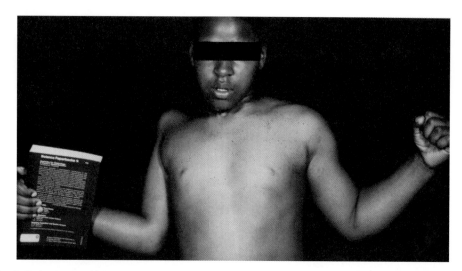

Fig. 9.50 A 13-year-old boy: avulsion of C5, C6 and C7. Repair at 2 months: accessory to suprascapular transfer, and one bundle of the ulnar nerve to the nerve to the biceps and the nerve to the medial head of the triceps; the medial cutaneous nerve of the forearm was transferred to the lateral root of the median nerve. Result at 18 months: full range of lateral rotation; abduction to 60°; power of elbow flexion, MRC grade 4; and power of elbow extension, MRC grade 3+.

RESULTS

Our late colleague Mark Dunkerton studied 154 cases of closed supraclavicular lesion operated on between 1975 and 1983, and developed a system of assessment, some elements of which are set out in Table 9.9; a note of his findings is given in Table 9.10 (Dunkerton, unpublished work, 1985). He allotted scores to different segments of the limb by their ability to perform tasks, and then scored the limb as a whole. Dunkerton's system was extended by Holt (1994) and by Patterson, Dunkerton et al (1990) in their analysis of shoulder function after grafting and nerve transfer, and we are grateful to our colleagues for releasing to us their accumulated data, much of which remains unpublished (Holt (1994) should be consulted). Their system is summarised in Table 9.11.

Amongst Algimantas Narakas' many contributions, one in particular is notable because it permits comparison of results between different units using different types of repair. He outlined the system in 1986 at a meeting held in Lausanne. It is set out in Table 9.12. We have incorporated this into our own method, which includes an analysis of the benefits of operations for reconstruction, the effect of operation on pain, and the extent of rehabilitation (Table 9.13). Over 600 cases have been entered into this system since 1988. Narakas was well aware of the defects of his system, which include a bias towards function at the shoulder and elbow at the expense of the hand, a bias in favour of motor recovery at the expense of sensation, and the lack of any assessment of pain. Nevertheless, it is an important contribution and most of the results which now follow are based on it.

We describe below the results obtained in: 65 cases of vascularised ulnar nerve graft; 149 consecutive repairs performed during 1991–1993; 403 nerve transfers performed during 1986–1992; and 15 older patients operated on during 1988–1994. We have already referred to Dunkerton's

Table 9.9 Method of assessment of outcome

1. Patient details	Including limb dominance and occupation
2. Accident details	Including analysis of force expended on forequarter
3. Clinical findings	Including directly related injury, distant injury; noting endocrine abnormality and Brown–Séquard syndrome
4. Ancillary evidence	Including physiological, histamine, sensory action potential, radiological, myelography
5. Findings at operation	Action
6. Progression of recovery	For sensation, muscle power, temperature sense, by individual spinal nerve
7. Usefulness of limb	Shoulder – holding objects against side; reaching above head
	Elbow – supporting objects
	Hand and forearm – writing
8. Overall limb function	Graded by such functions as brushing or combing hair, opening a door, taking food to mouth, holding objects, and scored from 0–10

Drawn from Dunkerton (unpublished material, 1984) and much abbreviated.

Table 9.10 Operated closed supraclavicular lesions ($n = 154$), 1975–1984*

Mean age	21 years
Motorcycle accident	92%
Repairs by graft	85 cases
No repair possible	37 cases
Lesions in continuity	32 cases
Rupture subclavian–axillary artery	12 cases

Drawn from Dunkerton (unpublished work, 1984).
*Excludes repair by vascularised ulnar nerve graft.

Comment on Dunkerton's study. From 38 patients with grafts for ruptures of C5 and C6, 17 regained shoulder control and elbow flexion, 18 more recovered elbow flexion, while 3 patients made no recovery at all. Dunkerton found no difference in outcome between the 11 cases repaired within 1 month of injury and the 27 cases repaired after 1 month. He also commented that early exploration was more reliable in predicting outcome of lesions in continuity: 6 of 7 cases explored within 2 weeks of injury with lesions deemed favourable went on to good recovery, whereas only 7 of 12 cases with lesions in continuity explored later did reasonably well.

Table 9.11 Suprascapular nerve function (Holt 1994)

Excellent	
Abduction	> 120
Lateral rotation	> 60
Supraspinatus	MRC grade 5
Infraspinatus	MRC grade 4 or better
Narakas gain	9 points
Good	
Abduction	> 60
Lateral rotation	> 30
Supraspinatus	MRC grade 4
Infraspinatus	MRC grade 3
Narakas gain	7–8 points
Fair	
Abduction	30–60
Lateral rotation	10–30
Supraspinatus	MRC grade 3 or better
Infraspinatus	MRC grade 3 or better
Narakas gain	4–6 points
Poor	
Abduction	< 30
Lateral rotation	< 10
Supraspinatus	MRC grade 2 + or less
Infraspinatus	MRC grade 2 + or less
Narakas gain	3 points or less

Table 9.12 Narakas' score chart

	0	1	2	3	4	5
Shoulder: 13 points						
Abduction and/or forward flexion (max. 5 points)	Flail	0–30 stable	30–60	60–90	90–120	>120
External rotation (max. 4 points)	0	0–10	10–30	30–60	60	
Thoracobrachial grasp (max. 2 points)	0	Can hold a file against chest	Can hold a bag weighing 1 kg or more against chest			
Posterior projection (max. 2 points)	Nil	Wrist can be brought to lateral aspect of hip	Wrist behind plane of glutei or better			
Elbow: max. 9 points						
Flexion (5 points)	0	Hand to pocket or belt	To 90° against gravity	To 90° with 1 kg in hand	To 90° or more with 3 kg	Flexes 90° or more with 3 kg
Extension (4 points)	Not possible	Full extension	Extends with 1 kg	Extends with 3 kg	Better than 3 kg	
Forearm, pronosupination: max. 3 points	None	10–50°	50° or better	100° or better		
Wrist: max. 8 points						
Extension (4 points)	None	Against gravity	With 1 kg in hand	With 3 kg	Better than 3 kg	
Flexion (4 points)	None	Incomplete against gravity	Complete against gravity	With 1 kg or against strong grasp	More than 1 kg	
Hand: max. 17 points★						
Long fingers motor (max. 5 points)	Total palsy	Passive hook	Active hook by finger flexion (primitive grasp)	Opening and closing fist power 1<3 kg	Power 3–8 kg	Independence of finger grasp >8 kg

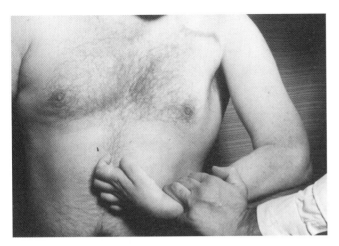

Fig. 9.53 Rupture of C5, avulsion of C6 to T1. One strand of vascularised ulnar nerve graft from C5 to the lateral cord. Outcome at 20 months.

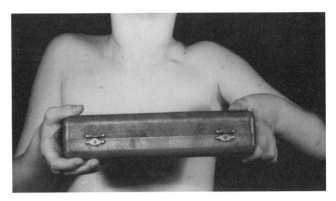

Fig. 9.54 A 3-year-old girl: rupture of C5 and C6, avulsion of C7, C8 and T1. Repair by 3 strands of vascularised ulnar nerve graft, with other grafts to the lateral and posterior cords and the medial root of the median nerve. Function at 3 years.

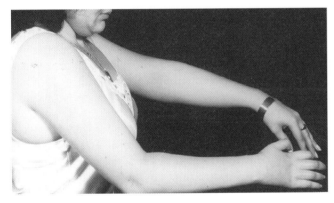

Fig. 9.55 A 17-year-old girl: result at 8 years.

Delay

There is an inexorable decline in results with delay (Tables 9.15 and 9.16).

Age

Repairs were performed in complete lesions in 15 patients aged between 46 and 73 years during the period 1988–1994. Results were poor but by no means worthless, and we do not think that older patients should be denied operation even if this does little more than establish prognosis (Table 9.17).

Table 9.15 Effect of delay on recovery: 147 cases of closed supraclavicular injury repaired 1991–1993; minimum follow-up 24 months (14 patients lost to follow-up)

	Repair within				
Gain in Narakas' points	14 days	3 months	6 months	12 months	>12 months
Partial lesion: (C7) (C8) T1 intact					
0–5	4	5	2	7	3
6–10	7	15	6	3	0
11–15	10	2	1	0	0
16–20	8	4	1	0	0
≥21	0	0	0	0	0
Complete lesion: ruptures or avulsions C5–T1					
0–5	11	9	4	2	2
6–10	8	6	4	1	0
11–15	11	1	1	0	0
16–20	2	0	0	0	0
≥21	2	0	0	0	0

(i)   In 6 more patients there was *no* recovery at all – no motor nor sensory improvement and no relief of pain.
(ii) 33 of 63 cases operated on within 14 days of injury gained 11 points or more.
(iii) 7 of 43 cases operated on between 15 days and 3 months from injury gained 11 points or more.
(iv) 3 of 19 cases operated on between 3 and 6 months from injury gained 11 points.
(v)   *None* of the 18 cases operated after 6 months from injury gained 11 points.
(vi) 55 of 153 cases achieved no *useful* function.
(vii) 43 of 153 cases achieved two-segment function. Of these, 33 were operated on within 14 days.
(viii) 3 patients regained useful hand function following repair. *All* were operated on within 14 days.
(ix) Vascularised ulnar nerve graft excluded.

Table 9.16 Recovery and interval from injury to repair: 367 "elements" (grafted roots, or transfers to trunk nerves) in 153 cases operated on during 1991–1993

	Interval from injury to repair			
Recovery	Within 14 days	To 3 months	To 6 months	To 12 months
Partial				
Useful	75	83	16	11
Failure	11	25	3	11
Complete				
Useful	43	15	3	7
Failure	22	17	6	19

(i) Intercostal transfers for pain relief, for hand sensation, and for medial cord function are not included.
(ii) Vascularised ulnar nerve graft excluded.

Table 9.17 Effect of age on recovery: 15 patients with complete lesions and partial lesions operated on during 1988–1994; aged over 45 years at the time of injury

Recovery	No. of patients
Useful*	5
None	10

* Useful recovery is defined as a gain of 6 points or more from the repair.

Table 9.18 Effect of extent of lesion on recovery of grafts of 153 roots,* 1991–1993

	Extent of lesion	
Recovery	Partial	Complete
Good	38	14
Fair	28	34
Poor	13	26

* These results for each *root* grafted: good, 6 points or more; fair, 3–5 points; poor, <3 points.

Table 9.19 Results of 403 nerve transfers, 1986–1992

Transfer	No. cases
Nerve to serratus anterior	28
Accessory to suprascapular	156
Intercostal to circumflex	6
Accessory to musculocutaneous	11
Oberlin's operation (ulnar to nerve to biceps)	17
Intercostal to lateral cord	138
Intercostal to nerve to biceps, or nerve to wrist extension	21
Intercostal to medial cord, or derivatives	26

Intercostal transfer solely for pain is considered in Chapter 15, and is not included here.

Extent of lesion

Recovery is less after grafts in complete than in partial lesions. It may be that some of the repaired roots were poor, but we think that this reflects a decline in the regenerative capacity of cells within the spinal cord and dorsal root ganglia (Table 9.18).

Nerve transfers

The results of 403 nerve transfers done during 1986–1992 are given in Table 9.19.

1. *Nerve to serratus anterior*. Results were useful in 26 of 28 cases. This seems to be the most reliable of our transfers (Table 9.20).
2. *Accessory to suprascapular*. The results of 74 of 96 transfers in partial lesions were fair or better, with function superior to glenohumeral arthrodesis (Table 9.21). Results for the complete lesions were much worse, an observation first made by Holt (1994). Patterson et al (1990) described 44 cases of reinnervation of the suprascapular nerve in patients with lesions of the upper part of the brachial plexus. In 14 cases the rupture of the upper trunk was grafted. In 16 more the trunk was repaired by graft but the suprascapular nerve was separately repaired by the graft passing between it and the anterior face of C5. Accessory to suprascapular transfer was performed in the last 14 patients, with repair of the ruptures of C5 and C6. The shoulder function was decidedly better in the last group than in the first two. The reasons for failure included a second lesion of the suprascapular nerve (2 cases), rupture of the rotator cuff (5 cases), stiffness of the glenohumeral joint from intra-articular fracture (11 cases) and paralysis of the serratus anterior and the shoulder adductors (18 cases).

Table 9.20 Nerve to serratus anterior transfer: 28 cases (intercostal 21, branch of dorsal scapular 7)

Result (MRC class)	No. cases
4 or better	22
3	4
Less	2

Table 9.21 Accessory to suprascapular transfer: 156 cases

Result	Partial lesion	Complete lesion
Excellent	16	4
Good	21	6
Fair	37	15
Poor	22	33

The operation is valuable in avulsion of the upper three roots. When it is combined with grafts to the posterior division of the upper trunk results are usually superior to those following repair of distal ruptures of the circumflex and suprascapular nerves (Figs 9.56 to 9.58).

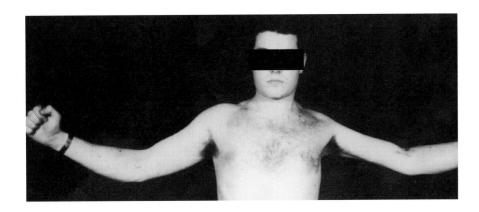

Fig. 9.56 A 26-year-old man: rupture at C5, avulsion at C6 and C7. Operation at 4 days: branch of dorsal scapular nerve to serratus anterior, accessory to suprascapular nerve, graft of C5 to upper trunk, and supraclavicular nerves to C7. Function at 28 months.

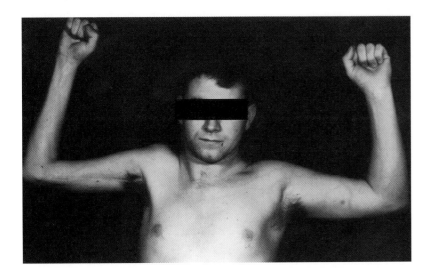

Fig. 9.57 A 22-year-old man: rupture at C5, avulsion at C6 and C7. Operation at 10 days from injury: accessory to suprascapular nerve and branch of dorsal scapular nerve to serratus anterior, graft of C5 to upper trunk. Function at 18 months.

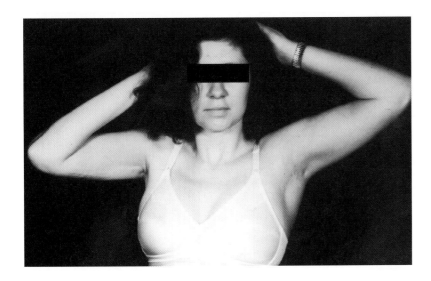

Fig. 9.58 A 26-year-old woman: rupture at C5, avulsion at C6 and C7. Accessory to suprascapular transfer, branch of dorsal scapular to nerve to serratus anterior, graft of C5 to the lateral cord and intercostal T3, and deep branch T4 and T5 to circumflex nerve. Function at 26 months.

Elbow flexion

We have used accessory to musculocutaneous transfer as an operation of last resort in 11 cases and found it useful in 9 (Table 9.22).

Oberlin's operation

Oberlin recommends this for avulsion of C5 and C6. Our own results were unsatisfactory when C7 was avulsed (Table 9.23). This is the most reliable nerve transfer for elbow flexion when used within the indications described by its originator.

Intercostal transfer

In common with our colleagues on the Continent, we have not matched the results of Nagano and colleagues (Table 9.24). Results are disappointing in the complete lesion. It is sometimes possible to separate the motor division of musculocutaneous nerve from the cutaneous branch as far proximally as the axilla, and this permits direct transfer to it of the deep divisions of T3, T4 and T5. This seems better than transferring the whole intercostal nerve to the musculocutaneous nerve.

The use of intercostal nerves in obstetric palsy is described in Chapter 10 and in the relief of pain in Chapter 15. Useful sensation was regained in the hand in only about 10% of cases, with ability to localise to the thumb and the index and middle fingers. Protective sensation was recovered in about 40%. In most patients, light touch is referred to the chest wall. It appears that transfer of the medial cutaneous nerve of forearm, when that is possible, is more reliable in restoring sensation to the thumb and index finger.

The role of intercostals in other transfers are set out in Tables 9.25 to 9.27. The occasional useful result following the transfer to the medial head of the median or ulnar nerves is interesting. In four patients the flexor digitorum profundus recovered power to MRC grade 4, there was recovery into intrinsic muscles sufficient to balance the posture of the digits, and light touch was accurately localised within the digits. All four of these patients were aged less than 21 years, and in three cases the operation was performed within a few days of the injury. Much has been achieved in 25 years. The advances include: the ability regularly to restore useful function in the proximal parts of the limb; greater accuracy in diagnosis; versatility of techniques of repair; and, as we think is shown beyond any shadow of reasonable doubt, urgency of repair. This leaves us with the complete lesion; about one-half of the total. The three approaches have been outlined. These are: limited reinnervation by graft and transfer, free muscle transfer, and contralateral plexus transfer. We think the way forward is through repair, by replantation, of the avulsed nerves.

Table 9.22 Accessory to musculocutaneous transfer: 11 cases

Result (MRC class)	No. cases
Elbow flexion 3 or better	9
Elbow flexion 2 or less	2

Table 9.23 Oberlin's operation: ulnar to nerve to biceps: 17 cases

Result (MRC class)	No. cases
Elbow flexion 4 or better	9
Elbow flexion 3 to 3+	4
Elbow flexion 2 or less	4

Table 9.24 Intercostal to lateral cord transfer – musculocutaneous: 138 cases

Result (MRC class)	Partial lesion	Complete lesion
Elbow flexion 3+ or better	24	6
Elbow flexion 3	15	18
Elbow flexion 2 or less	36	39

Table 9.25 Intercostal to circumflex transfer: 6 cases

Result (MRC class)	No. cases
Deltoid 4	2
Deltoid 3	2
Deltoid 2 or less	2

Table 9.26 Transfer of intercostal nerves to triceps or to radial wrist extensors

Result (MRC class)	No. cases
Triceps 3	4
Triceps 2 or less	11
Wrist extension 3	2
Wrist extension 2 or less	4

Table 9.27 Transfer of the intercostal nerves to medial cord or derivatives: 26 cases

Result (MRC class)	No. cases
FDP, 4; intrinsic muscles, 2	4
Protective sensation ulnar two digits FDP and FCU, 3	6
Some sensation FDP, 2 or less	6
No function	10

FCU, flexor carpi unlaris; FDU, flexor digitorum profundus.

REIMPLANTATION OF AVULSED SPINAL NERVES

(What follows is a transcript of the paper given by George Bonney at the Brachial Plexus Conference held in Edinburgh, at the College of Surgeons in February 1994.)

THE FIRST CLINICAL CASE
– GEORGE BONNEY, 1977

The complete supraclavicular traction lesion of the brachial plexus is perhaps the most shattering of all injuries of the peripheral nerves. Its high incidence is in young persons, in young men in particular; many of those injured are not educationally prepared for sedentary work; the results of treatment, though better than formerly, are still poor; many patients are subject to constant pain from early days after injury, and many of these continue for years to experience that pain. The principal cause of the poor results and of the pain is certainly the high incidence of avulsion of roots from the spinal cord. I use the term "avulsion" because that is the description in general use, but I shall later show that, in certain cases at least, the lesion is an actual rupture of roots near the spinal cord. In this respect – that of the proximity of the lesion to the spinal cord – the supraclavicular lesion of the plexus may be regarded as one not only of the peripheral but also of the central nervous system. From that extension of the lesion flow many of the difficulties surrounding its treatment.

Avulsion is more common in the lower than the upper roots. It usually affects both posterior and anterior roots of the nerve or nerves affected. The extent of movement of the avulsed roots depends on the degree of force to which the limb is subjected and on the amount of separation of the forequarter from the axial skeleton. Usually, the roots are dragged from the spinal cord, through the intervertebral foramen and into the supraclavicular region. In some they may be dragged as far as the space deep to the clavicle; in others, the separation is slight enough to permit the roots to remain in the intervertebral canal. At the time of injury, the dura-arachnoid of the root sleeve is torn, so that there is an outflow of spinal fluid. The amount of outflow depends on the extent of the tear in the dura-arachnoid: it may be so slight as to form no more than a small collection in the intervertebral foramen. As time goes by, the collection of fluid becomes encapsulated to form a pseudomeningocele.

When they are widely displaced, the avulsed roots soon become fixed in the position of displacement by longitudinal contracture of the nerves themselves, and by surrounding organisation of exudate and blood.

The actual level of the neural lesion is certainly in some cases, and in the case of the posterior roots, just distal to the surface of the spinal cord. In the case of the anterior roots, it has been reported that anterior horn cells have been avulsed with the roots, although limited observations seem to show that this is an exceptional circumstance. I dare say that the usual site of rupture of anterior roots is just distal to the surface of the spinal cord. I do not doubt that more study of the spinal roots is required to determine the level of separation. If indeed there are two categories of "avulsion" – separation just outside the surface of the cord, and true avulsion from the substance of the cord – important questions are raised about the different degrees of damage to the cord. In the first type of lesion, the damage to the cord would be slight; but in the latter case, extensive damage would be done to all the laminae in the posterior horn. It could be that the cases in which the separation has occurred outside the cord are those in which pain is not experienced. "De-afferentation" alone may not be enough to explain the whole of the pain in these cases.

Up to the present, high traction lesions of the brachial plexus have been treated, where possible, by graft repair of nerves ruptured outside the spinal canal, and by "neurotisation", according to art and to availability of donor nerves, of the distal segments of avulsed roots. The results have certainly been an improvement on those of former methods of treatment by waiting for natural recovery, by peripheral "reconstruction," and by amputation arthrodesis. In particular, relief of pain following reinnervation along a "neurotised" nerve has been seen too often for this phenomenon to be discounted as incidental.

The goal of many of those working in this field has for long been the reimplantation of avulsed roots. The idea is superficially attractive: in the case of many fibres of the posterior root in particular, the nerve cell is not far from its termination in the posterior horn, either at the level of entry or at a few levels up or down the cord. In a simplified mode of thought, the liability to confusion between afferent and efferent axons is diminished by the separation into anterior and posterior roots.

When the matter is viewed more deeply, many difficulties arise: practical difficulties, technical difficulties, and difficulties concerned with the microstructure of the elements concerned. First, reimplantation is, in most cases, possible only within the first 48 hours after injury: after that time the avulsed roots are so much fixed in the position of displacement that they cannot be drawn back through the intervertebral foramina into contact with the spinal cord. Next, such early intervention is rarely possible: lesions of this severity are often associated with other, life-threatening, injuries that require treatment before neural repair can be contemplated. Thirdly, surgeons capable of reimplanting an avulsed brachial plexus are so widely scattered as to make it unlikely that a suitable patient and suitable surgeon will meet at the rendezvous.

The next consideration concerns the spinal cord itself. In these cases the cord has been damaged by the avulsion of one to five roots. The risks of interfering, however marginally, on this damaged cord are clear. In the case of the anterior roots, reimplantation through a posterior approach is possible only if the cord is rotated. Certainly, the cord can, with care and for short periods, be rotated by means of small stays inserted in the denticulate ligaments, but any prolonged rotation or any clumsy rotation will surely damage (at least) the ipsilateral long tracts.

The posterior roots are, near the cord, represented as multiple rootlets that pose particular problems in repair. The stouter, usually single, anterior roots are, for reasons already advanced, difficult to access by the posterior approach. Although the roots have a collagen content, in comparison with the peripheral nerve they are intensely fragile and susceptible to surgical trauma.

As to the small scale, we are here proceeding in the transitional region between the central and the peripheral nervous systems, where the "matrix" changes from one of oligodentrocytes and astrocytes to one of Schwann cells and collagen. Indeed, it may be that in the case to which I shall later refer, the actual separation took place in that transitional zone. Axons are indeed continuous through this zone, though extensive arrangements take place near it; it may be that certain axons have smaller diameters in the central nervous system than they have in the periphery. There is, I think, a separation of the blood supplies of the two systems; Carlstedt and colleagues tell us that "no blood vessels are seen in the mantle zone" of the transitional region (Berthold et al 1993).

The separation of function implied by the division into anterior and posterior roots is not, of course, complete. There are many unmyelinated and small myelinated afferent fibres in the anterior root: there are in the anterior root of the first thoracic nerve the preganglionic fibres of the autonomic system. The variation of destination of the preganglionic fibres of the posterior root is extreme: many of the large myelinated fibres terminate in the first to the fourth laminae of the posterior horn; proprioceptive primary afferents terminate in the two deeper laminae. Great possibilities for confusion are present.

I describe my first experience of the "reimplantation" of cervical nerve roots to show that in certain cases this is technically possible. Since that time, experimental work has been done to show that the theory of this "reimplantation" was unsound; on the other hand, other experimental work has shown the validity of such reconnection in the case of the anterior roots, and that end to end anastomosis or reimplantation is not essential.

In 1977, my colleague Michael Laurence, then orthopaedic surgeon at Guy's Hospital, called me to see a young man who had been admitted to Guy's with all the signs of a complete avulsion of the right brachial plexus resulting from a motor cycle accident. There were no serious associated injuries; the patient's condition was very good. This patient was instantly transferred to St Mary's Hospital,

Paddington, where I was then orthopaedic surgeon. I confirmed Michael Laurence's diagnosis, and made arrangements for operation.

The operation, with anaesthetic given by Dr Clive Roberts, lasted 12 hours. It was done by Angus Jamieson and myself. Surgery was started about 24 hours after injury. With the patient in the left lateral position, I exposed the brachial plexus above the clavicle; the plexus had, as was expected, been completely avulsed. I marked the seventh and eighth cervical nerves and their roots. I then exposed the posterior elements of the cervical spine through a posterior incision, and went on to expose the right side of the cervical dura by hemilaminectomy. I opened the dura to expose the right side of the spinal cord and to show the avulsion of the roots. Now I passed fine forceps through the foramina between the sixth and seventh and seventh and eighth vertebrae, and with these caught hold of sutures tied to the cuffs of dura at the junction of roots with peripheral nerves. With these sutures, the roots were drawn back into the spinal canal. Forceful traction was not needed; the roots lay easily in the canal, offering themselves for reattachment. I decided, because of the dangers already mentioned, to reattach the posterior roots and to confine the reattachment to the seventh and eighth nerves. With some difficulty, I repaired the dural defects at the levels of avulsion in order to lessen later traction on the repaired roots.

Now, using the microscope, Angus Jamieson inspected the surface of the cord. It was clear that the rupture had taken place just distal to the surface of the cord: little stumps of the rootlets were visible. This observation may be of particular importance. With the microscope, and using 11/0 sutures, Angus was able to reattach the rootlets of the two nerves. The dura was closed; both wounds were closed in the usual way. I did not use any external splintage after operation (Figs 9.59 and 9.60).

Although the patient recovered easily and well from the intervention, there was no evidence of regeneration during the period of observation, which was unusually short (18 months). It is perhaps interesting that there was no pain during the period of observation.

Evidently, reimplantation, or perhaps reattachment, of avulsed (or perhaps ruptured) roots is possible. However, it is doubtful whether any regeneration is possible along posterior, afferent roots. Experimental evidence suggests that regeneration is possible along anterior, largely efferent roots; the experience of this single case suggests that such reattachment is possible, and that the hazard is not prohibitive.

If such reattachment were to be attempted, it might be preferable to approach the cord from the front, through the vertebral bodies and intervertebral discs. Not only is the cord accessible by this approach, but the line of avulsion or rupture is presented to the operator's vision. Further, such an approach would allow the whole operation

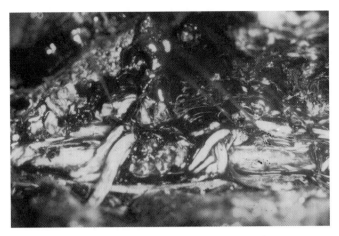

Fig. 9.59 Roots of C7 and C8 drawn back into the canal.

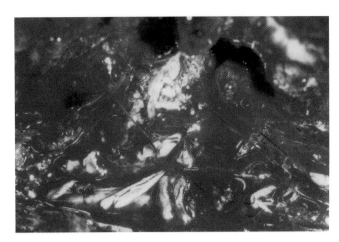

Fig. 9.60 The dorsal roots reimplanted.

to be done through a single incision and approach, with the patient in the semisedentary position.

Further work is, as I have suggested, necessary in order to attempt to confirm the level of separation or avulsion of the roots in humans after injury. The best evidence comes from inspection of the cord within 48 hours of injury, but opportunities for that are rare and may be getting rarer. It may be that more attention should be given to the proximal ends of avulsed roots found at supraclavicular exploration, in an attempt to determine whether the separation is in fact at the transitional zone between central and peripheral nervous tissue.

I have many people to thank for giving me this opportunity, and only myself to blame for the failure to take full advantage of it. Michael Laurence was sharp enough to recognise the opportunity, Clive Roberts saw the patient safely through a prolonged operation, the operation theatre staff provided the means, and Angus Jamieson did the difficult part of the procedure, adding at the same time a valuable insight into the level of separation. Sadly, the patient did not benefit, but he did not suffer damage.

SUBSEQUENT WORK – THE EXPERIENCE OF THOMAS CARLSTEDT

Prompted by these earliest attempts at reimplantation Jamieson and Eames (1980) demonstrated regeneration of axons through reattached ventral roots in the dog. Carlstedt et al (1900) went very much further in a lengthy series of experiments, and we are particularly grateful to Thomas Carlstedt for releasing his original material and for his open discussion of his work. In 1983, Risling, Culheim and Hildebrand showed regeneration into the ventral roots of peripheral nerves after axonotomy within the lumbar cord of the cat. Using this model, Linda et al (1993) showed that half of the motor neurons had survived and that axons grew into the ventral root within a

month of injury. Carlstedt et al (1986) demonstrated functional recovery after reimplantation of the ventral root in rats. Carlstedt and colleagues (Culheim et al 1989) confirmed functional integration of spinal cord circuit by intracellular technique and staining (Figs 9.61 to 9.63), and went on to work with monkeys, proving that functional recovery was possible after reimplantation of ventral roots of C5, C6, and C7 (Carlstedt et al 1993). However, useful hand function was not seen after reimplantation of C8 and T1. This regeneration, within the cord itself, was associated with laminin and low affinity neurotrophin receptor, which are known to be specific for regeneration within peripheral nerves (Risling et al 1993). In the early stages of recovery there was incoordination or co-contraction, but with maturation of the repair useful voluntary arm movements returned.

Carlstedt applied this knowledge to humans, and he has now operated on seven adults and two children with obstetric palsy. The outcome of his first five adult cases is shown in Table 9.28. He uses the posterior subscapular approach developed by Kline et al (1992) (see Ch. 7) to expose the brachial plexus. The spinal cord is then displayed by hemilaminectomy. The ventral roots or interposed grafts are inserted just below the surface of the cord through small slits in the pia, and secured with fibrin clot glue (Figs 9.64 and 9.65).

Case 2 in Table 9.28 was reported by Carlstedt, Grane, Hallin and Norén in 1995. Electromyographic evidence of reinnervation of muscles through the reattached ventral roots of C6 and C7 was evident at 9 months (Figs 9.66 and 9.67). The fifth cervical nerve was blocked with local anaesthetic. There was no effect on biceps function.

Carlstedt has made further observations and suggestions. He points out that myelography may be misleading. In case 1 (see Table 9.28) for instance, myelography suggested that C5 and C6 were intact while C7, C8 and T1 were avulsed. In fact, C5 and C6 were avulsed, T1 was

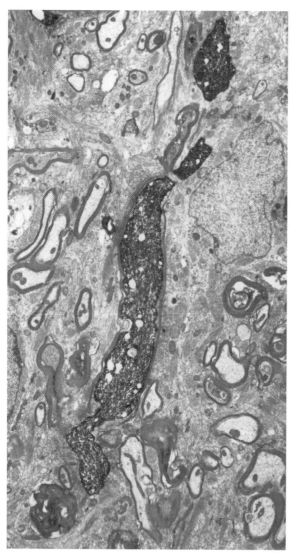

Fig. 9.61 Regenerating motor axons in the lumbar spinal cord of the cat. Horseradish peroxidase, tangential section, × 2700. (Courtesy of Mr Thomas Carlstedt.)

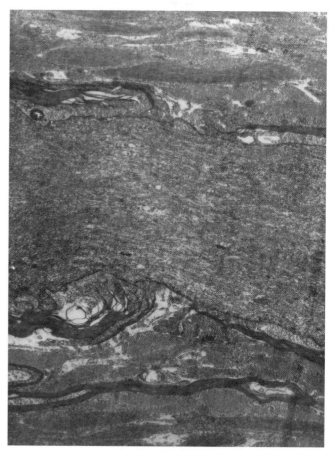

Fig. 9.62 Regenerating motor axon in the lumbar spinal cord of the cat. Horseradish peroxidase, tangential section, × 8000. (Courtesy of Mr Thomas Carlstedt.)

not. This operative finding had been predicted by the recording of sensory action potentials for the median and ulnar nerves. Carlstedt goes further: it may be the case that recovery is more likely in ruptures of roots peripheral to the transitional zone and the deviation of the cord in case 1 was an indication that the prognosis was singularly poor. These suggestions and findings add much weight to the concept of two fundamentally distinct types of preganglionic injury: central to and peripheral to the transitional zones.

Carlstedt's findings in two cases of birth lesion are significant. In one case, operated on at 8 months of age, the plexus appeared healthy in the posterior triangle. At hemilaminectomy the fifth and sixth cervical nerves were found avulsed; these were central lesions. The ventral roots were reimplanted through serial nerve grafts. By 1 year there was electromyographic evidence of recovery into deltoid and biceps, but this did not advance to functional gain.

We think that Thomas Carlstedt's work points the way to the future. There can be no doubt that functional recovery from the spinal cord to the periphery is possible. Much remains to be done – improvements in access to the spinal cord, the possibility of repair directly to the torn stumps of central roots and the problem of sensory recovery through the repaired dorsal rootlets.

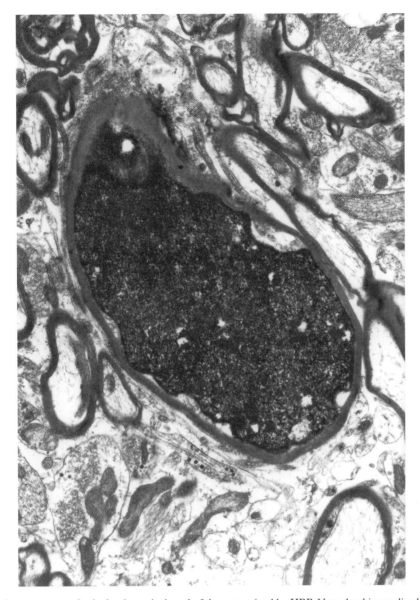

Fig. 9.63 Regenerating motor axon in the lumbar spinal cord of the cat, stained by HRP. Note the thin myelin sheath. The specimen was taken at 1 year from operation. Horseradish peroxidase, longitudinal section, × 30 400. (Courtesy of Mr Thomas Carlstedt.)

Table 9.28 Outcome after spinal cord implantation of avulsed ventral roots: the first five operated patients, with minimum 1 year follow-up

Patient No.	Age (years)	Delay	Avulsion	Implantation	Outcome (MRC class)
1	28	7 months	C5, C8	C5, C6	At 3 years: supraspinatus, 2; biceps, 1
2	26	1 month	C6, T1	C6, C7	At 3 years: supra and infraspinatus deltoid, triceps, brachioradialis, 2; pectoralis biceps, 4
3	46	3 weeks	C5, T1	C5, C6	At 2 years: no recovery
4	33	2 months	C5, C6	C5, C6	At 1 year: biceps, 1
5	25	2 weeks	C5, C7	C5, C6, C7	At 1 year: supra and infraspinatus deltoid, biceps 1; triceps, supinator, 2

Figs 9.64 and 9.65 Re-connection to cord (Thomas Carlstedt: Case 2). The left side of the spinal cord is shown.

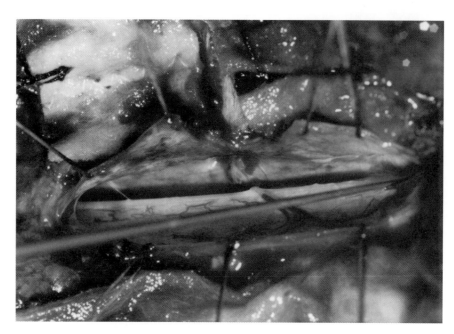

Fig. 9.64 Note the short stump of the dorsal rootlet of C6.

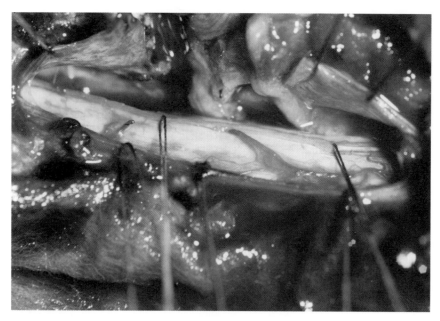

Fig. 9.65 Sural grafts implanted.

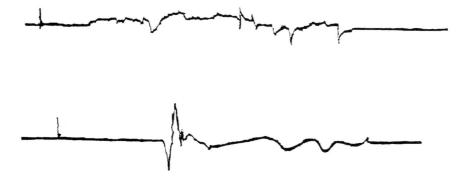

Fig. 9.66 Electromyogram of biceps muscle 3 months (top) and 9 months (bottom) after reimplantation. Note the return of the action potential. (Thomas Carlstedt's: Case 2).

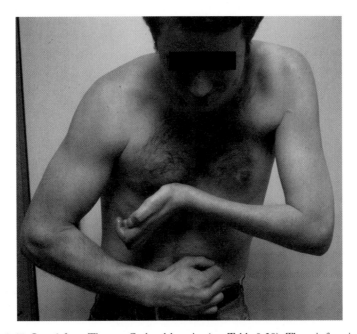

Fig. 9.67 Case 2 from Thomas Carlstedt's series (see Table 9.28). There is functional flexion at the elbow. There has been useful recovery in the deltoid and pectoralis major and some recovery into the brachioradialis and the extensor muscles of the wrist.

10. Birth lesions of the brachial plexus

Historical review; epidemiology; natural history; classification; diagnosis, treatment and after-care; measurement of outcome; absence of pain in children with traction lesion of plexus; deformities in obstetric brachial plexus palsy; classification; recognition and treatment.

Platt (1956) wrote elegantly of the birth lesion of the brachial plexus, describing it as "a vanishing condition". Seddon (1975) said: "the decline in the incidence of these injuries during the last 40 years, which is not confined to what we are pleased to call advanced countries, is one indication of widespread improvement of the standard of obstetrics. Whereas Sever, an American, writing in 1925 could report 1100 cases, my own experience is limited to under 50 cases over a period of almost 40 years." It is no longer true to say that obstetric brachial plexus palsy (OBPP) is a rare condition. We have seen a dramatic increase in cases over the last 5 years, and new cases now exceed adult referrals to our centre. Rational discussion of the British experience is marred by the inadequacy of our Central Statistical Service in the Office of Population Censuses and Surveys. Birth lesions of the plexus are lumped together with congenital deformities. The deterioration of our statistical service is further exposed by Power (1994), who commented: "it is regrettable that figures for birth weights were no longer kept in England and Wales from 1986". We start from two weak points in the British experience: the incidence is unknown, and one of the most important risk factors cannot be measured.

Serious study of the disorder began over 150 years ago, significantly earlier than equivalent work in the adult lesion. The history of this study is marked by controversy about causation, about the natural history and treatment, and about the causes of secondary deformity. These controversies persist. Smellie (1765) is credited with the first description of the birth lesion. He reported the case of a child born with bilateral weakness, who rapidly recovered. Danyou (1851) described the necroscopy findings in an 8-day-old baby: he found blood staining within the upper trunk of the brachial plexus. It fell to Duchenne (1872) to confirm that the lesion of the brachial plexus was caused during birth and that it was not a congenital lesion. Duchenne described four cases of complete paralysis involving loss of control of the shoulder and loss of elbow flexion caused by avulsion of C5 and C6, a rare injury (Fig. 10.1a). Erb (1875, 1876) defined the level of the lesion, at the formation of the upper trunk. Klumpke

(1885) described lesions of the lower nerves in the brachial plexus, and also emphasised the significance of the Bernard–Horner sign (Figs 10.1b and 10.2). The cause and the most important patterns of injury were clearly defined over 100 years ago. There followed important work which identified risk factors and mechanisms of injury. Trombetta (1880) found that two groups were particularly at risk: the heavy baby and the baby born by breech. Duval and Guillain (1898) showed that spinal nerves were stretched and that the 5th and 6th cervical nerves were prone to rupture when the shoulder was forcibly depressed. The involvement of the central nervous system was described by Boyer (1911) from necropsy findings in a 41-year-old woman. By the turn of the century there was a good deal of interest in operative repair. Kennedy (1903) described three cases of suture of the upper trunk, Clark et al (1905) reported seven more, and Taylor (1920) described 200 cases, operating in 80. Wyeth and Sharpe (1917) reviewed 81 cases, and recommended operation at 1 month of age if the lesion was complete and at 3 months if recovery was incomplete.

Postoperative deaths and the difficulty in demonstrating benefit following repair led to disenchantment with this pioneering work. Other writers, including Sever (1925) and Jepson (1930), described cases of complete paralysis in children who had undergone excision of neuroma and repair, commenting that these were the only examples they ever saw of complete failure of recovery. The following two generations saw a good deal of interest in palliative operations. We now acknowledge the work of those European colleagues who started again with detailed studies of the natural history of OBPP and who recommenced operative repair. Their work has stimulated much of our own. In the late 1970s, Morelli and Narakas, encouraged by their experience with adults, made a disciplined start in delineating the indications for, and the techniques of, operative repair (Narakas 1981a, Morelli et al 1984). Gilbert, who now has the largest experience of any, carefully described the natural history of an untreated population and, with his colleague Tassin, proposed a system of classification which is now widely adopted

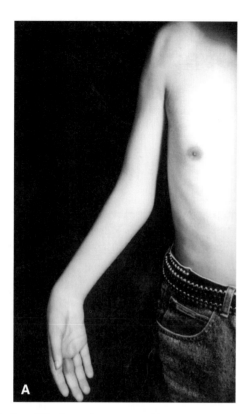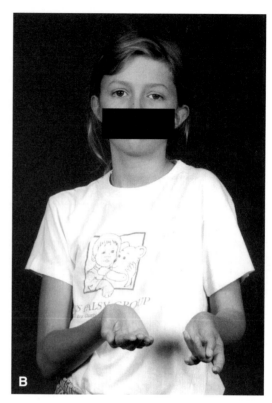

Fig. 10.1 (a) Lesion of Duchenne in a 17-year-old man. Poor function in the shoulder, atrophy of elbow flexor muscles, and ulnar deviation of the wrist indicate avulsion of C5 and C6. (b) Klumpke's lesion in a 12-year-old girl. The small muscles of the hand are atrophied: the extrinsic digital flexors and extensors are weak or paralysed, the wrist extensors are unopposed; note the Bernard–Horner sign.

(Gilbert & Tassin 1984). Gilbert and Raimondi (1993) have developed useful systems for measuring outcome for the shoulder, the elbow, and the hand. Zancolli & Zancolli (1993) continued with extensive and impressive analytic studies of the associated secondary deformities.

From Houston, Texas, Laurent et al (1993) reported on the cases of 116 infants with birth injuries of the plexus, and compared the results of early operation in 24 selected cases with those in four children whose parents refused recommended operation. Operation was successful in more than 90% of cases, whereas none of the children whose parents refused operation gained any improvement. The authors outline a scheme of treatment, and describe methods of treatment and findings at operation.

EPIDEMIOLOGY

Incidence

This is unknown in the UK. Published figures from other countries suggest a range from less than 0.1% to 4% of live births. Greenwald et al (1984) found 61 cases among 30 000 consecutive live births from a single group of hospitals in the USA. Levine et al (1984) saw 2.6 cases per 1000 deliveries, in a study of over 13 000 babies, and Rubin (1964) found 18 cases in a total of over 15 000 live births. Both these papers describe the associated bone injury and facial nerve palsy. Camus et al (1995) noted only 17 cases of OBPP from over 20 000 live deliveries at the Pitié hospital over a 10-year period; they stated that the bone injuries recovered better than the neurological ones. Specht (1975) thought the incidence was no more than 0.57 per 1000 deliveries; Tan (1973), in a study from Singapore, found it even lower, at 0.14 per 1000 in vertex deliveries, but that it rose to 24.5 per 1000 in breech deliveries. The significance of breech delivery was further depicted by Boo et al (1991), who found, in a survey of Malaysian patients, an incidence of 1.6 per 1000 of all live births, rising to 8.6 per 1000 in breech.

Risk factors

There are two risk factors of note. The birth lesion in breech delivery is severe and often bilateral. Gilbert (1995) found a high incidence of preganglionic injury, particularly of the higher spinal nerves. Slooff and Blaauw (1995) had 40 cases delivered by breech (23% of their total): in 11 cases there was bilateral palsy; in 12 there was phrenic nerve palsy. C5 and C6 were damaged in 24 cases, and C5, C6 and C7 were damaged in 14 more; the lesion was complete in two cases. At least one avulsion occurred in 35 of these 40 children. Both of these papers showed

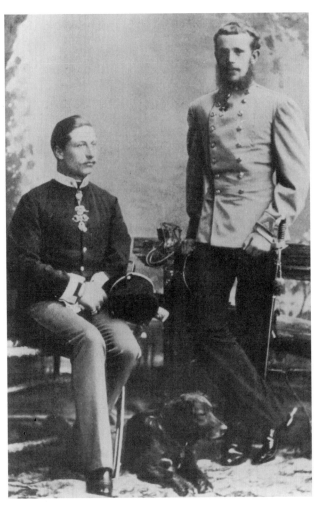

Fig. 10.2 Crown Prince Wilhelm with Rudolph von Habsburg (1881). The future German Emperor covers his withered hand; drooping of the left eye-lid is detectable. Wilhelm was born by breech; labour was prolonged, and there was anoxia (Ober 1992). His mother, Crown Princess Victoria (later Empress) was 5′2″ tall.

that birth weight was significantly less than the mean. Many infants were premature. They also emphasised the serious complication of phrenic nerve palsy, a problem noted earlier by Weigert (1920), Grenet et al (1937) and Bellini (1963).

Birth weight

It is plain that the heavy baby born by cephalic presentation is at risk. Zancolli & Zancolli (1993) found that 90% of his 512 patients weighed more than 4 kg at birth; the mean birth weight was 4.55 kg. Gilbert (1993) found a mean of 4.3 kg. Taggart and Giddins (1994) studied risk factors in 230 consecutive babies. They considered four main groups of factors: those affecting the parents, those occurring during pregnancy, those occurring during labour and those relating to the child. There was no significant correlation with social class. There was a trend towards

the mother being heavier and shorter than the national average, and also to excessive weight gain during pregnancy, but none of these factors was considered to be statistically significant. The one factor of obvious significance was the birth weight of the baby, with a mean of 4.5 kg set against the mean for the North West Thames Region of 3.88 kg. Furthermore these writers found that the birth weight increased with the severity of lesion. Shoulder dystocia was recorded as a complication of birth in over 60%, a finding similar to that of Gilbert. But shoulder dystocia is not a precise term: the *Lancet* leader (1988) showed marked disparity between the USA and Europe in the definition and diagnosis of cephalopelvic disproportion as an indication for Caesarean section. In one Irish hospital this was set at 1.7%, while in an equivalent American hospital it was set at 11% (Sheehan, 1987). Bottoms et al (1980) found that the indication of shoulder dystocia accounted for no less than 30% of the increase in Caesarean sections over a 10-year period, which is rather difficult to explain biologically! Sandmire and O'Halloin (1988) described 73 cases of shoulder dystocia; there were 12 cases of OBPP. These writers were unable accurately to predict shoulder dystocia, but birth weight is clearly significant as they found that 0.3% of babies weighing less than 4 kg were at risk of the complication: 4.7% of those weighing 4–4.5 kg and 9.4% of those weighing over 4.5 kg were so at risk.

Notwithstanding the ambiguity surrounding the diagnosis of shoulder dystocia, we believe that Power in his important paper of 1994 provides an explanation for the apparent increase in OBPP. He found a 0.4% average increase in birth weight between the years 1981 to 1992 in Scotland. In England and Wales separate figures were not kept after 1986 for babies weighing more than 4 kg, but Power found a mean annual increase of 0.35% in earlier years. Borellie and Raab (1997) confirmed the trend to heavier babies in Scotland, and analysed possible related factors. Bromwich (1986) discussed macrosomia, suggesting that a birth weight over 4 kg qualified for this definition. Big women have big babies; those who are heavy, or tall, or who gained more than 20 kg in weight during pregnancy, or are in the upper tenth percentile of weight for height are predisposed to macrosomia. Bromwich noted that in some countries there was definite relation between birth weight and social class; heavier babies for the upper classes.

Evidently there is one proven explanation for the increase in OBPP and that is the rise in birth weight. It seems odd that the incidence of this serious complication is rising when there are now so many aids to determine the size of the child, presentation and disproportion. It must be asked whether this increased incidence reflects a change in obstetric practice. Certainly, Slooff has had to treat a number of severely damaged children born at home in the Netherlands, and many of these children were born by breech. To the increase in birth weight, apparently a reflection of betterment of national health, must be added the question of ill-informed maternal choice. The direct physical cause of the lesion is the forced separation of the forequarter from the axial skeleton caused by obstruction at the narrowest point of the birth canal. When the shoulder is forward the separation is in a downward direction; when there is obstruction to breech delivery, it is in an upward direction.

The congenital lesion

The possibility of intrauterine causation is not only a matter of intellectual debate; increasingly, it is a factor in medicolegal dispute. Dunn and Engle (1985) described cases of birth palsy from abnormal intrauterine position associated with oligohydramnios. Jennett et al (1992) compared two groups of OBPP, 17 related to shoulder dystocia and 22 not so related, from a population of 57 000 live births. They found marked differences between the two: in the nondystocia group the babies were lighter and the mother younger, these features being adduced to support the hypothesis of intrauterine causation. In two of our cases the umbilical cord was seen, on ultrasound scanning, to be wrapped around the neck: both babies were born with a complete brachial plexus palsy with Bernard–Horner sign. In spite of this, recovery was *full* by the age of 6 months in one child, and impressive in the second by 12 months, a course much more favourable than might have been anticipated for this depth of lesion. In two more of our cases, oligohydramnios was a definite contributory factor. There have been a handful of reports describing aplasia of the spinal nerves. It must be admitted that there are occasional instances of intrauterine causation.

The report of Paradiso et al (1997) adds weight to these conjectures. They present persuasive electromyographic evidence of intrauterine injury in an 18-day-old infant with a lesion of the fifth and sixth cervical nerves after a difficult breech delivery. High voltage polyphasic motor unit potentials were found in the deltoid and biceps muscles – findings consistent with a lesion occurring several weeks before delivery. Comparison of these findings with those from 78 other children supports the authors' contention.

NATURAL HISTORY

Interpretation of the many papers describing the evolution of the condition is difficult because their conclusions are so variable. There are those that describe a favourable prognosis for the majority of cases. Our late colleague A. J. Harrold, a particularly astute clinician, reported a favourable outcome in over 80% (Bennet & Harrold 1976). Hardy (1981), Jackson et al (1988), Donn and Faix (1983), Gordon et al (1973) and Specht (1975) were

similarly optimistic. On the other hand, Sharrard (1971) found that recovery was poor in at least one-half of babies born with complete lesion. Adler and Patterson (1967) found full recovery in only 10% of their cases. Gjorup (1965) followed 103 patients for over 33 years, finding 22 with a poor result. Forty of those with useful recovery considered that they had some persisting significant disability. Wickstrom (1960) found 40% of the children he followed with persisting poor function at shoulder, elbow, and hand, noting that the outlook in the complete lesion was by no means good, an observation confirmed by Rossi et al (1982), who followed 34 cases and found severe persisting defect with complete or lower trunk lesions in 12 children. Eng (1971) and Eng et al (1978) made particularly detailed observations in a series of 135 children. There were severe, persisting problems in 30%; the deformities of the shoulder and elbow were resistant to conventional physiotherapy. A notable finding was the demonstration of neurapraxia in eight children with paralysed muscles, but a normal electromyogram. Narakas (1987a) analysed the outcome in 460 patients and found that few babies born with complete paralysis made good recovery at the shoulder. He did find that 90% recovered good hand function. Zancolli & Zancolli (1993) followed 512 cases from 1959 to 1987; in a more detailed study of 184 children they found that 82% of cases with damage to the 5th and 6th cervical nerves regained elbow flexion at or soon after 5 months. When the 7th nerve was damaged, one-half did not regain elbow extension. Of those with damage to the 8th cervical and first thoracic nerve, one-fifth made no recovery into the hand. They comment that if hand function was evident at 3 months the outcome was good, but if there was no recovery at all by 6 months then hand function would be poor or absent. A more cautious and less interventional posture is suggested by the work of Michelow et al (1994), who studied the natural history of spontaneous recovery in 66 children with OBPP (28 with involvement of the upper plexus and 38 with involvement of the whole plexus) and found that 61 recovered spontaneously.

A most detailed prospective study is that from Tassin (1983) and Gilbert and Tassin (1984), who followed 44 children at the Vincent de Paul Hospital in Paris. Fourteen (32%) made a complete recovery. These showed early and rapid improvement in deltoid and biceps at no later than 2 months. Eleven children (25%) showed useful recovery of the shoulder, but not of active lateral rotation. Nineteen babies (43%) made a far from full recovery. Their progress was slow, with biceps starting at between 6 and 10 months from birth. These writers proposed a new and relatively simple classification of OBPP, replacing earlier eponymous or regional systems, and we follow it. It is as follows:

Group 1 The 5th and 6th cervical nerves are damaged. There is paralysis of deltoid and biceps. About 90% of

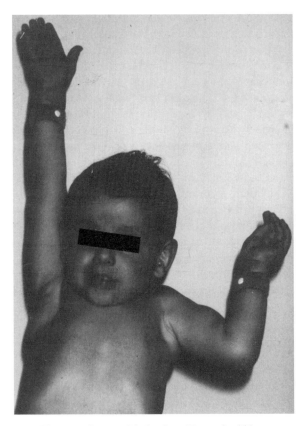

Fig. 10.3 A group 2 lesion in a 15-month-old boy.

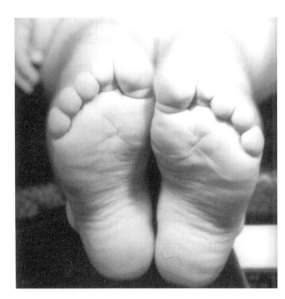

Fig. 10.4 The ipsilateral foot is smaller in this 8-year-old girl with a group IV lesion.

babies proceed to full spontaneous recovery, with clinical evidence of recovery at no later than 2 months.

Group 2 The 5th, 6th and 7th cervical nerves are damaged. The long flexor muscles of the hand are working from the time of birth, but there is paralysis of extension of elbow, wrist and digits. Perhaps 65% of these children make full spontaneous recovery, the remainder persist with serious defects in control of the shoulder. Recovery is slower, activity in the deltoid and biceps becoming clinically evident between 3 and 6 months (Fig. 10.3).

Group 3 Paralysis is virtually complete, although there is some flexion of the fingers at or shortly after birth. Full spontaneous recovery occurs in less than one-half of these children, and most are left with substantial impairment of function at the shoulder and elbow, with deficient rotation of the forearm. Wrist and finger extension does not recover in about one-quarter.

Group 4 The whole plexus is involved. Paralysis is complete. The limb is atonic, and there is a Bernard–Horner syndrome. No child makes a full recovery; the spinal nerves have been either ruptured or avulsed from the spinal cord, and there is permanent and serious defect within the limb.

The disparity in limb length ranges from up to 2% in group 1 to 20% in group 4. Damage to the spinal cord, which occurs in at least 2% of group 4 babies, presents as delayed and unsteady walking and smallness of the ipsilateral foot (Fig. 10.4).

Gilbert and Tassin's classification is very useful. It should be used at between 2 and 4 weeks from birth, when simple conduction block lesions *should have recovered.* Their classification permits clear definition of the extent of injury to the brachial plexus and offers a broad guide to prognosis. It is not, in itself, an indication for operation. It does not recognise Klumpke's lesion of damage confined to the 8th cervical and first thoracic nerves. We have seen two such cases. Different patterns of injury become apparent as the child recovers so that it becomes clear that the middle nerves, the 7th and 8th cervical, have been severely damaged, whereas those above and below have recovered. Brunelli and Brunelli (1991) described this as a fourth type of brachial plexus lesion, and it is not uncommon. In other children the injury of the 5th, 6th and 7th cervical nerves proves favourable. Injury to the 8th cervical and first thoracic is distinctly unfavourable; at maturity these cases show the features of Klumpke's lesion. We have seen six children with group 4 lesions who had made unexpectedly good recovery by the time they came to us. Paralysis persisted for at least the first 9 months of life. Function was not normal, but it was reasonably good, notably in the hand. It is clear that the Bernard–Horner sign, whilst suggestive of avulsion, is *not* an absolute indication. Furthermore, cases such as these remind us that every reasonable step towards accurate diagnosis should be made before recommending operation.

Our own experience using this classification is set out in Table 10.1. These children were referred because their lesions were unfavourable. They form a selected population, and care is required before inferring conclusions for OBPP as a whole.

Table 10.1 Lesions by Gilbert and Tassin grading: 680 babies, 1986–1995

	No. of babies
Group 1	118
Group 2	259
Group 3	200
Group 4	103
Brachial plexus explored	147
Palliative operations performed	347
No operation necessary	298
More than one operation necessary	112

DIAGNOSIS AND TREATMENT

Treatment of the condition falls into two parts. First and most important is description of the extent of neurological injury, and the central question here is whether the prognosis is favourable or not. There is, later, the problem of deformities secondary to the neural lesion. It should be said at the outset that palliative procedures for these are deeply unsatisfactory, and that results of musculotendinous transfers in OBPP are far inferior to those following good nerve regeneration, and on the whole they are inferior to those obtained for the treatment of poliomyelitis or simple peripheral nerve injuries. Indeed, the results are more uncertain than those of equivalent operations in adults. Reasons include: widespread weakness of muscle, which is at times not fully appreciated, from the diffuse nature of the injury to the nerves; inadequate cutaneous sensation and proprioception; and, later, skeletal deformities. The occasional outstanding result from free functioning muscle transfer is an exception. A major difficulty and point of persisting disagreement is the indication for operation upon the plexus. The close observations of our colleagues Gilbert, Slooff and Raimondi, together with the neurophysiological evidence given us by Dr Shelagh Smith, persuades us to side firmly with those who argue that operation for diagnosis and repair is amply justified in three circumstances:

- the natural history of group 4 lesion is bad and intervention is justified when electrophysiological evidence suggests multiple ruptures and avulsions
- we agree with Slooff & Blaauw (1995), who argues for similarly early operation in cases of damage to the upper portion of the brachial plexus associated with phrenic nerve palsy
- if there is no clinical evidence of recovery in deltoid and biceps in children falling into groups 1, 2 and 3 by 3 months, and if this is supported by adequate electrophysiological evidence, then operation is justified.

Diagnosis

This is usually straightforward. The characteristic posture of the C5/C6 (C7) lesion follows unrestrained activity through the lower trunk: the shoulder is adducted and medially rotated; the elbow is extended and the wrist flexed. The pronation posture is as much apparent as real; it is a consequence of full medial rotation at the shoulder. In the complete lesion the arm lies flaccid and the skin may be marbled. This, together with the Bernard–Horner syndrome, is indicative of multiple ruptures and avulsions. In the first weeks after birth the arm is painful to examine, and we have seen a hypersensitive skin rash in the dermatomes of C5 and C6 in cases of severe injury to these nerves. Discrepancy in size of the tips of the digits and nails is evident at about 6 weeks. The associated lesion of the spinal cord usually passes unnoticed until the child starts to walk, when the parents observe unsteadiness or disparity in the size of the foot. The opposite limb should always be examined, as birth lesions are bilateral in at least 2% of cases. Phrenic nerve palsy is a dangerous complication and may call for urgent plication of the diaphragm.

Differential diagnosis

Fracture of the clavicle or humerus may cause immobility mimicking paralysis. Neonatal sepsis of the glenohumeral joint has been recorded and has been mistaken for OBPP. We have seen cases of cerebral palsy, arthrogryposis and ischaemic injury to the cord mimicking OBPP.

The parents should be advised of the diagnosis once this is known: there will be anger, guilt, and, in most cases now, a suit for compensation. One of the advantages of separate centres for treatment is to ease clinicians of these emotional burdens. More to the point, perhaps, is that all involved can ensure that the child is given the best chance of recovery, a burden which must also be shouldered by the parents.

Physiotherapy

Parents must be involved in the treatment of the child from the outset. Regular and gentle exercises are essential in the prevention of fixed deformity, and the best physiotherapist is the mother or father or both. The role of the physiotherapist or attending doctor is to teach and then monitor progress. We have seen far too many examples of fixed deformity developing because parents sat passively at home awaiting the occasional visit by the community physiotherapist. Exercises must be frequent and gentle, and should not be performed if they cause pain. The chief aim is to maintain full passive rotation with full abduction at the glenohumeral joint. To achieve this both upper limbs must be worked together. This is particularly important, to work on one limb only merely moves the scapulothoracic joint and the twisting movements of the fretful child mislead the observer. A simple guide to parents is that these exercises should be performed for 2–3 minutes before every meal. For medial and lateral rotation the shoulder is first abducted; it is stretched in adduction; then in abduction. The inferior glenohumeral angle is maintained by gently holding the scapula against the chest whilst abducting the arm; the posterior glenohumeral angle is maintained by holding the scapula against the ribs, whilst flexing and medially rotating the arm. We believe that many fixed deformities can be prevented by this simple regime. We see no place at all for vigorous manipulation or for splinting. If gentle stretching movements cause pain then there must be fracture of clavicle or humerus, or posterior dislocation of the head of humerus.

The evolution of the paralysis

The progress of recovery or lack of it in the first 8 weeks is critical. In favourable lesions parents report powerful grasp at 2 weeks and then flexion at shoulder and at elbow at between 6 and 8 weeks. Return of a grasp within 4 weeks virtually guarantees that the child will regain good hand function. Gilbert and Tassin (1984) emphasise that early recovery signals a good prognosis, and in their cases with a favourable outcome all had elbow flexion and shoulder abduction at 3 months. We agree with these authors' argument that progress for the fifth cervical nerve is monitored by the deltoid muscle, and that for the sixth cervical nerve by the biceps. Persisting paralysis at 3 months confirms a deep lesion of these two nerves. Pitfalls include the spurious elevation of shoulder by the pectoralis major; the examiner should consider the child lying supine and seek true lateral elevation. Some children in groups 3 and 4 show recovery into the shoulder and arm by between 3 and 6 months, but never regain worthwhile hand function. They present, later, with supination deformity of the forearm, atrophy of the digits and very limited flexion. In these there has been useful recovery through C5, very limited recovery for T1, and ruptures or avulsions of C6, C7 and C8. Another group of children show very good recovery for C5 and for C6, and present with good function at the shoulder, elbow control and wrist extension, but they have no function in the hand at all. These have avulsion of C7, C7 and T1.

Evidence of anaesthesia is rare; sympathetic function usually returns, and self-mutilation is distinctly uncommon. Our experience of treating these unusual cases is related below. One child was 9 years old when we saw her. There had been no recovery for the first 8 months of life. Later, good recovery ensued in the arm and forearm; the distal extensors and flexors were powerful, and there was intrinsic balance. The Bernard–Horner sign persisted. This child constantly chewed her fingers, and had sustained unnoticed burns. Assessment of sensation showed remarkably good localisation and proprioception; recognition of shapes and textures was present but impaired. The hand was dry. This suggests that the sympathetic outflow did not recover, and that there was disproportionate impairment of Aδ and C fibre function, possibly indicating that there was damage to the anterolateral tract and descending autonomic fibres.

Other investigations

Gilbert (1995) noted from 79 myelograms that this investigation was particularly useful in detecting avulsion. Of the 395 roots examined there were three false-negative and 10 false-positive results. Slooff and Blaauw (1995) note the advantages of computed tomography (CT) scan and of magnetic resonance imaging (MRI) in showing haematoma within the spinal canal and atrophy and denervation of muscle. Francel et al (1995) give an indication of the value of a new method of MRI in the diagnosis of intradural injury in birth lesions. They use a special sequence of MRI called "fast spin-echo" (FSE MRI), which provides high speed noninvasive imaging and thus permits clinicians "to evaluate pre-ganglionic nerve root injuries without the use of general anaesthesia and lumbar puncture."

Both Gilbert and Slooff comment on the misleading nature of electromyographic evidence, finding these investigations unduly optimistic. Indeed, Vredveld et al (1994) suggest that the mixed interference pattern seen in electromyography (EMG) in children with clinical paralysis is a reflection of changes in the central nervous system rather than a consequence of a peripheral lesion. Molnar (1984) pointed out that EMG within 3 weeks of birth could be misleading, while Jaradeh et al (1994) advised serial EMG studies in their study of 13 cases. Our own experience differs. The investigations of our colleague Dr Smith (1996) have proved reliable as guides both to prognosis and to the extent of injury to individual spinal nerves. Above all, a specific injury of prolonged conduction block has been defined. Operation should not be performed in these. Why is there this difference? The nerve lesion in OBPP is not identical to that in the adult. Complete rupture of spinal nerves is unusual: a strand of tissue joining the nerve stumps is the rule and this conducts. In most of our children some active motor units were found in some muscles and nerve action potentials could be recorded across many lesions exposed at operation. This intraoperative electrophysiological evidence of recovery persuaded us against resection of lesions in 10 cases operated on before 1989. Recovery was good in only two cases; in four others recovery was so poor that repair was performed at a later intervention. Errors such as these are far fewer now that we have Smith's preoperative evidence.

Preoperative neurophysiological examination

The preoperative study requires two investigations. Nerve action potentials are recorded from median and ulnar nerves in the forearm, stimulating at the wrist and recording at the elbow. If the nerve action potential is close, in amplitude, to that in the healthy limb, then the lesion cannot be degenerative. There must either be conduction block or avulsion. These two are distinguished by EMG, sampling the deltoid (C5), biceps (C6), triceps or forearm extensors (C7), forearm flexors (C8) and the first dorsal interosseous muscle (T1). If there is poor motor unit activity with fibrillation then the root is avulsed. If there is no insertional activity and only normal units then the lesion is one of prolonged conduction block. The difficulty arises in the degenerative lesion: if the nerve action potential is significantly reduced to less than 50% and if there is a poor motor pattern exploration is indicated. If there is copious motor activity then operation is deferred (Table 10.2).

C5 and T1 are not amenable to nerve action potential study. The surgeon must balance the evidence from the investigation against the clinical progression. We have found that EMG of deltoid and biceps predicts, accurately, the state of C5 and C6, to the extent that rupture and avulsion may be distinguished and that favourable degenerative lesions (axonotmesis) may be distinguished from unfavourable lesions (rupture). Exploration is for diagnosis and for treatment; neurophysiological work is particularly valuable in the former role.

The operation

The child is supine. After induction of anaesthesia, recording electrodes are attached to the skin of the scalp and neck and sensory evoked potentials are recorded from the median and ulnar nerves at the wrist. The whole of the upper limb and one lower limb are prepared. The approach, by a transverse supraclavicular incision, is identical to that used in adult cases. Exposure of the plexus may be tedious, as scarring in the infant neck is often more severe than in the adult. Great care must be taken to trace and protect the phrenic nerve, which is often deviated laterally and involved in a neuroma of the upper and middle trunk. We have, on four occasions, found the phrenic nerve ruptured at the lower part of scalenus anterior. Regrettably, we have damaged the nerve on three more. The phrenic nerve having been defined, the fifth and sixth cervical nerves are found and followed. The suprascapular nerve is a useful guide to the lateral aspect of the upper trunk, and the extent to which it is pulled inferiorly, deep to the clavicle, indicates the violence of the traction force expended upon the plexus. Now the anterior and posterior divisions of the upper trunk are seen and marked with light vascular slings. Then the middle trunk is displayed. The proximal segments of C7, C8 and D1 are seen after section of scalenus anterior. The subclavian artery is a consistent and valuable guide to the lower trunk. We have never encountered rupture of the subclavian artery, but Gilbert has seen this once. We have demonstrated one double lesion of a distal rupture of the musculocutaneous nerve in a case of avulsion of C5 and C6.

Now the whole of the plexus is displayed with its lesions. If the middle and lower trunks are damaged the clavicle needs to be cut to permit adequate display. That can be done with bone cutters. Findings for each nerve are recorded: their appearance and texture; evidence of conduction by stimulation proximal to the lesion and recording from the scalp; by proximal stimulation and noting muscle response; by stimulation distal to the lesion and recording from the scalp; and noting muscle response.

Appearance

Avulsion. The dorsal root ganglion is often seen, especially for C6, C7 and C8. Separation of ventral and dorsal rootlets permits selective reinnervation by joining such nerves as the spinal accessory or lateral pectoral to these ventral rootlets. In other cases, however, the nerve is seemingly in place, albeit atrophic and yellowish (Fig. 10.5).

Table 10.2 Neurophysiological evidence

Group	NAP	EMG	Diagnosis	Pathophysiological	Action
A	Normal or near-normal	No spontaneous activity. Normal units	Prolonged conduction block	Neurapraxia	Observe. Prevent fixed deformity
B	(i) 50% or above of normal	Copious recruitment, mild axonal injury	Favourable rupture	Axonotmesis	Observe. Prevent fixed deformity
	(ii) Absent or less than 50% of normal	Limited recruitment, moderate axonal injury. Collateral reinnervation	Unfavourable rupture	Neurotmesis	Exploration and repair
C	Present in some cases; more often absent	Poor recruitment; fibrillation potentials; reinnervation, nascent units. Severe axonal injury	Avulsions or severe rupture	Preganglionic or total neurotmesis	Exploration and repair

Drawn from Smith S M J (1996).
EMG, electromyography; NAP, nerve action potential.

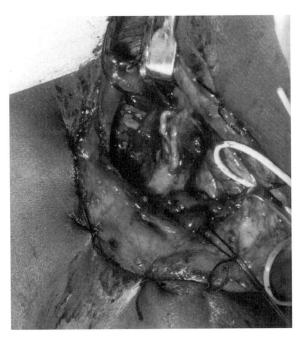

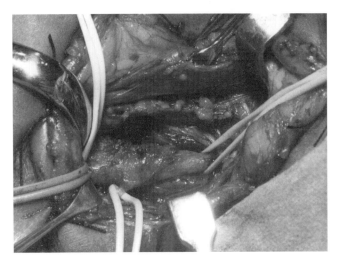

Fig. 10.6 Rupture of C5, C6 and C7.

Fig. 10.5 Avulsion of C5 and C6; the dorsal roots of C5 are displayed.

Lesion in continuity. This difficult injury is seen in C7 and sometimes C8. The nerve is elongated, tortuous and fibrosed, but not, evidently, ruptured or avulsed.

Rupture and neuroma. On occasion, a soft fusiform neuroma is encountered, the diameter of which is less than twice that of the upper trunk. Conduction is good. We regard these as "favourable" ruptures, or at least degenerative lesions of reasonable prognosis, and do not resect them. Smith found that the median nerve action potential was at least 50% of normal in these cases. The more typical neuroma is hard, and has a diameter more than twice that of the trunk. Smith found the median nerve action potential was absent or small in these cases. Some conduction is usual, but we take this as indicating an unfavourable degenerative lesion, axonotmesis combined with neurotmesis, and we resect them (Fig. 10.6). Lastly, the appearance is clearly a rupture: the neuroma has two swellings like a Bactrian camel, but even here some conducting tissue connecting the proximal neuroma and the distal glioma is usual (Fig. 10.7).

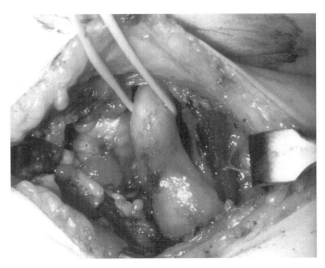

Fig. 10.7 Rupture of C5 and C6 at the formation of the upper trunk.

Neurophysiological factors

Now, sensory evoked potentials are recorded from each spinal nerve. If these are absent, and if there is no distal motor response, then avulsion is confirmed. We have seen a few examples of selective avulsion of the dorsal rootlets of C8 and D1, where there was no sensory evoked potential but a definite motor response was produced in forearm and hand. Sensory evoked potentials do not have any quantitative value, only qualitative. We have not found amplitude and latency to be useful indicators of the state of the nerve, but the waveform certainly is. If the shape of the trace is abnormal, then the nerve certainly has some intradural injury, an observation consistent with findings in adult lesions and confirmed by histological examination of biopsies from a number of stumps that showed ganglion cells.

There is almost always some distal muscular response on stimulation of spinal nerves proximal to the neuroma, and in some of our early cases this persuaded us to leave the lesion alone. As we have seen, this was a mistake, for useful recovery did not occur. For C5 the usual response is adduction at the shoulder, with some medial rotation and perhaps some slight response in deltoid. Stimulation of C6 causes powerful adduction of the shoulder; stimulation of C7 gives response in the pectoralis major and sometimes in the triceps. Nerve action potentials are recorded across the lesion and are detected in many cases even when the neuroma is plainly a bad one. The nerve action potential indicates that some conducting elements persist or have regenerated across the lesion. Rarely, conduction distal to the neuroma is better than the response to proximal stimulation, suggesting that there is an element of conduction block. Finally, sensory evoked potentials are sought by stimulation distal to the lesion, and, remarkably, these are often recordable (Fig. 10.8).

The decision to resect is guided by the preoperative evidence, together with the appearance and feel of the neuroma. Sensory evoked potentials are useful indicators of the state of the proximal stump, and so help in choosing the spinal nerve on which to base grafts. Our interpretation of the lesions displayed is set out in Table 10.3. In some of our early cases only time revealed the full extent of injury; we believe that there was selective rupture of either ventral or dorsal rootlets in some cases of avulsion, and we admit that other surgeons might treat some of our axonotmeses as ruptures.

Technique of repair

This is usually by conventional grafting. The proportions of the infant make it a tight matter to secure adequate donor cutaneous nerve. The injured upper limb is fertile ground, providing the medial cutaneous nerve of forearm, the superficial radial nerve and the cutaneous division of the musculocutaneous nerve. These suffice for one or two ruptures. If three nerves must be grafted then a sural nerve is also necessary. Groups 3 and 4 are mixtures of ruptures and avulsions. The aim must be to reinnervate the whole plexus, combining graft with transfer. In, for instance, ruptures of C5, C6 and C7 with avulsion of C8 and T1, the shoulder is reinnervated by accessory to suprascapular transfer and the other three nerves are spread about the whole of the plexus. When only two or even one rupture is found, with avulsion of the remainder, we now follow Gilbert (1994) in using the proximal stump to reinnervate the lower trunk. Gilbert argued that with loss

of hand function there was no real prospect of a useful upper limb, and we were so much persuaded by the force of his argument that we have abandoned our earlier approach of using intercostal nerves T3 to T6, or other transfers to reinnervate the lower trunk in avulsion of C8 and D1. In such cases the upper and middle trunks must

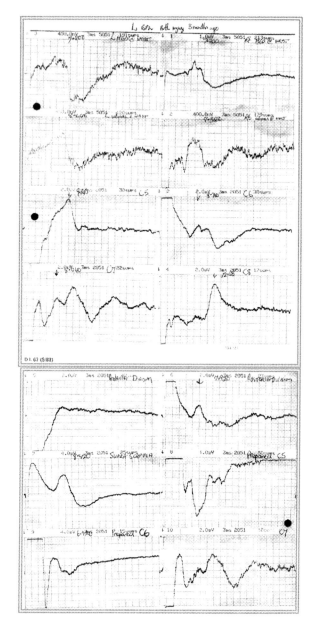

Fig. 10.8 Intraoperative sensory evoked potentials (SEPs) in a 3-month-old girl. Preoperative investigation predicted neurotmesis (unfavourable group B) of C6, with a more favourable motor pattern for C5. The upper trunk was ruptured distal to the suprascapular nerve. Normal traces are seen for C5, C6 and C7: there is no SEP for the anterior division, and a normal trace for the suprascapular nerve. SEPs were recorded from the unafflicted left median and ulnar nerves by transcutaneous stimulation at the wrist: that for the right ulnar was normal; it was diminished for the right median.

Table 10.3 The nerve lesion: 147 operated cases, 1986–1995

Nerve	No. intact	Axonotmesis (lesion in continuity)	Rupture	Avulsion
C5	0	35	101	11
C6	0	28	91	28
C7	21	60	36	30
C8	71	27	13	36
T1	77	30	6	34

There were 94 repairs and 53 neurolyses. Re-exploration and repair was later performed in 10 patients whose progress was disappointing after the first exploration.

be reinnervated either by selective transfer to the ventral and dorsal rootlets or by transfer of the accessory to the suprascapular nerve for the shoulder and of intercostal nerves for the lateral cord. In three early cases of severe lesion we used the ulnar nerve as a donor, but we do not recommend this. Other methods that have been described include that of Slooff, who recommends the hypoglossal nerve for transfer, and that of Gu, who has discussed using the ipsilateral phrenic nerve and the posterior division of the contralateral 7th cervical nerve. We are uncertain about the role of these techniques, which were developed for the severe adult case. Certainly phrenic nerve palsy is a serious matter in the young child.

Fibrin clot glue is used for the grafts, and suture and glue for the transfers. If the clavicle has been divided this is sutured before inserting the grafts. The infant is immobilised in plaster of Paris splint, controlling movements of the head and of the damaged upper limb. The splint must be carefully applied so that the mother can continue to feed the child without undue difficulty and to clean the skin about the neck and the chest. The plaster is retained for 4 weeks. Then, the parents return to their regime of gentle and regular stretching of all the joints of the upper limb.

Results

The remarkable feature of recovery through grafts in OBPP is its slowness. The rate of recovery is slower than in adults, so that a graft of the upper trunk is followed by: obvious function in deltoid and biceps no earlier than 9 months; wrist extension between 15 and 18 months; finger flexors at about the same time; and intrinsic muscles no sooner than 18 months. In three children, in whom the middle and lower trunks had been reinnervated, recovery of hand function was not seen until nearly 4 years had passed. In one, wrist extension recovered at 3 years, and finger flexion followed soon after. In two more, finger flexion and intrinsic function were undetectable for 42 months. In all three cases hand function was, ultimately, at least useful.

On the other hand, the trophic state of the limb improves much earlier, with vasomotor control and sweating becoming apparent at about 6 months from the repair. It is perhaps the case that this slowness reflects the prolonged maturation of the spindle and proprioceptive function. Another remarkable feature is the seeming preservation of the sensation to the skin of the hand, so that the atrophic denervation skin appearance, which is so common after damage to adult trunk nerves, is rarely seen in infancy. Conversely, the children change dominance. In almost every case of significant lesion the injured side becomes nondominant: only a few children change dominance after recovery, and never before the age of 4 or 5 years.

Measurement of outcome

We use four systems. The Mallett (1972) system (Fig. 10.9) is a useful guide to function at the shoulder. Our results are drawn by adding the sum for the five functions, so that a good shoulder merits 15 points and a bad one 5 points. This is complemented by Gilbert's (1993) classification (Table 10.4). Its originator is aware of the deficiencies of

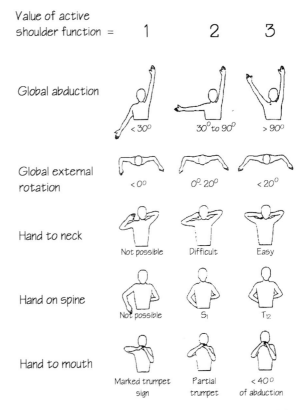

Fig. 10.9 The Mallet system of measuring function at the shoulder.

Table 10.4 Shoulder paralysis

Stage	Description
0	Flail shoulder
I	Abduction or flexion to 45° No active lateral rotation
II	Abduction <90° Lateral rotation to neutral
III	Abduction 90° Weak lateral rotation
IV	Abduction <120° Incomplete lateral rotation
V	Abduction >120° Active lateral rotation

From Gilbert (1993).
The suffix + is added to indicate sufficient medial rotation permitting the hand to come against the opposite shoulder.

the system (that medial rotation is underrated and that lateral rotation can exist without abduction), but there is a degree of consistency between the two systems. This method of analysis is on trial in five centres and awaits modification. Raimondi's (1993) classification is useful and consistent in defining hand function (Table 10.5). More recently, Gilbert and Raimondi (1996) have introduced an assessment for the elbow (Table 10.6; Figs 10.10 and 10.11). We think that over 2000 repairs of OBPP have been performed over the last 20 years, but results are difficult to analyse because of the length of time for recovery

and because of changes in technique, particularly the introduction of intraplexual transfer for the group 4 lesions.

Gilbert (1995) has the largest series, with 178 cases followed for 3 years or more. Sixty-five children had repairs for C5 and C6 lesions. Of these 80% achieved shoulder function at grade 4 or 5, and all but one regained elbow flexion. Of the 59 children who had repairs to C5, C6 and C7 lesions, 65% regained shoulder function to grades 4 or 5 and 70% recovered wrist extension. In the 54 children with total lesions, useful finger flexion was regained in 75%, and useful intrinsic function was obtained in 50%.

Table 10.5 Hand evaluation scale

Grade	Description
0	Complete paralysis or slight finger flexion of no use; useless thumb – no pinch; some or no sensation
I	Limited active flexion of fingers; no extension of wrist or fingers; possibility of thumb lateral pinch
II	Active flexion of wrist, with passive flexion of fingers (tenodesis); passive lateral pinch of thumb
III	Active complete flexion of wrist and fingers; mobile thumb with partial abduction – opposition. Intrinsic balance; no active supination; good possibilities for palliative surgery
IV	Active complete flexion of wrist and fingers; active wrist extension; weak or absent finger extension. Good thumb opposition, with active ulnaris intrinsics; partial pronosupination
V	Hand IV, with finger extension and almost complete pronosupination

From Raimondi (1993).

Table 10.6 Elbow recovery

	Score
Flexion:	
Nil or some contraction	1
Incomplete flexion	2
Complete flexion	3
Extension:	
No extension	0
Weak extension	1
Good extension	2
Extension deficit:	
0–30°	0
30–50°	−1
>50°	−2

From Gilbert and Raimondi (1996).

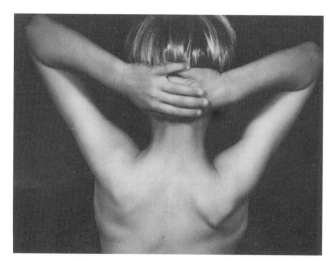

Fig. 10.10 Rupture of C5 and C6. Repaired at age 3 months. The results at age 6 years: shoulder, Gilbert 5+; elbow, 5; hand, Raimondi 5.

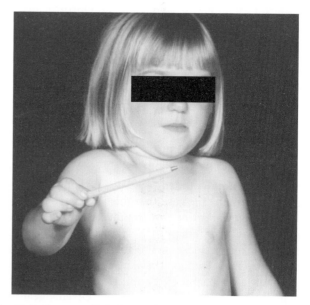

Fig. 10.11 Rupture of C5, C6 and C7; avulsion of C8 and T1. Repair at age 10 weeks: C6 and part of C7 transferred to C8 and T1; upper and middle trunks grafted from C5 and part of C7; accessory to suprascapular transfer. Result at age 5 years: shoulder, Gilbert 3+; elbow, 4; hand, Raimondi 4.

Our own results are summarised in Table 10.7. We believe, although we cannot prove it, that no child gained less function than if no operation had been performed. The phrenic nerve was damaged on three occasions, and in two children plication of the hemidiaphragm proved necessary. Avulsion of one or more roots brought about a generalised loss of function, which could only be mitigated by intra- or extraplexual transfer. All children in group C who regained hand function to grade 4 or 5 had some recovery through lesions in continuity of C7, C8 or T1. Later operations for the treatment of the medial rotation contracture and of posterior dislocation were necessary in 28 children, and the results set out in Table 10.7 indicate the final result after these operations. Subsequent muscle transfers were performed on 38 occasions and the results of these are not included in the table, which sets out neurological recovery. Nine of these were for the shoulder (one in group A, and four each in groups B and C). Ten muscle transfers to improve elbow flexion and active supination were done (one in group A, four in group B and five in group C), and 19 musculotendinous transfers were necessary for hand function, usually to regain extension of the wrist and the digits (five in group B and 14 in group C). An improvement in function of one grade was achieved in most cases.

Late reinnervation

What can be done for the child presenting late with severe defects so extreme that there is little or no chance of success from musculotendinous transfer? There is, of course, free muscle transfer, but this cannot restore intrinsic function or sensation. Accessory to suprascapular transfer was performed on three children, aged 4–7 years, who had poor shoulder function, but a good hand. EMG showed some activity in the supra- and infraspinatus muscles. The deltoid seemed quite powerful – in these three cases the defect lay in the muscles of the rotator cuff. The results were striking: all achieved Gilbert grade V+ (Mallett 14 or 15) within 12 months of operation. We have been similarly impressed by late nerve transfer to improve the trophic state of the hand, and to restore sensation in four cases. The most remarkable was that of an 11-year-old boy who presented with severe trophic disturbance of the little, ring and middle fingers, from untreated avulsion of C8 and T1. A small sensory action potential (SAP) was recordable from the ulnar nerve. The sensory divisions of intercostal 2 and 3 were transferred to the ulnar nerve. The boy's parents reported improvement in the appearance of the digits by 6 months. At 6 years from operation, he was able to localise light touch, sweating had returned and there was some return of gnosis. He now works full time as a car mechanic. In all four cases parents reported improvement in colour, an increase in growth and recovery of protective sensation. In one child, painful stimuli applied to the little finger were felt in the chest wall. These cases are summarised in Table 10.8.

We have performed three late cases of repair of the lower trunk of the plexus at the ages of $3^{1}/_{2}$, 4 and 5 years. There had been useful recovery to the shoulder through C5 in all three children, and two regained wrist extension. Electromyographic examination showed motor activity in the forearm flexor muscles, so that these were not hopelessly fibrosed. In these cases an upper spinal nerve was used to reinnervate the lower trunk, preserving the best functioning nerve, usually C5. Recovery is awaited. While

Table 10.7 Results of repairs: 65 cases, minimum follow-up 30 months

Lesion	Shoulder			Elbow		Hand	
	Gilbert	Mallett					
A. Group I (C5, C6)	1	6–7	0	1	0	1	0
One or two roots grafted	2	8–9	0	2	0	2	0
Six cases	3	10–11	0	3	0	3	0
	4	12–13	1	4	1	4	0
	5	14–15	5	5	5	5	6
B. Group II (C5, C6, C7)	1	6–7	0	1	0	1	0
Two or three roots grafted	2	8–9	0	2	0	2	0
Twenty-five cases	3	10–11	8	3	5	3	0
	4	12–13	11	4	9	4	12
	5	14–15	6	5	11	5	13
C. Groups III and IV (C5, C6, C7, C8, T1)	1	6–7	0	1	1	1	0
Two or three roots grafted, with	2	8–9	7	2	4	2	4
intra- or extraplexual transfer	3	10–11	13	3	6	3	10
Thirty-four cases	4	12–13	8	4	18	4	20
	5	14–15	6	5	5	5	0

This excludes four cases of avulsion of C5 and C6, and 11 cases of late reinnervation (older than 2 years).

Table 10.8 Late nerve transfer for sensation

Sex	Age at operation (years)	Lesion	Defect	Operation	Sympathetic return	Protective sensation	Localisation	Growth
M	7	C5, C6, C7	Thumb/index	MCF to lateral root median	Yes	Yes	Yes	Yes
M	11	C8, T1	Ulnar 3 fingers	ICN 2 and 3 to ulnar	Yes	Yes	Yes	Yes
F	5	C7, C8, T1	Ulnar 3 fingers	ICN 2 and 3 to ulnar	Yes	Yes	Yes	Yes
F	7	C7, C8, T1	Ulnar 3 fingers	ICN 2 and 3 to ulnar	Yes	Yes	No	Yes

ICN, intercostal nerve; MCF, medial cutaneous nerve of forearm.

late return of sensation can be expected, it is not yet clear whether the combination of peripheral or target organ change together with central motor neuron loss renders such late nerve repair a waste of time.

There are important differences between the adult lesion and OBPP, and lessons learnt from the adult are not necessarily applicable to the child. First, there are more partial intradural lesions in OBPP. We have demonstrated cases of partial function through ventral rootlets with proven avulsion of the dorsal rootlets. It is possible that the rarity of complete sensory loss reflects sparing of dorsal rootlets. Next, the definition of the injury to the nerves in the posterior triangle is less abrupt. There is a spectrum from the lesion in continuity to the neuroma and so to the rupture; that is in continuity from axonotmesis to neurotmesis. There is almost always some conducting tissue across the lesion, a fact which may have contributed to other workers' disenchantment with EMG. Next, the recognition of prolonged conduction block in about 15% of cases is a most important advance for it explains the unexpectedly favourable progression noted by other writers in children who start recovery late (no earlier than 9 months) and then go on to make a full recovery.

It does seem that pain is very rare in children. The central pain of avulsion injury, which is such an abomination in adults, has not been encountered in any child. Is this perhaps related to the rarity of complete sensory loss in the hand? The posterior columns are not, of course, myelinated in the neonate. A possible alternative explanation comes from the anatomical arrangement of the spinal cord in infancy; perhaps the transitional zone is more vulnerable than in the adult. In the infant, the spinal cord fills the cervical canal, and the spinal roots emerge at, or near to, a right angle from the cord; separation is more likely at the transitional zone than true avulsion. This may perhaps have something to do with the absence of pain: the adult's system for analysis of sensations has become accustomed to the input along the posterior columns, and so responds to its abolition or diminution by giving rise to pain, whereas no such acclimatisation has taken place in the neonate. In this context, we have treated three children who sustained severe closed traction lesions of the brachial plexus from road traffic accidents before the age of 4 years. None ever complained of pain. One patient *may* provide a key to understanding. A 7-year-old boy suffered complete preganglionic lesion of the brachial plexus. Repair was not possible. He adjusted well, and did well at school. He came back, at age 17, in severe pain, which had started a year before, at a time when he had more or less stopped growing. His description of pain was characteristic: constant crushing and burning in the hand, convulsive, shooting down the upper limb. Thankfully, pain was abolished by transcutaneous stimulation. It is perhaps significant that this boy's pain started quite suddenly 9 years after his injury, at a time when he approached maturity.

The rate of recovery is slow considering the distance through which new axons must grow. Furthermore, recovery, though usually good, is never complete. This may be a reflection of loss of ventral horn cells; such changes are more severe in the young than in the mature animal. Of itself this is a considerable argument for early intervention in those cases in which a secure diagnosis can be established. At present this is possible only in the two unfavourable types of lesion: groups 1 and 2 with phrenic nerve palsy, and group 4 with Bernard–Horner syndrome.

DEFORMITIES IN OBPP

These fall into two groups. In the first there has been a good recovery through lesions of C5 and C6, and C7, either spontaneously or following repair. It is in this group that treatment is most rewarding, for it unmasks the real potential for function. Two joints are affected. The most common and significant deformities afflict the shoulder, above all the medial rotation contracture described by Seddon as "this vicious contracture" with all the implications for the joint (Fig. 10.12), but there are allied contractures of the posterior and inferior muscles which, although of secondary importance, are no less annoying. Next, at the elbow, is the flexion and pronation deformity, which we believe is secondary to the deformity of the shoulder in most cases, although Aitken (1952) considered it a very difficult sequel in OBPP.

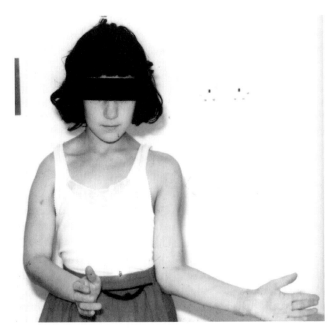

Fig. 10.12 Limitation of active lateral rotation caused by posterior dislocation of the head of the humerus in a 7-year-old girl.

It is the case that disability after partial recovery of these upper nerves, which leaves a supple but weak limb, is amenable to treatment by some muscle transfers. Two of these are noteworthy. The first is transfer of the latissimus dorsi to the supra- and infraspinatus muscles; this is indicated when the shoulder is reduced, and is supple, and when the deltoid works. The operation was described by L'Episcopo and Brooklyn (1939), and we have found useful results in 18 cases. The indications are narrow; the skeletal development of the shoulder must be normal, there must be no fixed deformity, the power of the deltoid should be at least MRC grade 3 and the subscapularis and pectoralis major should be sufficiently strong to maintain medial rotation. Gilbert et al (1988) described the indications, technique and results in 44 cases, and their results were good. The next useful operation is transfer of the pectoralis minor to the biceps when elbow flexion is weak and when there is limited active supination. The operation was recommended to us by Professor Laurent Sedel, and it is described in Chapter 17. Preoperative requirements include elbow flexion of MRC power grade 3, and an absence of fixed pronation deformity at the elbow. Ten of 14 cases made significant gains in the power of elbow flexion and in active supination.

The situation is very different, and very much worse, in the complete lesion, with poor recovery (shoulder, Gilbert 1–3; hand Raimondi 1–3). A flexed supinated elbow is a common and disabling deformity. We know of no useful muscle transfers for the paralysed shoulder. Free muscle transfer, an operation of last resort, can restore flexion to the elbow or extension of wrist. The results of tendon

transfers in the hand are unpredictable, and on the whole they are worse than those for any other neurological disorder. All our operations for dislocated head of radius have failed. We know of no useful operation for restoring active pronosupination in these cases, and have been disappointed by the results of rerouting the biceps tendon (Grilli 1959), which is described in detail by Zancolli & Zancolli (1993). Two operations are useful in palliation. Rotation osteotomy of the radius, in its middle part, places the hand in a more useful position, but wrist extension against gravity is essential. The desired position is described by the patient: about 30° of pronation is a useful compromise. Operation may have to be repeated as the child grows. The next useful operation does something to overcome the deformity in which the hand lies in ulnar deviation with the thumb in the palm. This is a common sequel in group 3 following poor recovery for C5, C6 and C7. The deformity is progressive and is deleterious both cosmetically and functionally. It is caused by muscle imbalance, through unopposed action of the flexor carpi ulnaris (FCU) and extensor carpi ulnaris (ECU) which overwhelm the weak radial muscles (the extensor carpi radialis (ECR), flexor carpi radialis (FCR), abductor pollicis longus (APL) and extensor pollicis longus (EPL)). The best technique is that developed by our colleague, David Evans, in which the ECU, which is often prolapsed to the anterior surface of the forearm, is transferred to one slip of the APL. If wrist extension is adequate, the muscle is transferred, subcutaneously, on the anterior aspect of the forearm. If wrist extension is poor and if there is a tendency to supination, ECU is better transferred to the extensor carpi radialis brevis (ECRB).

Medial rotation contracture of the shoulder and its consequences

We turn now to the most common and the most serious of deformities, the medial rotation contracture and allied deformities at the shoulder. There is a considerable difference in the literature about this problem, between those who find it a consequence of injury to bone, growth plate and muscle occurring at birth, and those who consider it a consequence of muscle imbalance following neurological injury. We believe that the latter is the explanation in most cases. Fairbank (1913) described luxation of the shoulder in infancy. Putti (1932) and Scaglietti (1938) and Zancolli & Zancolli (1993) described the bony lesion and considered damage to the growth plate (epiphysiolysis) as a major factor, and recommended methods of treatment that either attempted relocation of the shoulder or left it as it is was and did no more than palliate. Moore (1971) described posterior bone block for posterior dislocation. We did not find this satisfactory in two of our early cases in which it was attempted. Wickstrom (1962) related his considerable experience in treatment of the deformed shoulder.

Gilbert (1993) takes a different view, one with which we agree: "Contrary to traditional thinking, the surgeon should not wait to treat an internal rotation contracture. In the absence of surgical treatment, recovery is limited, abduction is impossible, the extremity is dysfunctional, and, most important, osseous and articular deformity occur. Posterior subluxation and deformity of the humeral head permanently worsens the prognosis. These anomalies, which have long been considered the result of obstetrical palsy, are in fact simply a consequence of untreated contractures." Goddard (1993) made a radiological study of 200 cases, and he uncovered only two instances of injury to the growth plate.

Our position is based on experience with over 400 operations at the shoulder in children with at least useful neurological recovery, and we are particularly indebted to the late Mark Dunkerton for his original observations, and to Dr Liang Chen, whose close analysis of 120 consecutive cases provides real insight into the problem.

CAUSATION

Table 10.9 sets out the material for discussion. We think that the dislocation occurred at or very shortly after birth in 11 cases, and one father gave a clear description of a mechanism. During a difficult vertex delivery the afflicted arm was pulled into abduction and then across the chest, into forced flexion with medial rotation. It is likely that dislocation occurred at this moment. In five more cases in which neurological recovery had otherwise been good, we found the subscapularis muscle densely fibrosed, and we think that this is a postischaemic or compartment syndrome lesion analogous to that described in the adult case by Landi et al 1992. We also believe that some cases of severe contracture involving the latissimus dorsi and teres major, which we term the inferior glenohumeral contracture, and of contracture of the deltoid and infraspinatus,

which we term the posterior glenohumeral contracture, are a reflection of direct damage to those muscles during delivery. With these exclusions, which are perhaps 20% of the total, we think that the deformity is provoked by muscular imbalance, and that the muscular imbalance is caused by the neurological injury. The subscapularis muscle, the most powerful muscle within the rotator cuff and the most powerful medial rotator of the shoulder, is innervated by the 7th and 8th cervical nerves. In lesions of C5, C6 and C7, the muscle either works from the outset, or it rapidly recovers and overwhelms the weaker abductors and lateral rotators innervated by the 5th and 6th cervical nerves. We have unwittingly, or in retrospect, seen progression from an uncomplicated medial rotation contracture to subluxation or dislocation in 27 cases following successful repair of the upper and middle trunks of the brachial plexus. Chen made the alarming observation that the shoulders of no less than 12 children, awaiting treatment for an uncomplicated medial rotation contracture, had progressed to dislocation whilst awaiting admission. In these cases, what was originally no more than a loss of 30–40° of passive lateral rotation had progressed to subluxation or dislocation. Furthermore, no less than 29 of 86 operations of subscapularis slide, which had initially restored full lateral rotation with secure relocation of the head of the humerus, later failed, and a second operation by anterior approach was necessary.

We define our terms below.

The medial rotation contracture. The contour of the shoulder is normal; the only abnormality is restriction of passive lateral rotation which is diminished by 30–40°. There is a mild flexion pronation posture of the forearm, but this is not fixed. Radiographs show a delay in ossification, but are otherwise normal. An uncommon, and interesting, cause of medial rotation contracture is overgrowth of the coracoid, which we have seen butting against the head of the humerus in five children. This was the only recognisable abnormality in these shoulders, and blocked lateral rotation beyond 10–20°. Shortening of the coracoid, and section of the upper one-third of the subscapularis tendon, restored full rotation and normal shoulder function in all five cases (Figs 10.13 and 10.14).

Posterior subluxation (simple). The head of the humerus is prominent to palpation; passive lateral rotation is restricted to about 10°. The flexion pronation posture of the forearm has advanced. The radiological appearances are characteristic – there is, as yet, no secondary deformity of the acromion, the coracoid, or the glenoid (Fig. 10.15).

Posterior dislocation (simple). There is obvious abnormality of the contour of the shoulder; the head of humerus can be seen and palpated behind the glenoid. It may be possible to click the humeral head in and out of the glenoid. There is a fixed medial rotation contracture, and by now there may be fixed flexion pronation posture of the forearm. Radiographs confirm displacement, and there

Table 10.9 Shoulder deformity in groups I, II and III, with potentially useful hand: 232 operations, 1988–1995

Deformity	No. cases
Medial rotation contracture	62
Coracoid elongation	5
Total	67
Simple subluxation	16
Simple dislocation	35
Total	51
Complex subluxation	16
Complex dislocation	47
Total	63
Inferior glenohumeral angle contracture	34
Posterior glenohumeral contracture	17
Total	51

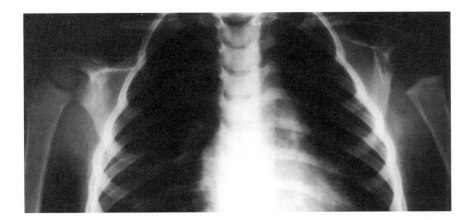

Fig. 10.13 Delayed ossification of the head of the humerus in a child aged 1 year with simple medial rotation contracture.

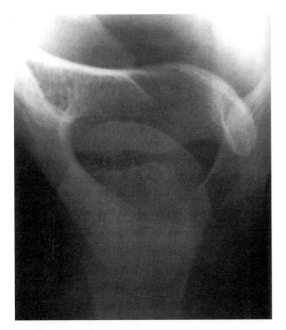 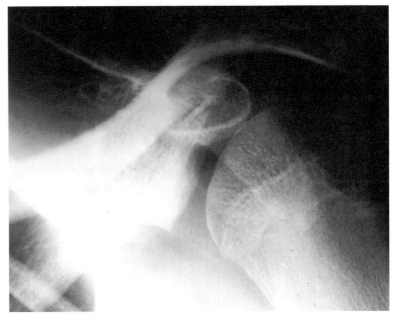

Fig. 10.14 (Left) Overgrowth of coracoid blocked lateral rotation beyond neutral in a 7-year-old boy. The head of the humerus was located. (Right) A gain of 50° of active lateral rotation followed shortening of the coracoid.

is a characteristic windswept or curved appearance of the proximal humerus (Figs 10.16 and 10.17).

Complex subluxation/dislocation. In this, the final stage, marked skeletal abnormalities are apparent to clinical and radiological examination. We have seen a number of young adults in this situation in whom function of the shoulder was extremely poor, and it was indeed impaired throughout the upper limb. These patients had pain, and the compensatory thoracoscapular movement seen in many young children had disappeared. There was fixed flexion at the elbow with pronation of the forearm, and in four cases the head of the radius was dislocated. We were unable to offer any useful treatment to these patients (Fig. 10.18). Lateral rotation osteotomy in these cases is useless.

We single out three skeletal abnormalities as significant. The coracoid is elongated and it may also be curved posteriorly, an abnormality easily detectable by palpation. Next, the acromion is elongated and hooked downwards. Last, there is a bifacetal appearance in the glenoid. The true glenoid lies above and anterior; the false glenoid lies below and inferior. In complex subluxation the articulation is between the head of the humerus and the false glenoid. In complex dislocation the articulation is between the lesser tuberosity and the false glenoid. Examination of the shoulder with image intensifier shows that the head of the humerus is forced downwards by the acromion when the arm is abducted. When the arm is brought to the side the head of the humerus rises and the lesser tuberosity

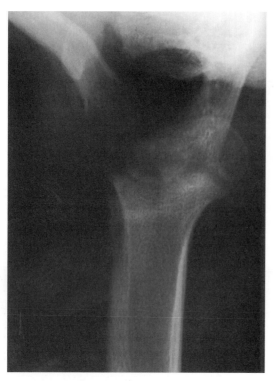

Fig. 10.15 A 3-year-old boy. There was still some contact between the anterior part of the head of the humerus and the undeformed glenoid.

slides into the superior facet. This leads to an apparent abduction contracture, because if the head of the humerus is held in the plane of the superior facet the arm can be fully adducted only by forcing the spine of the scapula upwards (Figs 10.19 to 10.21).

The inferior glenohumeral angle. We measure and record the inferior glenohumeral angle as that between the axis of the humerus and the lateral border of the scapula with the arm in abduction. In the normal shoulder this is at least 150°. In some children contracture of the inferior capsule of latissimus dorsi and of teres major is so tight that the angle is diminished to 30–40° (Fig. 10.22).

The posterior glenohumeral contracture. This was recognised by Putti (1932), who noted the winging of the scapula in flexion of the arm. We measure and record the angle as follows. The afflicted hand is placed on the opposite shoulder, with the axis of the humerus parallel to the ground. The angle between the humerus and the blade of the scapula is measured. In a normal shoulder this should be at least 70°, while in a severe contracture it may be reduced to 0°. Some of this contracture arises from capsular tightness and can be overcome by firm depression of the scapula onto the chest wall whilst holding the arm in the position described. This is one exercise the children tolerate well; they do not find it painful. However, some of the contracture arises from bone deformity, we presume of retroversion of the neck of the humerus, and it is an almost inevitable consequence of successful relocation in complex dislocation. The treatment for it, which is straightforward enough, is outlined below (Fig. 10.23).

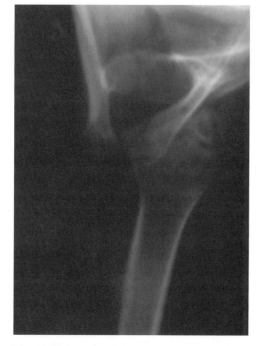

Fig. 10.16 Posterior dislocation in a 4-year-old girl. There appeared to be no secondary deformity of the coracoid or glenoid. The anterior face of the head of the humerus was flattened, and the articulation was between the lesser tuberosity and the glenoid.

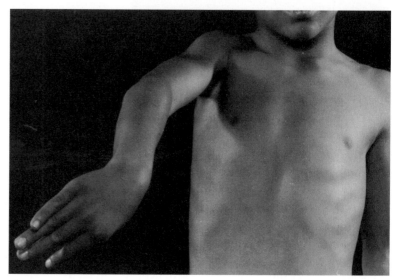

Fig. 10.17 Posterior dislocation in a 5-year-old boy, with no significant secondary deformity of the glenoid, coracoid, or acromion.

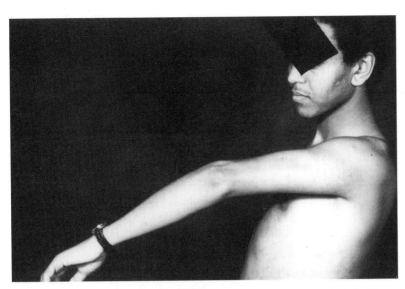

Fig. 10.18 A 21-year-old man with complex posterior dislocation. He had significant pain from the shoulder joint, the head of radius was dislocated, and function throughout the upper limb was substantially marred. Neurological recovery from this group II lesion was good. There is no place for lateral rotation osteotomy of the humerus here.

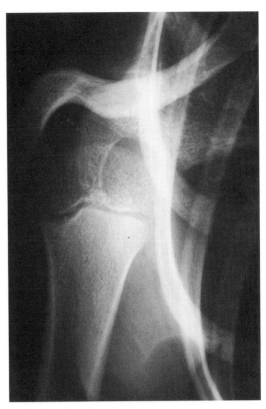

Fig. 10.19 Complex dislocation in a 9-year-old boy, showing hooking of the acromion, overgrowth of the coracoid, and a double facet appearance of the glenoid.

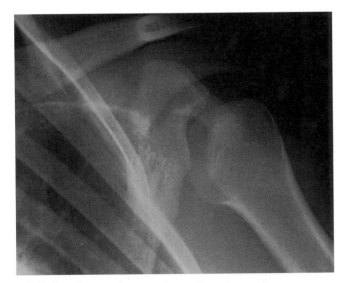

Fig. 10.20 A 17-year-old man with complex dislocation, with well-developed true and false glenoid cavities. In adduction the lesser tuberosity articulates with the true glenoid. (Mr Thomas Carlstedt's case.)

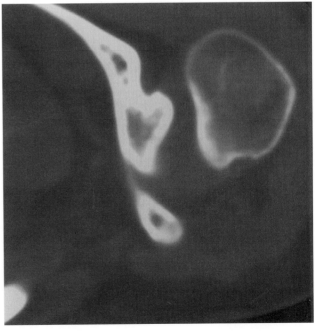

Fig. 10.21 CT scan of a posterior dislocation in a 5-year-old child. The lesser tuberosity articulates with a reasonably well-formed glenoid, but in other cases the glenoid is flattened or even slightly convex. (Mr Thomas Carlstedt's case.)

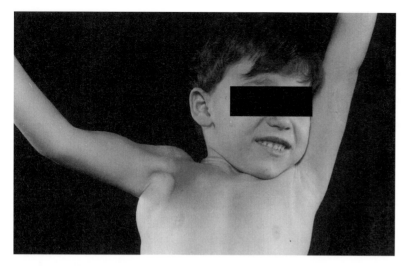

Fig. 10.22 Inferior glenohumeral contracture unmasked after relocation of the shoulder. The inferior glenohumeral angle (about 70°) is less than one-half of that on the normal side (180°).

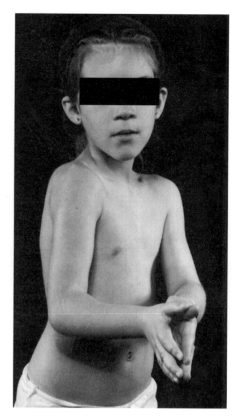

Fig. 10.23 Posterior glenohumeral contracture, unmasked after relocation of the shoulder, prevented this 5-year-old girl from bringing her hand into her body.

TREATMENT

Prevention is best and it is possible. Parents are taught a set of exercises that start soon after birth, and progress must be regularly supervised. Much physiotherapy that we have seen is valueless. Both arms must be worked simultaneously in adduction. The range of movements is recorded, paying particular attention to the arc of lateral rotation in abduction and adduction. Active treatment is indicated when lateral rotation is diminished by 40°. Our systems for prospective analysis are set out in Tables 10.10 and 10.11.

Table 10.10 Type of record kept at the Royal National Orthopaedic Hospital Peripheral Nerve Injury and Congenital Hand Unit: shoulder – nonoperated cases of OBPP

Name and number	DOB	Tassin	Date of clinic attendance	X-rays	EMG	Clinical diagnosis	Pathology of shoulder
							1. Dislocation 2. Subluxation 3. Contracture 4. Flail
Seen by OT			**Mallett chart**			**Gilbert grading**	**Raimondi grading (hand)**

DOB, Date of Birth; OT, Occupational Therapist.

Table 10.11 Type of record kept at the Royal National Orthopaedic Hospital Peripheral Nerve Injury and Congenital Hand Unit: shoulder operations in OBPP patients

Name	Tassin	DOO	X-rays	EMG	Operation	Surgical pathology
					On BP:	**Of plexus:**
					On shoulder:	**Of shoulder:** 1. Dislocation 2. Subluxation 3. Contracture 4. Flail

Seen by OT:		Mallett score		Gilbert grading (shoulder)		Raimondi grading (hand)
Before opn:		Before opn:		Before opn:		Before opn:
After opn:		After opn:		After opn:		After opn:

Range of movement

FF		ER		GH angle		ABD		IR		Rotation forearm		FF		ER		GH angle		ABD		IR		Rotation forearm	
Ac	Pa	Ac	Pa	Ac	Pa	Ac	Pa	Ac	Pa	Ac	Pa	Ac	Pa	Ac	Pa	Ac	Pa	Ac	Pa	Ac	Pa	Ac	Pa

ABD, abduction; AC, active; BP, brachial plexus; DOO, date of operation; ER, external (lateral) rotation; FF, forward flexion; GH, glenohumeral; IR, internal (medial) rotation; Pa, passive; opn, operation.

Subscapularis slide

This is indicated when the joint is reduced, when there is no hint of bone deformity, particularly of elongation of the coracoid, and when lateral rotation is diminished by 30–40°, no more. Results from the operation are a good deal better in children under the age of 18 months. The technique was described by Carlioz and Brahimi in 1986. The muscle is exposed by incision in the midaxillary line at its insertion. It is then detached from the inner face of the scapular, respecting of the neurovascular pedicles, and with care not to damage teres major and serratus anterior. Often the tightest part of the muscle is its upper part. Full lateral rotation is obtained, the capsule is not opened, and the shoulder is immobilised for 6 weeks with the arm adducted in full lateral rotation. Gilbert, who drew our attention to this useful operation, described his results in 66 patients with a follow-up of more than 5 years (Gilbert 1993). In 28 children there had already been repair of the brachial plexus. Results were good, the average postoperative gain in lateral rotation being 70° in children aged less than 2 years at the time of operation, and half of these patients recovered full active lateral rotation. Only eight required secondary muscle transfer. Our own results are set out in Table 10.12. In the long term, no less than one-third failed. In some cases this was because of inappropriate selection, but in others bone deformities developed even though the shoulder had been concentrically reduced at the first operation (Fig. 10.24).

Table 10.12 Results of operation for subscapularis recession: 86 cases, minimum follow-up of 12 months, 1988–1995

	Mallett grade					Gilbert grade					Raimondi grade				
	5–6	7–8	9–10	11–12	13–15	1	2	3	4	5	1	2	3	4	5
Preoperative (No. of shoulders)	36	39	8	3	0	51	12	9	5	0	0	10	12	42	22
Postoperative (No. of shoulders)	7	5	14	35	25	5	5	11	30	35	0	7	6	15	58

The deformity recurred in 29 of these cases, and a second operation through an anterior approach, with bone work, was necessary.

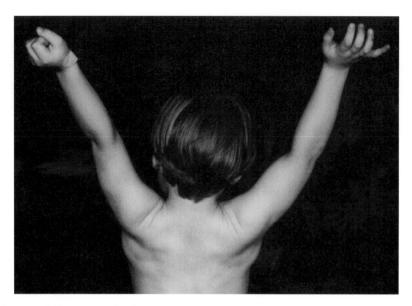

Fig. 10.24 A 3-year-old boy 18 months after subscapularis slide. There is a full range of movement at the shoulder.

Simple dislocation and subluxation

The extent of bone abnormality is determined by plain radiographs before operation and by screening the shoulder with image intensifier after induction of anaesthetic. The shoulder is approached through the deltopectoral groove, the coracobrachialis tendon is detached from the tip of the coracoid, and the subscapularis tendon is exposed and lengthened. A partial incision of the capsule is necessary to confirm that the head of the humerus is truly and fully reduced. With the shoulder fully located and in full lateral rotation, impingement from abnormality of the coracoid or acromion is sought. Subscapularis must be repaired; in a few of our earlier cases we neglected to do this and these children lost active medial rotation and required secondary operations to restore it. The limb is immobilised for 6 weeks. Results in 38 cases are described in Table 10.13.

Table 10.13 Simple dislocation and subluxation treated by the anterior approach with elongation of the subscapularis tendon: 38 cases, minimum follow-up 18 months, 1990–1994

	Mallett grade					Gilbert grade					Raimondi grade				
	5–6	7–8	9–10	11–12	13–15	1	2	3	4	5	1	2	3	4	5
Preoperative (No. of cases)	21	12	5	0		28	7	2	1	0			14	15	9
Postoperative (No. of cases)	1	3	15	8	11	1	2	10	15	10	0		8	5	25

The complex dislocation

The purpose of operation is to secure reduction of the head of the humerus into the true glenoid by removing obstructing deformities. There are two of these:

- the coracoid is always long and must be shortened by 1–2.5 cm
- there is overgrowth of the acromion.

Our experience of osteotomy of the acromion has been unsatisfactory: in fact we do not know what to do about this deformity. The subscapularis tendon is formally lengthened, and the capsule opened. It can now be confirmed that the lesser tuberosity is articulated with the false or inferior glenoid. The head of the humerus articulates with the true, superior, glenoid when the arm is in full lateral rotation, but tends to drop out at about the neutral position of rotation. The subscapularis tendon is repaired, the pectoralis minor and coracobrachialis are reattached to the stump of the coracoid, and the shoulder is immobilised for 6–8 weeks, as outlined above.

Results are described in Table 10.14. The operation has been performed in 48 cases, and adequate follow-up is available in 21. The oldest child in whom the operation was performed was aged 12 years and the functional improvement was substantial (Figs 10.25 and 10.26). We have encountered a number of difficulties. These include failure to hold reduction. In early cases we used a fine Steinmann pin passed across the glenohumeral joint, but abandoned this technique when one pin migrated. The major error is to immobilise the limb in any degree of abduction; the arm must be held in adduction. In a few cases with severe overgrowth of the acromion it is not possible to hold the head of the humerus into the true glenoid: it will do no more than articulate with the false glenoid. There is always an initial loss of active medial rotation, and in some children this never returns. It is in these cases that the posterior glenohumeral contracture, of winging of the scapula, the sign first recognised by Putti, is so prominent. In six children included in the data in Table 16 and in 17 children overall who have had successful relocation of the shoulder, operation has proved necessary to restore active medial rotation permitting the arm to come to the opposite shoulder and behind the back. The simplest way to achieve this is by medial rotation osteotomy of the humerus, to about 40°. A useful range of active lateral rotation was retained, at least 50°, and good medial active rotation was achieved in all cases except one. We do not know which children require this operation, and do not perform it within a minimum of 6 months after relocation.

The results of relocation of the dislocated shoulder in these children are, on the whole, impressive and we consider this to be the single most useful palliative operation in the treatment of OBPP. Many questions and difficulties remain. At what stage should relocation be abandoned because of deformity of the joint, and at what age is only a lateral rotation osteotomy possible? We do not know what to do about the overgrowth of the acromion, and at times it seems impossible to secure reduction of the humeral head into the true glenoid (Figs 10.27 and 10.28). Nonetheless, the overall improvement in function is impressive, and the outcome so far is far superior to that of the untreated cases presenting to us in late adolescence or early adult life.

Chen made a particularly important observation. In no less than 50% of all the children who had operations for medial rotation contracture or dislocation there was substantial improvement in the flexion deformity of the elbow and in the range of active supination. Furthermore, 20% of these children showed a remarkable improvement, which was unexpected and which we cannot explain, in function in the hand and notably in the power of extension of the wrist.

The flexion deformity of the elbow in the child with good neurological recovery

This is a particularly annoying contracture and one which we believe should be prevented in nearly every case by gentle but persistent stretching work. Operations have been performed in 12 cases, in which the lacertus fibrosus was divided and the sheath of brachialis muscle incised. This brought about a modest improvement. Elongation of the biceps tendon itself should be avoided, as this diminishes the range of motion. A far better approach is skilful serial plaster splinting. This technique, developed by Sister Evelyn Hunter RGN, is demonstrated in Chapter 17.

Table 10.14 Complex dislocation and subluxation treated by the anterior approach with shortening of the coracoid, osteotomy of the acromion in three cases, and elongation of the subscapularis tendon: 21 cases, minimum follow-up 24 months, 1991–1994

	Mallett grade					Gilbert grade					Raimondi grade				
	5–6	7–8	9–10	11–12	13–15	1	2	3	4	5	1	2	3	4	5
Preoperative (No. of cases)	14	4	1	2	0	14	6	1	0	0	0	0	7	10	4
Postoperative (No. of cases)	0	1	5	6	9	0	2	4	6	9	0	0	2	5	14

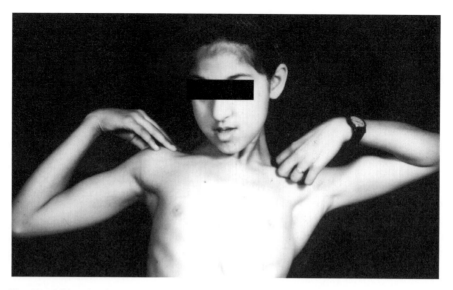

Fig. 10.25 Function in a 12-year-old girl at 6 years after relocation of complex dislocation of the right shoulder. There was virtually full range of movement at the shoulder.

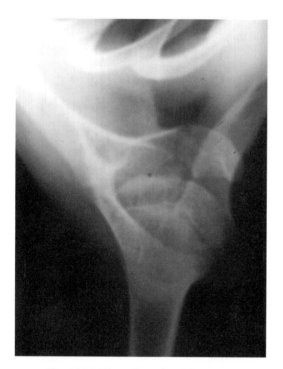
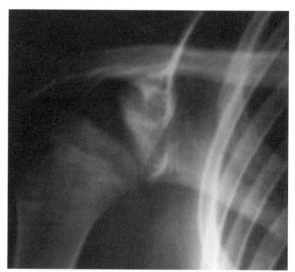

Fig. 10.26 The radiographs of the case shown in Figure 10.25. The contour of the glenoid is abnormal.

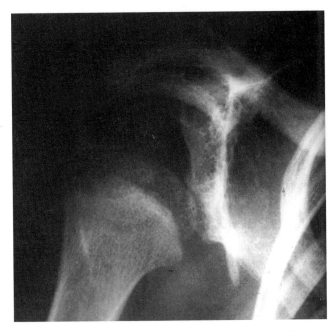

Fig. 10.27 A 9-year-old girl at 6 years after relocation of complex dislocation. The head of the humerus articulates with the false glenoid. The spur of bone seen below the glenoid is common after subscapularis recession, which was performed in this child at the age of 18 months. Function was good.

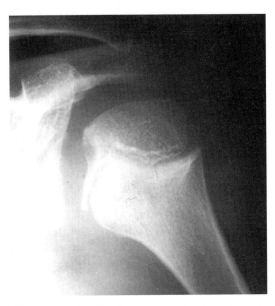

Fig. 10.28 A 7-year-old girl at 3 years after relocation of complex dislocation, showing persisting flattening of head of humerus. Function was good.

SUMMARY

We hope and think that the renewal of interest in the operative treatment of birth lesions of the brachial plexus initiated by colleagues in continental Europe and in North America, will extend to the UK. Certainly, practice here has lagged behind that in those countries, partly through a lack of awareness of the possibilities of operative treatment, and partly through a too facile optimism about the outcome of natural process. There seems to be no reason to think that the incidence of these lesions is likely to decline in the near future; rather, the indications are that the incidence is likely to rise or remain steady, and that the parents of the injured children will increasingly have recourse to legal process. Of course, as is the case in so many other fields, prevention is better than cure: it may be that with increasing awareness the maintenance of records will improve, that particular risk factors will be better defined, and that changes in obstetric practice will eventually lead to a decline in the incidence of this distressing lesion.

11. Results

Systems of measuring outcome: Seddon; Kline and Hudson; factors governing outcome after nerve repair; the spinal accessory nerve, the nerve to serratus anterior, circumflex and suprascapular nerves, the musculocutaneous and radial nerves, the median and ulnar nerves, the digital nerves. Results after repair of trunk nerves in the lower limb.

The results are set out here for over 900 repairs of trunk peripheral nerves followed for more than 2 years. Of course, recovery continues for longer than this in median and ulnar nerves, while the outcome after repair of nerves such as the spinal accessory or musculocutaneous is evident within 2 years.

We have used the systems developed by Seddon (1975) which were drawn from the Medical Research Council (MRC) system (Tables 11.1 and 11.2). In some nerves muscular function is a good deal more important than recovery of sensation, and for the spinal accessory, suprascapular, circumflex, musculocutaneous, radial, femoral and common peroneal nerves little significance is attributed to the extent of recovery of cutaneous sensation – *except when recovery was complicated by severe pain, when the result is considered a poor or bad one.* Recovery of sensation has been given equal importance to muscle function in the description of results for median and ulnar nerves and for the tibial division of the sciatic nerve and the posterior tibial nerve. One could argue that sensibility is the most important function of the median and posterior tibial nerves. Some allowance is made for the recovery of sympathetic efferent activity in these nerves and after repair of palmar cutaneous (digital) nerves. Results for repairs in the adult plexus and in obstetrical brachial plexus palsy (OBPP) are set out in the appropriate chapters.

Seddon's system has been modified for particular nerves; the method of assessment, which is often based on the work of colleagues who have studied some of these patients, is set out for each individual nerve.

Recovery of nerves after suture is a prolonged business. The rate of recall for children after repair in OBPP is over 90%, and for adults after repair of supraclavicular injury it is over 80%, but this proportion diminishes in other types of nerve. For nerves damaged in the axilla and arm and for those of the leg it is little over 60%, and for those after repair of nerves of cutaneous sensation in the hand it is no

Table 11.1 Medical Research Council System

Motor function

M0 No contraction

M1 Return of perceptible contraction in the proximal muscles

M2 Return of perceptible contraction in both proximal and distal muscles

M3 Return of function in both proximal and distal muscles of such degree that all *important* muscles are sufficiently powerful to act against resistance

M4 Return of function as in stage 3 with the addition that all *synergic* and independent movements are possible

M5 Complete recovery

Sensory function

S0 Absence of sensibility in the autonomous area

S1 Recovery of deep cutaneous pain sensibility within the *autonomous area* of the nerve

S2 Return of some degree of superficial cutaneous pain and tactile sensibility within the autonomous area of the nerve

S3 Return of some degree of superficial cutaneous pain and tactile sensibility within the autonomous area with disappearance of any previous overreaction

S3+ Return of sensibility as in stage 3 with the addition that there is some recovery of two-point discrimination within the autonomous area

S4 Complete recovery

Table 11.2 Grading of results

Grade	Description
Motor recovery	
M4 or better	Good
M3	Fair
M2	Poor
M1 and M0	Bad
Sensory recovery	
S4 (normal) or S3+	Good
S3	Fair
S2	Poor
S1 and S0	Bad

Drawn from Seddon (1975).

more than 25%. It would be nice to think that patients who failed to attend had got better; it is equally possible that their operations had failed.

All systems of measurement have their defects, and it seems that the more closely one looks at the result of a nerve repair the more defects are revealed. Kline and Hudson (1995) have developed the systems set out in Tables 11.3 and 11.4. They have developed an "excellent" result, a result which we have given to a small number of repairs of the median nerve in the forearm.

The outcome in our cases is set out according to the cause of injury: the "tidy" wound from knife, glass or scalpel; the "untidy" wound from axe, saw, penetrating missile, open fracture or dislocation, or burn; and the closed traction lesion. This reflects our view that the violence of the injury and the extent of damage to the nerve and adjacent tissues is the single most important determinant of outcome, closely followed by the delay between injury and repair, and our tables include an analysis of the effect of this too.

There are a number of other factors that are important in prognosis which were clearly defined in the MRC Special Report (1954) and by Seddon (1975), Sunderland (1978) and Kline and Hudson (1995) among others.

Table 11.3 Louisiana State University Medical Center grading system for motor and sensory function

Grade	Evaluation	Description
Individual muscle grades		
0	Absent	No contraction
1	Poor	Trace contraction
2	Fair	Movement against gravity only
3	Moderate	Movement against gravity and some (mild) resistance
4	Good	Movement against moderate resistance
5	Excellent	Movement against maximal resistance
Sensory grades		
0	Absent	No response to touch, pin or pressure
1	Bad	Testing gives hyperaesthesia or paraesthesia; deep pain recovery in autonomous zones
2	Poor	Sensory responses sufficient for grip and slow protection; sensory stimuli mislocalised with overresponse
3	Moderate	Response to touch and pin in autonomous zones; sensation mislocalised and not normal, with some overresponse
4	Good	Response to touch and pin in autonomous zones; response localised but sensation not normal; no overresponse
5	Excellent	Near-normal response to touch and pin in entire field, including autonomous zones

Table 11.4 Louisiana State University Medical Center grading system for whole-nerve injury

Grade	Evaluation	Description
0	Absent	No muscle contraction, absent sensation
1	Poor	Proximal muscles contract but not against gravity; sensory grade 1 or 0
2	Fair	Proximal muscles contract against gravity; distal muscles do not contract; sensory grade, if applicable, is usually 2 or lower
3	Moderate	Proximal muscles contract against gravity and some resistance; some distal muscles contract against at least gravity; sensory grade is usually 3
4	Good	All proximal and some distal muscles contract against gravity and some resistance; sensory grade is 3 or better
5	Excellent	All muscles contract against moderate resistance; sensory grade 4 or better

From Kline and Hudson (1995).

AGE

Some reference to outcome in children is made for each individual nerve, but we have not separated out this age group because of insufficient numbers. Let it suffice that the recovery of repair of a nerve in a child is, on the whole, a good deal better than in an adult, but it is not as good as has sometimes been assumed. Some of the most difficult problems in reconstruction (see Ch. 17) follow a failure of recovery of either the tibial or the common peroneal division of the sciatic nerve in the growing child, and we have already seen the unpredictability, and the limitations, of outcome after repair of the plexus in the birth lesion (see Ch. 10).

LEVEL OF INJURY

This is particularly important in the median and ulnar nerves, and results for these are set out for the axilla and arm and then for the forearm and hand. The level of injury is relevant in the radial nerve as well, but it seems to be less important for the sciatic nerve and its divisions.

The spinal accessory nerve

Paralysis of the trapezius causes profound disturbance of the function of the shoulder girdle. The shoulder droops and abduction is usually limited to less than 70°. The scapular wings, which may lead to an erroneous diagnosis of paralysis of the serratus anterior. Norden (1946) related a series of 16 cases, with persisting pain and inability to work. Valtonen and Lilius (1974) noted pain and severe disability in 11 of their 15 patients. Seddon described 14 cases. Osgaard et al (1987) repaired nine nerves: six repairs, within 4 months did well; three later cases did not. Kline and Hudson (1995) described 84 cases; nearly three-quarters of these were iatropathic. Useful improvement in function was usual in 33 nerves which were repaired.

Our material is set out in Table 11.5. Williams et al (1996) reported 40 of our cases, 23 of which were caused by surgeons working in the posterior triangle (Table 11.6). Delay in diagnosis was usual, ranging from immediate to 32 months. Twenty-six of these 40 patients had severe pain at rest, which disturbed sleep; in eight more there was significant pain brought on by movement of the shoulder.

In 24 cases the nerve was repaired by grafting, and useful recovery was seen in 19 of these, with relief of pain and improvement in the range and strength of shoulder movement. What are the causes of the severity of pain so characteristic of injury to this nerve? Traction upon the brachial plexus from the unsupported shoulder is not a wholly adequate explanation. The onset to pain is too early, and those patients who suffer damage to the nerve at operation with local anaesthetic describe a severe shooting pain coursing into the neck and shoulder. Some patients noted relief of pain within days of repair of the nerve, long before any return of function to the trapezius. Brown et al (1988) noted that sensory nerves were a potential source of pain, and Wetmore and Elde (1991) showed afferent neurons in the accessory nerve of the rat.

Case report. A 28-year-old woman suffered accessory palsy from lymph node biopsy high in the posterior triangle of the neck. Diagnosis was not made for nearly 2 years and no active treatment was proposed until we saw her at 32 months. She was still in pain, and abduction at the shoulder was limited to 70°. The nerve, which had been divided at the posterior margin of the sternomastoid, was repaired. She said that her pain had disappeared by about 2 weeks from operation, and by 9 months there was substantial recovery of the upper fibres of the trapezius muscle, with concomitant improvement in function.

Function was significantly improved in 39 of 46 repairs with adequate follow-up. Recovery was better in stab wounds, but these were younger patients and, in all except one, repair was effected within 3 months of injury.

It is remarkable that when this nerve is deliberately sectioned at the base of the posterior triangle to transfer to

Table 11.5 Operations on lesions of the spinal accessory nerve

Cause	No. of cases	
	Neurolysis	Repair
Stab wound	2	10
Penetrating missile wound	1	2
Traction	1	3
Iatropathic	12	31
Irradiation	2	0
Total	18	46

Table 11.6 Classification of recovery

Grade	Evaluation	Description	No. of cases	Treatment
A	Poor –	No change	7	Graft 4, neurolysis 3
B	Fair –	Pain and movement improved	10	Graft 6, neurolysis 4
C	Good –	Almost normal (difficulty with overhead work)	15	Graft 13, neurolysis 2
D	Excellent –	Normal (from patient's point of view)	4	Graft 1, neurolysis 3

another nerve, loss of function and pain are extremely rare, yet when the nerve is damaged 6–8 cm more proximally, pain with significant loss of function is almost inevitable. It is a shameful matter that the nerve is so commonly damaged during operations, that diagnosis is usually delayed and that only exceptionally are urgent efforts made to rectify the situation. As Williams et al (1996) say: "injury to the accessory nerve results in a characteristic group of symptoms and signs – reduced shoulder abduction, drooped shoulder and pain. Repair of the nerve improves symptoms in most cases. A sound grasp of the surgical anatomy, together with the use of a nerve stimulator, ought to prevent this serious complication of surgery in the neck".

The nerve to serratus anterior

This nerve is most commonly damaged in lesions of the brachial plexus (see Ch. 9), but it is particularly vulnerable to accidental damage where it crosses the first and second ribs. When the serratus anterior is paralysed, the inferior pole of the scapula does not move forward but slides medially and cranially. Deep aching pain is common and it is sometimes severe. When we have been given the chance to repair the nerve after a stab wound (five cases) or intraoperative injury (four cases), results have been very good, indeed better than for almost any other peripheral nerve. Operations for palliation for paralysis of the serratus anterior and the trapezius are described in Chapter 17.

Circumflex and suprascapular nerves

The results presented (Tables 11.7 and 11.8) are based on the findings of Spilsbury and Birch (1996) and the methods we used are described more fully in Chapter 8.

Results were bad when there was associated rupture of the rotator cuff, and results were poor in three cases in which the repair of the cuff was performed at the same time as grafting of the circumflex nerve. These three patients are not included in the tables. In two more patients with intra-articular fracture that led to post-traumatic arthritis, glenohumeral arthrodesis was necessary. Tight contracture of the capsule was a common contributory factor to the failure, especially after multiple ruptures of nerve trunks. All repairs of the circumflex nerve performed at more than 1 year from injury failed.

We think that the shoulder assessment system developed by Constant (1987 & 1997) is extremely useful, and we should use it in future work. Again, we draw attention to Spilsbury's measurements of endurance and power in the reinnervated deltoid, which fell far short of normal even in the "good" category.

Table 11.7 Grading of results of operation on the circumflex and suprascapular nerves

Grade	Description
Circumflex nerve	
Good	Deltoid, MRC 4 or better; abduction, elevation at least 120°
Fair	Deltoid, MRC 3+ or better; abduction, elevation 90–120°
Poor or bad	Less than above
Suprascapular nerve	
Good	Abduction, 120° or more; lateral rotation, 3° or more
Fair	Abduction, 90–120°; lateral rotation, 0–30°
Poor	Less than above

Table 11.8 Results obtained in operation on the circumflex nerve (56 cases) and suprascapular nerve (24 cases)

Result	No. of cases
Circumflex nerve	
Good	25
Fair	23
Poor	8
Suprascapular nerve	
Good	20
Fair	2
Poor	2

Table 11.9 Results of 154 repairs to musculocutaneous nerves (children and adults)

Grade	Description	Injury type (No. of cases)			
		Tidy	Untidy*	Traction	Total
Good	Flexion of elbow, M4 or better	21	26	55	102
Fair	Flexion of elbow against gravity	3	8	24	35
Poor	< MRC 3	1	6	10	17
Total		25	40	89	154

*Including penetrating missile injuries.

The musculocutaneous nerve

This is one of the best nerves to repair, so much so that repair was attempted even in extremely unfavourable cases with postischaemic fibrosis, after direct damage to the elbow flexor muscles, or after prolonged delay. Three sutures failed (included in Table 11.9). These were revised with grafts, achieving two "good" and one "fair" result.

Radial nerve (Table 11.10)

These results (Table 11.10) are not as good as one might expect, and they appear to be inferior to those reported by Seddon (1975). Useful wrist extension was regained in two-thirds of patients, but extension of the fingers and thumb was achieved in only one-third. In high lesions of the posterior cord the results have been graded as "fair" if useful elbow extension (MRC 4) followed repair.

As one might expect, recovery for the posterior interosseous nerve is usually good (Table 11.11).

Median and ulnar nerves

Intraclavicular lesions

The effect of age and of level of injury are very striking for these two nerves. Equally, or even more so, are the effects of the cause of injury and the delay between injury and repair. The clearest evidence for this comes from the study by Cavanagh et al (1987) of the complex infraclavicular injury in which several nerve trunks were ruptured, or torn by a knife or missile, an injury complicated by rupture of the axillary artery in over one-third of cases. Results for the injured nerves, by cause, and related to the interval between injury and repair, are set out in Tables 11.12 to 11.14. Only one of 22 cases of median and ulnar repairs achieved a good result in the delayed repair group. Results

Table 11.10 Results of 131 repairs to radial nerves (children and adults)

| Grade | Description | Injury type (No. of cases) | | | |
		Tidy	Untidy*	Traction	Total
Good	Extension of elbow, wrist and digits, MRC 4 or better	12	20	6	38
Fair	Extension of elbow and wrist against gravity	10	18	19	47
Poor	< MRC 3	5	16	25	46
Total		27	54	50	131

*Including penetrating missile wounds.

Table 11.11 Results of operation on the posterior interosseous nerve (11 cases)

Grade	Description	No. of cases
Good	Active extension of fingers and thumb, MRC 4 or better	8
Fair	Active extension of fingers and thumb, MRC 3 or 3+	2
Poor or bad	Less than the above	1

Table 11.12 Results for injured median and ulnar nerves in intraclavicular lesions

| Injured nerve | Result | | | |
	Good	Fair	Poor	Total
Median and ulnar	15	21	19	55
Radial and musculocutaneous	29	20	8	57
Suprascapular and circumflex	12	3	3	18
Total	56	44	30	130

Drawn from Cavanagh et al (1987).

Table 11.13 Results for injured median and ulnar nerves by cause in intraclavicular lesions

| Lesion | Result | | | |
	Good	Fair	Poor	Total
Closed				
Infraclavicular with suprascapular involvement	1	4	6	11
Infraclavicular only	31	30	19	80
Open	24	10	5	39
Total	56	44	30	130

Drawn from Cavanagh et al (1987).

Table 11.14 Results for injured median and ulnar nerves by interval between injury and repair in intraclavicular lesions

| Lesion | Result | | | |
	Good	Fair	Poor	Total
Early (within 14 days)				
Median and ulnar	14	13	6	33
Radial and musculocutaneous	19	10	1	30
Suprascapular and circumflex	7	2	2	11
Total	40	25	9	74
Late (after 14 days: 22 weeks on average)				
Median and ulnar	1	8	13	22
Radial and musculocutaneous	10	10	7	27
Suprascapular and circumflex	5	1	1	7
Total	16	19	21	56

Drawn from Cavanagh et al (1987).

were certainly worse when there was associated damage to the supraclavicular brachial plexus. These results provide ample justification for our policy of urgent primary repair whenever possible in these severe and complex injuries.

High lesions

The results after repair of high median and ulnar nerve lesions are, on the whole, much more modest than those following more distal repairs, and thus a less demanding

Table 11.15 Grading of results in high median and ulnar nerve repair

Grade	Description
Median nerve	
Good	Long flexor muscles, MRC 4 or better. Localisation to digit, without hypersensitivity. Return of sweating
Fair	Long flexor muscles, MRC 3 or 3+. "Protective sensation". Moderate or no hypersensitivity. Sweating diminished or absent
Poor or bad	Long flexor muscles, MRC 2 or less. "Protective sensation", but severe hypersensitivity, *or* no sensation
Ulnar nerve	
Good	FCU and FDP of little and ring fingers, MRC 4 or better. Intrinsic muscles MRC 2 or better. Localisation to little and ring fingers. No hypersensitivity. Return of sweating
Fair	FCU and FDP of little and ring fingers, MRC 3 or 3+. No intrinsic muscle function. "Protective" sensation in little and ring fingers. Moderate hypersensitivity. Little or no sweating
Poor or bad	FCU and FDP of little and ring fingers, MRC 2. No intrinsic muscle function. "Protective" sensation with severe hypersensitivity, *or* no sensation. No sweating

FCU, flexor carpi ulnaris; FDP, flexor digitorum profondus.

Table 11.16 Results in 85 repairs of median nerves in the axilla or arm (adults and children)*

Grade	Wound type (No. cases)			Total
	Tidy	Untidy†	Traction	
Good	6	4	3	13
Fair	8	8	15	31
Poor or bad	3	12	26	41
Total	17	24	44	85

*Includes 28 repairs of either the lateral or medial root of the nerve in the axilla.
†Including penetrating missile injury.

Table 11.17 Results of 60 repairs of the medial cord or ulnar nerve in the axilla and arm (children and adults)*

Grade	Wound type (No. of cases)			Total
	Tidy	Untidy	Traction	
Good	3	2	0	5
Fair	5	13	7	25
Poor or bad	2	10	18	30
Total	10	25	25	60

*All five good results followed repair within 48 hours of injury (two in children). Results of repair after 3 months of injury were always poor in the untidy and traction lesions.
†Including penetrating missile injury.

system of assessment is used for repairs of these nerves damaged in the axilla and arm (Table 11.15). Results are described in Tables 11.16 and 11.17.

Distal lesions

Results for median and ulnar nerves in the forearm and wrist were presented by Birch and Raji (1991). The method of assessment used in this series is set out (Table 11.18), and the results obtained in 254 nerves are given in Tables 11.19 and 11.20.

Digital nerves

Goldie and Coates (1992) made a detailed study of 27 of our patients. Thirty nerves were repaired, all but one by primary repair using sutures (we did not have access to fibrin clot glue at that time). The digital artery was repaired if it had been damaged. Examination for sensation was thorough and it was helped by using weighted (5 and 10 g) pins designed for us by Professor Ruth Bowden. The results were surprising in that they were rather disappointing, an indication perhaps that the more scrupulously one examines outcome of a nerve repair the more

one will find wrong. Normal two-point discrimination was regained in 37% of fingers, but only 27% of patients graded their overall results as "excellent," and 40% complained of persistent hyperaesthesia up to 2 years. Goldie and Coates concluded: "following repair of the divided digital nerve, normal sensation will never be regained. Hyperaesthesia may be present for months or years but will ultimately resolve. The final result will take two or three years to achieve". Fortunately, results do seem to be a good deal better in children. Results for 102 adult distal nerves and 27 children's digital nerves are set out in Tables 11.21 and 11.22. It does seem odd that recovery of sensation after a well-executed primary repair of the median nerve at the wrist is regularly better than that from repair of digital nerves more distally. It is only fair to add that a number of patients reported striking improvement in sensation, with rapid loss of cold sensitivity and hypersensitivity to touch, some years after repair. Plainly, recovery of sensation and improvement in sensitivity is a very prolonged business.

Case report. Primary repair of the median and ulnar nerves was performed in a 22-year-old staff nurse. Recovery was quite good, but marred by cold sensitivity, so that her result was considered only fair at 3 years after

Table 11.18 Method of grading results in median and ulnar nerves in distal lesions

Grade	Motor	Sensory	Equivalent on Seddon's grading
Excellent	Power, MRC 5. No wasting or deformity. No trophic changes	Function indistinguishable from normal hand. Good stereognosis, no hypersensitivity. 2PD equivalent to uninjured digits	Good: M5, S4
Good	Power, MRC 4 to 5. Abolition of paralytic deformity. Minimal pulp wasting	Accurate speedy localisation. Can recognise texture or objects. Minor cold sensitivity and hypersensitivity. 2PD < 8 mm at tips of fingers	Good: M5, S3+
Fair	MRC 3 or more. Some sweating. Pulp wasted	Accurate localisation to digit. No stereognosis. 2PD > 8 mm. Significant cold sensitivity and hypersensitivity	Fair: M3, S3
Poor or bad	MRC 3 or less. No sweating. Trophic changes	No sensation. Severe cold sensitivity or hypersensitivity	Bad: M 01 or 2 01 or 2

2PD, two-point discrimination.

Table 11.19 Repair of 119 median nerves in tidy wounds from distal wrist crease to elbow crease (adults; age 16–65 years)

	Repair type (No. of cases)			
Outcome	Primary repair	Delayed suture	Graft	Total
Excellent	5	1	0	6
Good	27	9	12	48
Fair	12	14	25	51
Poor or bad	2	7	5	14
Total	46	31	42	119

Table 11.20 Repair of 145 ulnar nerves in tidy wounds from distal wrist crease to elbow crease (adults; age 16–65 years)

	Repair type (No. of cases)			
Outcome	Primary repair	Delayed suture	Graft	Total
Excellent	8	1	2	11
Good	25	6	22	53
Fair	13	16	27	56
Poor or bad	0	9	16	25
Total	46	32	67	145

Table 11.21 Results obtained in repair of adult digital nerves

Outcome	No. of nerves
Repair within 48 hours of injury	
Excellent	1
Good	33
Fair	24
Poor or bad	16
Repair 2 weeks or more from injury	
Excellent	0
Good	9
Fair	11
Poor or bad	8
Total	28

14 digital *arteries* repaired at primary operation;
17 flexor tendons repaired at primary operation.

Table 11.22 Results obtained in 27 digital nerves repaired at varying intervals from injury: children (aged 15 years or less)

Outcome	No. of nerves
Excellent	17
Good	8
Fair	2
Poor or bad	0

operation. She came to see us 7 years after operation to report a striking improvement over the course of a few months. Oversensitivity had disappeared. The final result for the ulnar nerve was considered excellent, and it was very good for the median nerve.

Case report. A 39-year-old nursing sister wounded the digital nerves to her little and ring fingers. Recovery was marred by cold sensitivity, and overreaction to light touch, until there was quite sudden resolution of these difficulties, over a few weeks, 6 years after operation.

Trunk nerves in the lower limb

Most injuries to trunk nerves in the lower limb occurred in "untidy" wounds (penetrating missiles being the main cause), and all were associated with fractures and dislocations. Tidy wounds were unusual except in iatropathic cases, and there were quite a few of these. Associated arterial injury was common and had a particularly deleterious effect. Several of our repairs of the common peroneal nerve failed because earlier injury to the anterior tibial artery had been unrecognised and untreated, which always led to severe ischaemic fibrosis in the anterolateral muscles of the leg. However, it is clear that the sciatic nerve has an undeservedly bad reputation. We have seen four impressive results from primary repair of stab wounds of the nerve at the hip. Three of these were performed by orthopaedic colleagues on the day of injury, and one was treated by us. Sunderland et al (1993) have presented a very detailed account of one such case.

Clawson and Seddon (1960a,b) and Seddon (1975) wrote of the very large series of injuries to the sciatic nerves and its divisions. In speaking of the lack of correspondence between neurological and functional recovery, Seddon commented: "it is more pronounced in the case of the sciatic nerve than in any other. One of our patients with total sciatic paralysis continued rock climbing and tackles difficult routes. Another, with common peroneal paralysis, pilots jet aircraft and enjoys playing 18 holes of golf. These patients are not wildly exceptional. By contrast there are a few with only a slight neurological deficit who were very sorry for themselves". We follow Seddon in describing results for the two divisions of the sciatic nerve, irrespective of the level of injury or whether one or both had been damaged. The elements of our system for measuring outcome are set out in Tables 11.23 and 11.24. The system for the common peroneal nerve was developed by Wilkinson in his study of 27 elective repairs of the common peroneal nerve (Wilkinson and Birch 1995).

We have found severe pain and hypersensitivity to be a frequent complication of repair of the sciatic nerve, the tibial division or the posterior tibial nerve. It was not seen in any patient with clear evidence of recovery into the sympathetic efferents. Recovery into the small muscles of the foot was seen in all four of the good results of primary repair in tidy wounds at the hip, but it was rarely seen after repair in "untidy" wounds or after traction injuries (Tables 11.25 to 11.27).

The femoral nerve

We think our results of repair of this nerve are disappointing. Significant pain and hypersensitivity was common, indeed severe pain after injury to the femoral nerve is an underestimated problem. The injury was complicated by arterial lesion in three cases and by sepsis in two more, and results were poor in all of these cases (Table 11.28).

Table 11.23 Assessment of recovery of the common peroneal nerve

MRC grade and description		Assessment
M0	No contraction	Bad
M1	Perceptible contraction	Bad
M2	Contraction with gravity eliminated	Poor
M3	Contraction against gravity	Fair
M4	Contraction against resistance	Good
M5	Normal power, full recovery	Good

Table 11.24 Assessment of results for tibial division of the sciatic nerve and the posterior tibial nerve

Assessment	Motor recovery	Sensory recovery
Good	Heel flexors, MRC 4 or better. Tibialis posterior, flexor digitorum longus, and flexor hallucis longus, MRC 3. Return of sweating. No fixed deformity, no trophic disturbance. Normal shoes	Protective sensation with no more than mild hypersensitivity; no spontaneous pain
Fair	Heel flexors, MRC 3+ or better. No useful recovery in long flexor muscles. Incomplete return of sweating. No serious trophic disturbance, no fixed deformity. Normal shoes with or without foot drop splint.	Protective sensation; hypersensitivity not interfering with daily activities
Poor and bad	No useful motor recovery; and/or significant fixed deformity; and/or trophic ulceration	No return of sensation; and/or significant hypersensitivity interfering with daily activities

Table 11.25 Outcome of 70 repairs of the common peroneal division of the sciatic nerve or common peroneal nerve (adults and children)

| Grade | Wound type (No. of cases) | | | |
	Tidy	Untidy*	Traction	Total
Good	9	7	9	25
Fair	5	5	7	17
Poor or bad	3	9	16	28
Total	17	21	32	70

There were 16 repairs at the hip (4 good, 3 fair). All four good results followed urgent repair (3 in tidy wounds; 1 in untidy wound). Of 7 repairs in childrens' nerves, 4 were good, 2 were fair and 1 was bad
*Including penetrating missile wounds.

Table 11.26 Effect of delay on recovery in 70 common peroneal division nerve repairs

| Outcome | Delay* (months) | | | |
	0–6	7–12	>12	Total
Good	18	6	1	25
Fair	9	5	3	17
Poor	11	9	8	28
Total	38	20	12	70

*Interval between injury and repair.

Table 11.27 Repair of tibial division of the sciatic nerve or posterior tibial nerve (children and adults)

| Outcome | Wound type (No. of cases) | | | |
	Tidy	Untidy	Traction	Total
Good	6	3	2	11
Fair	3	9	11	23
Poor or bad	3	5	10	18
Total	12	17	23	52

Of the 11 good results, 8 were repaired within 2 months of injury (4 urgently; 3 of these were in children). Two of six repairs in children failed.

Table 11.28 Femoral nerve repairs (adults)

Outcome	No. of cases
Good	3
Fair	3
Poor or bad	5
Total	11

12. Entrapment neuropathy

Entrapment neuropathies: definition of entrapment; importance of suspecting an underlying cause; the three common entrapment neuropathies – thoracic outlet syndrome, carpal tunnel syndrome, ulnar neuropathy – consideration of each, with pathological changes, clinical features, operative treatment and results of operation; the rarer entrapment neuropathies, with brief description and account of experience; general caution about diagnosis and operative treatment of "entrapment syndromes".

The term "entrapment neuropathy" should probably be reserved for instances in which a small addition to the crowding produced by existing anatomical arrangements is liable to cause compression or constriction or distortion of a peripheral nerve or, by interfering with the ability of the nerve to glide, to cause traction injury.

The situation of the median nerve deep to the flexor retinaculum provides an obvious example of such an anatomical arrangement, and the causes of lesions there provide a microcosm of the wider field. Cros and Shahani (1991) reserve the term "entrapment neuropathy" for "situations in which constriction and/or distortion of the peripheral nerves are implicated". They distinguish "entrapment" neuropathy from "compression" and "constriction" neuropathies, indicating that "entrapment" "calls attention to certain anatomical locations at which peripheral nerves are vulnerable". Stewart (1993) defines entrapment neuropathies as "compression neuropathies that occur at specific places where nerves are confined to narrow anatomic pathways and therefore are particularly susceptible to constricting pressures". Comtet (1993) offers this definition: "In certain pathological situations, an incompatibility may develop between a peripheral nerve and an existing anatomic space. The term 'nerve entrapment' refers to such a condition."

Certainly, entrapment neuropathy is a variety and an extension of compression neuropathy; even a variety of traction neuropathy. In these, the lesion of the nerve may be produced anywhere along its course. In entrapment neuropathy precipitation of injury and hence of the onset of symptoms is provided by local causes, which may be external or internal.

A purely external cause is exemplified by the pressure on the ulnar nerve at the elbow that may initiate chronic ulnar neuropathy. Here, it may well be that the condition is prolonged after cessation of external pressure by interference with the gliding facility caused by perineural fibrosis resulting from the pressure injury.

Internal causes may be extraneural or intraneural, or a combination of both; they may be purely local, or part of a systemic disorder. Purely local extraneural causes are: the presence of a ganglion, a tumour, a congenital abnormality (Watson-Jones 1949); a deformity from past fracture; or anomalous muscles (Still & Kleinert 1973). Local extraneural causes may arise from systemic disorders such as: rheumatoid arthritis (Pallis & Scott 1965, Pallis 1966, White et al 1988); gout; pseudogout (Weinstein et al 1968, Spiegel et al 1976, Rate et al 1992); the endocrine changes of pregnancy (Soferman et al 1964, Tobin 1967, Nicholas et al 1971) and of the menopause (Confino-Cohen et al 1991, Hall et al 1992); treatment with oral contraceptives (Sabour & Fadel 1970); hypothyroidism (Martin et al 1983, Wise et al 1995); or acromegaly (Kellgren et al 1952).

Intraneural changes usually arise from general conditions causing or associated with neuropathy: hereditary susceptibility to pressure (Earl et al 1964, Behse et al 1972, Madrid & Bradley 1975); alcoholism; diabetes mellitus; uraemia; carcinoma; and, rarely, acute demyelinating polyneuropathy (Guillain – Barré syndrome). A purely local intraneural cause is the intraneural "lipoma", described separately in 1964 by Mikhail, Morley, Pulvertaft, Watson, Jones and Yeoman. Another is the condition of the nerve arising from a more proximal lesion; the "double-crush" syndrome of Upton and McComas (1973). In this, the susceptibility of the distal nerve is, no doubt, determined largely by interference with axonal transport (Hurst et al 1985). This interference and the effect of the proximal lesion on the neural elements produce endoneurial oedema with circulatory defect, loss of elasticity, abnormality of connective tissues, and a reduction in the number of neural filaments (Pfeffer et al 1986, Nemoto et al 1987, Osterman 1988, 1991, Augustijn & Vannesti 1992). Leffert (1972) comments particularly on the role of the double-crush effect in the production of symptoms from ulnar neuropathy at the elbow. Shimpo et al (1987) offered experimental evidence of the role of a more proximal lesion in producing a "double-crush" effect.

Both intra- and extraneural causes operate in rheumatoid arthritis, hypothyroidism and acromegaly, in which generalised neuropathy and extraneural changes in synovium and connective tissue are present. In many cases it appears at first sight impossible to distinguish a precipitating cause other than the anatomical situation of the affected nerve, but the more rigorously investigation is pressed the fewer such cases there will be. Investigation should be pressed, because the occurrence of an "entrapment syndrome" may be the first symptom of serious underlying disease, and both surgeon and patient may have cause later to regret a temporarily successful operation. Wide reviews of the field as a whole are given by Spinner and Spencer (1974) and Gelberman et al (1993).

NEURAL PATHOLOGY

In cases in which there is existing neuropathy, the primary pathology is that of the neuropathy (see Ch. 6). The neural lesion directly attributable to local causes or to the addition of local causes to an underlying condition concerns vascular supply, axonal transport mechanisms, the myelin sheaths, the axons and the connective tissues.

Vascular mechanisms

Interference with the blood supply of the nerve, at first episodic, is usually the start of the process. The effects of ischaemia on nerve and muscle were examined by Harrison (1976). We owe to Lundborg (1988b) the concept of fascicular vascular units, each with their endoneurial and perineurial vascular systems linked segmentally to the mobile epineurial vascular network. The integrity of the connection clearly depends on the facility with which the nerve glides in its surrounding connective tissues and the fascicles glide in the epineurium. So, any restriction of excursion in either plane could interfere with the blood supply. Commonly, such interference is caused by external compression. That aspect was investigated by Rydevik et al (1981), who observed the changes in the microcirculation, both intra- and extrafascicular, produced by graded compression applied to the tibial nerves of rabbits. As low a pressure as 20–30 mmHg interfered with vascular flow; at 60–80 mmHg pressure there was no blood flow.

Sunderland (1976) thought of the mechanism in carpal tunnel syndrome as intrafascicular anoxia caused by obstruction of venous return. That, in his view, produced oedema and further increase of the pressure. The reversibility of the changes is clearly shown by Gilliatt and Wilson's (1953) pneumatic tourniquet test for "carpal tunnel syndrome", and by Fullerton's (1963) demonstration of the median nerve's abnormal susceptibility to ischaemia in that condition. Indeed, Wilson-McDonald and Caughey (1984) showed the diurnal variation of nerve conduction in that condition. Interestingly enough, they found no such variation in hand volume: the concept of nocturnal accumulation of fluid may be flawed. Causey (1948) studied the effect of circumferential pressure on the nerve fibres of rabbits, and indicated the local reduction in endoneurial fluid and in the fibre diameter.

Axonal transport mechanisms

Weiss and Hiscoe (1948), whose work foreshadowed later investigations into axonal transport, noted the integration of the axon and perikaryon as a single unit. They observed that in some cases the volume of the axon was as much as 100 times as great as that of the perikaryon. Studying the regeneration of nerves through zones of constriction, they noted the "damming" of axoplasm in the proximal segment, and drew from that the conclusion that "the column of axoplasm is maintained in constant proximo-distal movement". The later studies of Rydevik et al (1980) and Dahlin et al (1984, 1986b) showed that continued compression at low pressure caused partial or even complete block to fast orthograde transport. There was similar though more slowly developing blockage of slow transport. Compression at low pressure may also affect retrograde transport. The implication of these findings with regard both to single and double lesions is obvious.

The myelin sheath

Thomas and Fullerton (1963) had the opportunity of examining the median nerves of a patient with known right "carpal tunnel syndrome" who died from the effects of an astrocytoma. They found during life a reduction of conduction velocity in the affected median nerve. The fibre size in the right median nerve in the forearm did not differ from that in the left nerve at the same level. However, there was some reduction of fibre size in the right nerve just above the flexor retinaculum, and there was "striking" reduction in the nerve deep to the retinaculum. These studies obviously indicate axonal change as well as change in the myelin sheath. The principal evidence for demyelination is, of course, the finding of diminished velocity of conduction across a zone of entrapment (Gilliatt & Thomas 1960). Furthermore, abnormality of the myelin sheath consistent with causation by pressure has been observed in man by Neary et al (1975), Neary and Eames (1975) and Jefferson and Eames (1979). Demyelination clearly occurs in acute compression (Ochoa et al 1972, Gilliatt 1981). To what extent it is possible to extrapolate from the findings of Ochoa and Marrotte (1973) in the guinea-pig or from those of Gilliatt (1981) is perhaps doubtful. Neary et al (1975) did indeed have the opportunity of examining a median nerve trapped at the wrist, and found changes similar to those seen in animals' nerves subjected to external pressure. However, Brown et al (1976) found that in the case of ulnar neuropathy at the elbow abnormalities of conduction could be found in no more than one-third of nerves examined at the time of operation. As Cros and Shahani (1991) point out, the situation is complicated by the development of changes proximal and distal to the site of entrapment.

The axons

The axons are the last to be affected, and it is the larger ones that suffer. The clinical evidence of that affection is of course wasting and the presence of fibrillation potentials in the wasted muscles. Thomas and Fullerton (1963) provided clear evidence of the presence and the nature of this axonal loss.

The connective tissue

Examining necropsy material from 12 patients without histories of symptoms, Neary et al (1975) found that enlargement of the ulnar nerve at the elbow and of the median nerve at the wrist from increase in connective tissue component was common. All the work seems to substantiate the sequence of events proposed in 1964 by Weisl and Osborne: partial obstruction of vessels; oedema; distal and proximal collection of axonal substance; and invasion of oedema by fibroblasts.

The sequence of events

The effect of all the processes described above is eventually to produce swelling above the level of constriction and wasting at the site of constriction. That swelling, at first due to oedema, later becomes more rigid because of collagenisation. The wasting, at first due to the loss of myelin, later becomes more permanent because of loss of axons. With loss of axons changes occur in the target organs. At some stage a point is reached at which both local and peripheral changes become irreversible.

CLINICAL FEATURES

The symptoms are motor and sensory; they are rarely, if ever, related to disturbance of autonomic function. When, as at the thoracic outlet, the main vessels are in close relation to the nerves at the site of entrapment, there may be vascular symptoms. These may be arterial or venous. Sensory symptoms predominate in the case of nerves containing many fibres mediating cutaneous sensibility; motor symptoms predominate in the case of nerves the fibres of which are distributed solely or almost exclusively to muscle. Sensory symptoms may of course arise from entrapment of a "purely motor" nerve: there are afferent fibres in all such nerves, some from the spindles and Golgi organs, and others from free endings in the muscle and tendon. Sensory symptoms are pain, other paraesthesiae and numbness. In the case of the median nerve in particular, sensory symptoms are at first, and sometimes throughout, episodic. Precipitation of symptoms is presumably due to ischaemia affecting a nerve already damaged. Indeed, Gilliatt and Wilson's (1953) diagnostic test depends on such a mechanism.

Motor symptoms are weakness, wasting, fasciculation and occasional "spasms" or cramps – "painful contractures of part of a muscle or of whole muscles related to active involuntary firing of motor units" (Thomas & Ochoa 1993). Extensive weakness and wasting are, naturally, associated with the circulatory changes of disuse. In the early stages of motor affection, abnormal sensitivity to cold is often noticed, taking the form of much increased weakness of the cold extremity.

THE THREE COMMON ENTRAPMENT SYNDROMES

THE THORACIC OUTLET SYNDROME AND COSTOCLAVICULAR COMPRESSION

The thoracic outlet syndrome as a whole is the mother of all entrapment syndromes with regard to the length of its history, and for complexity, importance, discussion concerning treatment and variability of results.

Narakas (1993a) assigns to Sir Astley Cooper (1821) the credit for the earliest identification of thoracic outlet syndrome. Cooper wrote (Cooper & Travers 1817): "I have seen an exostosis arise from the sixth or seventh cervical vertebra or perhaps from both." He went on to describe the case of a woman, whose age is not recorded, who came into Guy's Hospital with no pulse at the wrist or elbow and with "venous redness" of the upper limb, which was cold, "benumbed" and painful. There was a projection of the lower cervical vertebrae towards the clavicle, with consequent pressure on the subclavian artery. The condition of the limb improved with palliative treatment, but the pulses did not return. It would, perhaps, be right to credit Astley Cooper with the first description of the arterial outlet syndrome. Willshire (1860) reported the case of a right seventh cervical rib in a young girl, with at least distortion and perhaps aneurysm of the subclavian artery. A year later, Coote (1861) reported the removal of a left seventh cervical rib causing aneurysm of the subclavian artery. In 1905, J. B. Murphy reported a similar procedure in the case of a man aged 38 years. T. Murphy (1910) introduced the concept of interference with the neurovascular bundle by a "normal" first rib, and successfully removed such a rib in the case of a 28-year-old woman. Morley (1913) showed the case of a 42-year-old woman with "pressure neuritis" of the lower trunk of the left right brachial plexus from a "normal" first rib. Removal of the rib gave relief of symptoms. The appearance of the nerve at operation is not described. In discussing the causation of symptoms, Morley raised the question of treatment by "developing the trapezii and levators of the scapula by systematic exercises". Stopford and Telford (1919) expanded the concept and reported ten cases. Todd (1912) discussed "cervical rib" and factors controlling its presence and size, and in the same year described the descent of the shoulder girdle after birth. Wood Jones (1910, 1911) discussed variations of the first rib associated with changes in the constitution of the brachial plexus, and Ochsner et al (1935) introduced the conception of the "scalenus anticus" syndrome, giving the credit to Naffziger. Naffziger and Grant (1938) crystallised those views in their account of "neuritis of the brachial plexus mechanical in origin". By then, the separation of "vascular" or "arterial" and "neural" syndromes was established.

Two physicians, Lewis and Pickering (1934), pointed to the mechanism of production of the arterial lesion – namely, intimal breakage with local thrombosis and distal embolisation. Eden (1939) reviewed 48 cases of arterial affection at the outlet, and added two cases in addition to that of Lewis and Pickering. Eden noted that in his first case the local thrombosis extended even after removal of the distorting seventh cervical rib. In the same year, Hill added another case.

Falconer and Weddell (1943) introduced the concept of costoclavicular compression, and showed the mechanism of venous compression in this condition. In 1951, McCleery et al dealt in greater depth with the mechanism of venous obstruction at the outlet and behind the clavicle, and Adams et al (1968) extended these concepts. Roos (1971) showed that thrombectomy was possible by the axillary approach with removal of the first rib, and Sanders and Haug (1990) contributed a comprehensive review of subclavian venous obstruction at the outlet.

Walshe et al (1944) after reviewing "normal first rib" and "scalenus anticus" syndromes, suggested that the essential feature determining the onset of symptoms was dropping of the shoulder girdle. Adson (1951) regarded the scalenus anticus syndrome without seventh cervical rib as having been "established as an independent entity". Fernandez (1955) described the "scalenus medius sickle" acting in the same manner as the seventh cervical rib. Raaf (1955) recommended a "thorough exploration of the brachial plexus in preference to simple anterior scalenotomy". Rob and Standeven (1958) are almost certainly responsible for the concept of the "thoracic outlet syndrome"; they reported ten cases of major arterial lesion associated with seventh cervical or first thoracic ribs. In his review article of 1962, Clagett confirmed that assignment of credit. Wickham and Martin (1962) added further arterial cases, and in the same year Falconer and Li reported on the results of removal of the first rib in costoclavicular compression Eastcott (1962) reported four arterial reconstructions in five cases of arterial outlet syndrome. Among these was the case of a woman who underwent removal of a seventh cervical rib and 33 years later came with a saccular aneurysm of the second and third parts of the subclavian artery.

Brannon (1963) added further cases of neural affection, and Bonney (1965) reported good results after removal of the "scalenus medius band" (Fernandez' "sickle") in such cases. Roos (1966) introduced the valuable concept of transaxillary removal of the first rib: a concept later expanded and refined by Roos and colleagues (Roos & Owens 1966, Roos 1971, 1981, 1982). Roos' work continues (Earnshaw 1995). It was the paper by Gilliatt et al (1970) that finally established the "neural" syndrome as a true separate entity. The suggestion by Griffiths (1964), among others, that the neural syndrome did not exist received a blow from Bonney's (1977) finding that there was in fact slowing of conduction along the lower trunk at the site of distortion. Lascelles et al (1977) defined the concept of vascular, neural and neurovascular syndromes in their series of 29 patients.

We emerge now with the certain concept of arterial, neural and venous syndromes from obstruction at or near the thoracic outlet, recognising that the neural syndrome is often combined with an element of arterial obstruction.

Anatomy

The lower part of the brachial plexus, and the lower trunk in particular, joined at the first rib by the subclavian vessels, run a regular obstacle course on their way to the lower borders of the pectoralis minor muscle. The eighth cervical anterior primary ramus and most of the anterior primary ramus of the first thoracic nerve form the lower trunk. In front of this, on the first rib, is the subclavian artery; in front of that is the tendon of scalenus anterior muscle; and in front of that, the subclavian vein. Behind it is the scalenus medius muscle; from above it is joined by the anterior primary ramus of the seventh cervical nerve forming the middle trunk (Figs 12.1 to 12.3).

Lateral to the scalenus anterior, the upper trunk is added to the plexus. As the neurovascular bundle proceeds distally the trunks divide to form the cords disposed lateral, posterior and medial to the artery, all lying deep to the vein. In this posture the neurovascular bundle passes deep to the clavicle and subclavius muscle and across the edge of the first rib; it then passes deep to the upper part of the pectoralis minor muscle. It is then free to continue into the axilla.

The obstacles placed in the way of the first thoracic nerve and its successors may be: the trap between the edge of the suprapleural membrane, or a variant of it, and the first rib or the scalenus medius (Figs 12.4 and 12.5); a seventh cervical rib or a variant; a "scalenus sickle" – an aponeurotic band forming the anterior part of the scalenus medius muscle; the first rib itself; an abnormality of the first rib; an anomalous part of the scalenus anterior muscle passing between the nerve and artery (Fig. 12.6); the

Figs 12.1 to 12.3 The thoracic outlet, the first rib, and the costoclavicular interval.

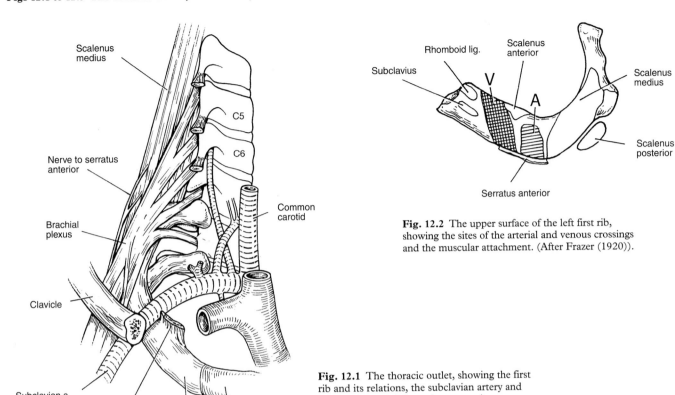

Fig. 12.1 The thoracic outlet, showing the first rib and its relations, the subclavian artery and the attachment of the scalenus anterior.

Fig. 12.2 The upper surface of the left first rib, showing the sites of the arterial and venous crossings and the muscular attachment. (After Frazer (1920)).

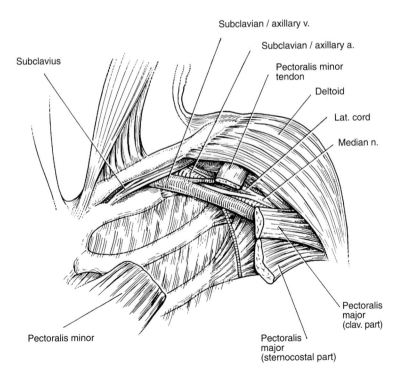

Fig. 12.3 The costoclavicular interval, showing the subclavius and its relation to the neurovascular bundle. (After Frazer (1920)).

Figs 12.4 and 12.5 Two cases of entrapment of the lower trunk through abnormality of the suprapleural membrane and scalenus medius.

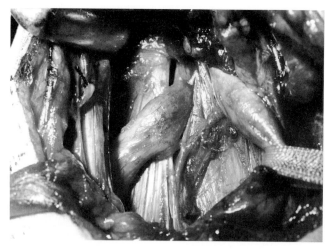

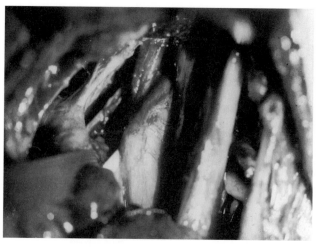

Fig. 12.4 The right lower trunk is trapped between the aponeurotic edge of the scalenus medius posteriorly and the suprapleural membrane anteriorly.

Fig. 12.5 The left lower trunk is trapped between a "scalenus sickle" and a scalenus minimus (pleuralis).

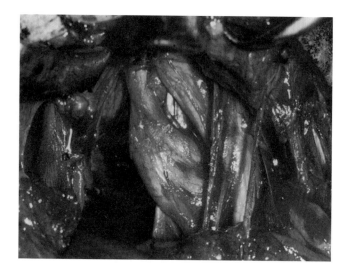

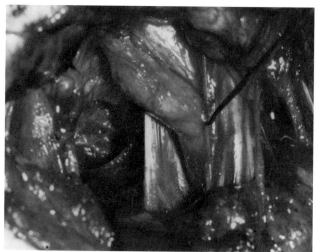

Fig. 12.6 A "scalenus sickle" and an anomalous scalenus anterior. The left lower trunk passes over the edge of the sickle and behind the part of the scalenus anterior that passes behind the subclavian artery. (Right) The trunk is elevated to show the lower part of the sickle.

costoclavicular space between the first rib and the clavicle and subclavius, where deformity of the clavicle, either congenital or acquired, may reduce the available space; crossing by the costoclavicular ligament; crossing by the superior part of the pectoralis minor; or, finally, crossing by an "arch of Langer" (Kasai & Chiba 1977) in the distal part of the axilla. In the most proximal part of this course, the first thoracic nerve is maximally affected; in relation to the first rib, the lower trunk and the subclavian artery are maximally affected; in the costoclavicular space, the subclavian vein is predominantly affected; and, most distally, the medial origin of the median nerve is maximally affected.

The suprapleural membrane (Sibson's fascia)

In its pure form, the suprapleural membrane is a thin, fan-shaped structure apically attached to the tip of the seventh cervical transverse process; peripherally, it is attached to the medial edge of the rib. The extent of its peripheral attachment varies. The deep part of the membrane may be quite tough and aponeurotic. The *scalenus minimus* is the muscle that sometimes replaces the deep or posterior part of the membrane (see Fig. 12.5). The muscle may be up to 10 mm in diameter in its widest part, but is usually much smaller than that. Fawcett (1896) described this as "Sibson's muscle": he described it arising from the transverse process of the seventh cervical vertebra and inserting on the medial border of the first rib. Fawcett seems to consider this to be a part of the scalenus anterior muscle, but he also seems to differentiate it from the anomaly of a slip from the latter passing behind the subclavian artery – "a well known fact". The posterior border of the membrane and the edge of the first rib form the foramen through which the first thoracic nerve escapes. The membrane covers the apical pleura and intervenes between it and the subclavian artery (see Fig. 12.4).

The first rib

The broad first rib, the surface of which is more horizontal than vertical, extends from the head at the vertebral body, the neck and the costotransverse articulation, over the apical pleura to curve round to the costochondral junction, and then to the manubrium. The apical pleura is, in the healthy state, easily separable from the head and neck and most of the underside of the first rib. Anteriorly, it becomes rather adherent to the underside of the rib, in relation to the costochondral junction. The scalenus medius is attached to the upper surface of the rib posteriorly. The upper part of nerve to the serratus anterior is usually formed in the muscle by branches from the fourth, fifth and sixth cervical anterior rami; it emerges from the lateral surface of the scalenus, where it is usually joined by the contribution from the seventh cervical nerve. In front of the scalenus medius the surface of the rib is, in the adult, grooved by the passage of the first thoracic nerve and lower trunk. There is a distinct tubercle at the attachment of the scalenus anterior, behind which is the slight depression for the artery. In front of the scalene tubercle the vein runs over the upper surface of the rib. The intercostal muscles are attached to the edge of the rib (see Fig. 12.2). The lower part of the cervicothoracic (stellate) ganglion lies on the head of the first rib, deep to the proximal part of the vertebral artery arising from the subclavian. The major part of the first thoracic nerve is at first below the rib, and then medial to its edge. The white preganglionic ramus of the first thoracic nerve connects it to the stellate ganglion; the grey ramus (postganglionic) is

less noticeable. The size and disposition of the scalenus anterior varies: it may bifurcate to include the artery; the muscle itself may be bulky; the tendon may curve posteriorly round the artery to form a kind of snare. Deep to the scalenus, a very thin fascia covers the artery. The phrenic nerve, chiefly derived from the fourth cervical anterior ramus, curves round the muscle to run down in front of it into the thorax, lying at first behind the internal jugular vein and crossing behind the subclavian vein. On the left the thoracic duct and on the right the right lymphatic duct enter the brachiocephalic (innominate) vein at the subclavian–jugular (triradiate) junction.

The seventh cervical rib

Parry and Eastcott (1992) and Narakas (1993a) credit the second-century physician and anatomist Galen with the first description of the seventh cervical rib. A little later, Gruber (1869) published his classification of such ribs according to their size and connections. Narakas (1993a) indicates an incidence of seventh cervical ribs of 0.004–1%, giving bilateral affection in half the cases and an incidence in women three times that in men. Adson and Coffey (1927) gave an incidence of 0.1%, with a preference for the left side. Narakas (1993a) says that cervical rib "is asymptomatic in 90% to 95% of persons". Adson and Coffey (1927) seem to indicate that, of their 303 cases in half a million new patients, 167 were asymptomatic. They operated on 36 ribs: 15 right, 18 left and 3 bilateral.

The extent of the rib, which is rarely bilaterally symmetrical, ranges from a prolongation and pointing of the seventh cervical transverse process to a complete rib, which is in all respects like a first thoracic rib. Sargent (1921) recognised five types: exaggerated "costal process"; short articulating rib with fibrous prolongation; jointed rib long enough to carry the eighth cervical nerve; jointed rib either fused at its end with the first rib or articulating with it; and, in effect, a complete seventh cervical rib with cartilaginous union to the first costal cartilage or to the manubrium (Figs 12.7 to 12.12). Unless it joins the first costal cartilage or manubrium by a costal cartilage, the seventh cervical rib is always connected in some way to the first thoracic rib, either by a band, bone or an articulation. This classification differs slightly from that of Gruber (1869), which was used by Narakas (1993b). Gruber (1869) classified seventh cervical ribs into four grades, ranging from an articulated rib extending beyond the end of the transverse process to a virtually complete rib extending to the manubrium through a cartilage blending with the first costal cartilage. He shows in his figure 2 a left cervical rib which is fused with the transverse process. The nerves and the vessel are most likely to be affected by ribs of Gruber's second and third grades and of Sargent's third and fourth types (see Figs 12.8 to 12.12).

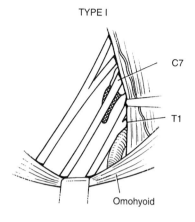

TYPE I

Fig. 12.7 Variations of the seventh cervical rib, ranging from elongation of the seventh cervical transverse process to a virtually complete additional rib. (After Sargent (1921)).

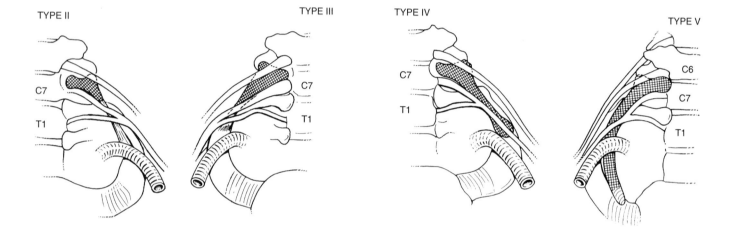

Figs 12.8 to 12.12 **Radiographs showing varieties of the seventh cervical rib.**

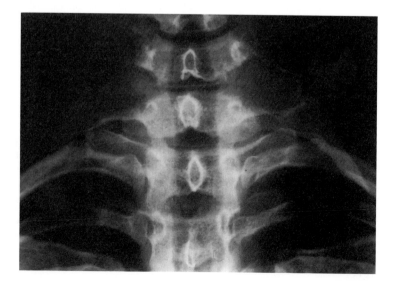

Fig. 12.8 Elongated transverse process (left) and partly formed rib (right). There was affection of the lower trunk on the right.

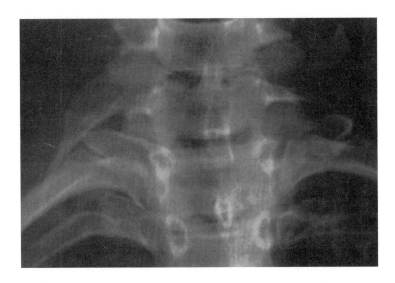

Fig. 12.9 Vestigial cervical rib (left). Note the downward (caudad) inclination of the seventh cervical transverse processes and the upward (cephalad) inclination of those of the first thoracic vertebra.

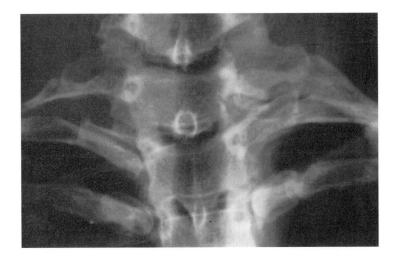

Fig. 12.10 Vestigial cervical rib (left) and, in effect, a first thoracic rib (right). Note the upper thoracic scoliosis.

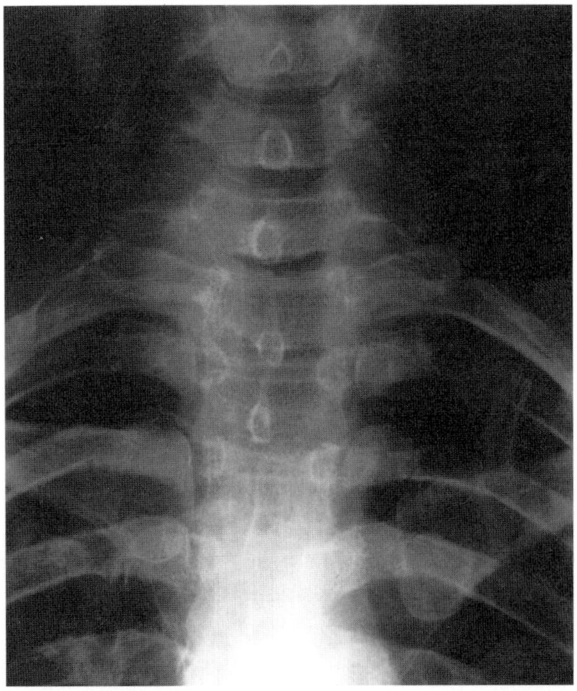

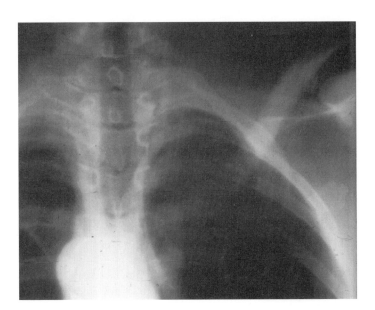

Fig. 12.12 Bilateral cervical ribs associated with arterial affection.

Fig. 12.11 A well-formed left cervical rib. This was associated with arterial affection.

Aetiology, symptoms and treatment

Symptoms vary according to the level of compression and the structure compressed. They are, as has been said, arterial, venous, and neural. Often, neural affection is associated with a degree of arterial obstruction.

Arterial affection

Arterial affection occurs as the subclavian artery crosses a "normal" first rib or a seventh cervical rib, commonly one with bony union to, or synchondrosis or synostosis with, a boss on the first rib at about its middle part. The vessel is distorted by the bone and constricted by a leash formed by the tendon of insertion of the scalenus anterior. The sequence of events is: intimal breakage; local thrombosis; peripheral embolisation; and complete axial obstruction (Figs 12.13 and 12.14). There is commonly dilation of the artery distal to the point of constriction: that dilation may proceed to the formation of a true aneurysm (Wickham & Martin 1962).

Symptoms are initially those of a Raynaud phenomenon with episodic blanching and temperature change, episodic pain with muscular activity and distal ulceration and necrosis. Complete obstruction of the main vessel with distal embolisation may lead to critical ischaemia. The most dangerous complication is that demonstrated by Symonds in 1923 – that of contralateral hemiplegia, doubtless from embolisation from thrombus extending proximally to the carotid vessel (Symonds 1927). The arterial form of outlet syndrome is a condition predominantly affecting young women; the occurrence of such symptoms in older persons must suggest a primary diagnosis of atherosclerosis (Joyce & Hollier 1984). We have seen a case of Takayasu's arteritis (Horwitz 1977, Lupi-Herrera et al 1977) diagnosed as "arterial outlet syndrome".

Signs. The extremity may be cooler than that of the unaffected limb; there is likely to be a pulse difference, even absence of a pulse. Even if the hands are the same colour at rest, slightly dependent, there is likely to be blanching of the affected hand on elevation (Fig. 12.15). When a seventh cervical rib is present it is usually palpable above the clavicle, where there may be a bruit or abnormal pulsation. Doppler ultrasound examination is likely to show abnormality: Parry and Eastcott (1992) name principally the finding of a clamped, monophasic velocity signal anywhere over the arterial tree of the upper limb. Radiographs will of course show a seventh cervical rib if one is present. In one case in which fully formed bilateral

---

Figs 12.13 and 12.14 Cervical rib associated with arterial affection.

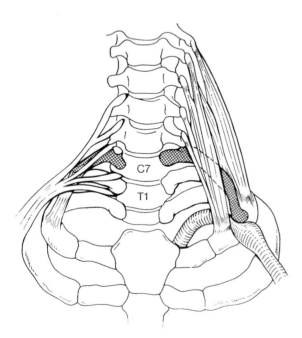

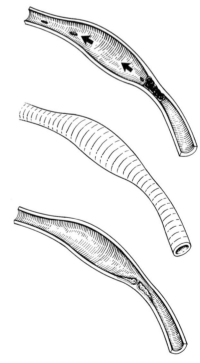

Fig. 12.13 Drawing shows (right) the type of the rib most commonly associated with arterial affection. Note the articulation with a boss on the upper surface of the first rib.

Fig. 12.14 The stages of arterial affection: intimal breakage with local thrombosis; stenosis with post-stenotic dilation; and thrombosis with distal embolisation.

seventh cervical ribs were present, the abnormality was missed because the radiologist thought that they were normal first thoracic ribs (Figs 12.16 and 12.17). The radiologist had omitted to observe the downwardly oblique form of the transverse processes to which they were attached. That form, contrasting with the upwardly oblique direction of the first thoracic transverse processes, is a sure guide to seventh cervical rib.

Imaging. Arteriography, preferably aided by digital subtraction technology, confirms the site and extent of the obstruction, the extent of stenosis and aneurysm formation, and the extent of distal occlusion. Other, noninvasive, methods of imaging are even now super-seding arteriography in this and other fields. The advantages of magnetic resonance angiography are shown by Friedman et al (1995) and by Bell et al (1995). Duplex

---

Figs 12.15 to 12.25 Arterial outlet syndrome.

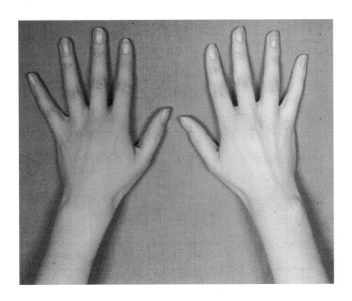

Fig. 12.15 Elevation in a case of affection of the right subclavian artery of a 19-year-old girl producing blanching of the right hand.

Figs 12.16 and 12.17 Bilateral well-formed cervical ribs in a 16-year-old girl who suffered affection of the right subclavian artery.

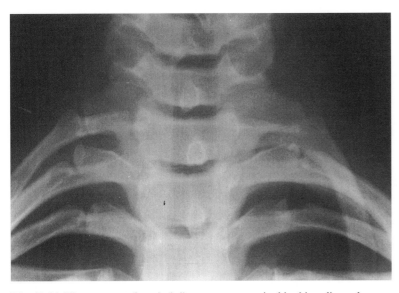

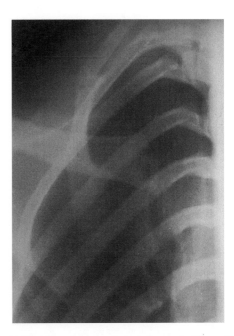

Fig. 12.16 The presence of cervical ribs was not recognised in this radiograph, although the inclination of the transverse processes is well shown.

Fig. 12.17 A later radiograph than the one in Figure 12.16 clearly shows the right cervical rib articulating with a boss on the upper surface of the first rib. In this case there was thrombosis and peripheral embolisation.

ultrasonography (Kreel & Thornton 1992, Rosfors et al 1993, Sumner 1993, Whiteley et al 1995) may emerge as the noninvasive method of choice. With arteriography in particular, it is often important to examine the vessel with the limb elevated or abducted at the shoulder (Figs 12.13 to 12.25).

Treatment. Operation is required urgently in cases of critical ischaemia, and soon in cases in which ischaemia is threatened. It is, we think, indicated when a cervical rib is present, causing no symptoms, but producing deformity of the subclavian artery sufficient to cause a steady bruit over the vessel. Eastcott (1973a) restricted this indication:

he then stated a belief that a preventive operation was "justified" if a patient has already had arterial reconstruction on one side and then showed minimal signs of vascular involvement on the other. We certainly think that the "prophylactic" operation is indicated in such a case if there is a persistent bruit over the contralateral subclavian artery. Such a bruit must surely indicate distortion of the vessel; that distortion is surely likely, in time, to cause intimal breakage and thrombosis.

The structures are exposed at the outlet by the supraclavicular approach and the scalenus anterior is divided. The subclavian artery is then mobilised with more than

Figs 12.18 to 12.21 Angiographic appearances.

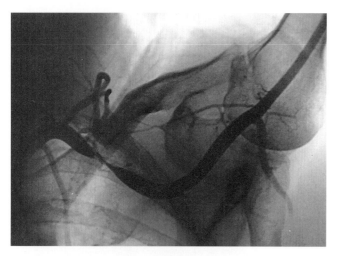

Fig. 12.18 Complete occlusion over cervical rib.

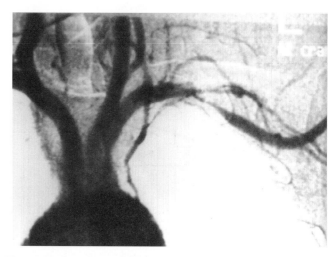

Fig. 12.19 Complete occlusion at the outlet in a 40-year-old woman, a heavy smoker.

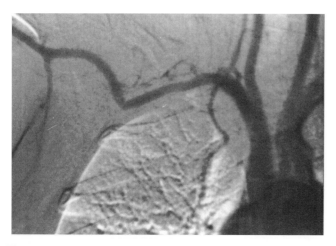

Fig. 12.20 Obstruction of the artery at the outlet with elevation of limb.

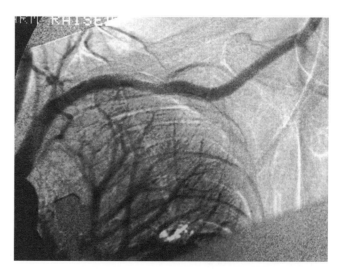

Fig. 12.21 Narrowing of the artery over the first rib, with elevation of the limb.

Figs 12.22 to 12.25 Appearance at operation in three cases.

Figs 12.22 and 12.23 Thrombosis, stenosis, and post-stenotic dilation of the subclavian artery, with periarteritis (and distal embolisation) in a girl with a cervical rib.

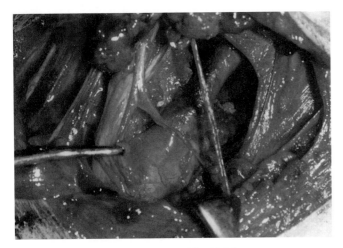

Fig. 12.22 The artery as first seen (see Fig. 12.23).

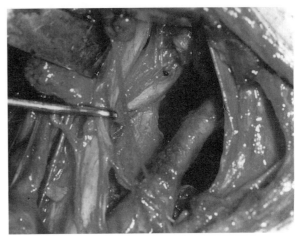

Fig. 12.23 The relation of the artery to the cervical rib (see Fig. 12.22).

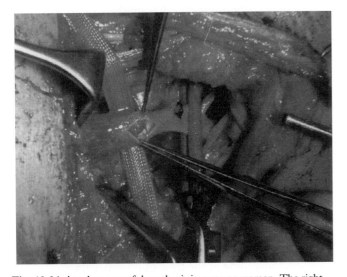

Fig. 12.24 Another case of thrombosis in a young woman. The right subclavian artery has been opened to show the detached intima.

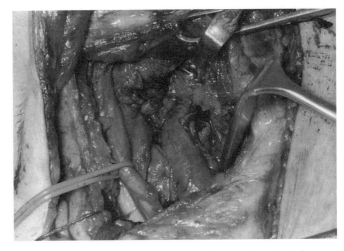

Fig. 12.25 Thrombosis and post-stenotic dilation of the subclavian artery in association with a cervical rib.

the usual degree of care. Peri-arteritis may make the mobilisation difficult; the artery is more than usually fragile (Figs 12.22 to 12.26; see also Plate section). Tapes are passed for control; branches are divided as necessary for the mobilisation. The lower part of the plexus is then defined, the middle and lower trunks are separated and the first thoracic nerve is carefully defined. Now, the main distorting agent – the seventh cervical rib or variant, or first thoracic rib – is defined and removed. The removal should be extraperiosteal, though it is sometimes difficult to achieve this. If additional exposure is required, the transclavicular approach (Bonney 1977, Birch et al 1990) is probably the most useful and the least damaging.

The arterial intervention. In cases with clear signs of arterial affection it is rarely sufficient simply to remove the seventh cervical or first rib and to rely on the decompression so afforded. Haug and Sanders (1991) follow Scher et al (1984) in defining four stages of arterial affection in

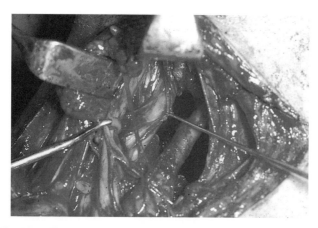

Fig. 12.26 Recent thrombosis of the subclavian artery. Note the periarteritis and post-stenotic dilation. Successful endarterectomy. (See also Plate section.)

connection with the seventh cervical rib. Their recommendations are as follows:

- Stage 0 Rib(s) with no symptoms and no aneurysm should be left alone, though the presence of a bruit is an indication for angiography
- Stage 1 Rib(s) with minimal stenosis and mild post-stenotic dilation are treated with arterial decompression by resection of the abnormal rib
- Stage 2 Rib(s) with aneurysm, intimal damage, and mural thrombosis should be treated by resection of the rib and excision and repair or ligation and bypass of the aneurysm
- Stage 3 Rib(s) with distal embolisation require distal embolectomy and cervicothoracic sympathectomy in addition to rib resection and arterial reconstruction.

Evidently, arterial reconstruction is necessary when there is thrombosis with or without distal embolisation, aneurysm formation or tight stenosis. When there is no more than a slight stenosis with similar post-stenotic dilation, without evidence of thrombosis or intimal damage, it may be sufficient to confine operation to simple decompression. If there is doubt, the artery should be opened between clamps and the intima should be inspected. If there is intimal damage with thrombosis, thrombectomy and endarterectomy will be sufficient. Parry and Eastcott (1992) recommend endarterectomy or resection and anastomosis for short stenoses; strip resection for a large aneurysm, and saphenous vein grafting for more extensive lesions. Distal thrombectomy with the Fogarty catheter is necessary when there has been distal thrombosis, and in such cases in particular cervicothoracic sympathectomy is a useful adjunct. In some cases in which operation is undertaken after there has been extensive distal thrombosis, a long bypass graft may be necessary. We have no personal experience of such cases, but have seen critical ischaemia relieved by this intervention.

The venous syndrome

McCleery et al (1951) examined in particular the role of the subclavius muscle and costo-coracoid ligament in causing venous obstruction, and reported the results of operation in five cases. Parry and Eastcott (1992) define two entities: acute thrombosis of the subclavian vein related to effort, and chronic intermittent venous obstruction. Acute thrombosis is rare; it may be associated with malignant disease; and it usually occurs in men, probably arising from a period of heavy work superimposed on an anatomical predisposition. It is associated with pain, swelling, discolouration and enlargement of superficial veins. Phlebography is confirmatory.

Episodic obstruction is seen in young women more than in men. They give a history of episodic pain in and swelling of one or both upper limbs related to activity and subsiding with rest. Bracing of the shoulders may produce prominence of superficial veins. Phlebography will show obstruction at the level of the first rib when the shoulder is braced back. Sanders and Haug (1990) published a comprehensive review of acute and chronic obstruction of the subclavian vein, both thrombotic and nonthrombotic. They indicated findings by other workers of an incidence of venous problems in 1.5–5% of patients with thoracic outlet syndrome, and drew particular attention to the role of the costoclavicular ligament in causing obstruction. Sanders and Haug also described the use and limitations of venous duplex scanning (Kreel & Thornton 1992) in diagnosis.

In episodic compression the most appropriate procedure is transaxillary removal of the first rib (Roos 1966, 1971, 1981, 1982, 1984, 1987, Roos and Owens 1966, Lord 1971, Urschel et al 1971). The decompression afforded is complete and lasting, and the results are good. Similar results could doubtless be obtained in cases of thrombosis if early intervention were possible and thrombectomy were added to the removal of the first rib. Certainly, Roos (1971, 1984) reported success after thrombectomy done at the time of transaxillary removal of the first rib. Parry and Eastcott (1992) are not sanguine about the results of other methods of treatment. They stress the limitations imposed by late recognition and delayed action. Sanders and Haug (1990) agree that in chronic obstruction resection of the first rib is the simplest and least complicated procedure. Dealing with treatment of the thrombosed vein by fibrinolysis, angioplasty, thrombectomy, "endovenectomy", bypass, and reconstruction, they conclude that "the data do not allow a definitive choice among these treatment options". We have not had the opportunity of operation early after thrombosis, but believe that the correct procedure in such a case may well be transaxillary removal of the first rib combined with thrombectomy. The instant success of early iliac thrombectomy in a case of venous thrombosis after anterior lumbosacral fusion reinforces that view (Fig. 12.27).

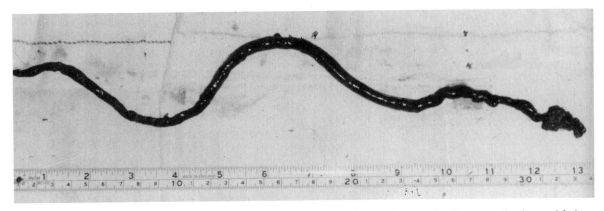

Fig. 12.27 A 40-cm thrombus removed from the left common iliac vein 36 hours after operation for anterior lumbosacral fusion. There was no subsequent morbidity.

Certainly, the dispersion of the thrombus by fibrinolysis should be followed soon by transaxillary removal of the first rib (Roos 1987).

The neural syndrome

Gilliatt et al (1970) stressed, what previous authors had emphasised, that the condition was overwhelmingly more common in women than in men (Wilson 1913, 1954). It was indeed this consideration that led Griffiths (1964) to deny the existence of the syndrome. All the patients studied by Gilliatt and his colleagues were female; their ages at onset varied from 13 to 73 years.

The question now to be asked is why symptoms should appear at a particular stage. In only one of our cases was the onset of symptoms related to an undoubted dropping of the shoulder girdle on the thorax. That was in a case of accidental damage to the spinal accessory nerve in a female nurse aged 30 years. Failure elsewhere of restoration by anchoring of the scapula to the vertebral spines and of "decompression" by removal of the clavicle led to transaxillary removal of the first rib, which was lastingly effective. In other cases, determination by "dropping" of the shoulder girdle on the thorax can only be surmised. Mulder et al (1973) proposed a traumatic origin, finding this in five men and two women after injuries to the clavicle, first rib, and cervical spine. Sanders et al (1979) proposed damage to the scalenus anterior muscle as in whiplash injury, with subsequent scarring and compression of underlying structures. This concept was expanded by Sanders and Haug (1991). In our experience a clear history of injury is obtained in a minority of cases, but the subject requires further examination, with particular attention to the incidence of injury in cases in which pain and paraesthesia are predominant.

The most common site of distortion or compression is in the proximal part of the outlet, either between the first rib and the suprapleural membrane or a scalenus minimus, or over a scalenus sickle, a seventh cervical rib or a first thoracic rib. At this level it is the first thoracic nerve and the lower trunk that are affected. It may be as well at this stage to distinguish patients coming with objective evidence of a lesion of the lower trunk from those coming with pain, paraesthesiae and mild disturbances of circulation. All the patients in the Gilliatt series came into the first category. The distinction was well made by Wilbourn (1988). He named the first category "true" or "classical" neurogenic thoracic outlet syndrome, and the second, "disputed" neurogenic thoracic outlet syndrome. The incidence of the "classical" syndrome was estimated by Gilliatt (1984) at 1 per 1 million.

In the "classical" form of the syndrome, the patient comes with pain and paraesthesia affecting the ulnar side of the forearm and the ulnar two digits, and with progressive weakness and wasting of the muscles innervated by the lower trunk of the brachial plexus. These are, predominantly, the intrinsic muscles of the hand, but also the long flexors of the fingers (Figs 12.28 to 12.33). The motor affection is nearly always more profound than is the affection of cutaneous sensibility. In these cases the diagnosis is suggested by the neurological findings; the task is to make sure that the lesion is indeed one of compression or distortion at the thoracic outlet, rather than one of affection of the spinal cord, the nerves in the intervertebral foramina, the ulnar nerve or the median nerve. The involvement of all intrinsic muscles and of forearm flexors suggests the lower trunk rather than the median or ulnar nerve; the finding of tenderness in the root of the neck or the production of radiated paraesthesiae on tapping suggests the lower trunk and the outlet (Morley 1913). The motor defect caused by osteoarthritis of the cervical spine usually affects the uppermost three nerves of the brachial plexus in preference to the lowest two. The presence of a scalenus medius band is suggested by an elongation of the seventh cervical transverse process, by the presence of a bruit over the subclavian artery at rest or with bracing, and by a certain fullness above the clavicle. The division of opinion about the value of electrophysiological examination, and in particular of measurement of sensory evoked potentials (Gilliatt et al 1970, Urschel et al 1971, Livingstone et al 1984, Veilleux et al 1988, Dawson et al 1990a, Wilbourn 1993), may stem as much from confused thinking about the type of lesion under investigation as from the difficulty of measuring conduction across the zone of the lesion. In our view, Wilbourn (1993) assigns to electrophysiological examination its true and important

---

Figs 12.28 to 12.33 The classical neurological outlet syndrome.

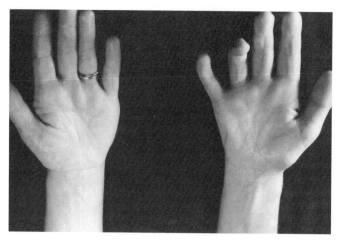

Fig. 12.28 Severe wasting of the intrinsic muscles of the right hand in a 35-year-old woman.

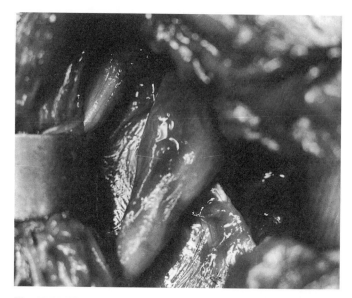

Fig. 12.29 The right lower trunk angulated over a "scalenus sickle". There is extreme attenuation of the trunk, which in the photograph appears to be rather lateral to the sickle. When the nerve was first exposed at operation, the zone of attenuation was in fact at the site of angulation. There was slow improvement after decompression.

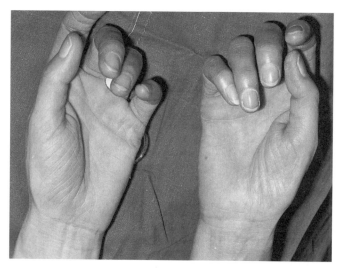

Fig. 12.30 Another case of wasting of the intrinsic muscles of the right hand, in a 40-year-old woman.

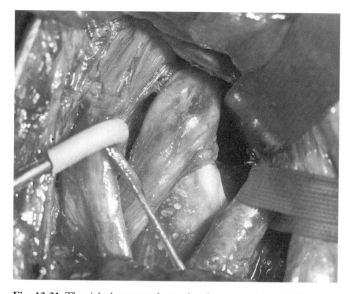

Fig. 12.31 The right lower trunk angulated over a scalenus sickle. Again, there was slow improvement after decompression.

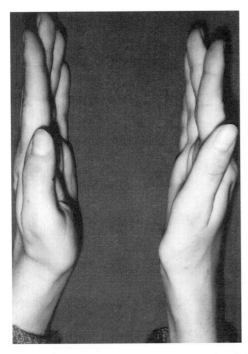

Fig. 12.32 A third case of wasting of the intrinsic muscles of the right hand, in a 45-year-old woman.

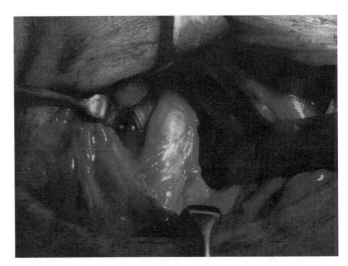

Fig. 12.33 The right lower trunk angulated over a scalenus sickle.

role in the confirmation of diagnosis in the "true neuro-genic" syndrome. The place of magnetic resonance imaging in diagnosis is discussed by Panegyres et al (1993); the finding of deviation of the plexus proved a fairly reliable predictor.

There is little doubt that operation is indicated in "true" neural outlet syndrome. The best approach, in our view, is supraclavicular exploration of the plexus with division of the scalenus anterior and removal of any and all compressing or distorting agents (scalenus band, seventh cervical rib, scalenus minimus and aponeurotic edge of suprapleural membrane) (see Figs 12.29, 12.31 and 12.33). Improvement in the power and bulk of the forearm flexors can confidently be predicted; recovery of power and bulk in the intrinsic muscles is less likely, and is certain to take 2 or more years.

Neural outlet syndrome without plain motor signs

This is much more difficult. A large variety of symptoms has been attributed to compression at the outlet in addition to pain, paraesthesiae and numbness affecting the ulnar side of the forearm and hand, and circulatory disorder of the hand. Thus, it has been proposed that the seventh cervical nerve can be involved; pain spreading to the neck and shoulder and upper limb has been attributed to distortion at the outlet (Raaf 1955) and headaches have

been attributed to "spasm" of the scalenus anterior (Cox & Cocks 1973). Sanders et al (1979) listed headache and pain in the neck and shoulder. Demos et al (1980) related vertebrobasilar insufficiency to arterial compression by the scalenus anterior. This widening of indications led, no doubt, to many operations on the outlet and even many resections of first ribs which were not really necessary. The idea must, however, occur to every thoughtful clinician that cases of "true" neural affection must begin with pain and paraesthesiae. If it were possible to identify such cases and act at this early stage the difficult problem of serious wasting of peripheral muscles would not be encountered. This thoughtful clinician must also reflect on the un-doubted morbidity associated with operations on the thoracic outlet (Horowitz 1985, Cherington et al 1986, Wilbourn 1988). He or she will also bear in mind reports of success after "conservative" treatment (Peet et al 1956, Smith 1979, Sällstrom and Celigin 1983, Novak et al 1995), and may be aware of the success of certain osteopaths in treating Richard Miller's (personal communication) "intercostobrachial syndrome". A number of tests depending on the effect on the neurovascular bundle of alteration of the position of the shoulder girdle on the thorax are available (Adson & Coffey 1927, Falconer and Weddell 1943, Adson 1947). Regrettably, none is specific: "positive" signs can be elicited in many healthy and symptomless persons. Narakas (1993a) offers the best evidence so far available concerning the correlation of the results of the various tests with findings at operation.

Case report. A 34-year-old woman had a left seventh cervical rib removed by the supraclavicular route without suffering any adverse consequence. The rib articulated with a bony prominence on the first thoracic rib. It was noted at the time that there was a vestigial seventh cervical rib on the right side. Three years later the patient began to get episodic cramp and alteration of sensibility in the right (dominant) upper limb. There were no clear objective signs of interference with the neurovascular bundle. The vestigial rib and a fibrous prolongation were removed. After operation there was severe pain in the limb, with associated paralysis in the distribution of the lower trunk. Thirty months after this operation persistent pain and electrophysiological evidence of severe chronic denervation led to re-exploration. The lowest three nerves of the plexus were found surrounded by dense fibrous tissue, and there was fusiform enlargement of the lower trunk proximal to the first rib. Its epineurium was swollen and thickened over about 3 cm of its length. There was no evidence of discontinuity. Evidently, during operation there had been traction and localised pressure on the lower part of the plexus sufficient to produce a deep lesion of the lower trunk.

The nerves were freed from scar tissue, and the thickened epineurium was divided throughout its length, to show bundles traversing the lesion. A small catheter was left in place for infusion of bupivavcaine. There was marked relief of pain after operation; later, there was progressive, though incomplete, recovery of motor and sensory function. A year after operation the relief of pain was maintained.

We think that the clinician, having excluded causes outside the thoracic outlet, should first attempt to identify conditions which are or could be precursors of the "true" neural syndrome. Here is a typical example: a woman in her twenties or thirties, with paraesthesia affecting the ulnar side of her forearm and hand, and mild circulatory changes in the hand. There is tenderness over the lower part of the plexus above the clavicle on the affected side, but none on the unaffected side. There is an impression of fullness in this site of tenderness; tapping produces radiating paraesthesia. There is a bruit over the subclavian artery at rest on the affected side, but not on the unaffected side. The radial pulse on the affected side is labile, disappearing with bracing of the shoulder or elevation of the limb. Radiographs show elongation of the seventh cervical transverse process or some degree of seventh cervical rib. Magnetic resonance imaging shows distortion of the lower part of the brachial plexus. Electrophysiological examination shows F-wave abnormalities in the ulnar nerve. Lucky is the clinician who is presented with so full a picture! But it does happen; when it does, a period of "conservative" treatment is given, but it is no more than a formality, and operation is recommended when that treatment fails.

Far more difficult is the case in which the symptoms are more diffuse and the signs less clear. The finding of a bruit over the subclavian vessel on the symptomless side as well as on the affected side is, at least, discouraging, as is lability of the radial pulse on the unaffected side. Failure to gain supporting evidence from electrophysiological evidence, from arteriography or from magnetic resonance imaging should encourage clinicians to give "conservative" methods a trial. We must, however, record that one of our best and most lasting successes was obtained in a case in which operation was undertaken on a speculative basis and in which no abnormality was found at operation.

Most difficult of all is the case in which operation, usually a simple section of the scalenus anterior muscle, has been undertaken on a largely speculative basis and has at first succeeded, and in which symptoms have recurred. All who operate regularly at the thoracic outlet know well the extraordinary amount of scarring that can follow even an operation as simple as anterior scalenotomy. No one should lightly recommend a first operation on the thoracic outlet; even the boldest may recoil from the prospect of doing a second operation in a scarred field. This may, however, be inevitable when:

- primary operation limited to scalenectomy has plainly for a time relieved symptoms
- there are true signs of recurrent interference with structures at the outlet
- damage to nerves has been inflicted during the primary operation.

Considerations about operation

Three routes are available for access to the thoracic outlet and neurovascular bundle:

- anterior supraclavicular
- transaxillary
- posterior.

The *anterior route* (Hempel et al 1981), if necessary extended by the transclavicular method (Bonney 1977, Birch et al 1990), offers the best exposure of the plexus, the artery and the sympathetic chain, and of the proximal structures likely to distort or compress them. Its disadvantages are the difficulty of access for removal of the first rib and the restricted access to the subclavian vein. The latter difficulty is, however, removed by adding the transclavicular extension; indeed, access to the first rib is greatly improved by that extension. The *transaxillary approach* is admirable for access to the subclavian/axillary vein and the middle and anterior parts of the first rib. Its use is, of course, mandatory on the rare occasions when there is distal obstruction in the axilla. We have never found this route easy (we have always found access to the posterior part of the first rib limited), and we are not alone in discerning the risk to the plexus imposed by the position of the limb (Roos 1981). It is an admirable approach for a second operation following recurrence after a supraclavicular procedure. It is the obvious approach for relief of costoclavicular compression causing predominantly "venous" symptoms.

The *posterior approach*, described for cervicothoracic sympathectomy by Adson and Brown (1929) and used by Longo et al (1970), gives the best access to the posterior ends of the first rib and a seventh cervical rib, and allows the operator to separate the first thoracic nerve from the neck of the first rib. On the other hand, access to the vessels, the anterior part of the first rib and the distal part of the plexus is restricted. We prefer to reserve this approach for the removal of a remnant of the first rib or a seventh cervical rib left after a previous operation by the anterior route

In all these operations the nerves in particular should be handled very tenderly: retraction should be with slings only or very fine skin hooks in the epineurium, and only for a few minutes at a time; and access to bony structures behind the plexus should be achieved by separating the component nerves rather than by forward retraction of the plexus. Colour coding of the slings adds pleasing variety to the proceedings and, more importantly, permits the surgeon to identify to the assistant the nerve to be retracted. When the transaxillary route is used, the elevation at the shoulder should be relaxed for a few minutes at 15-minute intervals, so as to avoid prolonged tension on the infraclavicular part of the plexus.

The supraclavicular route

The patient is put in a semisedentary position, with the affected limb painted and in the field. The line of incision is marked with Bonney's blue (Berkeley and Bonney 1920). The low supraclavicular incision is made and the flaps are raised deep to the platysma and sutured back. The external jugular vein and the supraclavicular nerves are identified, mobilised and protected. The posterior border of the sternocleidomastoid muscle is defined and the omohyoid muscle and tendon are identified. The tendon of the omohyoid muscle is divided between sutures, for later repair. The underlying fascia and fat are divided to show the internal jugular vein and the scalenus anterior and the phrenic nerve. The transverse cervical vessels will probably have to be ligated and divided. The fascia over the phrenic nerve is divided and the nerve is mobilised and protected. Now the scalenus anterior is displayed down to its attachment, and the subclavian artery is shown medial and lateral to it. With the phrenic nerve protected, the scalenus anterior is divided close to its tendon. It is important that this division should be complete and should include the fascia at the back of the muscle, so as to permit

display and later mobilisation of the subclavian artery. The suprapleural membrane is now visible. It is defined and divided so that the apical parietal pleura can be pushed away from the sides of the vertebrae and the inside of the chest wall. Once the vessel is mobilised, it is possible to display the plexus from the fifth nerve just lateral to the scalenus anterior to the first thoracic nerve winding round the medial side of the posterior part of the first rib to join the eighth cervical nerve and form the lower trunk.

At this stage it should be possible to see or feel any distorting or compressing agent: a scalenus minimus; a scalenus medius band; or a seventh cervical rib. A scalenus minimus or an aponeurotic thickening of the posterior edge of the suprapleural membrane should be divided. A scalenus medius band should be removed as follows. First, it is carefully cut at its attachment to the first rib below the first thoracic nerve and then it is traced up behind the lower trunk, and between the eighth and seventh cervical nerves, to its attachment to the seventh cervical transverse process. Its deep surface is separated from the muscular part of the scalenus medius, its attachment to the transverse process is divided and it is removed. If the underlying muscle appears to be distorting the lower part of the plexus, its prominent part should also be removed. The question will now arise of whether the decompression effected is adequate. Before the wound is closed the surgeon should certainly put his or her finger between the first rib and the clavicle and manipulate the upper limb to make sure the finger is not trapped in any position of the shoulder girdle. If there is clear evidence of costoclavicular compression the first rib should be removed; the opportunity to do this with relative ease will not occur again. If there is no such compression the rib should be left alone.

Seventh cervical ribs should be removed from the level of the tip of the transverse process to the attachment to the first rib wherever the latter may be and in whatever manner it may be formed. The posterior end is best reached between the seventh and eighth nerves; its middle between the eighth cervical and first thoracic nerves; and the lower end below the first thoracic nerve, either behind or in front of the artery. Any articulating bony boss on the first rib should be removed with the attached tendon of scalenus anterior.

The first thoracic rib should be treated in the same way, though it is more difficult to remove this whole than is the case with a seventh cervical rib. It is permissible to leave 1 cm projecting beyond the tip of the transverse process, so long as the tip of this fragment does not interfere with the first thoracic nerve. Particular care has to be taken with the removal of the anterior part of the rib: the subclavian vein can be nipped, and the pleura is often adherent here to the under surface of the rib. The rib is divided near the costochondral junction or separated from the costal cartilage. The importance of the extraperiosteal removal of ribs is again stressed.

It is a good plan regularly to try to confirm the diagnosis by stimulation and recording from the nerves of the plexus and by recording from muscle during stimulation of the nerve. This method may be used to measure the extent and duration of traction tolerated by nerves, but it is important to remember that at least some of the nerves seen may already be the subject of injury. Once all has been done that needs to be done, the wound is closed over a suction drain. A few stitches reunite the fatty areolar tissue, the omohyoid muscle is repaired, and the platysma and skin are closed. A subcuticular suture is neat, but a well-placed and well-sutured wound heals well, whatever type of suture is used.

Dangers of operation. As has been indicated, a number of important structures are in danger during the operation. The first thoracic nerve may be damaged during removal of the posterior part of the rib. Sometimes the nerve is so much attenuated over a scalenus medius band or seventh cervical rib that the surgeon may fail to see it and may accidentally divide it. It is difficult to avoid damaging the phrenic nerve by traction, so producing a temporary paralysis of the hemidiaphragm. It should be possible to avoid causing permanent paralysis; in one of our cases this led to what amounted to an eventration of the hemidiaphragm. The subclavian artery is sometimes fragile, even when symptoms are predominantly neural. The most serious immediate danger is that of wounding the subclavian vein behind the clavicle. It may be difficult to effect repair in this restricted space because of difficulty of achieving control. In these difficult circumstances it may be necessary, while bleeding is controlled by pressure, to extend the exposure by elevation of the manubrioclavicular flap. It is in the region of the vein and triradiate junction on the left side that the thoracic duct may be injured. If the duct and the defect can be identified it is as well to repair the hole, especially if the pleura has been opened. Damage to the pleura is a tiresome but sometimes unavoidable complication, usually necessitating the introduction of an intercostal catheter connected to a water seal. Sometimes the hole can effectively be repaired, the air aspirated and the lung expanded, and the necessity for pleural drainage avoided. Damage to the thoracic duct can usually be avoided, except in a scarred field. This damage is usually recognised because of the leak of milky fluid. It is best to identify and repair the leak, because if the pleura has been opened there is a real danger of the formation of a chylothorax. If the hole cannot be repaired, it can be plugged with a little muscle graft.

The principal delayed complication of operation is interference with conduction through the plexus and the development of a painful neuropathy, with extensive scarring around the nerves. Paraesthesiae in the limb for a few days after an extensive decompression are common. Interference with conduction is, or should be, temporary, dependent on a simple block to conduction caused by the handling and retraction of the nerves. In a proportion of cases, even when the utmost care is taken to avoid rough handling of the plexus, a painful and persistent neuropathy develops; this is resistant to treatment with analgesics and, in particular, to further nonspecific exploration for decompression. It is this complication which should be present in the mind of every surgeon about to propose operation for thoracic outlet syndrome, and in particular for outlet syndrome not associated with a clearly defined lesion. The cases for and against such intervention have already been examined.

The transaxillary route

This is the method of choice in cases of costoclavicular and axillary compression, in particular in cases of venous compression or obstruction. It is also the approach of choice in cases of recurrence of symptoms after supraclavicular intervention.

The operation is not easy: no one has obtained results to match those of Roos (1966, 1971, 1979, 1981, 1987, 1995), and few will be able to claim the 90% good results reported by Wood et al (1988). The positioning of the patient is very important. Best is a lateral position, with the table slightly rolled towards the surgeon. The assistant holds the affected limb at an angle of 90° to the axial line; he or she should not hold it in lateral rotation, and should be prepared to relax the position for a few minutes every 15 minutes. The incision is in the skin crease at the level of the third rib, just below the hair line. The flaps are raised, and the chest wall and neurovascular bundle are displayed.

As with all transaxillary procedures, it is as well early to define with the stimulator the position of the nerve to serratus anterior in the posterior part of the wound. The intercostobrachial nerve running down the axilla is seen and preserved. Later, the superior thoracic artery and vein are tied and divided to allow access to the upper part of the axillary tunnel. With swab dissection the operator follows the chest wall, under the neurovascular bundle and into the apex of the axilla, until the lateral edge of the first rib is felt. It is as well at this stage to verify identification of the rib on the screen: the second rib has been mistaken for the first.

Roos has said that with abduction of the shoulder the axilla opens up like an oyster. He may perhaps, in writing this, have forgotten that for the unpractised hand opening an oyster is very difficult. Access does indeed depend critically on abduction of the shoulder, but the surgeon must at all times bear in mind the limits of tolerance of that position by the nerves of the plexus. We have found Deaver retractors useful, but Roos (1981) prefers the Heaney vaginal retractor, it being less liable to damage the vein and muscles.

The first rib, the lateral margin of which is at first the only part easily visible, is cleared by swab dissection to reveal the upper surface crossed by the first thoracic nerve and subclavian artery and receiving the attachment of the scalenus anterior. In front of this is the crossing of the subclavian vein. Anterior to the vein is the tendon of the subclavius muscle. Laterally, the edge of the first rib receives attachment of the intercostal muscles. Once these have been cleared from the rib, the apical pleura can be separated from its lower surface. The tendons of the subclavius and the scalenus anterior muscles are divided, and the nerve, artery and vein are very carefully mobilised from the upper surface of the rib. The scalenus medius muscle is cleared from the upper surface of the posterior part of the rib, and then the suprapleural membrane can be freed from the medial surface of the rib. In these proceedings the Howarth dissector and the small Doyen raspatory are useful. The aim is to remove the rib extraperiosteally from anteriorly, just in front of the subclavian vein, to posteriorly, behind the crossing of the first thoracic nerve. The anterior division is the easier: with the vein held up and the pleura depressed, the rib can be divided with fine bone cutters or simply separated from the costal cartilage. The posterior division is more difficult, because of the presence of the first thoracic nerve. This can be held and pushed out of the way during the division of the bone – usually, just distal to the costotransverse joint. A long instrument rather like the device used for removing meat from lobster claws is useful for this. The fork of the instrument is run posteriorly along the medial edge of the rib so that the nerve is pushed out of the way. The rib is strong here: it can rarely be divided with a single bite of the bone cutters. The proximal end almost always needs trimming with the rongeurs; Roos' (1981) detailed description of the procedure is required reading for all operators in this field. Bleeding is checked before closure. The wound comes together very well with the lowering of the limb. Subcutaneous fascia and skin are closed over a suction drain; if the pleura has been opened, an intercostal catheter should be added.

Dangers and complications. The chief immediate danger is that of wounding the subclavian vein. Bleeding is very severe. It must be checked with local pressure until the vein is sufficiently accessible proximally and distally to permit isolation of the segment and repair of the tear. The lesion most often suffered by the plexus during the operation is that inflicted by prolonged abduction and lateral rotation, neither of which should be permissible. The lesion so inflicted is usually a conduction block, but recovery may take weeks or even months. No surgeon should attempt this operation who is unable with certainty to avoid cutting the plexus or any part of it. It must be remembered that the first thoracic nerve is very vulnerable during the exposure and division of the posterior part of the rib. Horowitz (1985) describes damage to the plexus during operation; even causalgia arising from that damage. He makes recommendations concerning intermittent

relaxation of the position of abduction. The vulnerability of the nerve to serratus anterior has been mentioned (Wood & Frykman 1980).

The posterior approach

The posterior approach, developed from the one used by Adson and Brown (1929) following Henry (1924), for cervicothoracic sympathectomy is the route of choice for the removal of a seventh cervical rib or the posterior part of such a rib or the posterior part of a first thoracic rib after a previous intervention. Although Adson and Brown describe it as "easy", we have found it too difficult and too traumatic and bloody to be suitable as a primary route for the removal of a seventh cervical or first thoracic rib. It is, in effect, a cervical extension of lateral rachotomy or "anterolateral decompression". Its extended version has been shown in Figures 7.36 to 7.40.

The lateral position is best, with the affected side uppermost. The curved paravertebral incision is centred on the seventh cervical or the first thoracic rib and the flaps are raised. Now the superficial muscles (chiefly the trapezius, rhomboids and splenius capitis) are divided near the midline and are retracted laterally as a flap. The posterior paravertebral muscles are retracted medially to expose the transverse processes, and in particular those of the seventh cervical and first thoracic vertebrae. The seventh cervical or the first thoracic rib or the posterior remnants are now exposed and freed from their soft tissue attachments. The eighth cervical and first thoracic nerves are related to the posterior part of the seventh cervical rib; the first thoracic nerve is related to the posterior part of the first thoracic rib. Each has to be identified and pushed away from the rib before any bone is cut. The seventh cervical or the first thoracic transverse process is nibbled away. It should be possible with this approach to remove virtually all but the head of the seventh cervical or the first thoracic rib. With perseverance and care it is possible to remove the whole of the posterior part of such ribs. The incision closes nicely: the paravertebral muscles are allowed to regain their original position and are there sutured. A suction drain is inserted here. The superficial muscles are drawn back over them and are sutured. The subcutaneous tissues are sutured before the skin is closed. Pain is common after this operation, doubtless because of the amount of muscle cutting and retraction necessary. Neural, vascular and pleural complications are rare.

Results

Dunnet and Birch (1994) analysed results in 47 of our patients (40 women and 7 men) operated on by the supraclavicular route for the neural type of thoracic outlet syndrome between 1982 and 1992. There were 55 procedures, including 25 removals of the first rib and 11 removals of a seventh cervical rib. Eight patients were completely relieved of symptoms and 35 were improved. There was, however, a 32% incidence of recurrence, at an average of 19 months (range 1 month to 6.5 years) after operation. Worryingly, there was no correlation between outcome and findings at operation. Indeed, in one of our most completely and lastingly successful cases (not included in those analysed by Dunnet and Birch), neither neural nor arterial abnormality was found at operation.

The necessity for operation in the arterial type of thoracic outlet syndrome is not in doubt; in such cases the results of operations that are carefully planned and well executed are good, so long as the condition has not been allowed to advance too far. The same necessity obtains in the rare instances of the venous type of outlet compression; here too, the results of operation are good. With the neural type of outlet syndrome the results are less reliable, and it may be that in some of these cases we have erred in not removing the first thoracic rib at the time of removal of a scalenus sickle or other soft tissue obstruction. In cases in which there are no important objective neurological abnormalities, it is important, before advising operation, to be very sure that everything possible has been done to locate the site of the lesion, and that the hazards of operation in this field are known to the patient.

THE CARPAL TUNNEL SYNDROME

The carpal tunnel syndrome is not quite the oldest but it is certainly the commonest of entrapment syndromes. It is also the entrapment syndrome in which it is most often possible to demonstrate an underlying cause, in the nerve, in its surroundings, or in both. Although in their extensive study of the condition Rosenbaum and Ochoa (1993a) state that "most cases of carpal tunnel syndrome are unrelated to a causal anomaly or systemic illness", they go on to show that in a combined series of 2705 patients there were 321 with rheumatoid arthritis, 166 diabetics, and 94 with hypothyroidism: altogether 581 patients. In another 30 the condition was related to pregnancy or to an oral contraceptive. That is almost one in four cases related to one of the four most common associated conditions. Rosenbaum and Ochoa's table 5.1 lists the other, less common, associated factors. Clearly, the clinician should initially regard "carpal tunnel syndrome" as a symptom rather than as a diagnosis.

Tubiana and Brockman (1993) assign the credit for the first description of the syndrome to Putnam (1880). Schulze (1893) was responsible for the term *akroparästhesie*. He described eight cases (four men and four women) in at least some of whom paraesthesiae were caused by compression of the median nerve.

Marie and Foix (1913) described necropsy findings in a case of wasting of the muscles of the thenar eminence, showing the role of the flexor retinaculum in compressing the median nerve. Learmonth (1933) was probably the first to divide the flexor retinaculum for compression of the median nerve. He did a "blind" division in a case of compression due to arthritis of the wrist following injury. Zachary (1945) described two cases of carpal tunnel syndrome in which decompression was done by Seddon. In the case of a man with post-traumatic arthritis of the wrist and of a woman with malunion of a lower radial fracture, paraesthesiae were relieved and there was recovery of motor power and muscle bulk. The credit for the first decompression of the median nerve for "idiopathic" carpal tunnel syndrome probably goes to Cannon and Love (1946). It was, however, the paper by Brain et al (1947) that opened British eyes to the existence of the condition and to the benefits of treatment by operation. The senior author of this book is happy to recall that the last of this famous trio is a contemporary; that he was house surgeon to the second and later his colleague, and that for some years he sat beside the first author at meetings of the Council of the Medical Defence Union. Brain and his colleagues did not deal only with clinical features and results of operations, they also made measurements of variations in pressure in the carpal tunnel. It is interesting to note that those measurements showed that extension of the wrist produced in the carpal tunnel a rise in pressure much greater than that produced by flexion.

Since 1947 the carpal tunnel industry has expanded enormously; so too has the understanding of the underlying causes. However, practice has tended to run ahead of the systematic search for an underlying cause. Decompression is, after all, superficially a simple and generally successful operation; the systematic source for a cause is often long and sometimes fruitless.

We owe to Gelberman et al (1981), Hamanuka et al (1995) and Seradge et al (1995) further knowledge about the role of raised pressure in the carpal tunnel and to Hongell and Matsson (1971) information about the early improvement of conductivity after decompression. All aspects of the carpal tunnel syndrome have been illuminated by the work of Phalen (1966, 1972, 1981), to whom we owe an important diagnostic test depending on the production of symptoms by forced flexion of the wrist. Nerve conduction has been studied by, among others, Phalen (1972), Harris et al (1974), Spindler and Dellon (1982), Wilson-Macdonald and Caughey (1984) and Hamanuka et al (1995). Fullerton (1963) studied the effects of ischaemia on conduction along the median nerve at the wrist in cases of carpal tunnel syndrome, and found that the nerve was "abnormally susceptible to ischaemia. There was rapid failure of motor conduction." Wilson-Macdonald and Caughey (1984) sensibly tested conduction velocity over periods of 24 hours, and found a significant reduction at night in affected hands.

Gelberman et al (1988a) defined three classes of carpal tunnel syndrome: early (including acute), intermediate and advanced. The acute type, rare though it is, certainly is a distinct entity. Adamson et al (1971) indicated eight causes in nine cases, including haematoma after operation for Dupuytren's disease, and swelling following a burn. More specific causes of the acute syndrome are pseudo-gout and hyperparathyroidism (Weinstein et al 1968), pseudo-gout alone (Spiegel et al 1976, Rate et al 1992), infection (Williams & Geer 1963) and spontaneous haemorrhage into the nerve (Hayden 1964, Flynn et al 1995). Lanz and Wolter (1975) have reviewed the whole field.

The underlying causes of carpal tunnel syndrome were considered at length by Phalen (1966) in his magisterial review of the experience of 17 years in dealing with diagnosis and treatment in 654 hands, on 212 of which operation was done. The most common associated conditions were diabetes mellitus and rheumatoid arthritis, but it is interesting to observe that in almost 50 cases the symptoms of carpal tunnel syndrome were associated with "arthritis" of the shoulder or "tennis elbow". Phalen's experience of the preponderance of female sufferers from the condition reflects the general experience of a 6:1 female/male ratio. The predominance in the age range 40–60 years also reflects the experience of others. Phalen's (1981) observation of thickening of the synovium from various causes as a precipitator of symptoms is confirmed by Lanz (1993). Lanz goes on to list various causes of thickening of the paratenon, and proceeds to discuss other causes of compression, including malformation of the carpus from hereditary metabolic or developmental disuse (Watson–Jones 1949). Lanz considers simple thickening of the flexor retinaculum, often from repeated occupational stress, to be a rare cause of carpal tunnel syndrome. We attempted to distinguish "thick" from "normal" retinacula at operation, but after some years recognised that this subjective distinction could hardly be valid.

At St Mary's Hospital we had the opportunity of observing several patients with carpal tunnel syndrome associated with uraemia and haemodialysis. This aspect is well considered by Allieu et al (1983), who had the opportunity of studying 31 affected hands in 20 uraemic patients subjected to haemodialysis. They discuss the change in the synovium, the role of the arteriovenous fistula, and the response to operation. In particular they note that the changes in the synovial membrane are due to amyloid deposits of type AL (amyloid protein light chain related). We are much indebted to Dr Barry Hulme, consultant nephrologist to St Mary's Hospital, for the following note on the current (1995) position regarding carpal tunnel syndrome in patients undergoing dialysis: "It is now unusual for patients to receive haemodialysis with a forearm shunt, and most patients have arteriovenous fistula created by anastomosing the radial artery at the wrist to an adjacent vein. Carpal tunnel syndrome is seen in dialysis patients with increasing frequency. The carpal tunnel

syndrome in these patients is due to a deposition of amyloid associated with excessive levels of β_2 microglobulin. It occurs particularly in patients who have been on haemodialysis for longer than ten years and it occurs whether the patients are treated by haemodialysis or peritoneal dialysis and irrespective of the form of vascular access."

Dr Hulme drew our attention to the work of Aoike et al (1995) directed at the problem of removing β_2 microglobulin. They studied the effect on the incidence of joint pains, carpal tunnel syndrome and bone cysts of using a β_2 microglobulin removing membrane. Plasma β_2 microglobulin was maintained at a lower level, and the incidence of bone cysts and carpal tunnel syndrome fell with it, as did the incidence of haemodialysis-related amyloidosis. There may be lessons in this for carpal tunnel syndromes of other aetiologies. Fitzgerald (1978) describes what must now be a very rare cause: ergotism. Kellgren et al (1952) discussed the incidence in acromegaly, finding three cases of bilateral affection in 25 cases. Inglis et al (1972) narrated a variety of causes in this large series.

The role of hormonal changes in women has been known for years. Soferman et al (1964) studied 18 women with symptoms of median nerve compression during pregnancy, finding that in 13 of these symptoms subsided after delivery. Wilkinson (1960), however, related the case of a 74-year-old woman who had suffered from the symptoms of carpal tunnel syndrome for *36 years*, ever since the onset at the sixth month of pregnancy. Tobin (1967) reckoned that up to 45% of pregnant women suffered from numbness and tingling in the fingers. Nicholas et al (1971) studied 100 women in the third trimester of pregnancy and found that 18 had signs or symptoms of median nerve compression at the wrist. In most cases symptoms abated in the postpartum period. Although Wilkinson (1960) thought that weight gain with fluid retention was the cause of compression in pregnant women, Nicholas and his colleagues failed to find in the women affected any gain in weight greater than expected in normal pregnancy. Sabour and Fâdel (1970) noted the influence of the oral contraceptive in determining the onset of symptoms. Confino-Cohen et al (1991) and later Hall et al (1992) noted the effect of hormone replacement therapy in reducing the symptoms of carpal tunnel syndrome.

Clinicians dealing with children are likely to encounter the rare diseases due to inborn errors of metabolism, and to find compression of the median nerve in some of these cases. Thus, Moxley (1991) draws attention to the occurrence of carpal tunnel syndrome in certain mucopolysaccharidoses – namely, MPS I S (Scheie), MPS II B (Hunter) and MPS VI A, B, and C (Maroteaux–Lamy). Doubtless, the mechanism of interference in this disorder of storage is the lack of space resulting from the accumulation of polysaccharide.

A more proximal lesion

In carpal tunnel syndrome the question of a more proximal lesion is perhaps raised more often than it is in any other entrapment neuropathy. The question of the affection of cervical nerves in the intervertebral foramina or of the trunks of the brachial plexus at the thoracic outlet is raised. Hurst et al (1985) studied 1000 affected hands in 888 patients and found a significant increase in bilateral affection in patients with cervical spinal osteoarthritis. They attributed this "double-crush" effect partly to interference with axoplasmic transport, and partly to "disruption" of nerve transmission. Studying over 500 patients with "carpal tunnel syndrome", Pfeffer et al (1986) defined three groups: cervical radiculopathy, pure carpal tunnel syndrome and elements of both conditions. They hazarded the suggestion that in the third group an association with cervical radiculopathy could be the cause of failure after operation. The experimental work of Nemoto et al (1987) confirmed the mechanism of the "combined" lesion, in which the loss of nerve function after a double lesion is greater than the sum of the deficits from each single lesion. Osterman (1988) related the carpal tunnel syndrome not only to cervical radiculopathy but also to the thoracic outlet and pronator syndromes. Finally, Narakas (1993b) reviewed the history of affection of nerves at two or more levels, and particularly considered the relation between carpal tunnel syndrome and thoracic outlet syndrome. He concluded that the association causing a double-crush syndrome was "difficult to demonstrate with certainty in all cases in which it seems to exist". Narakas also mentioned the alarming concept of the "triple-crush" syndrome – an association of radiculopathy, outlet syndrome and a distal entrapment. In one thought-provoking case which came to our attention, decompression of the median nerve of the left (nondominant) hand of a woman in her forties was done for symptoms of episodic paraesthesiae in the distribution of the nerve. A particularly long and thick retinaculum was indeed found and divided. Operation had no lasting effect on the symptoms. Shortly after operation, the patient drew attention to the presence in the left axilla of a lump, pressure on which reproduced the symptoms. Magnetic resonance imaging showed a tumour in the line of the neurovascular bundle (Fig. 12.34). The tumour was later removed: it was shown histologically to be a benign schwannoma. Here, the "primary" symptom-producing lesion was in the axilla rather than in the carpal tunnel, and the "compression" in the latter site played no role in the production of symptoms.

The role of repetitive strain

We have certainly seen carpal tunnel determined, in men as well as in women, by repetitive use of the fingers, as

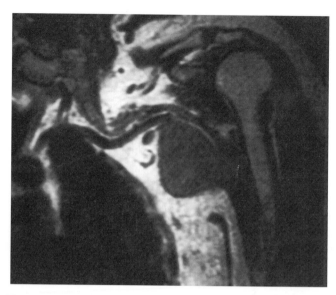

Fig. 12.34 Magnetic resonance image showing a schwannoma of the median nerve just below the axilla in a 55-year-old woman initially treated for "carpal tunnel syndrome".

in stripping insulation from wires, assembly-line work and even knitting.

Anatomy

The "bottleneck" (Lanz 1993) of the carpal tunnel is formed posteriorly and laterally by the concavity formed by the carpal bones: in particular the scaphoid, lunate and hamate, and pisiform bones. It is roofed by the flexor retinaculum and anchored medially to the pisiform and hamate bones and laterally to the scaphoid bone and the trapezium. The width of the retinaculum is about 2.5 cm; its length is about the same (Fig. 12.35). Proximally it blends with the antebrachial fascia, and distally it blends with the palmar aponeurosis. The tendon of the palmaris longus muscle is attached to it anteriorly. A deep lamina on the radial side is attached to the medial lip of a groove on the trapezium. Between this layer and the more superficial part lies the tendon of the flexor carpi radialis muscle in its synovial sheath. On the ulnar side a localised thickening of the antebrachial fascia extends laterally from the pisiform bone as a superficial part of the retinaculum, crossing superficial to the ulnar nerve and vessels to blend with the retinaculum lateral to them.

In the tunnel are accommodated the median nerve, the tendons of the deep and superficial flexor muscles of the fingers, the tendon of the long flexor of the thumb, and the synovial membrane. Sometimes, especially in persons who do repetitive work with their fingers, the most proximal parts of the lumbrical muscles, attached to the tendons of the flexor profundus, extend into the carpal tunnel (Siegel et al 1995).

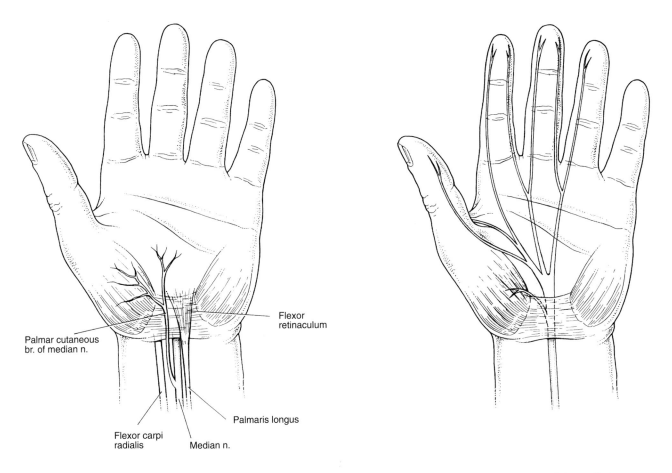

Fig. 12.35 The flexor retinaculum. Note the palmaris longus and the palmar cutaneous and motor branches of the median nerve.

The positions of the motor and the palmar cutaneous branches of the median nerve are very important for the surgeon. Lanz (1993) illustrates 12 variants of the main nerve and its motor branch. In most cases the motor branch arises from the radial side of the nerve in the carpal tunnel and runs laterally, soon branching to supply the opponens and short abductors of the thumb, and often part of the flexor brevis. A particular hazard for the surgeon is produced by an origin from the ulnar side of the nerve and a course across it, either deep or superficial, to the retinaculum. Ogden (1972) describes a retrograde branch, probably motor, actually traversing the retinaculum. Wadsworth (1984a) shows an excellent illustration of the variations in origin and course of the motor branch of the median nerve.

The palmar cutaneous branch arises from the median nerve about 7 cm above the wrist crease and runs distally medial to the tendon of the flexor carpi radialis to innervate the skin over the thenar eminence and the radial side of the proximal part of the palm. Semple and Cargill (1969) drew attention to the higher incidence of tenderness of and around the scar when a transverse incision was used, and attributed this damage to the palmar cutaneous branch. Carroll and Green (1972) and Taleisnik (1973) draw attention to the need to avoid damage to this branch during the operation. Damage can cause a profound and persistent painful state, with very troublesome hyperaesthesia and hyperalgesia, and even hyperpathia and allodynia.

Clinical features

Typically, a woman in her fifties presents with pain and paraesthesiae and even numbness in the fingers of both hands, present particularly at night and on waking from sleep. Symptoms are usually worse in one hand than in the other. During attacks the fingers feel swollen. Relief is obtained by shaking the hands or by hanging them down. Symptoms may be provoked by work with the hands, in particular by repetitive activity such as knitting. There may be proximal radiation of the paraesthesiae. As time goes by, the paraesthesiae become more constant; numbness becomes established. Weakness becomes apparent, and thenar wasting is noticed. Some patients report subsidence of symptoms over long periods, with recurrence and, later, shortened periods of freedom. Loss of sleep and progressive defect of function bring such patients to seek advice.

Local physical signs range from virtually none to severe alteration of sensibility in the area of the median nerve and wasting of the opponens. Brain et al (1947) commented on an apparent weakness of the extensor longus pollicis, and canvassed possible reasons for this odd finding. One of us noticed this curious weakness many years ago and forgot all about it. Now we wonder whether the "weakness" of the extensor could be caused by the loss of the stabilising action of the short muscles of the thumb.

The median nerve is often tender at the upper margin of the flexor retinaculum; tapping there produces radiating paraesthesiae. Symptoms may be produced by a short period of ischaemia (Gilliatt & Wilson 1953) or of flexion of the wrist for 60 seconds (Phalen 1966, 1972, Gelberman et al 1993). Electrophysiological examination shows defect of conduction in many cases. Spindler and Dellon (1982) found abnormalities on electrophysiological examination in more than 80% of these patients. Fullerton (1963) showed rapid failure of motor conduction in response to ischaemia. Buchtal and Rosenfalck (1971) drew attention to the defect of conduction localised to the palm–wrist segment of the nerve. However, as Rosenbaum and Ochoa (1993b) remark: "the correlation between symptoms, signs and electrodiagnostic findings is imperfect". Certainly there are cases of carpal tunnel syndrome with well-marked symptoms in which no electrophysiological abnormalities are found. There are other cases in which electrophysiological abnormalities are found in the absence of present or past symptoms. Nevertheless, it is almost certainly right to test electrical reactions before starting treatment on a diagnosis of carpal tunnel syndrome, and it is certainly right to do so before deciding on operation. The tests depend on the measurement of motor and sensory nerve conduction: refinements can be added, such as the ischaemia test of Fullerton (1963), corrections designed to give residual motor latency, and palmar serial sensory studies (Kimura 1979). In the case in which the symptoms arising from a schwannoma of the left median nerve in the axilla were mistaken for those of carpal tunnel syndrome, antidromic sensory conduction velocity across the wrist was not reduced, but there was a small reduction of amplitude on the affected side. The absence of abnormality of conduction velocity in the presence of thenar wasting should, no doubt, have warned the clinicians that they were not dealing simply with "carpal tunnel syndrome". Computed tomography (Dekel & Rushworth 1993, Lanz 1993) and magnetic resonance imaging are perhaps better considered as methods of research than as clinical investigations, though Mesgarzadeh et al (1989a,b) clearly have indicated the usefulness of magnetic resonance imaging in primary diagnosis and in recognition of causes of failure.

Differential diagnosis

In this entrapment more than in any other it is necessary to be sure that the symptoms arise from the fact of the particular entrapment and that they are not in the end those of a systemic disorder or a more proximal neuropathy. Enough has already been said to indicate the need to think about the possibilities of systemic disease and of more proximal neuropathy at the thoracic outlet or the intervertebral foramen. We have several times seen the early symptoms of radiation neuropathy of the brachial plexus diagnosed as those of carpal tunnel syndrome. Indeed, in at least one of these cases, operation succeeded in relieving symptoms for a while. It is particularly important too, to distinguish symptoms primarily caused by compression in the carpal tunnel from those of compression in the intervertebral foramen or at the thoracic outlet. Of course, the precipitating or proximate cause may be in the carpal tunnel when there is more proximal compromise of function.

A distinguished clinician brought his wife for consultation. She had paraesthesiae in the fingers of both hands, predominantly affecting radial digits, and present particularly at night and aggravated by use. There was slight wasting of the thenar muscles, but no clear alteration of sensibility. The evidence from electrophysiological examination was unconvincing. There were bilateral seventh cervical ribs articulating with the middle parts of the first thoracic ribs. The question of intervention on the ribs was raised, but the evidence of the nocturnal paraesthesiae was decisive. Division of the flexor retinaculum was followed by instant and lasting relief of symptoms.

Treatment

Although the question of operation comes to the minds of many clinicians dealing with carpal tunnel syndrome, many patients can do without this ultimate deterrent. In most cases associated with pregnancy, symptoms subside spontaneously after delivery (Tobin 1967, Nicholas et al 1971); in many other cases of "idiopathic" affection, symptoms subside spontaneously and do not recur. Cessation of a particular activity provoking symptoms often leads to remission. Harris et al (1974) reserved operation for cases in which there were electrophysiological abnormalities. The only absolute indications for operation are, perhaps:

- acute carpal tunnel syndrome
- persistent and progressive symptoms with alteration of sensibility and weakness of the thenar muscles.

In most other cases it is permissible to wait or to observe the effect of treatment short of operation. Thus, hormone replacement treatment (Confino-Cohen et al 1991, Hall et al 1992) is applicable in menopausal women not already receiving it. In cases in which there is clear hypothyroidism, treatment with thyroid supplement is often enough to produce remission. Ellis et al (1982) reported a regular response to treatment with pyridoxine (vitamin B_6), though later Amadio (1985) concluded that there was no place for such treatment. The question of injection of steroids into the carpal tunnel is often raised. Foster (1960) described the results of hydrocortisone injection in 20 patients, five of whom suffered from diabetes mellitus. The duration of observation ranged from 11 to 16 months; there was recurrence of symptoms in 14 cases. Perhaps the best study of the results of injection is that contained in the larger review by Kulick et al (1986). They found that the average duration of benefit after injection was 27 weeks. Accidental injection of steroid into the median nerve can be avoided by placing the needle medial to the line of the nerve and giving a trial injection of local anaesthetic before the steroid is introduced. We do not think that this half-way house on the road to treatment should be used routinely, though it may find a place in patients wholly averse to operation or physically unfit for it. At various times splintage of the wrist has been tried and has in some cases been successful. When all reasonable methods have been tried and have failed, and when symptoms are persistent and disabling, there is a case for operation. There may sometimes be a case for operation as a diagnostic procedure, when there is doubt about the site of origin of symptoms. The use in such cases of operation rests on the rather insecure assumption that the commitment involved is slight. That assumption may not always be justified (Semple & Cargill 1969).

Operation

Tubiana and Brockman (1993) credited Cannon and Love (1946) with the first "liberation" of the carpal tunnel after "spontaneous" compression of the median nerve. Learmonth (1933) had shown the way with his "blind" division of the retinaculum through a short incision, and this method was used, with modifications, by Kremer et al (1953). Zachary (1945) reported open division of the retinaculum in two cases, and this method was followed by Brain et al (1947). The operative mason in that partnership used a straight vertical incision 2 in. long, ending distally at the distal transverse crease. Such an incision would nowadays be considered too high, and the reservations about leaving a scar in the palm would be considered invalid. Since that time, opinion has steadily come round to the use of an incision like that described by Lanz (1993), in which exposure is made through a palmar incision. If more proximal exposure is required, an antebrachial limb can be connected to the palmar incision by a transverse limb in the wrist crease (Fig. 12.36).

Three methods are available:

- open exposure and division of the retinaculum
- division of the retinaculum under vision through a short incision in the wrist crease
- division by an endoscopic method.

Each method has its advantages and disadvantages. We now prefer the first technique.

Open exposure

Anaesthesia may be general, local or regional for a primary operation, but general anaesthesia is necessary in operation after failure of a primary operation or after recurrence following a primary operation. If a bloodless field is used the cuff should always be released and bleeding checked before closure. We now rarely use a bloodless field in primary operations, preferring to rely on the effect of elevating the hand on pillows. The incision should be planned to avoid damage to the palmar cutaneous branch of the median nerve. It starts in the palm, just to the ulnar side of the midline, and curves ulnarward at the wrist crease (Fig. 12.36). The incision is deepened and the flexor retinaculum is exposed (Fig. 12.37). The retinaculum is divided from top to bottom under vision, and the nerve, tendons and synovial membranes are exposed. The state of the nerve, tendons and synovial membrane is recorded. If there is proliferative synovitis, the membrane is carefully and completely removed. For this removal it is necessary to extend the incision distally and into the forearm. If there is any doubt about the condition of the synovial membrane, a piece is removed for histological examination. If a cuff is used, it is released at this stage and particular note is taken of the reperfusion of the nerve. Very often, the nerve distal and proximal to the retinaculum will flush up, while the part formerly beneath it will stay white for a few seconds before flushing up (Fig. 12.38). Bleeding is checked and the skin is closed. We have not thought it necessary to resort to ligamentoplasty (Kapandji 1988); there is no case for internal neurolysis; and external neurolysis is only done if the nerve is adherent to adjacent structures. After the closure a padded dressing is applied. This is supplemented with a plaster slab with the wrist extended, to be retained for 72 hours. Splintage is retained longer after operations for "revision".

Restricted exposure

One of us has long experience of this method, derived from Learmonth (1933), but it is not recommended to surgeons who are less than patient or for cases in which any difficulty is apprehended. A headlight or an easily adjusted spot light is necessary. General or regional anaesthesia is necessary: so is a bloodless field. A 2-cm transverse incision is made in the wrist crease and the skin flaps are elevated

Figs 12.36 to 12.38 Open operation for decompression of the median nerve.

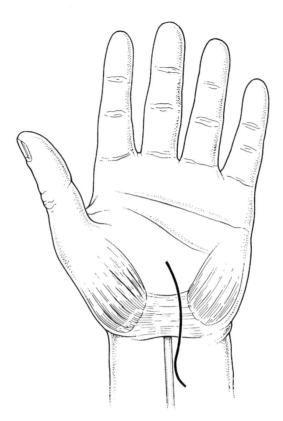

Fig. 12.36 The incision.

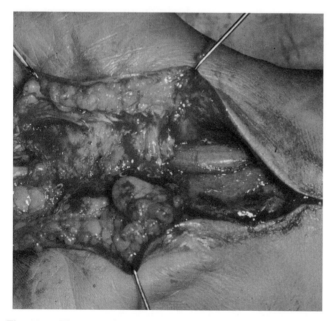

Fig. 12.37 The retinaculum exposed.

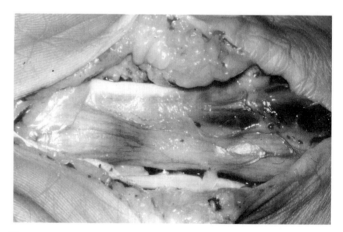

Fig. 12.38 The nerve "flushing up" after release of the cuff. Note the zone of constriction formerly deep to the retinaculum.

and undermined so as to show the anterior surface of the retinaculum and the antebrachial fascia. The palmar cutaneous branch of the median nerve is seen and spared, though it cannot be protected from retraction. With small retractors the proximal skin is lifted and the antebrachial fascia is divided along 2 cm. The distal skin is then lifted with retractors and, with the light illuminating the tunnel, the palmaris longus tendon is detached from the front of the retinaculum on its radial side and retracted medially. Then, with the palmaris longus retracted medially, the flexor retinaculum is divided under vision along the line of the ulnar border of the nerve with fine straight blunt-ended scissors. Both nerve and retinaculum are under vision throughout; the completion of the distal division is signalled by an unmistakable feeling of a "snap". If there is any doubt about completion, an incision must be made in the palm, the distal part of the retinaculum must be inspected, and, if necessary, the division must be completed under vision. The cuff is released and firm pressure is maintained over the incision and the palm for not less than 3 minutes. This pressure is almost always sufficient to check all bleeding, so that the operator can proceed to close the skin. If haemostasis is inadequate, pressure is maintained for a further 2 minutes.

Endoscopic division

We have no experience with the primary use of this method; we have experience only in dealing with some of the results of uninstructed use. Christian Thomas et al (1993) ascribe to Chow (1989) and Agee et al (1990) the credit for suggesting and developing the endoscopic method. It was, presumably, Okutsu (1987) who, with his description of a "universal endoscope", adumbrated the feasibility of this procedure. Thomas et al describe a two-portal approach requiring a grooved stylet and trochar, a knife with a reversed blade, a guide retractor, an endoscopic camera and video equipment and a splint designed to hold the wrist in extension. They go on to describe the method and its difficulties, and the advantages for the patient. They list among contraindications cases in which complete synovectomy is required, cases of infection, acute compression from any cause and cases of recurrence after operation. They note too that exposure is necessary when it is impossible to obtain good and full endoscopic visualisation.

Since that time Van Heest et al (1995) have studied in the cadaver the workings of single portal endoscopic release and have shown incomplete division of the retinaculum in no less than 24 of 43 operations. The results of two-portal endoscopic release have been compared with those of conventional operation: the only clear advantage of the former method has been found to be that of earlier restoration of the power of grip (Dumontier et al 1995). The results of endoscopic operation have been compared

with those of open operation by Bandi et al (1994) and Futami (1995). The findings were broadly similar. Futami (1995) compared results in a series of 10 patients with bilateral affection. The "conventional" release was done on one side; endoscopic release on the other. All patients preferred the latter mode because of the small skin incision, the absence of a painful scar, the short operation time, the reduced postoperative pain, the early return to work or other activity, and the short stay in hospital. Futami warned, however, that endoscopic release is a "technically demanding procedure, and major iatrogenic complications have been reported". There are no free lunches. De Smet and Fabry (1995) report a case of division of the motor branch of the ulnar nerve during two-portal endoscopic release. The endoscopic operation is, evidently, a method which could bring certain advantages to patients, in particular in shortening the period of convalescence. It is a method which the aspiring surgeon must learn and practise thoroughly before he or she starts to use it on patients. It is clear that the inexperienced and uninstructed surgeon can do as much damage in the palm of the hand with a knife and an endoscope as can be done elsewhere in the body by similar surgeons similarly equipped. Thomas et al (1993) conclude their study with a phrase which bears repeating here and elsewhere: "Endoscopic surgical technique requires rigorous training to avoid dangerous pitfalls: it must be performed by experienced hand surgeons." The phrase sounds better still in French. De Smet and Fabry (1995) repeat this admonition: "We should be wary about yielding to pressure to use endoscopic carpal tunnel release from instrument makers, medical supply houses, insurance companies, and patients." The British surgeon now must add "managers" to that list; unfortunately, he or she is no longer able always to resist pressure from such a source.

Difficulties, dangers and complications

The most comprehensive list of complications is that given by Kessler (1986): he records no less than 14, and follows that with the comment: "If one were to name the basic factor for the cause of the complications, it would have to be an inappropriate incision."

In the operation by restricted approach in particular, there is some danger of damage to the superficial palmar arch. This is probably of no great matter if the vessels are cleanly divided: bleeding will cease if pressure is maintained for 5 minutes. If the arterial division is only partial, so as to interfere with the retraction of the ends, bleeding may continue. That will usually be noticed at the time and the vessel will be exposed and ligated. Rarely, a false aneurysm forms in the palm of the hand and requires removal.

More serious is damage to the motor branch of the median nerve; the branch may follow an unusual course making it liable to injury (see p. 269). We have once divided the motor branch during an operation by restricted approach. The approach was at once extended, the damage was seen and the nerve repaired. There was full recovery.

More serious still is damage to the trunk or to the sensory branches of the median nerve. We have seen such damage inflicted elsewhere: remarkably enough, during the course of an operation with full exposure. Even more remarkably, the damage was not noted during operation nor fully appreciated until 3 months later. Nahabidian et al (1995) warn about the danger to the median nerve by the use of YAG laser without a protective shield. Davlin et al (1991) warn about a sensory neural loop arising from the median nerve at the carpal tunnel. We have, alas, seen a patient whose ulnar nerve was divided above its terminal bifurcation during endoscopic division of the flexor retinaculum.

Damage to the palmar cutaneous branch of the median nerve can sometimes produce a painful state, with spontaneous pain and hyperaesthesia of the palm and of the scar (Taleisnik 1973, Carroll & Green 1978). Louis et al (1985) found that damage to the palmar branch was the single most common cause of failure. They noted too, damage to the terminal branch of the radial nerve, abnormal hypertrophy of the scar, persistent dysaesthesia, incomplete division of the retinaculum and joint stiffness as other causes of failure. There may be allodynia or hyperalgesia and there may be hyperpathia. In some cases, the painful state develops the features of true causalgia; in some, a reflex sympathetic dystrophy seems to be produced (Nahabidian et al 1995). The methods of treatment of such states, and their limitations, are discussed in Chapter 16.

Early failure may be expected when the division of the retinaculum is incomplete (Langloh & Linschied 1972). Re-exploration should not be delayed. In other cases, of course, failure to relieve symptoms may indicate that the original diagnosis was mistaken. In making the distinction, much depends on the clinician's knowledge about the competence of the operator. It is, perhaps, when the clinician and the operator are combined in the same person that decision is most difficult. If error has to be made, it should always be on the side of further intervention: delay of completion of release is likely to be followed by marring of the result, even by further failure.

Late failure probably indicates re-formation of the retinaculum with recurrence of compression, indicating further operation. The accuracy of the original diagnosis should, however, be questioned, and the possibility should be borne in mind that recurrence of symptoms arises from changes intrinsic to the nerve.

The complication of prolapse of the structures through the opened retinaculum is, fortunately, rare. When one considers the anatomical arrangements of the carpal tunnel it may seem remarkable that prolapse is not more common. Yet, in practically all cases, the division of this important "pulley" does no more than produce a transient weakness of grip. It was, doubtless, the apprehension of this complication that led Narakas to the practice of a modified ligamentoplasty. It occurs to us now to wonder whether in one case there was any suggestion of an abnormality of connective tissue such as that of Ehlers–Danlos or Marfan syndromes.

Case report. A 54-year-old woman, otherwise healthy, showing no sign of peripheral neuropathy or other predisposing cause, presented with bilateral symptoms of carpal tunnel syndrome. Because symptoms were persistent and severe, the left and, 6 months later, the right median nerves were decompressed by the open method. Symptoms in the left hand subsided completely and did not recur. In the right hand (that of the dominant upper limb), however, there was early recurrence of pain. The nerve was re-explored 6 months after the primary operation. It was found to be embedded between the divided parts of the retinaculum, and was released. Relief was only temporary.

When the patient was seen 18 months after the second operation she had severe local and radiating pain, worst in the palm, present at night and with some burning element. There were intense paraesthesiae, and the digits of median nerve supply were numb. The Tinel sign was strongly positive in the middle of the scar; there was slowing of conduction, but there was no serious denervation of the abductor brevis pollicis. Symptoms had failed to respond to guanethidine infusion, transcutaneous stimulation or other methods.

At re-exploration, the median nerve was again found embedded in scar; as before, in the flexor retinaculum. Some epineurial vessels were intact. The nerve was freed, but there still did not seem to be room for it in the carpal tunnel. So, one tendon of the flexor carpi superficialis was removed, with preservation of the synovium. The nerve was then able to fall back into the carpal tunnel. The night pain subsided 48 hours after operation; the burning pain soon after that. Paraesthesiae were reduced. Six months after operation the result was still satisfactory.

The surgeon should no doubt be especially cautious about advising operation in any patient suffering from any general disorder of connective tissue. In particular, the propriety of decompression in any of the relevant polysaccharidoses must be canvassed. It occurs to one of us (R.B.) that the proper operation – therapeutic or even prophylactic – in such cases is the simple removal of one or two of the tendons of the flexor superficialis.

Results of operation

It is unfortunate that this operation, which is potentially among the least harmful and most beneficial of all elective operations (in the UK at least), is far too often done badly or done for the wrong indication or on an incorrect diagnosis. We have seen over 100 patients suffering persistent symptoms after such operations.

The most recent examinations of results are those by Katz et al (1995) and Higgs et al (1995). The former workers examined 35 patients before and after operation: they found that, though the strength of pinch grip returned to preoperative levels 3 months after operation and was actually improved at 24 months, two-point discrimination mained abnormal in more than half the cases after 2 years. Higgs et al (1995) examined the effect of compensation status of patients on results. They found that residual symptoms were significantly more common in the workers' compensation group.

Our experience is that when the median nerve is properly decompressed at the wrist for the correct indications, the result is lastingly good in 90% of cases. The great majority of the bad results that we have seen were due either to faulty diagnosis or to imperfect techniques of operation.

ENTRAPMENT OF ULNAR NERVE AT THE ELBOW

The third common entrapment syndrome has the special characteristic of rather frequent relation to external pressure or other trauma. The sex incidence is different from that in the thoracic outlet and carpal tunnel syndromes. In Gilliatt and Thomas' (1960) series, 13 of 14 patients investigated and treated were men.

As the ulnar nerve approaches the elbow, it runs behind the medial intermuscular septum and then passes subcutaneously behind the medial epicondyle of the humerus in the retrocondylar groove. It then passes superficial to the medial capsule of the elbow joint and deep to the arcade joining the two origins of the flexor carpi ulnaris muscle (the arcuate ligament). This is the "cubital tunnel". The nerve then runs between the flexor carpi ulnaris and flexor digitorum profundus muscles, joining the ulnar artery in its course down the forearm (Fig. 12.39). The muscular branches arise just below the elbow. The nerve is vulnerable to external pressure; it may be compressed between the arcuate ligament and the medial capsule; with relaxation of this ligament it may become hypermobile, dislocating forward when the elbow is flexed; because of the excursion required of it during movement of the elbow, it may be stretched during flexion if that excursion is restricted by changes due to the damage from external pressure. Wadsworth (1977) dealt with the "external compression" syndrome of the ulnar nerve, drawing on Osborne's (1970) exposition of the role of the arcuate ligament in different positions of the elbow. Compression, either acute or subacute, occurs with direct trauma or with long continued pressure, such as that which occurs in the unconscious patient, in those confined to bed or partly immobile, and in those who have over a short period of time lost much weight. From this beginning local swelling of the nerve accentuates compression between the arcuate

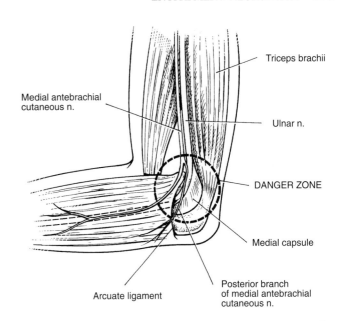

Fig. 12.39 The ulnar nerve at the elbow. Note the "arcuate ligament" and the posterior branch of the medial cutaneous nerve of the forearm.

ligament and the medial aspect of the elbow joint to produce a chronic localised neuropathy (Figs 12.40 and 12.41).

The same situation may arise without external compression or trauma. Osborne (1970) made clear the role of the arcuate ligament as a cause of entrapment. He showed how with flexion of the elbow the ligament's grip on the ulnar nerve was tightened. Liability to compression is increased if the space between the elbow and the ligament is further reduced by marginal osteophytosis or by chronic effusion in the joint with bulging of the capsule. Valgus deformity of the elbow may further increase the effect, as in the "tardy ulnar neuritis" that follows malunion of elbow fractures in children or similar damage in adults. The site of the lesion was investigated by Campbell et al (1988), who used intraoperative electroneurography. The usual site was the retrocondylar groove; the next most common, the cubital tunnel. In 3 of 17 cases there were lesions in both sites. Schuind et al (1995) showed how the elongation of the ulnar nerve produced by flexion of the elbow was largely confined to the section above the elbow. It may well be that in those cases in which the nerve lesion is in the retrocondylar groove, it is produced by restriction of excursion causing pressure against the back of the epicondyle in flexion of the elbow.

Inadequacy of the arcuate ligament may be a cause of ulnar neuritis: laxity may contribute to recurrent subluxation of the nerve over the medial epicondyle with flexion of the elbow. Indeed, Childress (1975) gave an incidence of subluxation of 16%. As is the case with other nerves in restricted spaces, ganglia or benign tumours situated here can produce affection of the nerve disproportionate to their size and intrinsic importance.

Figs 12.40 and 12.41 The ulnar nerve entrapped at the elbow.

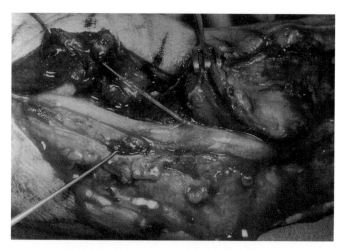

Fig. 12.40 The right ulnar nerve of a 40-year-old man entrapped below the elbow. The arcuate ligament has been divided. Note the narrowing of the nerve just below the origin of the first muscular branch, and the suggestion of swelling just below the medial epicondyle.

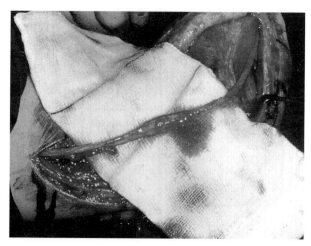

Fig. 12.41 The ulnar nerve mobilised with as many vessels as possible in a second transposition. Note the pseudoneuroma.

Rare causes of compression here have been described: "snapping" of the medial head of the triceps (Rolfsen 1970, Dreyfuss & Kessler 1978, Reis 1980, Hayashi et al 1984); the presence of an anconeus epitrochlearis (Dahners et al 1984); and stretching over a supracondylar spur (Fragiadakis & Lamb 1970). The evidence for causation by the "snapping" of the medial head of the triceps in Rolfsen's and Hayashi's cases remains unclear. Spinner (1993) describes entrapment following prolonged flexion of the elbow beyond 90° in connection with a pectoral flap procedure. We have seen this complication after capsulotomy of the elbow done to restore passive flexion, when after operation the elbow was held in a similar position, and also after Steindler flexorplasty, in spite of careful exposure and decompression of the nerve during operation. In the former case, certainly, the nerve was affected by a traction lesion. Dawson et al (1990a) classify the cause of ulnar affection at the elbow as: external pressure, compression by scar or by bone, recurrent subluxation and cubital tunnel syndrome.

The nature of the affection was explored by Gilliatt and Thomas (1960). In 14 patients they found substantial reduction in conduction velocity in the forearm and elbow regions. It is likely that initial episodic ischaemia is followed by demyelination of large fibres and later by axonal affection. The nerve itself is constricted at the site of compression and swollen into a pseudoneuroma above it. In this condition, the incidence of causation or precipitation by a local extra- or intraneural manifestation of a systemic condition is far lower than it is in carpal tunnel syndrome. Nevertheless, Upton et al (1978) found four instances of ulnar neuropathy at the elbow in 34 patients with rheumatoid arthritis. We have seen it as a complication of the start of treatment in leprosy (Hansen's disease) (Palande 1973): in that case, swelling of the nerve in response to antileprotic drugs precipitated entrapment beneath the arcade of the flexor carpi ulnaris. Now that leprosy is less common in the UK than it was in the late 1950s, this complication is unlikely to be seen in this country. Excessive use of the elbow is a recognised cause in manual workers. Godshall and Hansen (1971) even found two adolescents in whom neuropathy at the elbow had been provoked by pitching in baseball.

Clinical features

The patient, usually a man, presents with paraesthesia and alteration of sensibility in the distribution of the ulnar nerve. As in other lesions caused by compression, the modalities of sensation conveyed in the large fibres are at first affected. Thus, perception of pain is for long spared, whereas light touch and discrimination are early affected. The area affected includes that of the distribution of the dorsal branch. At a later stage there is weakness of the muscles of ulnar supply – the flexor carpi ulnaris and the ulnar part of the flexor profundus digitorum, and the muscles of the hand with the usual exception of the abductor brevis and the opponens pollicis.

The most common local signs are the tenderness over the ulnar nerve at the elbow, the production of paraesthesiae by tapping the nerve as it passes beneath the arcuate ligament, enlargement of the nerve at and above the medial epicondyle and hypermobility of the nerve. Wadsworth's (1982, 1984b) test relies on the production of symptoms and alteration of sensibility by holding the elbow fully flexed for not less than 5 minutes. Associated signs are those of deformity of the elbow, osteoarthritis or other joint disorder causing effusion and synovial thickening.

Diagnosis

Diagnosis may be easy, as in the case of a patient in his thirties with serious deformity of the elbow the late result of injury, with motor and sensory signs in the distribution of the ulnar nerve, with tenderness of an ulnar nerve thickened at the elbow, and with marked slowing of conduction along the ulnar nerve at the elbow. However, diagnosis may be difficult, as in the case of a man in his sixties with weakness and wasting of the small muscles of both hands and with marked degenerative changes in the cervical spine. An easily made, though rare, error is to confuse "snapping" of an enlarged or abnormal medial head of the triceps over the medial epicondyle with abnormal mobility of the ulnar nerve. The more important and much commoner difficulty is to determine the level, or even the levels, at which the nerve cell is being compressed, distorted or otherwise damaged. Is it in the anterior horn cell, in the spinal canal, in the intervertebral foramen, at the thoracic outlet, at the elbow or in the wrist or hand? Is there a dual or even a treble lesion? Enough has been said at the beginning of this chapter to impress on the clinician the importance of bearing in mind the possibility of a systemic cause of neuropathy.

Diagnosis is reached by:

- clinical examination
- electrophysiological investigation (Payan 1986)
- imaging.

Unfortunately, none of these methods is a wholly reliable predictor; even the sum of their combination may not be exact. The situation is further clouded by the possibility of lesions at more than one level, with a lesion at one being the determinant of the clinical affection.

1. The absence of a sensory component of the paralysis must suggest a lesion proximal to the junction of the motor and sensory roots, either in the cord or in the canal. The extension of the motor paralysis to the thenar muscles suggests a lesion of the lower trunk or more proximally. The absence of a sensory component combined with absence of affection of the ulnar-innervated muscles of the forearm suggests a lesion distal to the separation of motor and sensory branches at the wrist in the proximal part of the palm. In any case, the whole limb should be examined to exclude a more proximal lesion of the nerve or medial cord. So too should the lower limbs; the presence of long tract signs must indicate the probability of a lesion in the spinal canal or cord.

The presence of bilateral affection in a nonmanual worker ought to suggest a cause proximal to the elbow level, unless there are obvious local signs. Hypermobility, swelling and tenderness of the ulnar nerve at the elbow and a positive Tinel sign over it all suggest a lesion at the elbow level. Deformity of the elbow or the presence of polyarthritis causing effusion in the elbow also suggest a local cause of neuropathy.

2. Slowing of conduction along the ulnar nerve at the elbow suggests a lesion at that level, either solitary or as a determinant of symptoms from a dual lesion. However, such evidence is not confirmatory: the lesion at the elbow may be no more than a precipitating cause of symptoms and clinical signs, and may be no more than a coincidental finding. Evidence of axonal degeneration may fit in with a diagnosis of neuropathy at the elbow, but if the extent of affection is wider than the distribution of the ulnar nerve it is suggestive of damage in the anterior horn. Special techniques are of course available for the detection of motor neuron disease (De Lisa et al 1994). Strong clinical evidence of affection of the cord clearly raises the question of proceeding to measurement of evoked cortical responses.

3. Radiographs of the elbow may show obvious deformity, or encroachment on the cubital tunnel by osteophytes. In cases of doubt, radiographs of the neck are necessary to exclude a seventh cervical rib. The finding of degenerative changes in patients aged over 60 years is not necessarily significant, though that of osteophyte encroachment on the spinal canal or on one or more of the lower cervical intervertebral foramina is suggestive of a lesion in one of those sites. The ultimate investigation in cases of doubt is of course magnetic resonance imaging, which has probably superseded myelography and computed tomography with contrast enhancement. Not only is it possible to visualise the brachial plexus at the outlet (Panegyres et al 1993), but the cord, the canal and the foramina with their contents can also be seen. It should be possible with these investigations to settle diagnosis in most doubtful cases: certainly, it should be possible to separate all varieties of motor neuron disease and syringomyelia from the rest. In a small proportion of cases the answers to the questions of the level of the lesion and the presence of a dual lesion will remain uncertain. In these cases simple decompression is justifiable as a partly diagnostic procedure, so long, of course, as there is no hypermobility of the nerve. Of course, if there were such hypermobility, the diagnosis would hardly be likely to be in doubt.

Treatment

The object of treatment is to intervene before axonal degeneration has begun, but to hold off in cases in which spontaneous recovery can be expected. In early cases, and particularly in the case of thin patients, it is always worth trying a 3 month period of protection with the "cubital sleeve". Spontaneous resolution is unlikely if there is:

- chronic affection of the elbow joint leading to osteophytosis, effusion or synovial thickening
- serious valgus deformity of the elbow or local bony abnormality
- deep affection of the nerve with loss of sensibility
- recurrent subluxation of the ulnar nerve over the medial condyle, weakness, wasting and abnormal electrical reactions in the muscles.

Treatment by operation

Methods short of surgery really have no place in this condition. Three methods are available:

- simple decompression by division of the arcade of the flexor carpi ulnaris (Osborne 1970)
- removal of the ulnar nerve from the area of danger
- removal of a cause of danger; namely, the medial epicondyle of the humerus.

Simple decompression (Osborne 1957, 1970) is adequate in most cases. A recent study by Nathan et al (1995) showed good or excellent relief after decompression of 164 nerves in 131 patients. Over 0.8–12 years (average 4.3 years) good relief was maintained in 79%. Their predictors of good outcome were: absence of subluxation after operation, greater body weight and normal two-point discrimination before operation. The ulnar nerve is displayed through a short medial incision running distally from the level of the medial epicondyle. The arcuate ligament is divided and fibres of the flexor carpi ulnaris are separated (Fig. 12.42). The nerve is inspected before and after release of the cuff, and the area is inspected to exclude the possibility of a compressing agent such as a ganglion. The cuff is released and haemostasis secured. Osborne (1970) sutured the arcuate ligament deep to the ulnar nerve to provide a bed for it, but we have not followed this practice. The skin is closed. There is no need for any immobilisation; indeed, immobilisation could lead to tethering and to later trouble.

Transposition is necessary when there is:

- severe deformity
- extreme osteophytosis
- recurrent subluxation over the medial epicondyle
- recurrence of signs of nerve compression after simple decompression.

Both the surgeon and the patient must recognise the limitations and hazards of this procedure. A bloodless field

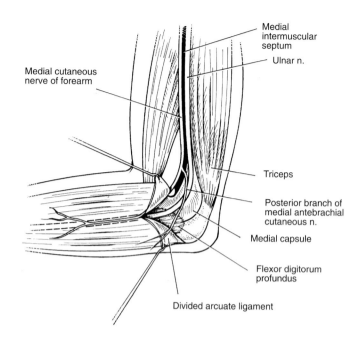

Fig. 12.42 Simple decompression of the ulnar nerve.

and general anaesthesia are necessary. The long posteromedial incision starts 10 cm above the medial epicondyle and ends 10 cm below it. The anterior skin flap is raised in its full thickness. Special care must be taken to identify and preserve the posterior terminal branch of the medial cutaneous nerve of the forearm, which runs obliquely in an awkward position distal to the medial epicondyle. Now the flexor origin and the undisplaced ulnar nerve are displayed. In the next step the ulnar nerve is mobilised, with its extrinsic axial vessels, from about 8 cm above to 6 cm below the epicondyle. Above the epicondyle mobilisation is effected simply by division of the overlying fascia; below it, the arcuate ligament has to be divided and the two parts of the flexor carpi ulnaris separated. In the lower part the uppermost muscular branches are displayed and mobilised, either with the main nerve or away from it. Now the medial intermuscular septum is excised (Fig. 12.43).

Subcutaneous transfer is recommended in most cases. The nerve is lifted from its bed and rerouted in front of the medial epicondyle and the flexor origin, care being taken to avoid kinking or obstruction at either end of the altered course. The cuff is deflated and bleeding is controlled. The two heads of the flexor carpi ulnaris can be brought together above the point of re-entry of the ulnar nerve, but there must be no constriction at that point. It is quite a good plan to put two or three sutures between the subcutaneous fat and the underlying aponeurosis of the flexor origin in order to retain the nerve in its new course. The skin is closed over a suction drain. In order to lessen adhesions around the transposed nerve, gentle movement of the elbow is encouraged after 24 hours.

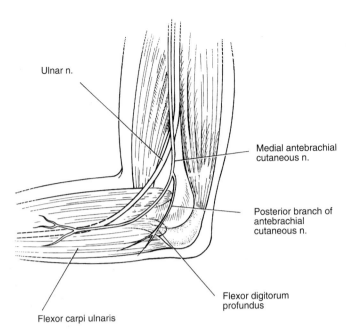

Ulnar n.

Medial antebrachial cutaneous n.

Posterior branch of antebrachial cutaneous n.

Flexor digitorum profundus

Flexor carpi ulnaris

Fig. 12.43 Anterior subcutaneous transposition of the ulnar nerve.

We are sure that there is no place for intramuscular transposition; we are increasingly unsure whether there is a case for submuscular transposition as advised by Seddon (1975h). That was, in effect, the technique described by Learmonth (1942), in which the ulnar nerve is laid alongside the median nerve. This is the technique described and used by Leffert (1972), who acknowledged its attribution to Learmonth and commented on its limitations. We have seen constriction, adhesion and distortion of the nerve in the submuscular bed, just as we have seen them in the intramuscular bed. Clearly, recurrence of neuropathy after intramuscular transposition is likely to require submuscular placing: adhesion would be inevitable if the intramuscular course were altered to a subcutaneous one. For submuscular transposition the superficial flexor muscles are divided about 2.5 cm distal to the medial epicondyle, and any tendinous connections are divided to provide an even, straight bed for the nerve. The nerve is raised and placed in this bed, so as to lie straight with the elbow flexed to a right angle. The cuff is deflated and bleeding is checked. The aponeurosis over the flexor origin is repaired with interrupted sutures. The mobility of the nerve in its new bed is checked and the skin is closed. A plaster is applied to hold the elbow at a right angle and to prevent extension of the wrist. It is retained for 2 weeks.

Difficulties and complications. Although generally good results after transposition are recorded by Vanderpool et al (1968), Campbell et al (1988) and Santa et al (1991), there are serious potential drawbacks.

The most serious early complication is devascularisation of the nerve by the mobilisation. This may be followed by complete and permanent paralysis. Seddon (1975h) did not perhaps stress sufficiently the risks or the severity of this complication, relying too much on the conception of the intrinsic axial blood supply of the nerve. This possibility of devascularisation is the single greatest argument in favour of restricting operation to simple decompression whenever possible. Devascularisation is followed not only by paralysis but often by severe and persistent pain. The pain is causalgic in nature; sometimes, it is shown to be dependent on sympathetic activity. Evidently impressed by the danger of devascularisation, Messina and Messina (1995) went to great lengths to preserve not only the axial extrinsic blood supply but also the segmented vessels. Their results were excellent, apparently in no way marred by the use of intramuscular placing of the nerve.

If haemostasis is inadequate, a large haematoma can accumulate under the flap and is liable to cause fibrosis, adhesion and constriction. Later consequences are failure to relieve symptoms and recurrence of symptoms after a period of relief. Early failure may, of course, be due to misdiagnosis; it may also be due to technical defect in transposition leaving the nerve kinked or trapped by an intramuscular septum. Late recurrence is most often caused by distortion by fibrous tissue, sometimes associated with intraneural fibrosis. In these cases, in which a lesion of the nerve at the elbow is plainly confirmed by clinical and electrophysiological evidence, there is a case for one further local intervention. The re-exploration and neurolysis of an ulnar nerve after a previous transposition is often difficult, time consuming and unrewarding.

Removal of the medial epicondyle

King and Morgan (1959) reported on late results of removing the medial epicondyle for traumatic ulnar neuritis. They had good results in 50% of their 20 cases. Magalon et al (1993) include this method as one of the three in current use. They describe it as an extension of simple decompression. The periosteum and the relevant part of the flexor origin are stripped from the epicondyle, which is then removed. The flexor origin is then sutured to the periosteal flap. The nerve is allowed to slide forward into the bed formed by the periosteum. Clearly, the danger of devascularising the nerve is much less in this procedure than it is in transposition.

Results

The results of transposition, and to a lesser extent of simple decompression of the ulnar nerve, are less predictable than are those of decompression of the median nerve. Even if transposition is properly done, with the correct indications, lasting success is obtained in scarcely more than three out of four cases.

THE LESS COMMON ENTRAPMENT SYNDROMES

There are a number of entrapment syndromes which, though much less common and sometimes less well defined than the three leaders, ought to be recognised and treated. In some, treatment is rapidly and remarkably successful. We shall take the syndromes in descending order: first down the upper limb, then down the lower limb. We have in fact put all the lower limb syndromes into this category, though we are uneasily aware that "Morton's metatarsalgia" has a claim to a place among the leaders. Some of these lesions arouse particular interest because they affect nerves that have no cutaneous sensory distribution. Yet in many cases entrapment of such nerves produces pain, sometimes as the sole presenting symptom. We stress again the afferent component in peripheral nerves commonly regarded as being "purely motor"; we stress too the point that not all the afferent fibres in those nerves convey impulses from the muscle spindles. Some – perhaps those reaching the centre by the anterior roots – are capable of conveying the sensation of pain.

THE UPPER LIMB

The nerve to the serratus anterior

The distinction between a true entrapment syndrome of the nerve to the serratus anterior and neuralgic amyotrophy or true traction injury is very difficult. Certainly, there are cases of sudden pain associated with paralysis of the serratus anterior which seem to depend on pressure from without. There are also cases in which there seems to be an element of traction by sudden or repeated depression of the forequarter. Gozna and Harris (1979) described 14 cases of such injury followed by "traumatic winging of the scapula". Gregg et al (1979) described 10 cases of "traction injury to the nerve to serratus anterior". Kaplan (1980) indicated the role of electrodiagnosis in such cases.

In one of our cases, a 21-year-old man presented with persistent paralysis of the right serratus anterior (that of the dominant upper limb) which had been present for 3 years. It had begun suddenly, with pain, after lifting heavy weights above shoulder level. Over the years the discomfort lessened, but the winging of the scapula persisted. The nerve to the serratus anterior was explored: it was found to be compressed by a small band of muscle which did not conform with the usual anatomy; it was also tethered at this level (Fig. 12.44). There was progressive recovery in the serratus anterior.

We have gradually come to the view that there is a true syndrome of entrapment of the nerve to the serratus anterior, arising in people who lift heavy weights or push heavy objects. Both these avocations require stabilisation of the forequarter on the chest wall and are commonly associated with a strong sustained inspiration. Both actions

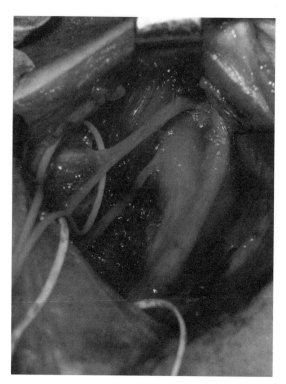

Fig. 12.44 The nerve to serratus anterior (centre) compressed near its origin.

bring the scalenus medius into action to stabilise the first rib and the thoracic cage; in both, there is a liability to trapping of the nerve to the serratus at or near its point of emergence from the muscle. Repeated actions of the type described are likely to confirm the entrapment.

The suprascapular nerve

Hadley et al (1986) ascribe the first description of entrapment of the suprascapular nerve to Kopell and Thompson (1959). They reported the cases of seven patients whose predominant symptom was pain. In 1981, Ganzhorn et al described a case in which the nerve was compressed by a cyst at the lateral border of the scapular spine. Sjöstrom and Mjöberg (1992) described a case associated with arthrodesis of the shoulder (scapulohumeral) joint. Mizuno et al (1990) described a case in which entrapment was apparently secondary to paralysis of the trapezius muscle from section of the spinal accessory nerve. Decompression produced relief. This important case certainly raises the question of how often the pain experienced after division of the spinal accessory nerve is caused by entrapment of the stretched suprascapular nerve.

The suprascapular nerve, which contains mainly fibres from the fifth and some from the fourth and sixth cervical nerves, arises from the upper trunk of the plexus and runs caudally and laterally to reach the supraspinatus muscle through a notch in the upper border of the scapula, completed into a foramen either by a ligament (the upper transverse, scapular, or suprascapular ligament) or by a bridge of bone. Supplying the supraspinatus it goes on to supply the infraspinatus muscle. It has no cutaneous sensory distribution. The scene is well set for entrapment: the scapula is very mobile on the thorax and axial skeleton; any local cyst or lipoma is likely to produce compression. Narakas (1993a) records that in 6 of his 12 cases pain was the primary complaint; in the other 6 there was progressive wasting of the spinati. He found a "huge spindle form pseudoneuroma … in front of the ligament that crosses the notch".

It is, evidently, necessary to be aware of this lesion in dealing with patients with scapular pain and in particular those with wasting of the spinati. Operation for decompression is described by Hadley et al (1986), Birch (1995) and Copeland (1995b). The approach is considered in Chapter 7. We have seen and treated three cases of entrapment of the suprascapular nerve: all were in men whose work involved lifting or working with heavy weights. There was, in all cases, electrophysiological evidence of involvement of the nerve. In all, pain was relieved by operation; in one, function was improved.

Quadrilateral space syndrome

Formerly, all aspirants in medicine in the UK were taught about the "quadrilateral space" formed medially by the long head of the triceps, laterally by the humerus, above by the subscapularis and teres minor, and below by the teres major amd latissimus dorsi (Fig. 12.45). The space transmits the circumflex nerve and the posterior circumflex humeral artery. Doubtless this antique teaching has been superseded by more important concepts; nevertheless, the quadrilateral space still makes itself felt. Cahill and Palmer (1983) recognised in young adults a syndrome of pain and paraesthesiae in the region of the shoulder. Their attention was first drawn to the syndrome in patients in whom operation for presumed thoracic outlet syndrome had failed to give relief. They noted provocation of symptoms by flexion of the shoulder and by abduction and

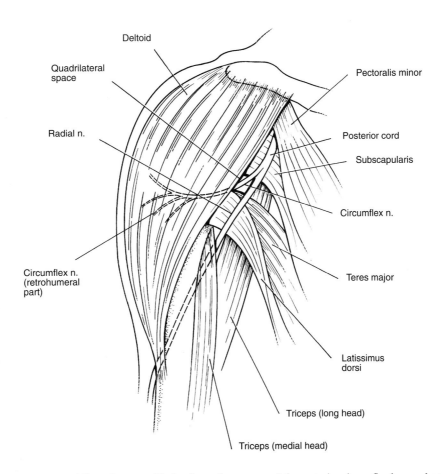

Fig. 12.45 The quadrilateral space, with the circumflex nerve and the posterior circumflex humeral artery.

lateral rotation, discrete local tenderness posteriorly and occasional nocturnal symptoms. In 2 of 18 patients the deltoid muscle was affected. Decompression, if necessary with detachment of teres minor, gave relief.

Redler et al (1986) reported the case of right-sided affection in a 20-year-old right-handed baseball pitcher "capable of a 95 mph fastball". It is perhaps fortunate for British clinicians and sportsmen that baseball has not yet caught on in the UK. This patient complained of a numb shoulder, with radiation of the pain down the arm. Hyperabduction and lateral rotation of the shoulder produced severe pain. Electromyographic and nerve conduction studies gave normal results, but arteriography showed occlusion of the posterior circumflex humeral artery with full abduction and lateral rotation of the shoulder. The athlete altered his pitching action, and for a time at least obtained relief. Cormier et al (1988) described another case in a baseball pitcher, and Dawson et al (1990b) observed the condition in "a member of a rowing team". Clearly, both artery and nerve are compressed, especially when there is hypertrophy or swelling of the muscles forming the boundaries of the space. It seems likely that most of the symptoms arise from compression of the nerve, which of course has a cutaneous sensory distribution. The principal importance of this syndrome may lie in the necessity to distinguish it from thoracic outlet compression and from disorders of the rotator cuff. This must be a rare condition. We have seen and treated only one patient with true compression of the neurovascular bundle in the quadrilateral space. In this case, and in two or three cases in which operation was not done, constriction was primarily caused by fracture through the neck of the humerus. In another case a terminal neuroma of the circumflex nerve ruptured in association with humeral fracture was resected. There was relief of symptoms in both cases.

The "supracondylar spur"

Bland-Sutton (1920) illustrated the "supracondyloid foramen" of the lion's humerus with the median nerve and brachial artery passing through it. He wrote "In Man the most frequent condition of this foramen, when existing, is to have the upper part of the ring formed by an osseous overgrowth from a humeral shaft, named the supracondylar process; the lower part of the ring is completed by a band of fibrous tissue extending to the internal condyle" (Fig. 12.46).

In 1966, Kessel and Rang reported two cases in which the presence of a supracondylar spur had produced symptoms. In the first case, the median nerve and brachial artery, and the ulnar artery, accompanying the median nerve through the "foramen", was chiefly affected. In 1972, Symeonides reported two further cases, in both of which the median nerve was affected. He gave a wide range

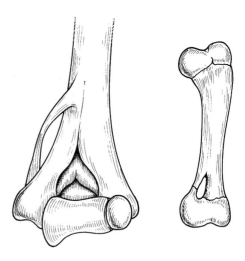

Fig. 12.46 Bland-Sutton's (1920) drawing of the supracondylar foramen in man (left) and the humerus of a fetal lion (right). Note the formation of the foramen in the fetal specimen.

for the incidence of the supracondylar spur (0.28–2.7%). Evidently, the presence of the spur is only rarely associated with symptoms of interference with neural and arterial function. Affection of the ulnar nerve by the spur is even less common than are those of the median nerve and ulnar artery.

Kessel and Rang (1966) ascribed to Struthers (1848) the early description of the supracondylar ligament and spur. Struthers himself found seven instances, and found the records of seven more. In one-third of his cases there was a high division of the "humeral" (Brachial) artery. Bland-Sutton (1920) seems to regard the "ligament of Struthers" as the vestigial lower part of "a climbing muscle conspicuous in most arboreal mammals", the dorsoepitrochlearis.

The possibility of the production of symptoms by a supracondylar spur and ligament must evidently be borne in mind when a young patient presents with symptoms of affection of the median nerve, ulnar artery or both, or even affection of the ulnar nerve

The radial nerve in the arm, at the elbow and below the elbow

Lotem et al (1971) described three instances of acute onset of weakness and alteration of sensibility in the distribution of the radial nerve following strenuous muscular effort. All three patients were manual workers; in all, short-lasting conduction block of the radial nerve followed a period of strenuous muscular effort. Lotem et al showed rather convincingly a probable site of entrapment against the bone by the arch of the origin of the lateral head of the triceps muscle. Wilhelm (1993) examined the matter further, adding 27 cases, at least two of which, and perhaps as many as seven, were similar to those reported by Lotem and colleagues. Most of the lesions in his series were, however, caused by chronic trauma. Although the cases of acute compression of the trunk of the radial nerve against the bone form a separate category, the syndrome seems always to shade into the "radial tunnel syndrome" postulated by Roles and Maudsley (1972). In 1979, Lister et al explored the matter further, and exactly defined their conception of a "radial tunnel".

Roles and Maudsley (1972) introduced the concept of entrapment of the radial nerve as a cause of "resistant" tennis elbow. They named this condition "radial tunnel syndrome", and described 36 cases to illustrate their point. The radial nerve enters its tunnel as it pierces the lateral intermuscular septum to lie between the brachialis muscle medially and the brachioradialis and later the long radial extensor muscles laterally. The nerve divides into a superficial (cutaneous sensory) and a deep (posterior interosseous; no cutaneous sensory distribution) branch at or about elbow level. At elbow level the nerves are, say Roles and Maudsley, "tethered to the capsule of the radio-humeral joint". Further distally the origin of the extensor carpi radialis brevis forms the lateral wall of the tunnel. Then the posterior interosseous nerve enters the supinator muscle under the "arcade of Frohse" (Frohse & Fränkel 1908). These authors give details of their 36 patients with "resistant tennis elbow", most of whom obtained a good or excellent result after operation for decompression of the radial nerve and its branches. In one case there was electromyographic evidence of severe entrapment, with fibrillation potentials; in six others, the diagnosis was "confirmed by EMG". In their electromyographic studies in cases of "epicondylalgia", Bence et al (1978) found a much higher incidence of electromyographic abnormalities. On the basis of conduction studies they classified cases as follows: arising from affection of nerve, either radicular or distal; arising from a humeroradial joint or the epicondylar muscles; and arising from a general disturbance of neuromuscular function.

Nakano (1978) confirmed this impression of entrapment by the fibrous edge of the extensor carpi radialis brevis, but Gelberman et al (1993) refer to this syndrome as "dubious". Narakas and Bonnard (1993) discussing "epicondylalgia" assigned the most prominent role to a tendinopathy at the epicondylar insertion, and indeed those who have seen acute calcific deposit in this site have little doubt about this. He named entrapment of the radial nerve or its terminal branches as a cause in 5–10% of cases. That seems to us to be a sensible view of the situation. It is indeed likely that the detachment of the extensor origin practised for "resistant tennis elbow" would in many cases relieve an unsuspected entrapment of the radial nerve at and below epicondylar level. However, clinicians confronted with "resistant tennis elbow" should be ready to stop and consider whether the cause may be entrapment, and whether operation should go further than simple release of the extensor origin.

The posterior interosseous nerve

The syndrome of entrapment of the posterior interosseous nerve is well established. Woltmann and Learmonth (1934) described five cases of "progressive paralysis of the nervus interosseus dorsalis," in one of which operation was done. The nerve was found to be lying between the supinator and its aponeurosis. It was released, but after 10 months there was no improvement. Thirty-two years later the matter was brought back to the attention of clinicians by four papers in the *British Journal of Bone and Joint Surgery* (Capener 1966, Bowen & Stone 1966, Mulholland 1966, Sharrard 1966). In Capener's case the entrapment was produced by a lipoma; in Bowen and Stone's case the cause was a ganglion. In two of Sharrard's six cases a benign tumour was responsible for the entrapment, and in Mulholland's remarkable case paralysis occurred years after recovery from a "wrist drop" produced by an injection. Spinner (1968) defined the role of the "arcade of Frohse" (Frohse & Fränkel 1908) in causing compression of the nerve. The role of rheumatoid synovitis in precipitating compression was noted by Marmor et al (1967), and later by Millender et al (1973) and White et al (1988). In 14 of Cravens and Kline's (1990) series of 32 lesions of the posterior interosseous nerve, "entrapment" was the cause. The "supinator channel syndrome" described by Blom et al (1971) seems to be an acute variant. Other causes of compression have been described: an enlarged bicipital bursa (Spinner et al 1993); vasculitis of the nerve (Hashizume et al 1993); intraneural ganglion (Hashizume et al 1995a); synovial haemangioma (Busa et al 1995); and multiple constrictions (Kotani et al 1995). The case of "delayed posterior interosseous nerve palsy" described by Hashizume et al (1995b) seems not to have been associated with any identified precipitating factor.

Clearly, compression of the posterior interosseous nerve is, in many cases, determined by an identifiable cause such as a benign tumour or swelling of the underlying synovial membrane and associated effusion in the joint. It is perhaps in less than half of cases that there is a simple "entrapment" at the arcade of Frohse over the nerve at its entry into the supinator muscle. Because the nerve is affected below the origin of the branches to the radial extensor muscles of the wrist, paralysis is confined to the extensors of the fingers and the ulnar extensor of the wrist. Thus active extension of the wrist is possible, but the extended hand tends to deviate radially. The entrapment can be entirely painless, but evidently in a number of cases there is radiated pain. The posterior interosseous nerve has no cutaneous sensory component, so pain presumably arises from compression of small myelinated afferent fibres or from supramaximal stimulation of large afferents from muscle spindles.

Treatment and results

There seems to be little evidence that the lesion of the posterior interosseous nerve, once begun, is spontaneously reversible. Indeed, the evidence is that there is a case for early intervention to:

- prevent deterioration to the point at which axonal degeneration has progressed to cause affection of the motor end-plates
- establish or deny presence of a clear cause such as rheumatoid arthropathy or benign tumour.

We think that the nerve is best exposed through a postero-lateral incision with forward reflection of the extensor muscles from their origin on the lateral epicondyle. Roles and Maudsley (1972), aiming for both terminal branches of the radial nerve, preferred to gain access to them on the other side of the extensor muscles, but we have preferred the older way. The nerve should be exposed from its origin to as far down in the supinator muscle as is necessary to ensure that there is no residual compression. Any lesion of the elbow joint or in the course of the nerve is, of course, dealt with *secundum artem*. In two of our cases, in neither of which pain was a symptom and in both of which the "silent" paralysis had progressed to paralysis and wasting, there was no recovery after operation in which the nerve was simply decompressed. It is evidently necessary to be aware of this syndrome and to be prepared to act before the changes in the muscle are irreversible. In cases of rheumatoid arthritis, paralysis of the extensors of the fingers may wrongly be attributed to tendon rupture. We have seen and treated three other patients with this condition: a 77 year old with symptoms starting 50 years after a Monteggia fracture–dislocation, and two children (a boy aged 14 and a girl aged 8 years) with hypertrophic neuropathy.

The median nerve in the forearm

The "pronator syndrome"

This, like the "quadrilateral space syndrome", is an affection of nerve apparently brought about by muscular effort, independent of any underlying abnormality of the nerve or the adjacent tissues.

Seyfarrth (1951) described "primary myosis" in the pronator teres as cause of "lesion of the N. medianus (pronator syndrome)". Marris and Peters followed in 1976 with a description of seven cases, describing clinical and electrophysiological features. All their cases occurred in men, all were related to muscular effort, and all manifested motor and sensory symptoms. Johnson et al (1979) were able to report on 71 cases, in 51 of which operation was required. The sites of compression were at the aponeurosis of the biceps (lacertus fibrous) the pronator teres or the arch of origin of the superficial flexor muscles.

King and Dunkerton (1982) presented four cases and dissected 40 limbs. Operation was done in all four cases.

The history is of paraesthesiae and numbness in the distribution of the median nerve, usually in the dominant upper limb, provoked by muscular effort such as writing, repetitive actions with the limb and similar activity. The important site of compression is in the median nerve's passage between the heads of the pronator teres muscle, where there may be a fibrous band. In one of King and Dunkerton's cases the compression was quite clearly caused by the aponeurosis of the biceps, and in another the junction of the two roots of the median nerve was below the level of the pronator teres. In that case it was the medial root that was compressed by a fibrous band in the pronator teres. In well-marked cases there is weakness, wasting and alteration of sensibility in the area of distribution of the median nerve. Weakness may be brought about by a period of exercise. When the compression is at the level of the biceps aponeurosis, there is weakness of the pronator teres, with a positive Tinel sign over the median nerve at this level.

Although steroid injection may give temporary relief (even lasting relief according to Seyfarrth), it seems that most patients with this trouble will need operation if they are to continue with the activity that provoked it. The median nerve must be exposed above, at and below elbow level, and traced through the pronator teres. Any constricting band or bands must be divided; if this seems necessary, the deep head of pronator teres can be divided.

Our experience with this syndrome is limited to three cases, in none of which was decompression followed by motor recovery.

The anterior interosseous nerve

As the median nerve passes between the deep and superficial heads of the pronator teres, it gives off from its deep surface the anterior interosseous nerve. This nerve then passes down the deep compartment of the forearm anterior to the interosseous membrane and deep to the deep flexors of the thumb and fingers. It supplies the long flexor of the thumb and the radial part of the deep flexor of the fingers. The nerve finishes deep to the pronator quadratus, supplying its deep part and the distal radioulnar and radiocarpal joints. There is no cutaneous sensory distribution.

Parsonage and Turner (1948), writing on the larger subject of "neuralgic amyotrophy", included one case of affection of the anterior interosseous nerve. Kiloh and Nevin (1952) described two cases of "isolated neuritis of the anterior interosseous nerve", and the term "Kiloh–Nevin syndrome" has since then from time to time been attached to this entrapment. Fearn and Goodfellow (1965) described the case of a 9-year-old boy with complete paralysis of the flexor longus pollicis and the deep flexor of the index finger. Operating, they found the nerve compressed 1 cm below its origin by a crescentic band continuous distally with the aponeurosis in the deep surface of the superficial (humeral) head of pronator teres. Three years later Sharrard (1968) and Vichare (1968) recorded between them five more cases, and confirmed that this was indeed a true entrapment, not apparently dependent on muscular effort. Spinner (1970) added 10 cases, and made anatomical studies of the region in 25 cadavers. The impression is that the constriction is either by a tendinous origin of the deep (ulnar) head of pronator teres, by thickening of the fascia over the deep flexors or by tendinous fibres in the deep part of the superficial (humeral) head of the pronator teres. The symptoms are predominantly motor, affecting the long flexor of the thumb and the radial part of the deep flexor of the fingers. Indeed, Marris and Peters (1976) claimed that "the anterior interosseous nerve entrapment syndrome [was] unique in lacking sensory symptoms". They were not quite right: no one is ever quite right; nothing is ever unique in medicine. There was pain in one of Kiloh and Nevin's cases. Why not? The anterior interosseous nerve presumably has its full complement of afferent fibres from muscle spindles and from endings in muscle. In an important paper, Seror (1996) describes findings in 13 patients with lesions of the anterior interosseous nerve referred for electrodiagnosis. Seror's conclusion that "operation is not to be considered for a year" because late spontaneous recovery may occur, may need modification. The extent of recovery was "unknown" in six cases; spontaneous recovery was seen chiefly in those cases in which paralysis had been produced by an "unusual effort". It may be that there are two forms of this disorder:

- an acute, recoverable, form in which the lesion is produced by a mechanism similar to that in "pronator syndrome"
- a chronic progressive form in which the lesion is caused and perpetuated by a persistent local abnormality.

Evidently, operation could be deferred in the acute form, but should not be delayed in the chronic progressive variety. Seror's comment on diagnosis is apposite: in only three cases was the correct diagnosis made before referral for electrodiagnosis.

Operation to expose the anterior interosseous nerve involves lifting the superficial flexors from their radial origin and retracting them and the pronator teres to show the deep compartment. The median nerve is usually attached loosely by areolar tissue to the deep surface of the flexor superficialis. The anterior interosseous nerve must be exposed from its origin and freed from any constricting agent in either head of the pronator teres or in the fascia over the deep flexors.

Two of our patients with entrapment of the anterior interosseous nerve presented at a late stage, with severe weakness and wasting. Both were male; one was in his teens and the other was in his thirties. Operation was done in both cases, and in both the constricting agent was thought to be a tendinous band in the deep (ulnar) head of pronator teres. In both cases, it seems, operation came too late: there was no improvement during the period of observation. In this as in other entrapment syndromes it will not do to wait until there are irreversible changes in muscle.

The ulnar nerve at the wrist and in the hand

Although Harrelson and Newman (1975) and Holtzmann et al (1984) have described entrapment of the ulnar nerve in the forearm, the level next most common after the elbow is at the wrist and in the hand.

Harris (1929) drew attention to "occupational" pressure neuritis of the deep palmar branch of the ulnar nerve. He described two cases, both in men, in which repeated external trauma had damaged the deep branch of the ulnar nerve. The situation of the ulnar nerve, and of its deep (motor) branch in particular, at the wrist and in the proximal part of the hand, is such as to predispose to compression if there is an additional occupant of "Guyon's space" (Guyon 1861). Seddon (1952) drew attention to affection of the deep branch by ganglia here, and in the same years Brooks' article on nerve compression by ganglia included three cases in which the ulnar nerve was affected at the wrist or in the hand. Shea and McClain (1969) defined the syndromes and described their various causes, and Lamb (1970) contributed 18 cases of compression of the ulnar nerve at the wrist and in the hand. Vanderpool et al (1968), in a general review of ulnar nerve entrapment, included cases of distal affection, and defined "Guyon's tunnel". Dupont et al (1965) described four cases, in one of which the lesion was caused by acute thromboangiitis of the ulnar artery. In the second case a ganglion was found, and in the other two there was persistent oedema after injury.

At the wrist the ulnar nerve, having given off its dorsal sensory branch, first passes superficial to the flexor retinaculum, deep to its superficial layer, medial to the ulnar artery. Here it divides into superficial (sensory) and deep (motor) branches. Both enter Guyon's (1861) space. Denman (1978) provides a good description and a good drawing of this space, which is floored by the pisohamate and pisometacarpal ligaments, roofed by the palmaris brevis muscle and the distal part of the superficial layer of the retinaculum, bounded medially by the pisiform bone and laterally by the hook of the hamate bone (Fig. 12.47). Denman (1978) suggests the term "pisoretinacular space" to replace the eponym. The nerve divides into its terminal branches. The deep branch passes between the flexor brevis and abductor muscles, pierces the opponens muscle, runs across the deep compartment of the palm to supply

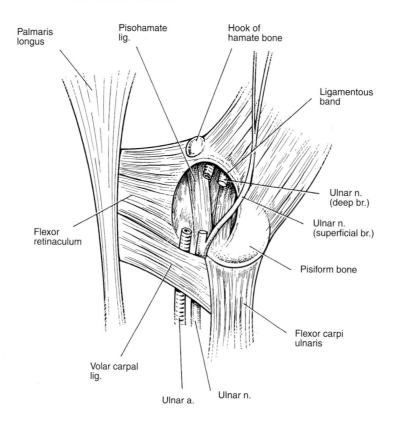

Fig. 12.47 Guyon's space. Note the possibilities for entrapment at and distal to the volar carpal ligament.

interossei and terminates in the adductor pollicis. It usually supplies part or all of the flexor brevis pollicis (Rowntree 1949). The superficial branch emerges over the hamate attachment of the flexor retinaculum to enter the palm, where it branches into digital nerves supplying the skin of the little finger and of the ulnar side of the ring finger.

Shea and McClain (1969) usefully define the ulnar nerve compression syndromes here according to the level of affection. In the first category there is compression in or proximal to the pisoretinacular space, so that both motor and cutaneous sensory functions are involved. In the second category, compression in the distal part of the space produces motor affection only. In the third category, caused in this case by nonunion of a fracture of the hook of the hamate bone, there is sensory affection only.

The causes of affection are variously described. The most common lesion is a ganglion (Brooks 1952, Seddon 1952, Shea and McClain 1969). McFarland and Hoffer (1971) reported a lipoma. Upton et al (1978) sought a neuropathic cause in rheumatoid arthritis, but could not find any instance of this in this site. Kalisman et al (1982) found compression by a false aneurysm. The finding of thromboangiitis of the ulnar artery by Dupont et al (1965) has been mentioned. Budny et al (1992) describe a case of entrapment by a nodule of "localised nodular synovitis".

It is easy to recognise the lesion when the patient presents with motor and sensory symptoms and signs, the alteration or loss of sensibility sparing the distribution of the dorsal branch. Presentation with weakness and wasting alone can cause difficulty; we have seen cases in which the signs were taken as those of the early stages of motor neuron disease. When there is a local cause apart from external trauma, there is usually tenderness and even a positive Tinel sign over the site of compression. Electromyography is confirmatory. Lesions of the deep branch of the ulnar nerve are famously recoverable, so long as the noxious agent is removed. Victor Horsley noted this as long ago as 1899; we have seen it in a case in which the deep branch was severed by plate glass and never formally repaired, yet regenerated sufficiently to restore bulk to the previously paralysed and wasted intrinsic muscles. There is in fact a case for exploration in all cases in which an external cause has been excluded and in which there is serious and persistent motor affection. The nerve is exposed from just above the wrist and right through the pisoretinacular space, and any causative lesion is found and removed. In three instances in which this was done and a ganglion was found and removed, there was full recovery. We have also found two lipomata, one schwannoma and one aneurysm of the ulnar artery.

THE PELVIS AND LOWER LIMB

"Meralgia paraesthetica"

Entrapment of the lateral cutaneous nerve of the thigh at the level of the inguinal ligament has a long and distinguished history. Seddon (1975h) assigned to Roth (1895a and b) and Bernhardt (1895) the credit for the original description. The last was not, alas, related to the divine Sarah, but, as Williams and Trzil (1991) remind us, it was his description which prompted Sigmund Freud (1895) to relate his own experience. It was indeed in this year, as the historian Claudio Magris and the monument in the Himmelstrasse remind us, that the secret of dreams was revealed to the Viennese physician (Magris 1989). Freud had observed "five to seven" cases; the knowledge of the syndrome brought to his notice the symptoms from which he had suffered intermittently over 5–6 years. Freud used the term *Bernhardt'sche Sensibilitätsstörung*, and noted possible causes such as "ileotyphus", lead poisoning, cold damage by the use of "very cold douches" and compression by the trouser band. Roth (1895) proposed the name "meralgia", derived from μηρος (meros, thigh) and αλγος (algos, pain).

Stookey (1928) noted many aetiological factors, and drew attention particularly to the role of standing and walking in the production of pain.

During the 1939–1945 war, the syndrome became familiar to medical officers who saw service men particularly exposed to the rigours of drilling on the barrack square. Ghent (1959) went very thoroughly into the varieties of passage of the lateral cutaneous nerve through the inguinal ligament (see Fig. 12.38). Nathan (1960) described a "fusiform enlargement" in the lateral cutaneous nerve of the thigh, and went very thoroughly into the wide variety of possible causes of pain and paraesthesiae affecting the lateral side of the thigh. In drawing attention to the change of course of the lateral cutaneous nerve as it negotiates the inguinal ligament, Edelson and Nathan (1977) examined Ghent's (1959) classification of the routes traversed. They found that passage through the sartorius was rare; they found too a high incidence of "gangliform" enlargement, noting that the thickening was caused by collagenisation rather than by mucoid degeneration. Jefferson and Eames (1979) examined 12 femoral cutaneous nerves taken at necropsy from persons dying without known disease of the peripheral nervous system. They found changes in five nerves: local demyelination, Wallerian degeneration, internodal swellings and endoneurial vascular thickening. The last was particularly seen in the nerve in the region of the inguinal ligament. Proposals regarding treatment have ranged from transposition (Keegan and Holyoke 1962) to resection of a length of nerve (Williams and Trzil 1991).

It is in its character as a symptom of underlying disease that this "entrapment" is particularly important. Krikler

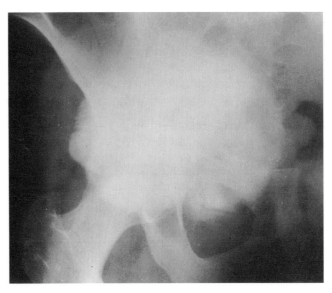

Fig. 12.48 Pelvic chondrosarcoma in a 17-year-old girl, who was initially treated for "meralgia paraesthetica".

and Grimer (1993) record the case of a pelvic chondrosarcoma presenting with "meralgia paraesthetica", and indeed that was the mode of presentation to us in 1960 of a young girl with that affliction (Fig. 12.48).

The symptoms are of pain, paraesthesiae and alteration of sensation affecting the lateral side of the thigh, made worse by standing and walking, and relieved by rest. There may be tenderness over the nerve in its transit of the inguinal ligament; there is an area of altered or absent sensation on the lateral side of the thigh. Conduction velocity along the nerve is affected (Savala et al 1979). Dawson et al (1990d) rightly remark that "differential diagnosis consists of an anatomic exercise to establish whether the lateral femoral cutaneous nerve is the only structure affected". The possibilities that must be excluded are:

- a general neuropathy
- a local manifestation of some other generalised condition
- a more proximal lesion of the second and third lumbar nerves
- local condition affecting the lumbar plexus or the lateral cutaneous nerve within the abdomen.

Perhaps in no other entrapment syndrome are there so many possibilities of missing an important and potentially serious underlying condition.

Treatment

Symptoms are, in most cases, mild. Often, particularly in pregnancy, they subside spontaneously. If symptoms are persistently troublesome, operation is probably the best course, though there is an incidence of failure with all methods. Dawson et al (1990c) recommend simple decompression by release of the entrapment in or under the inguinal ligament. Williams and Trzil (1991) favour resection of a length of nerve. We see this syndrome in its true form increasingly seldom; our preference is for simple decompression, having unavailingly sought to relieve intractable pain in four patients sent to us after section of the nerve.

Pudendal nerve entrapment

We have seen one instance of entrapment of the pudendal nerve at the entry to the perineum. In 1983, a 35-year-old woman presented with pain in the right side of the perineum, mostly present with sitting, but not associated in any way with visceral or sexual activity. There was a feeling of alteration of sensibility of the skin of the right side of the perineum. Pelvic examination showed no abnormality, though on rectal examination there was some tenderness on the right side. There was no objective sensory alteration. Radiographs showed no abnormality. Persistence of symptoms over a 6-month period of observation led to operation. The right pudendal nerve was exposed in the perineum by a right perineal incision. It was found undoubtedly compressed in the pudendal canal (Alcock's canal), and was released. There was no other lesion. The patient's symptoms were relieved and did not recur.

Our impression from this rapid and complete cure was that a speculative operation had proved a stroke of luck for the patient, rather than that a "new" entrapment syndrome had been revealed. It was only later that we became aware of the work of Amarenco et al (1987, 1988) and Robert et al (1989), and realised that we had forfeited a chance of lasting fame. The chagrin was shared by our colleague Mr Alasdair Fraser, whose advice on gynaecological aspects had been sought and who was present at the operation. Amarenco et al (1987) first described the syndrome of entrapment of the pudendal nerve in "Alcock's canal" or "perineal paralysis of the cyclist". They described five cases, the first, bilateral, in a 38-year-old man who had travelled "several hundred kilometres" on a cycle with a new saddle. Amarenco and colleagues expanded this description in 1988, reporting 15 cases of "perineal neuralgia" or "Alcock's canal syndrome" and adding the results of neurophysiological examination. Treatment was by steroid injection, with localisation by computed tomographic guidance. Robert et al (1989) made clinical, neurophysiological and anatomical studies, and reported on the results of nine operations aided by the use of a microscope.

The pudendal nerve, arising from the second, third and fourth sacral nerves, leaves the pelvis through the great sciatic foramen, and soon re-enters it through the lesser sciatic foramen. In its course on the medial side of the ischium it may be trapped between the ischial spine and the sacrotuberous ligament. Later the nerve or its branches may be trapped by the falciform edge of the ligament. Its vulnerability to external pressure during cycling is obvious; less obvious is a mechanism determining entrapment in the absence of such external pressure. Eight of Robert et al's (1989) patients were women; only one of these was a cyclist.

"Alcock's canal syndrome" or "perineal neuralgia" is, in our view, a true bill, easily explicable when it occurs in those who cycle long distances, but less easily explicable when there is no such association. General practitioners, orthopaedists and gynaecologists in particular should be aware of its existence and features, and of the possibilities offered by treatment. In the absence of this knowledge, sufferers may be dismissed, uncharitably and unfairly, as "a pain".

The piriformis syndrome

The piriformis syndrome is, like the quadrilateral space and pronator syndromes, dependent on muscular activity and hypertrophy. The sciatic nerve, with the inferior gluteal and pudendal nerves and the inferior gluteal vessels, leaves the pelvis through the lower part of the great sciatic foramen deep to the piriformis muscle running from the inner face of the bony pelvis to the great trochanter. The nerve passes over the tendon of the obturator internus muscle with the gemelli. There is an obvious liability to entrapment with hypertrophy or excess activity of the piriformis muscle. Solheim et al (1981) credited Yeoman (1928) with the first suggestion that the piriformis muscle had a role in the production of sciatica. Writing 6 years before Mixter and Barr (1934), Yeoman (1928) examined in particular the role of the sacroiliac joint in the production of sciatica. One of his conclusions was that "the symptoms are due to a periarthritis involving the anterior sacro iliac ligament, the pyriformis [sic] muscle,[1] and the adjacent radicals [sic] of the sciatic nerve, chiefly the first and second sacral nerves". Robinson (1947) raised the matter more definitely in his paper "Pyriformis [sic] syndrome in relation to sciatic pain", describing two cases of sciatica caused, apparently, by hypertrophy of the piriformis and relieved by section of the muscle. Mizuguchi (1976) enlarged the concept, describing division of the piriformis for the treatment of sciatica in 14 patients. In the same year, Pace and Nagle described the "piriform syndrome" as an entity to be distinguished from lumbar and sciatic pain of truly spinal origin. Their patients

---

[1]*Pirum* is Latin for pear; "piriformis" indicates "pear-shaped". πυρ (pur or pyr) is Greek for "fire"; the prefix "pyro-" signifies a connection with fire, as in pyrotechnics, pyromania, and so on. Pyrum was indeed an uncommon variant of *pirum*, but it is, we think, better to use the root "piri-" in order to avoid confusion.

(31 women and 6 men) showed no objective evidence of damage to the sciatic nerve. Adams (1980) added four cases, in one of which the nerve lay superficial to the muscle. Solheim et al (1981) described two cases of true "piriformis syndrome", both in women presenting with pain, paraesthesiae and local tenderness, and relieved by section of the muscle. Synek (1987) reviewed the literature and added one case. In our single case, a young man presented with pain, paraesthesiae and motor weakness. There was supporting electrophysiological evidence (Dr Nicholas Murray). At operation, there was clear evidence of entrapment at the level of the crossing of the sciatic nerve by the piriformis muscle. Division of the piriformis muscle was followed by complete and lasting relief.

Entrapment of the sciatic nerve at lower levels in the thigh has been reported by Banerjee and Hall (1976), Søgaard (1983), Venna et al (1991) and almost certainly by others. Banerjee and Hall described entrapment by a myofascial band in the lower thigh: Søgaard described entrapment by a similar band 10 cm distal to the fold of the buttock, and Venna and colleagues showed entrapment by a fibrovascular band in the thigh of a 12-year-old boy. Evidently, the clinician must be aware of these possibilities in dealing with otherwise unexplained cases of pain and paraesthesia in the distribution of the sciatic nerve.

The common peroneal nerve at the knee

The common peroneal nerve as it winds round the neck of the fibula is clearly as vulnerable to external trauma as is the ulnar nerve at the elbow. It is also vulnerable to pressure by a ganglion arising from the upper tibiofibular joint or other space-occupying lesion. It may truly be entrapped by the arch of origin of the peroneus longus muscle.

Ellis (1936) and Brooks (1952) wrote about the curious ganglia that affect this part of this nerve and seem rarely to affect similarly any other nerve. There is no evidence that these ganglia represent cystic degeneration of Schwannomata; rather, the histological evidence indicates that they are simple, often multilocular, ganglia. In the first of Parkes' (1961) cases, histological examination showed that the cysts were "situated between fascicles of nerve fibres". Ellis' description of them as cystic degeneration of nerve sheath was probably incorrect, but he rightly pointed to the hazards of removal. Brooks differentiated the ganglion that was separate from the nerve from that seemingly intrinsic to it, and warned of the dangers of removal of ganglia of the latter type. Gurdjian et al (1965) described one case of ganglion in the common peroneal nerve and one of ganglion in the ulnar nerve. In both, there was impairment of motor function, which was reduced after operation. Cobb and Moiel (1974) added two cases of ganglion affecting the common peroneal nerve. There were motor signs in both; both were improved

after operation. They reviewed 26 other cases, and had the impression that most improved or recovered after operation.

Seddon (1975e) says that the "cyst causes more or less paralysis", but in fact the presentation is as likely to be with pain or swelling as with motor deficit. All Parkes' (1961) seven patients presented with pain; there was apparently only one with serious motor affection. In that case the anterior tibial muscles were affected. Clark (1961) analysed the cases previously reported and three new ones: there was a high incidence of motor affection in the 15 cases collected. On the other hand, Stack et al (1965), reporting on nine cases, found pain the most common presenting symptom and paralysis the presenting symptom in one case only. Parkes (1961) draws attention to the important differential diagnosis from central nerve root irritation.

The diagnosis of ganglion of the common peroneal nerve must be borne in mind when a patient presents with a pain in the leg, a swelling in the region of the nerve and possibly weakness of the anterior tibial muscles. There is no alternative to the recommendation of exploration, but the risks to conducting tissue attaching to removal must be exposed to the patient. Exploration will soon reveal the extent of the attachment of the ganglion to the nerve. If it is clear early that

- the swelling is a ganglion
- the ganglion is intimately associated with the nerve,

it is sufficient to act as Parkes recommends and ablate the pedicle and decompress the ganglion by incision and expression of contents. Failure to identify and remove the pedicle is likely to lead to recurrence.

Maudsley (1967) was the first to describe the true entrapment syndrome of the peroneal nerve, presenting nine patients with pain down the lateral side of the leg, paraesthesiae and tenderness over the nerve at the level of the fibular neck. At operation a tight crescentic band at the origin of the peroneus longus was found constricting the nerve, which was swollen proximal to it. Symptoms were relieved in six cases. Nakano (1978) relates entrapment of the common peroneal nerve to entrapment by ganglion, hereditary compression neuropathy and leprosy (Hansen's disease). Baker and Scotland (1995) described "entrapment" by a fabella – rather, episodic distortion of the nerve over the sesamoid bone. It is plainly important to distinguish this syndrome from an affection of the fifth lumbar nerve. Singh et al (1974) make this point.

Banerjee and Koons (1981) describe two cases of entrapment of the superficial branch of the nerve as it passes obliquely through the deep fascia. In one case pressure was exerted by a fatty herniation. Kernohan et al (1985), Lowden (1985) and McAuliffe et al (1985) described similar entrapments, with paraesthesiae and alteration of sensibility. In all Kernohan's cases symptoms were relieved by the simple operation of releasing the nerve from the trap in the fascia. We have no experience of this condition, but we recognise that it is something to be remembered in cases of pain and paraesthesiae affecting the leg, in which no other explanation can be offered. Indeed, the same considerations apply in the case of other cutaneous nerves: for instance, the saphenous, which may be trapped on emerging from the femoral canal, and the sural, which may be trapped below the lateral malleolus (Montgomery et al 1989).

The tarsal tunnel syndrome

It was probably Lam (1962) who introduced the concept of entrapment of the tibial nerve beneath the medial retinaculum at the ankle. We should state that we have no real experience of dealing primarily with the syndrome; only that of dealing with the ill effects of operation on the basis of that diagnosis. Lam (1962) described the case of a 46-year-old man with sensory symptoms and signs, in whom decompression produced relief and return of sensibility. He later (1967) described 10 cases, in all of which decompression gave relief, though "no abnormality" was found in seven. Keck (1962) described the case of a 20-year-old man with bilateral numbness of and paraesthesiae in the soles of the feet, in whom decompression gave relief. Di Stefano et al (1972) reviewed the literature and provided two further cases; in one compression was caused by a ganglion; in the other it was caused by a neurilemmoma. They listed trauma, abnormal bands, ganglion and neurilemmoma as causes. Janecki and Dorberg (1977) provided another case in which a neurilemmoma of the medial plantar nerve was responsible for symptoms, and Kaplan and Kernohan (1981) identified as many as 21 patients with plantar pain and paraesthesiae indicating tarsal tunnel syndrome. In an extensive study of the condition in children, Albrektsson et al (1982) identified 10 cases with sensory symptoms. Exploration showed localised swelling of the nerve, narrowing of the tunnel, adhesions, constriction bands and even distortion of the nerve. Takahura et al (1991) operated on 50 feet of 45 patients, finding ganglia in 18, bony prominence in 15 and tumours in 3. In five cases "injury" was responsible.

Augustijn and Vannesti (1992) described three cases of "tarsal tunnel syndrome", in which the underlying cause was a more proximal lesion: in two cases an arterial lesion, and in one a tibial fracture. They invoked the "double-crush" hypothesis to explain the determination of symptoms. We reserve our position in this matter. Plantar pain, paraesthesiae and numbness may indeed be caused by compression of the tibial nerve under the retinaculum (Fig. 12.49), but the possibility of a more proximal cause must be excluded, and the diagnosis should be supported by the results of electrophysiological examination. When operation is done, the possibility that there may be a

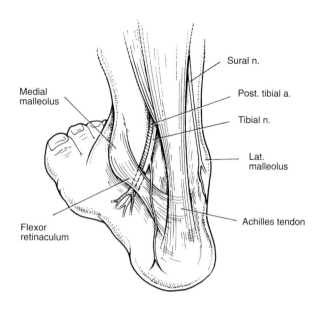

Fig. 12.49 The situation of the tibial nerve at the ankle under the flexor retinaculum.

tumour or ganglion near the nerve or a tumour in it must be borne in mind. In one of our cases the cause of "tarsal tunnel syndrome" was a synovioma occupying the medial plantar nerve at the level of the malleolus. In that case the pain and the numbness of the great toe had led to a primary diagnosis of multiple sclerosis. In another case we found an aneurysm of the posterior tibial artery. Our experience of dealing with the failures of operation for tarsal tunnel syndrome is very discouraging: two of the most severe pain states we have ever seen followed such procedures, and posed very difficult problems of treatment.

Plantar digital nerve entrapment

Seddon (1975f) included plantar digital nerve entrapment in entrapment neuropathies, and so, with slight misgiving, do we. "Morton's metatarsalgia" (Morton 1876) is singular in affecting principally the third intermetatarsal space. Women are affected more often than men: this incidence may relate to differing tastes in footwear. The pain is characteristically produced when the patient walks in shoes; it becomes progressively more severe, and is associated with radiation into the third and fourth toes. It does not cease when the patient stands still; it is only relieved, and then only slowly, when the shoe is removed. Then symptoms subside slowly. It is different from the pain of intermittent ischaemia of the muscle in its failure to respond to rest alone. Claustre and Simon (1978) show a good picture of the relations of the digital nerve in the "metatarsal canal": the nerve and artery are shown traversing the canal with the tendon of the lumbrical muscle and its synovial bursa, between the sheaths of the flexor tendons laterally, the transverse metatarsal ligament dorsally and the interdigital arcade ventrally.

The history of the matter is well related by Nissen (1948) and Seddon (1975h). Nissen (1948) clearly attributed the pathological changes to underlying arterial disease, but, as Seddon (1975h) pointed out, the interfascicular collagenisation seen in excised specimens of digital nerves is by no means characteristic of ischaemia. Much better, in our view, is the proposal of Claustre and Simon (1978) that the pain of "Morton's disease" is due to the presence of a neuroma caused initially by microtrauma against the transverse metatarsal ligament. The later formation of a neuroma produces compression in the canal, with secondary effects on the accompanying artery.

The common symptoms have been narrated. Examination shows tenderness of the plantar surface of the distal part of the third intermetatarsal space. There may be hyperalgesia and hypoaesthesia of the related sides of the third and fourth toes. Often enough, when the forefoot is squeezed in the hand, a feeling is experienced by the patient and the examiner of something jumping in the space between the metatarsal heads. The patient may feel pain while this is being done. Mulder (1951) noted that pressing on the sole over the point of tenderness helped to elicit the feeling.

Treatment

In early cases local injection of steroid may suffice. It is likely that once a neuroma has formed operation will be necessary in order to give relief. Betts (1940) was bold enough to incise the sole and remove such neuromata: the dire warnings about the production of a hypersensitive scar were shown to be overdone. Most scars of most operations done for removal of plantar digital neuromata heal well and are painless. On the other hand, Claustre and Simon (1978) indicate a course less drastic than neurectomy: they follow Gauthier and Dutertre (1975) in practising simple division of the metatarsal ligament through a dorsal incision.

CONCLUSION

Turner et al (1990) list 31 different entrapment syndromes. The concept of the entrapment syndrome is attractive; the belief that symptoms from such syndromes are easily relieved by a simple operation is specially attractive to operative masons. In practice, the matter is not so simple because, when things go wrong, symptoms are likely to be severe, persistent, and resistant to treatment. No letter fills us with such gloom and apprehension as one requesting an opinion on symptoms persistent after operation for entrapment neuropathy. The proffered case is indeed likely to prove a poisoned chalice.

13. Iatropathic injury

Iatropathic lesions of nerves: the legal situation; changes caused by legislation of 1990; rise in incidence of medical negligence claims; the nine main categories of iatropathic injury; neurotoxic drugs; anticoagulants; injection injury; unrecognised ischaemia; pressure and traction during general anaesthesia; traction during manipulation, including birth injuries of the brachial plexus; direct damage in the field of operation; ionising radiation; failure to recognise nerve injuries; objects of risk management.

Mit der Dummheit kämpfen Götter selbst vergebens

(J. C. von Schiller 1801)

When a patient enters hospital or starts medical treatment without a nerve injury and leaves hospital or completes treatment with one, the question is likely to be raised of whether medical negligence has been responsible for all or part of the lesion and the disability flowing from it. The determination of whether there has been medical negligence and the extent of damage flowing from it rests in the last resort with the Courts. There it will be determined whether the clinician concerned has "fallen short of the standard of a reasonably skilful medical man" (Finch & Cowley 1994). That standard is to some extent modified by a judgement of Mr Justice McNair in 1957, which was followed and confirmed by a ruling of the House of Lords in 1981 (Watt 1995). This ruling confirmed the earlier judgement that "a doctor is not guilty of negligence if he has acted in accordance with the practice accepted as proper by a responsible body of medical men skilled in that particular art". This test, named after Mr Bolam, the plaintiff in the original action, has had a continuing effect on legal process, and indeed on medical practice, in this country.

Similarly, a standard has been set by which the extent of information to be given about the risk of a proposed procedure may be judged. As a result of the judgement in the Sidaway case (1985) "it is now firmly settled as a matter of English law that when a doctor decides what he ought or ought not to tell his patient about the risks of the proposed procedure, the lawfulness of what he does will be principally judged by tests founded on evidence of appropriate contemporary standards of professional care. It will not be held against him that he has committed an unlawful battery because he did not make adequate disclosure of the possible risks" (Brooke and Barton 1994).

It will be seen that the odds are from the start stacked against a patient who is unable to command the services of the most skilful lawyers. The balance has further been shifted in the UK in recent years by three events:

- restriction of the availability of legal aid in civil cases
- the 1990 "reforms" of the National Health Service
- the shift, in 1990, of responsibility for indemnification in cases arising in the national hospital and community services, from the defence organisations to individual health authorities and "Trusts".

The effect of the first needs no explanation. As to the second: one effect of the 1990 "reforms" of the National Health Service was altogether to remove the conduct of affairs from the hands of clinicians and to place it in the hands of managers. So, the clinician who admits to a mistake which may cost his or her authority or "Trust" money, may face at least suspension and at worst dismissal. The fear of such process undoubtedly increases the difficulty that many clinicians experience in admitting fault, and leads too often to the defence of the indefensible. Sadly, expert testimony may be perverted by the same apprehensions. Clinicians called on to give expert evidence should bear in mind the words of Hodgkinson (1990a): "[The] principal and over-riding duty [is] not to the party by whom he is retained, but to the Court." They should not allow themselves to be persuaded to connive in the deceptions of the lawyers, though, sadly for the reputation of their profession, they do so more often than is seemly. Hodgkinson (1990b) has some words to say about this too: "Undoubtedly, however, there are occasions when experts depart from this ideal, whether because of a conscious or unconscious desire to help one party or because their personal or professional pride renders them unwilling to be dislodged from particular positions they have adopted within the discipline". To these factors other constraints are now added: the desire to please the officers of the body that is the source of reward and honour; the wish to be asked again; and the fear of provoking the resentment of persons in high position.

The second relevant effect of the "reforms" was to fragment the hospital service and to remove the management of the "Trust" hospitals from any form of supervision. Ministers are no longer responsible for the actions or decisions of Trust Boards; the abolition of Regional Health

Authorities has removed the sanction of supervision by a directly superior body.

The removal from the defence organisations of the responsibility for indemnification in cases occurring in the national hospital and community services, placed upon individual authorities and trusts burdens which they were ill prepared to bear. One observer at least foresaw this hazard (Bonney 1990). Sadly perhaps, Cassandra's fate had long been his: no one then or later believed his prophecies. "Cash limited" trusts have found it difficult to meet unbudgeted awards of large sums of money; the existence of a hidden liability from past events constitutes a formidable threat to the financial stability of these bodies. Hence, many claims are resisted which formerly would have been settled. Many of the patients so affected, condemned to wait for periods of from 5 to 10 years for resolution of their claims, tend to perpetuate their disabilities and to magnify their extent. So, treatment of such patients is often unrewarding and disappointing.

The transfer of responsibility for indemnification also destroyed the central databank of information on cases of medical negligence operated by the defence organisations, and so made the task of risk management more difficult. The possibility of a systematic analysis of the causes of action in respect of medical negligence and the identification of patients intrinsically likely to take action was destroyed. The tardy recognition of these drawbacks led in 1995 to proposals for the formation of a Special Health Authority (the "Litigation Authority") to oversee the operation of a central fund to spread the burden of indemnification. Unfortunately, this attempt to re-create the mechanism formerly operated by defence organisations was vitiated by the refusal to make adherence to the central fund mandatory. Further harm was done by making claims involving a total cost of £10 000 or less ineligible for support from central funds. There is no obligation on Trusts or Health Authorities to report such cases to the Litigation Authority. Thus, the possibility of the creation of a comprehensive central bank of evidence about the cost and causes of claims in respect of clinical negligence has for the present, and perhaps permanently, been removed.

The possibility of improvement of the system for determining the validity of a claim in respect of an alleged medical negligence and for compensating patients so injured is raised again in the report arising from the review of civil legal procedure in England and Wales undertaken by Lord Woolf, at present (1996) Master of the Rolls (Burn 1996, Dyer 1996, Richards et al 1996, Woolf 1996). If in the event the recommendations of Lord Woolf's report are implemented, the method for dealing with small claims at least will greatly be improved; it may even be that in large cases it will be more difficult than it is now for lawyers abetted by their clients and expert witnesses to delay, obfuscate and magnify costs. The task is formidable: the massed forces of reaction will, no doubt, combine to resist the assault on profitable practices and abrogation of accountability. Those who see that a change is necessary but lack the will to take the plunge should reflect that any new system is certain to be better than that currently in operation.

The present situation in medical negligence claims

In spite of all discouragements the incidence of claims alleging medical negligence and the cost of those claims have continued to rise. Harris (1995) observes that: "In 1978, settled cases of malpractice in the UK amounted to 1 in 1000, and in 1988 it was 13 in 1000". Harris goes on to say "although figures are not available for the current position – mainly due to the fact that these cases have been dealt with by health authorities under the Crown Indemnity Scheme since 1990 – the incidence is undoubtedly much higher". These are sombre words. An annual cost to the Health Service of £200 million has been admitted. It has to be recalled that in the absence of a central register that estimate is certain to be on the low side. The problem of medical negligence is likely to remain and to increase as public awareness grows and standards of medical practice decline. Whether actions in respect of negligence increase depends of course on whether legal assistance continues to be available, either through the legal aid mechanism or through a system of conditional or contingency fees.

We are indebted to the Medical Defence Union and in particular to Mrs Suzanne Collinge and Dr Michael Saunders, for the provision of information, carefully "anonymised", about cases concerning peripheral nerve injury either current during or settled in 1986. Of a total of 95 instances of nerve injury, the facial nerve led all the rest, with 17 cases, followed by the common peroneal (14 cases), the sciatic (9 cases), the radial, median and digital nerves (8 cases each), and the brachial plexus (5 cases). The remaining cases involved other nerves, including, surprisingly, the pudendal. Most of the damage was done in the field of operation; there were, however, nine cases in which action was taken because of delay in diagnosis of nerve damage. Curiously, there was only one case of birth injury of the brachial plexus, and only one of damage to the spinal accessory nerve during the biopsy of a cervical lymph node. Birch et al (1991a) narrated their experience of iatropathic lesions of peripheral nerves. They dealt with 14 lesions of the radial nerve; 10 each of the spinal accessory nerve, of the brachial plexus and of the common peroneal nerve; 8 of the ulnar nerve; 4 of the musculocutaneous nerve; 3 each of the median and femoral nerves; 2 of the tibial nerve; and 1 of the sciatic nerve. The delay in diagnosis ranged from seconds to *40 months*. Since that time, experience in this unit has greatly been expanded.

It has been traditional to describe injuries produced by doctors as "iatrogenic". We have for long disliked this usage, believing that the term indicates "doctor-producing" rather than "produced by or derived from a doctor". One of us suggested substitution by "iatrogenous" (Bonney 1986), and we continue to think that is the correct term. However, the difference between "iatrogenic" and "iatrogenous" may be too slight to be appreciated by the generality of clinicians. It may have been caviare to the general. Peter Malyan-Wilson (personal communication, 1994) suggests the use of "iatropathic", a form which he recalled from the work and writings of Dr H. St H. Vertue, formerly a physician at Guy's Hospital in the Borough. We now propose the use of this term.

IATROPATHIC NERVE INJURY

Iatropathic injury of peripheral nerves is a persistent and probably growing problem. The incidence of damage during operation is almost certainly increasing as a result of the subordination of the professional to the managerial ethos: the principle of consultant responsibility has been jettisoned; a "subconsultant" grade of operator is on the increase; the virtual imposition of "day case" operating has meant delegation to persons of inadequate knowledge and experience (Birch 1992, Bonney 1992); and the rush to "minimal access" and "endoscopic" methods in order to reduce hospitalisation has exacted its own toll of damage.

The distress and damage caused to patient and clinician by the legal process are so severe that all possible steps should be taken to avoid causing damage which might give rise to litigation and to mitigate the rigours of litigation when it becomes inevitable. However intelligent, alert, informed, compassionate and communicative a clinician may be, none can hope wholly to avoid complaint, and few can hope wholly to avoid legal process. The horrors of the last are very greatly mitigated if the clinician can rely on a well written, well ordered and comprehensive clinical record supplemented by properly completed charts and a well ordered nursing record. Sadly, Health Authorities and Trusts appear to accord a low priority to records systems; the record-keeping systems in the "private sector" are often worse. The defence organisations continually exhort their members to keep good records, but the exhortations seem too commonly to be disregarded. The keeping of a good record is a matter for self-discipline and care on the part of the clinician, supported by the availability of good systems for recording and retrieval.

METHODS OF IATROPATHIC INJURY OF NERVES

Nerves are injured by doctors in many ways:

- by administration of drugs likely to cause neuropathy
- by administration of drugs inhibiting coagulation of the blood and so capable of causing intraneural or extraneural haemorrhage
- by injection of a tissue-damaging substance into or near a main nerve
- by pressure from extraneural haemorrhage caused by accidental or deliberate arterial puncture
- by the production of or failure to recognise and treat ischaemia of a limb
- by closed pressure or traction during general anaesthesia
- by traction during manipulation under anaesthesia or during delivery
- by direct damage by pressure, traction, heat, clamping or cutting in the field of operation
- by ionising radiation.

The damage done by nerve injury, iatropathic or otherwise, may be compounded by failure of recognition and consequent delay in treatment.

DRUGS

Many drugs are neurotoxic. Le Quesne (1993) lists 21, of which the most commonly used are amiodarone, sodium aurothiomalate, isoniazid, phenytoin and vincristine (Donaghy 1996). The reintroduction of the neurotoxic drug thalidomide, for the treatment of, inter alia, erythema nodosum leprosum, discoid lupus erythematosus and rheumatoid arthritis (Chapon et al 1985, Sampaio et al 1991, LeQuesne 1993, Gardner-Medwin & Powell 1994, Powell 1996), may initiate a new wave of drug-induced neuropathy unless very careful observation is maintained. Orthopaedic surgeons in particular should be aware of the use of the drug in rheumatoid arthritis and of the possibility of subclinical neuropathy in patients so treated. Recently, Ellis and colleagues (1994) have drawn attention to neuropathy caused by bezafibrate. Most of these drugs seem predominantly to affect the axons. In most cases recovery slowly follows cessation of treatment, so it is important that early signs of neuropathy should be recognised. Delay in recognition may lead to failure of or delay in recovery, and so to legal process.

Drugs reducing the coagulability of blood

The use of these drugs has increased with recognition of the need to prevent deep venous thrombosis after operations in which this is a relatively common complication – notably, replacement arthroplasty of the hip. Intraneural bleeding may occur in or near the site of operation – in the sciatic nerve after replacement arthroplasty of the hip – or without association with operation, as in the after-treatment of myocardial infarction or deep vein thrombosis (Leonard 1972). The onset is sudden: fibres of all sizes are affected so that there is paralysis of all sensory modalities and of motor functions, including vasomotor and sudomotor action. The last feature distinguishes the lesion of the sciatic nerve from one of pressure or traction during operation.

Our experience of such injury is confined to lesions of the median nerve during the after-treatment of myocardial infarction with warfarin, and of the sciatic nerve during treatment with heparin for or prophylaxis against deep vein thrombosis after arthroplasty of the hip. In one of our cases, a 63-year-old man showed evidence of deep vein thrombosis 72 hours after arthroplasty of the hip by a posterior approach. Intravenous heparin was instantly started (30 000 units/24 hours). Thirty-six hours later there was a sudden onset of paralysis in the distribution of the ipsilateral sciatic nerve. All modalities were affected; pain was not severe. There was no evidence of bleeding into the wound cavity. Heparin was stopped. Over the next 2 weeks there was progressive and complete recovery. We are indebted to Mr Peter Baird for the details of another case, in which haemorrhage into the sciatic nerve was precipitated by the use of low-molecular-weight heparin for prophylaxis against thrombosis after arthroplasty of the hip. Twenty-four hours after operation there was severe burning pain in the foot, with sudden onset. Over the succeeding 4 hours there was progressive paralysis in the distribution of the sciatic nerve. The next day the nerve was explored (Mr Peter Baird). There was a haematoma within the epineurium of the sciatic nerve, more extensive in the common peroneal component. This haematoma was drained. Eighteen months later there was good recovery in the distribution of the tibial component, when electrophysiological examination showed virtually normal responses. In the common personal component there were a few surviving fibres, but there was no evidence of regeneration. In this case, doubtless, the function of the tibial component was saved by the prompt intervention, but the damage done by the haemorrhage to the common peroneal component was so severe as to be irreversible from the time of the incident.

It is likely that in such cases the chief indication for exploration and decompression is the presence of severe pain, indicating an acute and persistent irritative lesion. The second indication for operation is, we think, failure of early recovery. Thirdly, if a lesion were observed to deepen in spite of cessation of treatment with anticoagulants there would be a case for exploration. In those cases without pain and with early evidence of recovery, intervention is not indicated. It goes without saying that treatment with heparin should be discontinued as soon as such lesions declare themselves.

Simeone et al (1977) describe lesions of the lumbar plexus in two patients receiving anticoagulants who suffer haemorrhage into the psoas sheath. Sedel (1987) comments on six cases of damage to peripheral nerves caused by pressure from without by haematoma arising from the use of anticoagulant drugs. Three of these were not associated with any surgical procedure. Such lesions can, of course, complicate arthroplasty of the hip, when the involved nerve is usually the sciatic. Sedel comments that

decompression is effective if done within 6 hours at most. He goes on to say that "if the patient cannot be operated on within twelve hours, it is better not to attempt surgery. Generally, recovery will take place within one or two years". Our experience is rather similar to Sedel's, though we think that decompression can still be helpful up to 48 hours after the bleeding incident. Mr Barry Fearn, Mr George Raine and Mr John Strachan have each contributed details of sciatic nerve affection from massive haematoma in the buttock after arthroplasty of the hip combined with prophylactic treatment with anticoagulant. Haematoma was drained 4–48 hours after the initial bleed. In all cases there was severe pain, and that pain was relieved by decompression. In two of the three cases there was good recovery; electrophysiological examination (Dr N. Murray) confirmed regeneration. Evidently, clinicians should be aware of the possibility of this complication and of the distinct advantages of early operation.

Clearly, no blame can be attached in such circumstances if treatment with anticoagulant drugs is properly indicated and, when necessary, properly monitored, so long as the nerve lesion is promptly recognised and if necessary treated, and treatment with anticoagulants is stopped. The failure promptly to recognise that a haematoma was causing a lesion of a nerve could be held to indicate an inadequate standard of care; the failure to act in the face of severe pain and deep paralysis would almost certainly deserve censure. Lastly, it is important to recall that nonsteroidal anti-inflammatory drugs, which are likely to be in use in patients subjected to arthroplasty, are liable to potentiate the action of warfarin and heparin (*British National Formulary* 1993).

INJECTION INJURY

The damaging substances commonly injected into nerves are: steroid preparations; anaesthetic agents for intravenous use such as thiopentone; nonsteroidal anti-inflammatory drugs; anxiolytic agents such as diazepam; antibiotics; and local anaesthetics. The nerves most commonly affected are the radial in the arm, the median at the elbow and the sciatic in the buttock. Usually, the occurrence of severe local and radiated pain makes it plain that the drug has been injected into the nerve. The onset of motor and sensory paralysis may, however, be delayed for some hours. Although Hudson (1984) suggests that the ill effects arise from intraneural injection rather than from injection near the nerve and later diffusion, it is hard to resist the speculation that the latter must sometimes be the responsible mechanism. This suggestion is indeed supported by Kline and Hudson's latest (1995d) thoughts.

The ill effects of intraneural injection are produced by:

- mechanical disturbance of the nerve bundles
- the direct action of the drug on nerve fibres.

Extrafascicular

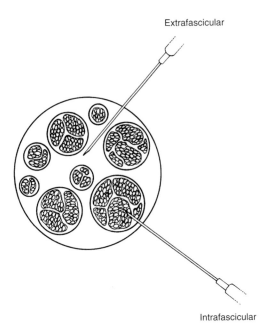

Intrafascicular

Fig. 13.1 Diagram showing intra- and extrafascicular injection.

Because in so many of these cases a veil of discretion is drawn over the proceedings, not so much is known as should be about the pathology of the lesion in the human being. Clark et al (1969) did electrophysiological studies of injection injury of the sciatic nerves of cats, and also made clinical studies. They found instant changes with intraneural injection of paraldehyde, at that time a drug in regular use for control of manic states. Paraldehyde was the only drug to cause disturbance when injected round rather than into the nerve. They further showed the different reactions to different drugs, and hazarded the view that the principal cause of damage was chemical. Asked about the possible benefits of instant action, Dr Clark replied: "I do not think that you could get there fast enough". That judgement may still be correct. Gentili et al

(1979) made a careful study of the effects of injection into the sciatic nerves of rats. They injected 11 different agents and used equal volumes of saline as controls, testing the effects of intra- and extrafascicular injection (Fig. 13.1). They found that the site of injection was critical: whereas extrafascicular injection caused only slight damage, intra-fascicular injection invariably produced injury. The agents most likely to do damage were penicillin, diazepam and chlorpromazine; those least likely were iron, dextran and cephalothin. Mackinnon and Dellon (1988c) add dexamethasone. Large myelinated fibres were more susceptible to damage than were smaller myelinated fibres. Axons, Schwann cells and myelin sheaths were all affected. There was, however, a regular tendency to regeneration, even in the most severely affected fibres.

Experience with injection injuries in human beings does not always match that with injection into the nerves of rats, just as the behaviour of the former is not regularly matched by that of the latter. Full recovery is by no means invariable; noxious injection is often followed by epineurial fibrosis, and sometimes by dense intraneural scarring (Fig. 3.2). It may be that there are three modes of injury:

- injection beneath the sheath of a neurovascular bundle
- injection adjacent to a nerve
- true intraneural injection.

Injection beneath the sheath of a neurovascular bundle as practised in brachial plexus block may produce the sort of effect caused by leakage from an arterial puncture site. Initial intraneural compression is succeeded by fibrosis, tethering to surrounding tissues and epineurial thickening. Early intervention is necessary if the effect of the initial block does not subside; later intervention with decompression can also be helpful.

Injection adjacent to a nerve, particularly one passing through a site of possible constriction, may cause an inflammatory reaction which later spreads to involve the nerve or later causes perineurial fibrosis. Late operation seems to be of little help in such cases.

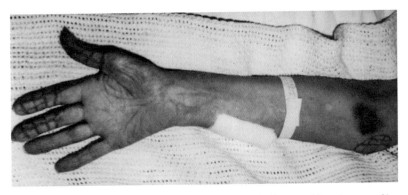

Fig. 13.2 Injury of the median nerve at the elbow by injection of anaesthetic agent. Note the area of loss of sensibility.

INTERSCALENE BLOCK

Winnie (1970) introduced the concept and practice of "interscalene block", in which a relatively large volume of local anaesthetic is injected into the interscalene space, through which pass, at least, the uppermost four nerves of the brachial plexus. He recorded success in 94% of the first 200 patients, and reported personal communications indicating a high percentage of success and absence of complications. However, there are in this site a number of structures of importance equal to or greater than that of the nerves of the plexus: the phrenic nerve; the vagus and recurrent laryngeal nerves; the cervical sympathetic chain; the vertebral artery; and the spinal canal, with the epidural and subarachnoid spaces and the spinal cord. The studies of Chakravorty (1969) indicated that, although the contribution of the vertebral artery to the anterior spinal artery did not extend below the third cervical level, radicular branches maintained the blood supply of the cord below that level by contributing to the longitudinal anastomosis.

Wedel (1994) indicates the possibility of damage to one or more of the structures adjacent to the interscalene space; the warning is repeated by McConachie and McGeachie (1995).

We have seen three patients who suffered serious neurological damage from interscalene block. Their histories are not yet complete, but it is appropriate to outline the case of a 4-year-old boy who suffered such damage.

The previously fit young patient fell 3 or 4 feet from the steps of a slide, sustaining a fracture through the extreme lateral end of the right clavicle. There was no loss of consciousness. The clavicular fragments were markedly displaced, with dropping of the forequarter, but there was no evidence of neural affection. Six days after injury, operative reduction and internal fixation were done. The distal clavicular fragment had pierced the trapezius and platysma; after reduction the fragments were united by two sutures. A right interscalene injection of 10 ml of 0.5% marcain (bupivacaine) was done. It was early clear that there was a lesion of the cord and brainstem, with right facial weakness, deviation of the uvula, left abducens paresis, right Bernard–Horner syndrome, and sensory and motor paralysis of the right upper limb. Probably, there was also recurrent laryngeal nerve paralysis; later collapse of the lower lobe of the right lung indicated the probability of paralysis of the right phrenic nerve.

Magnetic resonance imaging 2 days after operation showed swelling of the right side of the brainstem and cervical spinal cord. Vertebral angiography showed no abnormality.

It seems likely, in view of the absence of abnormal findings on angiography, that the responsible lesion here was a true spasm of the right vertebral artery, causing an ipsilateral lesion of the cervical cord and brainstem. The finding of central neurological damage in the other two cases indicates a similar mechanism there. Evidently, interscalene block is not lightly to be undertaken: the price of avoidance of general anaesthesia or of relief of pain after operation may be too high. The damage most to be feared is that to the vertebral artery: the suggestion is that the placing of the tip of the needle should always be confirmed by screening. Failure to aspirate blood may be misleading; even electrical stimulation at the time of injection may fail to elicit a response.

Intraneural injection: treatment

The key is avoidance. Noxious injection into the sciatic and radial nerves of the adult should be avoidable if the sites chosen are, respectively, the upper lateral quadrant of the buttock and the upper part of the middle fibres of the deltoid muscle. It should be possible to avoid injection of steroid into the median nerve at the wrist by inserting the needle to the medial side of the midline. Hudson (1987) suggests that local anaesthesia should not be used in this procedure, so that the injector can be warned by the patient's complaint of pain if the needle tip approaches the nerve. He suggests too, that in the performance of brachial plexus block with local anaesthetic, the agent should be injected round the nerve trunks rather than intraneurally. It is usually possible to avoid the median nerve during intravenous injection in the cubital fossa, but perfect safety cannot always be guaranteed with refractory children and struggling adults. Probably the cubital fossa is best avoided in such patients. In dealing with conscious patients, a complaint of pain and paraesthesia on injection should always lead to cessation.

In spite of all precautions there is a steady toll of noxious intraneural injection in general, hospital and community practice. Hudson (1984) and Mackinnon and Dellon (1988c) advise a policy of observation, with intervention if at the expected time there is no evidence of recovery. Kline and Hudson (1995d) later speculated on the possible benefits of early intervention, noting the constraints narrated below. We believe that, in some cases at least, a more active policy is indicated. We realise, however, that it is difficult to pursue such a policy when the injection is done in the home or in the surgery and when no clinician with special experience is available. Such conditions are only too likely to obtain. It has been noted that the discretion of the protagonists generally draws a veil over the early proceedings in these cases. No doctor or nurse is ever particularly likely to admit in the early stages that he or she has made an injection into a main nerve. When the onset of symptoms is delayed, the patient may reassure him- or herself with the thought that the symptoms are only to be expected. There is, surely, a case for early intervention when:

- the substance injected is known to be particularly neurotoxic (see p. 297)

- injection instantly causes severe local and radiated pain
- there is within 3 hours of injection a complete paralysis of all modalities of conduction in the distribution of the nerve concerned.

Under these circumstances the nerve should within 6 hours of injection be explored over a length of not less than 5 cm at the site of the damage; the epineurium should be opened along the length and the nerve should be irrigated with normal saline. Intraneural procedures are probably harmful. This is of course a counsel of perfection: in most cases intervention within 6 hours is hardly possible. The critical indication for operation is, we think, the presence of pain. If pain persists there is an indication for operation at 1 hour, 24 hours or even a week after the incident. One thing that operation can do is to relieve pain; the introduction of a tissue catheter through which an 0.25% solution of bupivacaine can be infused is a very valuable procedure.

Delayed exploration, at a time when little or no recovery is apparent, is likely to show epineurial fibrosis. The epineurium should be divided longitudinally over the length of the lesion. If bundles are seen traversing the zone of damage and if there is conduction across this zone, no more need be done. In the rarer cases of dense intraneural fibrosis with destruction of neural elements, without evidence of recovery and without electrical conductivity, resection and repair by graft are indicated.

Injection producing arterial bleeding

In four sites in particular, leakage after arterial puncture can cause nerve damage. These are the brachial artery in the arm, the ulnar artery at the elbow, the radial artery at the wrist and the femoral artery at the groin. In the first, arterial catheterisation for the purpose of angiography may be followed by bleeding into the fascial sheath enclosing the brachial vessels and the median nerve. In the second, the venepuncturist may pass the needle through the vein, into and through the median nerve, and into the ulnar artery, which at this level is separated from the nerve by the deep head of the pronator teres muscle alone. There follows bleeding into the deep compartment of the forearm, with affection of the ulnar nerve below the elbow (Fig. 13.3). We have seen five cases of affection of the median nerve at the wrist after radial arterial puncture, and four cases of affection of the femoral nerve after puncture of the femoral artery at the groin. We have also seen bleeding into the psoas sheath with affection of the lumbar plexus after aortography by direct puncture.

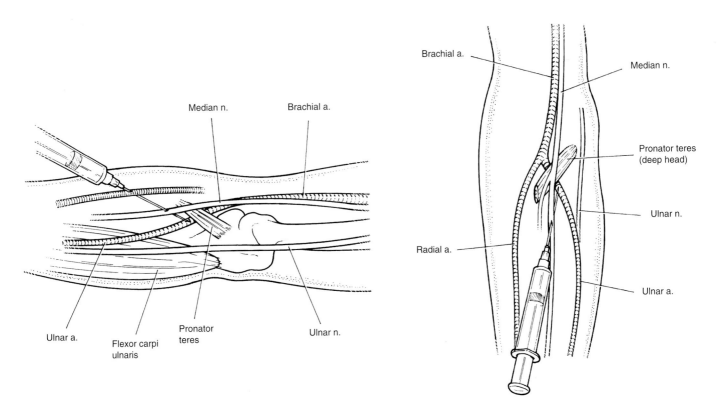

Fig. 13.3 Diagrams show mechanisms of injury to ulnar nerve during venepuncture. The needle traverses the vein, the median nerve, and the deep head of the pronator teres, and enters the ulnar artery. Bleeding into the medial deep compartment of the forearm causes damage to the ulnar nerve. (Right) Anteroposterior view; (left) lateral view.

In the first two cases there is pain and swelling with later bruising and obvious affection of the nerve. In the case of the ulnar artery the bleeding may not, because of its deep situation, be apparent for several days. In the case of the radial and femoral arteries there is usually early evidence of local haematoma. Avoidance is the best policy. The arteriographer should recognise that arterial puncture may be followed by leakage, and should ensure that pressure is applied locally for several minutes after withdrawal of the catheter. The venepuncturist should know that severe local and radiated pain indicates puncture of the median nerve, and should desist. If avoidance fails and nerves are injured, decompression should be done as soon as possible (preferably within 12 hours). In the case of the ulnar nerve, a simple decompression at and below the elbow usually suffices.

ISCHAEMIA

It is the accident and orthopaedic surgeon who is most often confronted with ischaemic lesions of peripheral nerve caused accidentally or by lack of care, or allowed to deepen and become irreversible through failure of recognition. It is in this field that some of the most catastrophic mistakes are made. The common errors are:

- failure to recognise ischaemia caused by interruption of main axial blood flow or by pressure within a fascial compartment
- accidental intra-arterial injection of a noxious agent
- accidental infusion into a fascial compartment
- production of "tourniquet paralysis".

Unrecognised peripheral ischaemia

When flow through a main artery of a limb is interrupted by laceration or thrombosis, with or without associated fracture of the adjacent long bone, there is, in the absence of adequate collateral circulation, distal ischaemia. The common sites for the combination of bony and arterial injury are the lower end of the humerus, the lower end of the femur and the upper end of the tibia. The effect of ischaemia is most marked in the case of muscle, and least marked in the case of skin. Muscle will not survive total ischaemia for longer than 6 hours; nerve will not survive for longer than 12 hours. One of the effects of anoxia is to increase capillary permeability, so that to the ischaemia caused by cessation of axial supply is added that caused by rising pressure within the fascial compartments. That process alone may be responsible for serious ischaemia when it is produced by local damage to bone and muscle, as in cases of displaced fracture of the bones of the forearm or leg (Parkes 1945, 1959, Holden 1975, Wiggins 1975, Patterson & Boddie 1977, Mubarack & Carroll 1979, Triffit et al 1992). If ischaemia is allowed to persist, muscle

dies and is replaced by fibrous tissue (Volkmann 1882); all neural elements are affected to a degree which may bar any later recovery through regeneration; finally, skin and bone die. The avoidance of these complications depends on early diagnosis and swift decisive action.

Because of the early affection of peripheral nervous tissue, one of the earliest signs of peripheral ischaemia is alteration of sensibility of the extremity. Mackinnon and Dellon (1988b) recognised that the earliest fibres to suffer were the largest – those conveying the sensation of vibration. The alteration affects all nerves in the ischaemic part of the limb, so that its pattern does not conform to the area of supply of any particular nerve or nerves. These facts are or should be well known to all who deal with injured patients, yet clinicians continue to:

- fail to grasp the urgency of the affair
- ignore warning signs
- attribute peripheral numbness and even pallor and temperature change associated with fracture to "arterial spasm"
- adopt a waiting policy
- rely on sympathetic block or sympathectomy to relieve "spasm" of a main artery and restore peripheral circulation
- rely on "capillary return" in the finger tips as an indication of adequate deep circulation.

All the lessons of the past are here to guide clinicians. "Spasm" alone is never a cause of obstruction of a main artery of an adult, though it may be associated with intimal damage and subsequent thrombosis (Collins & Jacobs 1961, Bergentz et al 1966, Eastcott 1973b, Rosental et al 1976, Samson & Pasternak 1980, Barros d'Sa 1992b,c). In children, spasm alone is sometimes the cause of main arterial obstruction (Barros D'Sa 1992d). We have seen no more than four cases of arterial spasm in children causing by itself circulatory impairment. Many have written stressing the urgency of the situation, the folly of waiting and seeing, and the need for early and decisive action (Hardy & Tibbs 1960, Connell 1962, Eastcott 1965, 1973b, Brewer et al 1969, Perry et al 1971, Rosental et al 1976, Reynolds et al 1979, Barros D'Sa 1982, 1992b). As long ago as 1968, Gorman indicated the unreliability of capillary and venous filling as signs of adequate peripheral circulation. Kinmonth et al (1956) plainly showed that spasm of main arteries was myogenic and independent of nervous control. Although Nicholson et al (1994) reported improvement after cervicothoracic sympathectomy for distal digital gangrene, there is no evidence that this procedure has any place in the treatment of ischaemia of deep issues resulting from obstruction of a main artery. As long ago as 1963, Bonney and Kirkup separately added to the literature cases of successful revascularisation of limbs by early intervention on damaged arteries. The former went so far as to write: "Surgeons who treat fractures have to be prepared to deal with associated lesions of the main vessels". No one took any notice: too often still, surgeons treating limbs with combined bony and arterial damage seem content to treat the fracture and to call in the "vascular surgeon" when signs of ischaemia have persisted for 12 or more hours. By that time intervention on the artery comes too late; indeed, re-establishment of axial flow may actually do harm (Braithwaite et al 1995) (Fig. 13.4).

The early symptoms and signs of dangerous peripheral ischaemia are pain, pallor, coolness, alteration of sensibility, absence of pulse and tenderness of muscle. If damage is to be avoided the circulation must be restored and the muscles must be decompressed within, at the most, 8 hours of injury. The only excuse for failure to act is the presence of a life-threatening condition forbidding early operation. To wait for a surgeon competent to deal with an arterial lesion is as unjustifiable as is a wait for a surgeon competent to deal with an associated lesion of bone or joint. In combined lesions of bone and vessel, the fragments must be fixed in order to protect the arterial repair, and the artery – or artery and vein – must be repaired in order to protect the extremity.

Accidental intra-arterial injection

The substances likely to be injected are thiopentone and diazepam; the recipient vessel is likely to be the brachial artery. The results are immediate and serious: pain and severe distal ischaemia are caused by initial spasm and later by widespread thrombosis (Cohen 1948). Although avoidance is better than any treatment, the penalty paid by the patient and the operator can be minimised by instant action. Barros D'Sa (1992e) recommends the administration through the injecting needle of 20 000 units of

heparin, 40–80 mg papaverine in 10–20 ml saline, 10–20 ml procaine hydrochloride and 5 ml of 1% tolazoline. Failure to improve indicates exploration and fasciotomy, but both are in vain unless undertaken within 48 hours of the damaging injection.

Infusion into a fascial compartment

Although the vigilance of nurses has up to the present usually prevented the infusion of a large volume of fluid into a fascial compartment when a needle or cannula becomes displaced from its position in a vein, cases of iatropathic compartment syndrome have been reported. Maor et al (1972) reported one case of Volkmann's contracture of the forearm from the infusion of no less than 3 litres of blood. Hastings and Misamore (1987) reported three cases with a rather different aetiology: here, the agent used for regional intravenous anaesthesia was accidentally diluted with hypertonic saline, and the increase in pressure was produced by osmosis. In unfortunate cases such as these, prompt fasciotomy offers the only chance of reducing the amount of damage.

Tourniquet paralysis

The use of the occluding cuff to produce a "bloodless" field is very common in orthopaedic work and indeed in work on the nerves of limbs. Without it, some procedures would hardly be possible, and others would certainly take an inordinately long time. It must not, however, be forgotten that in many cases in which the cuff is used the neural tissue may already be unduly susceptible to pressure: there may be a lesion of the nerve itself; there may be a neuropathy from rheumatoid arthritis or alcohol

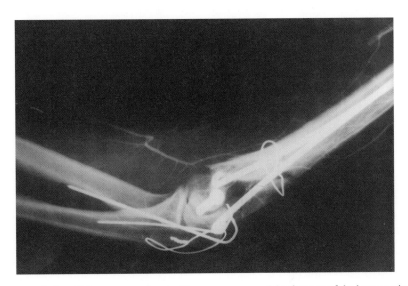

Fig. 13.4 Damage to the brachial artery associated with severe supracondylar fracture of the humerus in a 20-year-old woman. There is extensive occlusion of the brachial artery caused by intimal damage, thrombosis and spasm. There was infarction of all the flexor muscles of the forearm.

or diabetes or other causes; and wasting of muscle may have lessened the protection of nerves from pressure. It must not be forgotten, either, that the inflation pressure, the width of the cuff in relation to the size of the limb, the duration of application and the site of application are all of critical importance.

Evidently, a paralysis is always produced when an occluding cuff is in position for 30 minutes or longer. It nearly always recovers spontaneously within a few minutes of the release of the pressure. Sometimes the paralysis is longer lasting; rarely, some of its effects are permanent. The reversible paralysis is that of transient ischaemia; the long-lasting paralysis is that of damage to the myelin sheath; the permanent paralysis is that of damage to all elements of the nerve, including the axon, with ischaemic damage to muscle.

Józsa et al (1980) studied the effect of tourniquet ischaemia on human muscle; its effect on the muscles and nerves of humans and monkeys was studied by Klenerman (1980) and Klenerman et al (1980). Aho et al (1983), describing a case of tourniquet paralysis, discussed the subject in general and made recommendations about the pressure to be used and stressed the importance of checking the accuracy of gauges. Trojaborg's (1977) very important study of electrical reactions in a case of tourniquet paralysis showed a combination of conduction block and axonal degeneration. It stressed the important point, now rather often forgotten, that in cases of simple conduction block there is normal conduction below the level of the lesion. Rudge (1974) stressed the element of conduction

block in a similar case; he too stimulated both above and below the level of the lesion.

The dominant role in determining damage is clearly the inflation pressure, but the other factors should not be forgotten. In a case which came to our attention operation was done for reconstitution of the cruciate ligaments of the knee of a man in his forties. An occluding cuff, properly placed and correctly inflated, was in position for no more than 75 minutes. There followed a paralysis in the distribution of the common peroneal nerve. Later examination and investigation showed that the instability of the knee for which operation was done was caused by weakness of the muscles of the lower limb, the result of the presence of a dermoid tumour in the conus medullaris. The consequent wasting of muscles had so much reduced the protection of the nerves of the limb that they were seriously damaged by pressure of a degree and duration that would not have damaged nerves protected by healthy musculature (Fig. 13.5).

The occurrence of the "tourniquet paralysis" is often the cause of legal proceedings. Avoidance is the best policy; it must also be possible for the clinician to show that due care has been taken. We think that a cuff at least 12 cm wide should be used for the adult arm, and one at least 20 cm wide for the adult thigh. The cuff should be applied to the upper part of the arm or thigh. Padding should be applied between cuff and skin. Inflation pressure for the upper limb should be 50–75 mmHg above systolic pressure, and that for the lower limb 100–150 mmHg above systolic pressure. Aneroid gauges should be checked

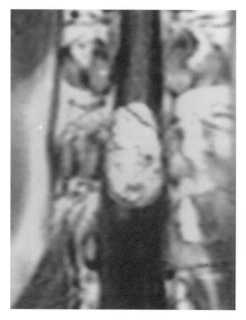 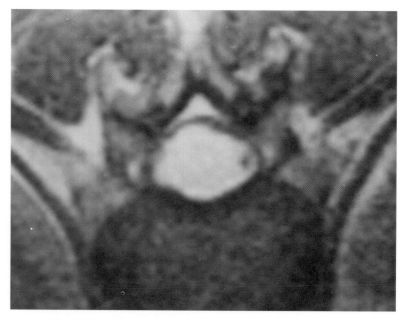

Fig. 13.5 Magnetic resonance imaging shows dermoid of the conus medullaris. This was associated with bilateral pes cavus, weakness and wasting of both lower limbs, and alteration of sensibility over the sacrum. "Tourniquet paralysis" followed application of a systolic cuff for operation to repair cruciate ligament. (Clinical diagnosis by Dr Christopher Pallis; operative diagnosis and removal by Professor David Thomas.)

regularly for accuracy against mercury gauges. The times of application and release should be recorded on a board in the operation theatre and in the notes. In the case of the arm, the surgeon should be told when the cuff has been in place for 1 hour; at this stage a further half hour's application is, if necessary, permissible. In the case of the thigh, the surgeon should be warned at 1 hour and again at 90 minutes; a limit of 2 hours should be imposed. These figures, derived from our own observations and experience, are broadly in line with "Bruner's 10 rules" (Bruner 1951), which were "revisited" by Braithwaite and Klenerman (1996). These figures are for limbs without serious wasting, and for nerves which are not abnormally susceptible. For patients with rheumatoid arthritis, diabetes mellitus, alcohol addiction or other possible causes of neuropathy the times must be reduced. In many such patients it is best to avoid altogether use of the tourniquet. We are indebted to Professor Averil Mansfield for the observation that the use of a tourniquet on a limb in which an arterial prosthesis has been inserted is absolutely contraindicated. It seems that the implant is insufficiently elastic to dilate after release of the cuff; also, collateral circulation is likely to be defective.

Experimental evidence has suggested that there is no advantage in releasing the cuff, allowing bleeding and then reinflating. However, anyone who has experienced the rapid return of power and sensibility when the blood is allowed to flow again after half an hour's occlusion is likely to think differently. This view seems to receive support from the comprehensive work of Sapega et al (1985). In any case, a "bleed" of a few minutes gives a helpful interval for rest and haemostasis and helps to limit desiccation of the tissues.

The perusal of hospital medical records confirms the impression that too few clinicians are aware of the importance of accurate recording. Too often the duration of application of a tourniquet is not recorded; almost always inflation pressure and site of application go unrecorded. When a tourniquet is used, this information should always be recorded in an ordered operation note. If there is no record and a tourniquet paralysis follows, no Judge can be blamed for thinking that the responsible clinician was less than serious about his or her work.

CLOSED PRESSURE AND TRACTION DURING GENERAL ANAESTHESIA

This has been discussed by Payan (1987).

Pressure from without

Too often in time-consuming operations insufficient attention is paid to the protection of nerves lying between skin and bone against pressure from without during anaesthesia, and too little attention is paid to avoidance of stretching, distortion and pressure from within. The ulnar nerve at the elbow, the radial nerve in the arm, the brachial plexus in the neck and the common peroneal nerve at the knee are all vulnerable to external pressure. All are particularly vulnerable if there is an existing neuropathy, even if the condition is symptomless. They are especially vulnerable too in patients who for any reason have lost weight and so have lost some natural padding.

The ulnar nerve. Wadsworth (1977) and Wadsworth and Brooks (1982) have drawn attention to the sequelae of external pressure on the ulnar nerve at the elbow. Wey and Guinn (1985) describe the lesion as a sequel of open-heart surgery. Typically, a few days after regaining consciousness after general anaesthesia a patient becomes aware of numbness of and paraesthesia in the little finger of one or both hands and of dysfunction of that hand or those hands. He or she will not necessarily complain at once: often, he or she will think that such symptoms necessarily accompany the proceedings. Complaint is later made to a nurse or a junior doctor, neither of whom is aware of the significance of the symptoms. Eventually the limb is examined and signs of a lesion of the ulnar nerve are found; often, the nerve is swollen and tender behind the medial epicondyle. Electrophysiological examination usually shows reduction in conduction velocity, indicating a lesion of the myelin sheath. Often enough "conservative" treatment is given. The principles of this are rather similar to those of Conservative government: nothing is done until the situation has righted itself or is beyond remedy or hope of recovery. In fact, the anatomical arrangements at the elbow make likely the continuation of the lesion originally caused by pressure from without. Excursion may be restricted, so that a small traction lesion is inflicted with each flexion of the elbow. In most such cases, clinicians have been content to await the outcome of natural process. However, the outcome may not be at all favourable. We believe that operation is indicated if:

- the initial lesion is deep and complete
- a lesion involving sensory and motor conduction shows no sign of recovery at 2 weeks
- the lesion deepens under observation.

The simple release described by Osborne (1970) is adequate.

The radial nerve. The nerve is vulnerable as it winds round the humerus, even though in most of this course it is protected by the triceps muscle. The most common cause of damage is compression between the bone and the side of the table or trolley when the arm is allowed to overhang the side of either. Usually these lesions are spontaneously recoverable.

The brachial plexus. The use of shoulder rests to support patients in the Trendelenburg position was formerly a common cause of lesions of the brachial plexus (Bonney 1947). The reduced incidence of such lesions indicates that this method of support has been modified or abandoned.

The common peroneal nerve. The common peroneal nerve is very vulnerable in its course behind and round the neck of the fibula. It was formerly a common casualty in gynaecological surgery through the use of slings maintaining limbs in the lithotomy position. It is still injured by prolonged recumbency when the backs of the knees are inadequately padded. The resulting foot drop usually recovers, though sometimes imperfectly. It may be that, as in the case of the ulnar nerve, surgeons should be readier than they are to explore and decompress.

The sciatic nerve. Tait and Danton's (1991) two cases of affection of the contralateral sciatic nerve during femoral nailing were, presumably, the result of external pressure.

The debate continues on whether patients should be compensated for these inconveniences arising from medical care. It may be that these injuries represent the price inevitably paid for the advantages of general anaesthesia; on the other hand, it can be argued that most are preventable if adequate care is taken. We think that if it can be shown that adequate care has been taken in the matter of protection of sensitive points, the occurrence of such a lesion should not be taken to indicate lack of care. Elbows should be well padded and well placed; prolonged flexion of elbows should be avoided; pressure over the brachial plexus should be avoided; unconscious patients should be well supervised during the recovery period; and the backs of the knees should be well padded. Lastly, the limbs of patients with known neuropathy should be treated very tenderly indeed. The Royal National Orthopaedic Hospital has developed a policy of prevention of damage by compression to the ulnar and common peroneal nerves before, during and after operation. The direction of this policy lies in the hands of senior nursing staff, whose work should be noted and emulated.

Closed pressure and traction from within

The brachial plexus. The brachial plexus above and below the clavicle is vulnerable during operations in which the upper limb is abducted and laterally rotated at the shoulder. The upper trunk may be compressed by the rising clavicle; the infraclavicular part of the plexus may be stretched over the front of the shoulder joint. The position is used in operations on the abdomen, to allow the anaesthetist access to the upper limb; it is used too in transaxillary operations on the sympathetic chain and in operations for removal of the first rib. Clausen (1942) was one of the first to draw attention to such lesions and to analyse their causes. Po and Hansen (1969) recorded six cases, two of which were associated with cardiac operation. Ewing (1950) and Kiloh (1950) added more cases. Cooper et al (1988) added more cases and drew attention

to the role of congenital anomalies in predisposing to injury. The lesions themselves, nearly always caused by transient ischaemia or by local demyelination, are generally recoverable, though the period of recovery may be long and the disability tiresome. Care must be taken not to maintain 90° abduction at the shoulder for longer than 20 minutes at a stretch, and if possible to avoid a position of lateral rotation at the glenohumeral joint. Whenever possible, abduction at the shoulder should be limited to 70°. It is fortunate that the development of the endoscopic transthoracic method (Kux 1978, Weale 1980, Gôthberg et al 1990, Nicholson et al 1994) has shortened the time required for cervicothoracic sympathectomy, and so has reduced the time during which the limb is abducted.

With the development of open heart surgery, further possibilities of damage to the brachial plexus, and in particular to its lowest part, have emerged. The mechanism of damage to the plexus during operations in which the chest is split open and the circulation is maintained by artificial means was examined by Graham et al (1981), Hanson et al (1983) and Cooper (1991). In Parks' (1973) huge 13-year study of peripheral neuropathy after 50 000 operations, the brachial plexus was found to be the most common site of injury. Twenty-three of the 28 cases of injury to the plexus followed open heart operations. Doubtless, it is the movement of the upper hemithorax on the axial skeleton that determines injury; it is hard to see how this movement could be avoided. Most of these lesions are recoverable; few are deep, and fewer still are complete.

DAMAGE BY TRACTION OR DISTORTION DURING MANIPULATION UNDER ANAESTHESIA

The practice of manipulation under anaesthesia by orthopaedic surgeons of spinal and other joints has declined with the gradual realisation that the methods used by qualified osteopaths are not only safer but also more successful. New methods involving traction have, however, appeared: for instance, arthroscopy of the hip requires traction on the limb, and such traction, when prolonged, may damage the sciatic and femoral nerves (Villar 1992). Indeed Rodeo et al (1993) showed that the widening of the indications for arthroscopy had opened up a whole new field of danger for nerves. They named four general types of neurological injury secondary to arthroscopy as: direct injury to a nerve; compression secondary to compartment syndrome; tourniquet-related conduction block; and reflex sympathetic dystrophy. In the course of their discussion they gave helpful advice about permissible pressures in occluding cuffs. The manipulation of any joint which has been fixed for some time in a position of deformity always carries the risk of damage to nerves passing across it and accustomed to the position of deformity. Aspden and Porter (1994) reported just such a case, in which the sciatic nerves were damaged by straightening knees that had long been flexed because of spastic diplegia. The authors do not relate whether any allegation of medical negligence was made in this case. Birch et al (1991b) reported on three cases in which the brachial plexus was damaged during manipulation of the shoulder for "frozen shoulder". In one of these cases, manipulation had caused anterior dislocation. The plexus was explored in this case; there was no interruption of continuity, and recovery followed.

Similar circumstances obtain in limb lengthening operations, even though it is usual to effect change slowly, over a period of weeks. It has been argued that, if during the process signs or symptoms or actual or impending neural damage appear, the process can be stopped to permit recovery. Galardi et al (1990) are less reassuring: they studied events in the limbs of five patients whose tibiae were lengthened at a rate of 1 mm/day over a period of 53–107 days. The ages of the patients ranged from 3 to 24 years. These workers examined the conduction velocity of nerves and the electrical activity in muscles during lengthening, and found evidence of damage to myelin sheaths and axons in all cases. Their findings evidently raise the question of whether nerve function should always be monitored during correction of major deformities of long standing. We think that this should in fact always be done when it is proposed to correct such a deformity in one stage at operation. Monitoring is evidently desirable during slow correction in the conscious patient.

The matter of birth injuries of the brachial plexus is considered in Chapter 10. Nowadays there are legal implications for paediatricians and orthopaedic surgeons, as well as for obstetricians and midwives. The growth of knowledge about the pathology of these lesions and the possibilities of repair have made it mandatory for all clinicians with responsibility for the newborn to be aware of changed circumstances. It is no longer sufficient to rely on spontaneous recovery and to limit treatment to advice about passive movements. In each case the nature and extent of the lesion should be determined by examination, extended observation and ancillary investigations. In appropriate cases operative repair should be advised. We hope that steps will be taken to remedy the present unsatisfactory situation in which the national incidence of birth lesions of the plexus cannot accurately be determined, and in which there are "inadequate arrangements for the investigation and treatment of infants who have suffered these lesions" (Birch 1995b).

DIRECT DAMAGE IN THE FIELD OF OPERATION

The most serious damage suffered by nerves at the hands of clinicians is usually that inflicted in the field of operation by cutting, stretching, compression and burning. It is with such injuries that surgeons are chiefly concerned, and it is in this field that the most serious mistakes are made. Evidently some operators are insufficiently familiar with topographical anatomy; some are unaware that nerves may be distorted or displaced by pathological changes and that there are anomalies of position and size; many are unaware of the concentration of function in the peripheral nervous tissue and of the vulnerability of that tissue relative to that of bone and muscle. The use during operation of agents acting on the neuromuscular junction ensures that transmission is usually blocked, so that accidental section or pinching of a nerve is not signalled by a contraction of muscle. Under such circumstances too, electrical stimulation for identification becomes unreliable. Section of a main nerve does not produce the instant, obvious and catastrophic effect produced by section of a main artery or vein. Lastly, the enforced revival of "day case" operations in the interests of economy has too often led to operations being done by inadequately qualified persons, under conditions inimical to the maintenance of proper standards of care (Birch 1992, Bonney 1992). When mistakes are made by such persons under such conditions, the onus is, or should be, as much on managers as on clinicians, though in practice it is always the clinicians who are obliged to justify their actions in open court.

Nerves are damaged in operation fields when:

- the object of operation is to relieve a condition affecting a particular nerve or nerves
- a nerve is closely associated with or embedded in a tumour affecting another organ or tissue
- a nerve is simply in the field of operation.

Operations for conditions affecting nerves

The conditions of nerves for which operation is done include: tumour; entrapment and other compression neuropathies; injuries of various types; lesions causing painful states; radiation neuropathy; and leprosy. In all these conditions neural function is liable to be impaired before operation, even though that impairment may not be clinically perceptible.

Tumours of nerves

This subject is discussed in Chapter 15. In the case of malignant tumours, further damage to neural function during removal is often inevitable; indeed, such tumours commonly come to notice through their effect on function. The surgeon's duty here is to warn and to do his or her best to balance for the patient the probable risks of failure to intervene against those of intervention. Birch (1993a) examines the factors governing the difficult decisions on whether and when to intervene on a solitary neurofibroma. The inexperienced surgeon who causes permanent neural deficit by ill-advised intervention on such a tumour is asking for trouble.

It is with schwannoma that the most common and most disastrous mistakes are made. Although this tumour is one of the few conditions that can successfully be treated by operation, many clinicians seem to be unaware of its existence. Kehoe et al (1995) studied the cases of 104 solitary benign tumours of peripheral nerves and found that the correct diagnosis had been made in only a few cases before operation. Schwannoma is indeed uncommon, as of course are conditions that can successfully be treated by operation. Most schwannomata are associated with main nerves of the limb, though their occurrence in the psoas muscle and elsewhere is recorded from time to time (Downey et al 1989, Hennigan et al 1992, Ross and Schaffer 1992, Vazquez-Burquero et al 1994). Clinicians should be aware that a small rounded laterally mobile tumour in the line of a main nerve of a limb, tapping on which gives rise to paraesthesia in the distribution of the nerve, is likely to be a schwannoma and is treatable by operation (Figs 13.6 to 13.8). When such a tumour is found in a person with the stigmata, however slight, of neurofibromatosis, the diagnosis becomes even more likely. Regrettably, schwannomata in the upper limb are diagnosed as "ganglia", in the axilla as "enlarged glands", in the neck as "enlarged lymph nodes" and in the lower limb quite often as "neuromata" or even "neuromas". Operation is delegated to a practitioner with restricted

Figs 13.6 to 13.8 Schwannoma of the median nerve.

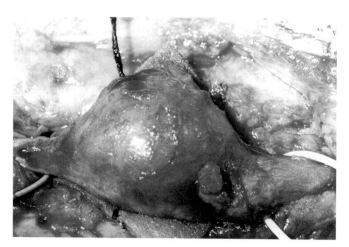

Fig. 13.6 Lateral schwannoma of the nerve in situ.

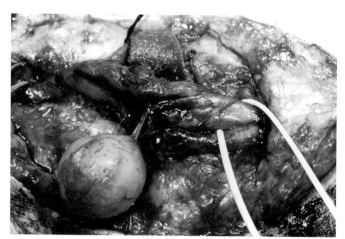

Fig. 13.7 The schwannoma enucleated.

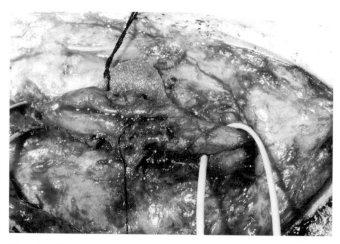

Fig. 13.8 The nerve after operation. There was no neurological deficit before or after operation.

experience; he or she finds a tumour and removes it, or recognises a nerve trunk swollen by an apparently invasive tumour and removes that (Figs 13.9 and 13.10). In either case a main nerve is damaged or a length of the nerve is removed. Recovering from anaesthesia, the patient notices motor and sensory defect; too often, he or she is not seen by any responsible person before leaving hospital, and the motor and sensory defect is ascribed to "neurapraxia" or, increasingly and horribly, to "neuropraxia". As Birch et al (1991) found, it may be weeks or months before the nature of the lesion is recognised and repair is undertaken. This is very sad: usually, a schwannoma can with little difficulty be enucleated from its parent nerve without any damage to conducting tissue (Figs 13.11 and 13.12). It is, of course, the laterally placed schwannomata that at operation are thought to be "ganglia", and the centrally placed ones that are thought to be malignant tumours. We have seen parts of many nerves removed by resection of a trunk bearing a central tumour, and many nerves damaged by the removal of a peripherally placed schwannoma. The upper trunk of the brachial plexus and the radial, ulnar and median are the nerves most commonly damaged in this way (Figs 13.13 to 13.15). It is important for the surgeon who comes to treat such lesions, and who may be required to provide evidence, to ask to see the sections taken from the material removed at the primary operation. Often enough, a cross-section of a trunk nerve is included in the specimen.

Correct diagnosis and skilled action are important factors in the avoidance of needless maiming. The patient with a suspected schwannoma should be sent to a clinician with experience in the field of peripheral nerve surgery, even if that referral causes budgetary problems for management. The problems are liable to be even more severe if unskilled proceeding causes permanent disability. If at operation the insufficiently skilled surgeon finds a tumour attached to or occupying a main nerve, he or she should close the wound and later make the appropriate referral. It is inadvisable to take a specimen for examination: the resulting fibrosis is bound to make enucleation needlessly difficult. If the unthinkable happens and a nerve is damaged or a length removed, the patient should at once be referred to a clinician with knowledge of these problems. The diagnosis of "neurapraxia" should be used only with the greatest of caution: that of "neuropraxia" never. No patient complaining after operation of symptoms of neural defect should be permitted to go home unseen by someone with suitable knowledge.

There are further pitfalls. Needle biopsy of, for instance, a lump in the neck may be unreliable unless the examiner is highly skilled. In one of our cases of schwannoma affecting the upper trunk of the brachial plexus, the specimen removed by a needle biopsy was said to show the features of "sarcoma". The upper trunk was removed; examination of the specimen plainly showed the characteristic features of schwannoma (see Ch. 15). The removal was a mistake; worse, it was a folly: a purely local removal of such a "sarcoma" could hardly be expected to be curative; if the tumour had been malignant, there would have been evidence of interference with conduction. It is, we

Figs 13.9 and 13.10 Forty years on: the upper trunk of the brachial plexus removed with a schwannoma. The situation 3 months later, at operation in 1952 by Donal Brooks and G.B.

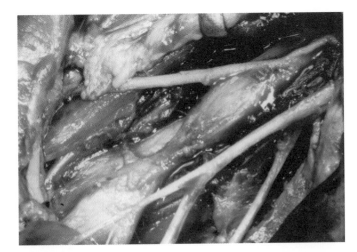

Fig. 13.9 Large gap in the upper trunk. Note the supraclavicular nerves.

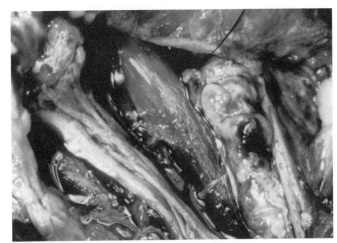

Fig. 13.10 The supraclavicular nerves have been used, with plasma clot suture, to bridge the gap after resection.

Figs 13.11 and 13.12 Lateral schwannoma of the sixth cervical nerve in a 50-year-old with neurofibromatosis.

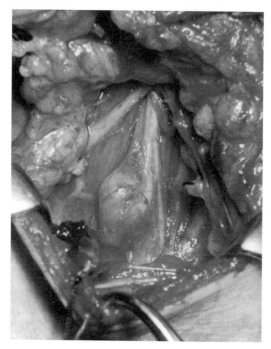

Fig. 13.11 The tumour in situ.

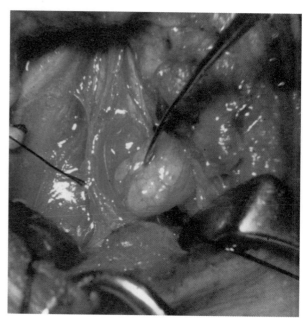

Fig. 13.12 The tumour being shelled out.

Figs 13.13 to 13.15 Damage to the upper trunk of the brachial plexus by resection of conducting tissue with schwannoma ("lymph node").

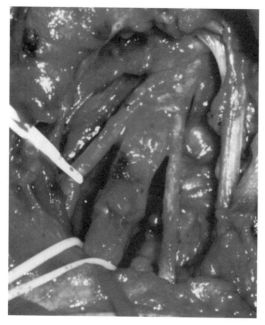

Fig. 13.13 Three months after damage to the posterior division of the upper trunk.

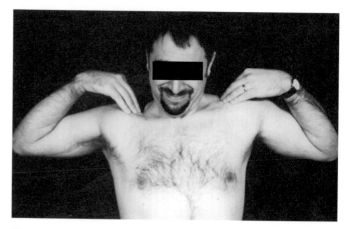

Fig. 13.14 Function 18 months after resection and graft (same case is in Fig. 13.13).

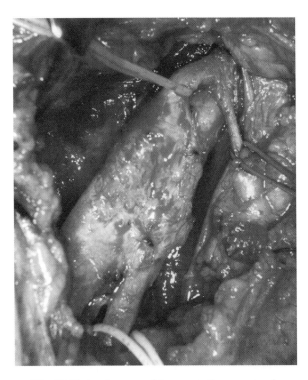

Fig. 13.15 Another case of damage to the upper trunk.

think, doubtful if biopsy of any type has any place in the diagnosis and treatment of tumours of neural origin. Needle biopsy or similar removal of a restricted amount of tissue may miss an area of malignant change; open biopsy is certain to scar the field and to make later enucleation unnecessarily difficult.

Rarely, a perfectly benign schwannoma appears at operation to be diffuse and invasive. In one of our cases a schwannoma of the seventh cranial nerve appeared at operation as a substance of the consistency of paste, infiltrating all conducting elements. A partial removal was done, with preservation of conducting elements. Histological examination showed plainly the characteristic features of schwannoma. There was no suggestion of malignant change. Six months later the tumour had wholly disappeared and the patient was symptomless. Wright and Bradford (1995) note a similar indolence or possibly regression in the case of certain acoustic "neuromata". As these workers remark, these tumours are in fact more properly called vestibular schwannomata.

Very rarely, perhaps even never, a benign schwannoma becomes malignant. We discuss this and related aspects in Chapter 15. It is sufficient here to say that the possibility of malignant change in a schwannoma is never sufficient basis for a "radical" excision of the tumour with a length of main nerve.

Lastly, schwannoma of the extracranial part of the facial nerve can be mistaken for "mixed parotid tumour", which is after all the most common tumour in this site. Very special care is needed in the enucleation of schwannoma in this site if permanent damage to conducting tissue is to be limited or avoided.

OPERATIONS FOR OTHER CONDITIONS OF NERVES

Most of the damage is done during operations for "entrapment syndrome", in particular to the brachial plexus at the thoracic outlet, the median nerve at the wrist and the ulnar nerve at the elbow and wrist.

The thoracic outlet

This subject is considered in detail in Chapter 8. The mistakes that we have encountered are:

- direct damage to the lower part of the plexus by rough handling and retraction
- section of an upper trunk mistaken for the tendon of the scalenus anterior
- damage to the white ramus of the first thoracic nerve causing Bernard–Horner syndrome

- damage to the phrenic nerve causing permanent paralysis of the hemidiaphragm and subsequent "paralytic eventration".

In addition, as Cherington et al (1986) and Wilbourn (1988) warn, decompression of the plexus in the root of the neck always brings the risk of producing a troublesome neuropathy. This may occur even when the handling of the conducting tissue is as gentle and restricted as is permissible within the limits imposed by the demands of full decompression.

A particular risk attaching to transaxillary operation is that of damage to the nerve to serratus anterior, running down the chest wall in the posterior part of the field. Since the development of endoscopic transthoracic sympathectomy the risk has greatly diminished, but it is still there in operations for removal of the first rib (Roos 1966, 1971, 1981, 1982). Here, of course, the aim must be avoidance. The nerve should be located with the stimulator and very gently retracted with its surrounding fat and areolar tissue from the field of operation. Whenever the axillary approach has been used, the function of the serratus anterior muscle should be tested as soon as possible after operation. The finding of complete paralysis indicates exploration and repair. Fiddian and King (1984) analysed the cases of 25 patients with scapular winging, and discussed types of winging and causes.

Neuralgic amyotrophy

It is in particular with lesions of the nerve to serratus anterior that the differential diagnosis of neuralgic amyotrophy is often canvassed. This is as convenient a place as any in which to introduce the subject.

Lederman and Paulson (1987) and Wilbourn (1993) give good accounts of this singular and rare (annual incidence 1.64 per 100 000 population (Beghi et al 1985)), disorder. As Parsonage and Turner (1948) remarked, "remarkably little was published about this condition before 1942". They refer to the cases of paralysis of the serratus anterior muscle after operations and infections reported by Bramwell and Struthers (1903), noting the paucity of references to the disorder in standard textbooks. Struthers (1903) drew attention to the vulnerability of the upper part of the nerve to serratus anterior as it emerged from the scalenus medius. Spillane (1943) brought the condition to general notice with his description of a "localised neuritis of the shoulder girdle" occurring in British, Australian, New Zealand and American troops in the Middle East and the UK. The details of 46 patients were available to him. Spillane noted the features that are now familiar to us: the linkage with infection and wounding; the onset with pain; and the common affection of the serratus anterior, the spinati, the deltoid and the trapezius. He noted too the particular vulnerability of the suprascapular nerve and the nerve to the serratus interior. Our speculations about aetiology are hardly more advanced than were Spillane's. A little earlier, Wyburn-Mason (1941) had noted a similar "outbreak" of brachial neuritis among civilians. It is to Parsonage and Turner (1948) that we owe the term "neuralgic amyotrophy", which so well indicates the combination of pain with paralysis and wasting. Martin and Kraft (1974) described the condition in 20 patients seen at the Philadelphia Naval Hospital between 1967 and 1969.

The association of neuralgic amyotrophy and its protean manifestations with precipitating events such as cold, injection, infection and operation is now well known. There is pain followed by motor paralysis, sometimes with alteration or loss of sensibility (Favero et al 1987). The muscles most commonly involved are the serratus anterior, the spinati, the deltoid and the trapezius. When paralysis occurs after an operation during which the nerve to one of these muscles might have been damaged, it may be very difficult, particularly in retrospect, to distinguish neuralgic amyotrophy from direct damage to the nerve. That difficulty is increased if the particular nerve has not been explored for evidence of damage. Indirect evidence collected years after the event is hardly ever decisive; the best method of distinction – early exploration of the affected nerve – is all too rarely done. The distinction is, of course, important for the patient and the operating surgeon, and could be important for the lawyer. To inflict serious damage on the nerve to the serratus anterior or the spinal accessory nerve during operation for a non-malignant condition would be considered careless; on the other hand, a surgeon could hardly be blamed for precipitation of an attack of neuralgic amyotrophy. Electrophysiological examination gives limited assistance (Petrera & Trojaborg 1984, Petrera 1991); the best late guide is the extent of recovery. As Wilbourn (1993) says: "Overall, neuralgic amyotrophy has a good prognosis. A retrospective series of 99 cases found that more than 80% of patients recovered functionally within two years of onset and more than 90% by four years. In contrast, serious and permanent defect of function usually follows a deep lesion of either the accessory nerve or the nerve to serratus anterior."

Median nerve at wrist

The most common hazards of decompression of the median nerve at the wrist are:

- inadequate decompression because of failure to divide the most distal part of the flexor retinaculum
- damage to the motor branch, to the palmar cutaneous branch, or to one or more terminal sensory branches
- prolapse of the nerve through the gap in the retinaculum

- damage to the superficial palmar arch causing haematoma, compression, pain and, later, fibrosis or even a late false aneurysm
- haematoma arising from defective haemostasis, leading to fibrosis around the nerve and to painful state.

We have even seen damage to the terminal branches of the ulnar nerve; even, after "endoscopic" decompression, damage to the distal part of the ulnar nerve itself. De Smet and Fabry (1995) record a case of damage to the motor branch of the ulnar nerve during two-portal endoscopic decompression.

The introduction of endoscopic operation to this field (Thomas et al 1993) offers new possibilities for incomplete decompression and damage to nerves. The particular advantages of endoscopic operation are, or should be, well known. It is, however, very important that all who use these methods should be thoroughly familiar with the techniques. Thomas et al (1993) give a warning which is applicable over the whole field: "Endoscopic surgical technique requires rigorous training to avoid dangerous pitfalls".

Lanz (1993) rightly says: "Incomplete division of the retinaculum, a common complication, can be avoided easily". It can, but the operator must know his or her business, an adequate exposure must be made, the occluding cuff must be released and haemostasis secured before skin closure, and the wrist should be splinted for a few days after operation. Inexperienced surgeons should not be required to tackle operation for symptoms persistent or arising after a primary operation. If in spite of all precautions the motor or a sensory branch is divided at the time of operation, it should instantly be repaired. The hand should be examined 12–24 hours after operation to confirm integrity of the motor and other branches, and action should be taken without delay if there is any evidence of damage.

Ulnar nerve at the elbow

Little harm can come to the ulnar nerve compressed at the elbow when operation is confined to decompression (Osborne 1970), though we have once seen the nerve divided with the skin incision. The common mistakes associated with transposition are:

- inadequate decompression, including failure fully to remove the medial intermuscular septum
- damage to the posterior branch of the medial cutaneous nerve of the forearm, which runs across the line of incision
- devascularisation of the nerve by excessive stripping of branches or failure to take axial vessels with the nerve
- imperfect placing either in subcutaneous or submuscular transposition, causing kinking of the nerve

- failure to mobilise the elbow sufficiently soon after subcutaneous transposition, leading to tethering
- haematoma after operation, especially after submuscular transposition, caused by imperfect haemostasis or imperfect drainage or by both.

Of these complications the most serious is devascularisation, which can lead to irremediable and painful loss of function.

We have seen "snapping" of the medial head of triceps over the medial epicondyle incorrectly diagnosed as subluxation of the ulnar nerve. There was initially no evidence of interference with conduction. The nerve was transposed subcutaneously. The "snapping" continued, now with paraesthesiae in the distribution of the ulnar nerve. At a second operation the nerve was found much adherent by fibrous tissue to adjacent structures, but the true cause of the "snapping" was not even then recognised. This experience recalls that of Rolfsen (1970), in whose cases the evidence concerning the extent of initial affection of the ulnar nerve is unclear. We have also seen the ulnar nerve severely damaged in "Guyon's space" in the proximal palm during operation undertaken in the mistaken belief that the lesion was there rather than at the elbow.

Operations on the sympathetic chain

The development of endoscopic techniques (Kux 1978, Weale 1980, Gôthberg et al 1990, Salob et al 1991, Nicholson et al 1994) has, in most cases, rendered obsolete open operation for cervicothoracic sympathectomy. The supraclavicular route will presumably remain the method of choice in cases in which sympathectomy is done as an adjunct to arterial reconstruction. The chief indication is likely to be hyperhidrosis of the palms and axillae of young girls. The latter are precisely the patients who are most likely to be bothered by the production of a Bernard–Horner syndrome. Damage to the cranial sympathetic supply can almost always be avoided by making the upper division of the chain below the stellate ganglion or through its lowest part. It is usually possible to identify the white ramus of the first thoracic nerve; possible even to stimulate it and observe the dilation of the ipsilateral pupil. So long as the section is made below the entry of the ramus into the stellate ganglion, a Bernard–Horner syndrome can almost always be avoided. Occasionally, doubtless because of traction on the chain, a transient Bernard–Horner syndrome is produced. Patients must always be warned of the possibility of this complication, because none can guarantee that in any particular case the cranial sympathetic supply enters the chain through the white ramus of the first thoracic nerve.

The proximity of the brachial plexus and of the lower trunk in particular to the target of operation renders them susceptible to injury. Adar (1979) commented on the incidence of damage to the lower trunk: he found 22 plexus injuries in 456 cervicothoracic sympathectomies by the supraclavicular approach in 228 patients. The damaged nerves seem to have recovered spontaneously in all cases. We have so far avoided this peril, but have seen not less than 10 instances of degenerative lesion of the lower trunk following cervicothoracic sympathectomy by the supraclavicular route. We have even seen the upper trunk of the plexus mistaken for the scalenus anterior and divided. The supersession of the supraclavicular by the transthoracic approach will surely make these injuries of historical importance only.

Lumbar sympathectomy

The practice of lumbar sympathectomy in occlusive arterial disease declined with the advance of arterial surgery; its use for the circulatory disorders of disuse has declined with the conquest of poliomyelitis. If in men the sympathetic outflow is interrupted either by bilateral excision of the first lumbar ganglia or by serious injury to the hypogastric plexus, there will be permanent failure of ejaculation through the penile urethra. Nowadays such interruption is more likely to arise from intervention on the lumbar spine by the anterior route than from deliberate intervention on the sympathetic chain. We have seen it after osteotomy at the level of L2/3 for severe deformity from ankylosing spondylitis. The subject has been examined by Whitelaw and Smithwick (1951) and May et al (1969).

Nerve damage during operation for neoplastic disease

It is rarely necessary to damage peripheral nerves during operation for benign neoplasm, but locally invasive conditions such as deep musculoaponeurotic fibromatosis may present particular difficulty (Fig. 13.16). Birch (1993a) relates that in two of his cases it was necessary to resect the main nerve in order to remove the tumour. Plainly, warning about the possibility or even probability of nerve damage must be given to such patients before operation. Equally plainly, no blame attaches to the surgeon who is obliged to resect nerve in order satisfactorily to remove this troublesome tumour. Latitude has to be granted to surgeons operating for removal of primary or secondary malignant tumours: the removal of a section of a trunk nerve may be necessary if the resection of the tumour is to be adequate. Thus, the spinal accessory nerve has to be sacrificed in radical clearance of lymph nodes in the neck (Maran 1994).

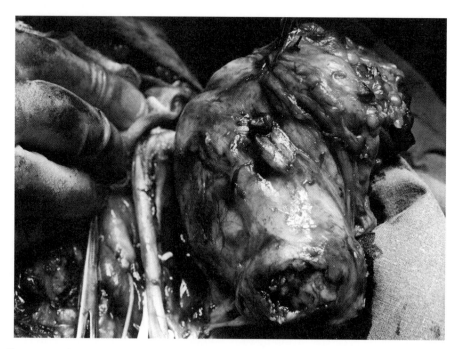

Fig. 13.16 Large musculoaponeurotic fibromatous tumour arising from the upper end of the left humerus and involving the nerves of the upper arm. The radial nerve passed through the tumour.

Nerve damage in the field of operation in general

In certain operations and in certain sites trunk nerves are in or close to the field of operation. Usually, the wounding or severance of such a nerve indicates a standard of care less than acceptable, though allowance has to be made in cases in which the field of operation is much scarred because of previous intervention or past infection. Some allowance has to be made in cases in which the nerve takes an abnormal course or, because of an anomaly, occupies an altogether unusual site. In some cases, even damage to a cutaneous nerve indicates an inappropriate level of care.

Although some allowance has to be made for the damage itself, little or no allowance should be made for failure to recognise the fact of nerve injury, failure to diagnose depth of affection and nature and extent of injury, and failure to take appropriate action. The early paper on this subject by Birch et al (1991a) showed a delay in diagnosis of from seconds to *40 months*, and in nearly half the patients diagnosis was delayed for *more than 6 months*. It is indeed hard, as Bonney (1986) commented, for the operating surgeon to credit that he or she has been responsible for the production of a serious nerve lesion, a feeling which may cloud vision and inhibit action. Nothing that has happened since that time has altered that perception.

The nerves principally at risk are those of the brachial plexus, the spinal accessory, the radial, the common peroneal and the ulnar. Birch et al (1991a), dealing with iatropathic injuries of nerves in all types of operation, found that these five led all the rest.

The spinal accessory nerve is too often divided during lymph node biopsy. Its superficial position in relation to the superficial lymph nodes makes it very vulnerable to the attentions of surgeons with inadequate knowledge of topographical anatomy (King & Motta 1983, Vastamäki & Solonen 1984). We have dealt with 49 cases of such damage to the spinal accessory nerve. In 38 of these repair was possible; in the remaining 11 muscle transfer or other procedure was used. We have seen at least another 30 cases in connection with legal process being taken by victims. In only a very few of these had repair even been attempted. The consequences of division are serious: there is nearly always persistent pain and dysfunction (Olàrte & Adams 1977, Sàeed & Gatens 1982, Nelson & Bicknell 1987) (Figs 13.17 and 13.18). The marring of function from the loss of the trapezius muscle is serious. Even if the lesion is quickly recognised and repaired, symptoms are likely to persist. The pain is of two types: a purely neuralgic pain from the damage to the sensory fibres in the nerve, and a constant dragging pain from the loss of one of the principal muscles sustaining the forequarter. In addition, the alteration in the posture of the shoulder girdle may initiate

distortion or compression of the suprascapular nerve at its foramen in the upper border of the scapula (see Ch. 12). A patient described to us the sensation of having his spinal accessory nerve clamped and cut during a "day case" operation under local anaesthesia for lymph node biopsy. It felt, he said, "as if someone had put a balloon under the skin of my neck and shoulder and suddenly inflated it". Osgaard et al (1987) relate similar experiences: they found that in similar circumstances patients experienced a sharp painful "electric shock" pain at the time of injury to the nerve. In the case reported by Barkhaus et al (1987) the lesion was produced by two ligatures round the nerve. Pain and paralysis followed. Although exploration and removal of the ligatures was not done until 10 weeks after injury, there was rapid diminution of pain and recovery of motor power.

Delay is common in the diagnosis and treatment of iatropathic lesions of the spinal accessory nerve: the patient may consider the pain a natural consequence of the operation; the complaint of weakness of the shoulder is likely to be delayed; without specific examination of the muscle the clinician will not make the diagnosis; even when the diagnosis is made, the clinician may think the nerve lesion to be spontaneously recoverable – so time is lost; a pattern

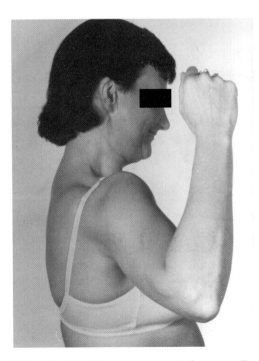

Fig. 13.17 Paralysis of the right trapezius muscle from wounding of the spinal accessory nerve during "lymph node biopsy". Note the difficulty in abducting the upper limb.

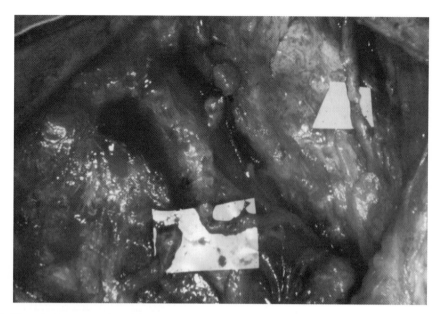

Fig. 13.18 The spinal accessory (top right) and the transverse cervical nerves damaged during "lymph node biopsy". The accessory nerve was in fact transected.

of pain is established; and the scene is set for litigation and for the unsatisfactory consequences of operation for repair undertaken in the shadow of litigation.

As if to make things more difficult, isolated paralyses of the spinal accessory nerve certainly occur in the absence of local trauma. Such cases are reported by Laha and Panchal (1979) and Doriguzzi et al (1982). In the former case, the trapezius alone was affected; in the latter, both the sterno-cleidomastoid and the trapezius muscle were paralysed. Laha and Panchal's case was probably an instance of neuralgic amyotrophy. In Doriguzzi's case, however, the affected muscles showed "continuous spontaneous activity of pseudomyotonic type characterised by bursts of action potentials". Evidently, some cases of accessory nerve paralysis after intervention on the neck may not be due to local damage to the nerve but rather to an affection similar to that of neuralgic amyotrophy. Early exploration offers the best chance of establishing diagnosis.

The brachial plexus is another common target for the sampler of lymph nodes: we have seen part of the upper trunk removed, and the upper trunk seriously damaged in this way. In former days, before the advent of endoscopic techniques, the upper trunk of the plexus has been divided in mistake for the scalenus anterior, and the first thoracic nerve and lower trunk have been removed, mistaken for the sympathetic chain. We have twice seen, at second hand, injury to the lateral cord of the brachial plexus during insertion of a pacemaker by a cardiologist through the subclavian vein. In both cases pain was a serious and persistent sequel; in the first, sensory affection predominated, and in the second, motor fibres were equally affected. We find it difficult to account for this damage: regrettably, the record of proceedings was, in both cases, defective, and in neither was exploration done. Both patients came to us after an interval so long that the possible benefit of exploration was, at least, doubtful. The occurrence seems to be rare: Murphy (1996) records only one instance of damage to the brachial plexus in 194 "temporary pacings", most of which were done by senior house officers. The mechanism of damage is not, however, explored.

The radial nerve is particularly at risk during operation for fixing the fragments of a broken humerus (Figs. 13.19 and 13.20), and its posterior interosseous branch is vulnerable during operation on the elbow by the posterolateral route. The ulnar nerve is at risk during operations for fixation of fractures about the elbow; we have seen it plated to the bone and so sharply kinked over the end of a plate that a degenerative lesion was produced. The musculocutaneous nerve, even the lateral cord of the plexus, and even on three occasions known to us the axillary artery, are at risk during operation for recurrent anterior dislocation of the shoulder (glenohumeral) joint (Figs 13.21 to 13.23). The risky parts of the procedure are those involving the isolation, detachment and mobilisation of the coracoid process and the short head of the biceps muscle, and the

Figs 13.19 and 13.20 Two cases of damage to the radial nerve during operation for fracture of the humerus.

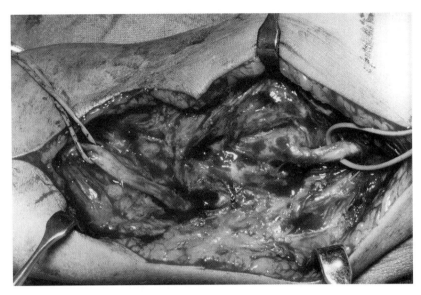

Fig. 13.19 The left radial nerve was left between the fragments of the humerus when the fragments were fixed with a plate.

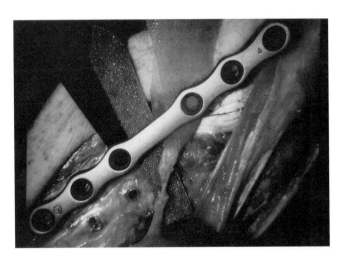

Fig. 13.20 The plate was fixed over the radial nerve. (Operation for removal of plate and repair of nerve by Mr Campbell Semple).

suture of the divided subscapularis muscle. The musculo-cutaneous nerve, or an upper component, may enter the biceps no more than 2 cm below the coracoid process, and can be damaged by traction or by the knife. In particular, when the coracoid process is transposed to the front of the neck of the scapula beneath the subscapularis muscle, it is possible to catch the lateral cord, and even the axillary artery too, in the stitch reuniting the subscapularis muscle. Digital nerves are, of course, at risk during operations for Dupuytren's disease. The vulnerability of the nerve to the serratus anterior during transaxillary operations has been stressed.

Figs 13.21 to 13.23 Three cases of damage to the musculocutaneous nerve during operation for recurrent dislocation of the shoulder.

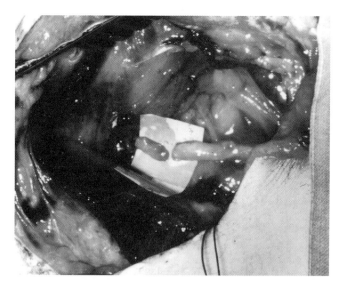

Fig. 13.21 The right musculocutaneous nerve divided during operation.

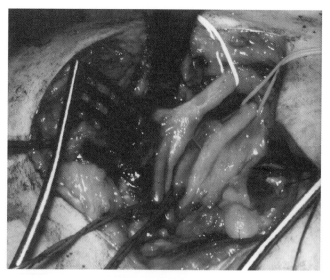

Fig. 13.22 Another division of the musculocutaneous nerve.

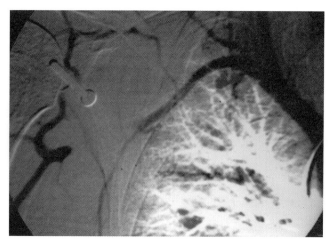

Fig. 13.23 Digital subtraction angiography shows occlusion of axillary artery in a case in which both artery and nerve were included in a suture.

The chest and abdomen

We have seen the lower trunk of the brachial plexus divided during removal through a thoracotomy of a benign tumour above the apex of the left lung (Figs 13.24 and 13.25). The femoral nerve is, from time to time, injured in its intra-abdominal extraperitoneal course during appendicectomy; it is sometimes damaged, probably by retraction, during hysterectomy (Winkelman 1958, Vosburgh & Finn 1961).

Figs 13.24 and 13.25 Damage to the lower trunk of the brachial plexus during operation for removal of an apical tumour.

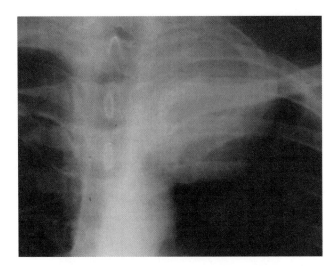

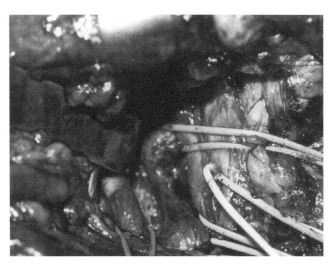

Fig. 13.24 Radiograph shows tumour at the apex of the right lung. It was a hamartoma. After operation there were signs of damage to the lower trunk.

Fig. 13.25 The lower trunk seen divided 4 months after primary operation.

The lower limb

The femoral nerve is vulnerable in its position lateral to the femoral artery, below the inguinal ligament (Figs 13.26 to 13.28). It and the sciatic nerve in its position behind the hip are vulnerable during operations on that joint. In former days, when femoral osteotomy was in common use for the treatment of osteoarthritis of the hip, the sciatic nerve was at risk from osteotome or chisel. Still, from time to time, the nerve is damaged during insertion or removal of a medullary nail in the femur (Fig. 13.29).

The common peroneal nerve is particularly vulnerable near the head of the fibula during operations for varicose veins (Fig. 13.30); even the tibial nerve is vulnerable during such operations. Before arthroplasty of the knee gained respectability, osteotomy through the upper part of the tibia offered, in many cases, alleviation of the symptoms of degenerative arthritis of the knee. Jackson and Waugh (1974), the chief proponents of this operation, drew attention to the associated risk to the common peroneal nerve. The risk remains, though the operation is now done much less commonly than in the 1970s. Fortunately, with the virtual disappearance of poliomyelitis in Europe and North America, the need for operations such as "triple arthrodesis" of the tarsus has virtually disappeared. Wounding of the plantar nerves was a hazard of that operation; it remains a hazard of arthrodesis of the ankle.

Damage to nerves during replacement arthroplasty of the hip

Replacement arthroplasty of the hip is pretty commonly done nowadays in the UK. Pike and Hollingsworth (1995) give a figure of 40 000 such operations done in one year. All three main nerves around the hip can be injured during this operation; the sciatic most frequently and the obturator least frequently. Both gluteal nerves are, from time to time, injured.

Interest in damage to the sciatic nerve during arthroplasty of the hip has been renewed. The additional disability caused by a deep and extensive lesion of the nerve is great; it is even greater when a lesion of the inferior gluteal nerve is added. The results of repair of so proximal a lesion of so large a nerve are liable to be imperfect. The sciatic nerve, emerging from the pelvis with the gluteal nerves through the great sciatic notch, passes under the piriformis muscle with the inferior gluteal nerve to run at the back of the hip joint separated from it by the tendon of obturator internus muscle and the gemelli. It is already in its two parts, the tibial and common peroneal, running side by side and forming one large nerve.

The nerve is vulnerable throughout and immediately after operation: by the knife or scissors during exposure; by traction during dislocation or after insertion of the implant; by crush from pressure forceps or retractor point; by burning by diathermy; by the heat of polymerising

Figs 13.26 to 13.28 The femoral nerve divided at groin level during "lymph node biopsy".

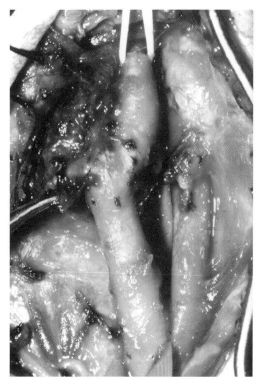

Fig. 13.26 The divided nerve 10 months after operation.

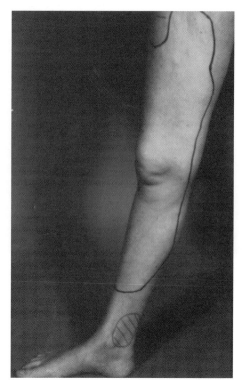

Fig. 13.27 The area of loss of sensibility.

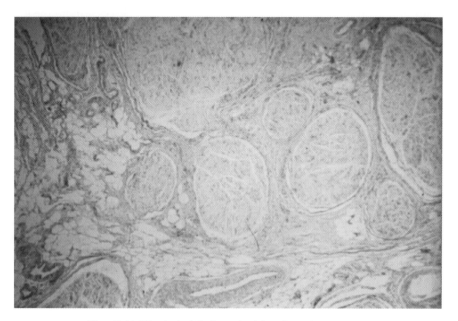

Fig. 13.28 Histological findings: fascicles of a main nerve.

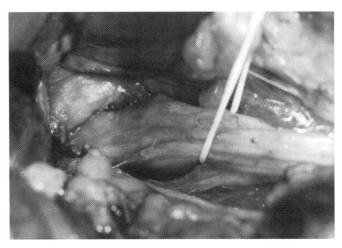

Fig. 13.29 The right sciatic nerve damaged by a chisel just below the foramen during removal of a medullary nail from the femur. The common peroneal nerve division has sustained severe damage.

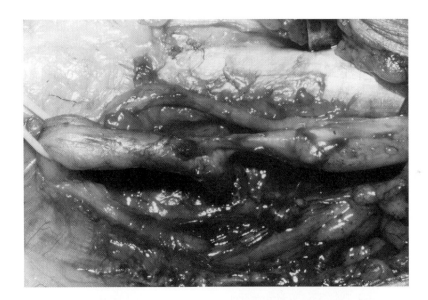

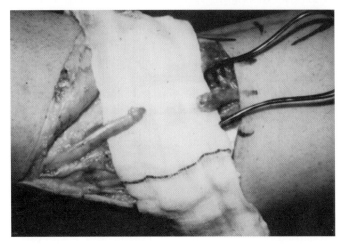

Fig. 13.30 Two cases of damage to the common peroneal nerve during operation for stripping of varicose veins.

cement by mangling by a drill or reamer which has escaped from the bone; or by external compression by haematoma or an encircling wire used to reattach a detached greater trochanter. Harkess (1992) reminds us that in cases of "protrusio acetabuli" the position of the sciatic nerve is so much altered in relation to the hip that the nerve is particularly vulnerable.

Weber et al (1976) commented on "peripheral neuropathies" associated with total replacement of the hip, and Ratliff (1984) reported on a series of 50 patients with this complication. Weber et al (1976) gave an incidence of only 0.7%, but indicated that in many more cases there was subclinical damage. The role of extruded cement in causing pressure was demonstrated by Casagrande and Danahy (1971), and later by Oleksak and Edge (1992). Calandruccio (1980) gave an incidence of injury to the sciatic nerve of 0.7–3%. He recommended exposure of the sciatic nerve during a posterior or anterolateral approach "where the anatomy of the hip is distorted as in external rotation deformity, intrapelvic protrusion of the acetabulum, shortness of the femoral head and neck, revision of a failed total hip arthroplasty and especially congenital dislocation". He repeated this caution in 1987. Kim and Kline (1995) studied lesions of the femoral nerve in particular: the most common mechanism of injury of this nerve was "iatrogenic complications due to various operative procedures in the vicinity of the nerve". Iatropathic damage accounted for 47 of 78 lesions, and in 12 of these the damage was done during arthroplasty of the hip.

Koka et al (1996) reported eight cases of "femoral neuropathy" in a series of 985 arthroplasties of the hip done through an anterolateral approach. There was good spontaneous recovery in all cases. They remarked on the ease with which the anterior retractor could be placed so as to compress the femoral nerve. Doubtless, the lesions in this series were caused by compression and distortion.

In the UCLA series reported by Schmalzreid and Amstutz (1991) there were 53 involved extremities in 3126 patients – an incidence of 1.7%. The sciatic nerve was involved in 43 cases, the sciatic and femoral in 7, and the femoral alone in 5. The cause of the lesion was unknown in as many as 55% of these cases. The incidence was highest (5.8%) in arthroplasty done for the late effects of congenital dislocation. That impression is confirmed by Fabre et al (1996), whose two cases of section of the femoral nerve occurred during arthroplasty for the late consequences of congenital dislocation. So high is the incidence in such cases and in other conditions of difficulty that the question of intraoperative monitoring in such cases (Nercessian et al 1989, Kennedy et al 1991) is seriously raised. Solheim and Hagen (1980) found an incidence of six major nerve injuries in 825 operations: four sciatic; one femoral; and one femoral and sciatic. In two of these cases the lesion was caused by haemorrhage associated with anticoagulant treatment.

Traction is undoubtedly the cause of the lesion in cases in which paralysis follows lengthening of the limb in operation for osteoarthritis secondary to dysplasia and subluxation or dislocation. Our findings in five cases of damage to the sciatic or femoral nerves of attenuation of longitudinal blood supply and partial epineurial rupture suggest that lengthening of 2 cm or more produces a lesion which, though degenerative, is recoverable. There is in all cases of sciatic nerve injury in which lengthening has exceeded 1 cm a case for instant revision of the arthroplasty and replacement of the components so as to relieve the strain on the nerve.

Birch et al (1992) were perhaps the first seriously to investigate the mechanism of damage by the heat of polymerising cement. They reported a case of pain and paralysis after such a thermal lesion of the sciatic nerve. Sixteen months after the event they explored the nerve and found it embedded in extruded cement. Two bundles only were intact and conducting. A 7-cm length of nerve was resected and the gap was bridged by grafts: the lesion was in effect localised to the part of the nerve exposed to heat. In a later investigation the same workers examined the effect of the heat generated in polymerising cement on the median nerve of an upper limb recently amputated for irrecoverable preganglionic injury of the plexus. They found here too a localised lesion with destruction of axoplasm, disruption of myelin and coagulation of endoneural collagen (see Figs 13.31 to 13.33).

Case report. A 56-year-old woman underwent cemented replacement arthroplasty for uncomplicated osteoarthritis of the left hip. She awoke from anaesthesia with severe pain and with complete paralysis in the distribution of the left sciatic nerve. No exploration was undertaken. When she was seen 18 months after the event there was virtually complete paralysis in the distribution of the sciatic nerve below the knee. There was some recovery of the hamstring muscles. Pain was persistent. Radiographs indicated extrusion of cement into the great sciatic notch (see Fig. 13.34). These were later supplemented by magnetic resonance imaging, which plainly showed the extrusion and its relation to the sciatic nerve (see Fig. 13.35). This patient refused operation; she took what was perhaps the wiser course of accepting £60 000 by way of compensation.

We have seen over 100 cases of damage to the nerves about the hip during hip arthroplasty and other procedures. Tables 13.1 to 13.4 summarise data about 54 re-explorations of nerves damaged during arthroplasty.

The gluteal nerves can be damaged during arthroplasty of the hip, either together with the sciatic nerve or alone. Jacobs and Buxton (1989) examined the course of the superior gluteal nerve, and drew attention to its vulnerability in lateral approaches to the hip. Baker and Bitounis (1989) added clinical observations concerning these conclusions. In later correspondence, McClelland (1990)

Figs 13.31 to 13.35 Two cases of damage to the sciatic nerve by cement during operation for arthroplasty of the hip:

Figs 13.31 to 13.33 Case 1.

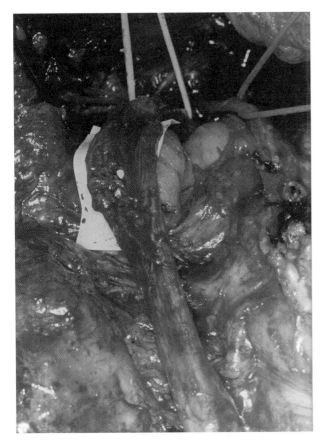

Fig. 13.31 The sciatic nerve seen at operation a year after initial operation. The extruded cement can be seen in relation to the nerve.

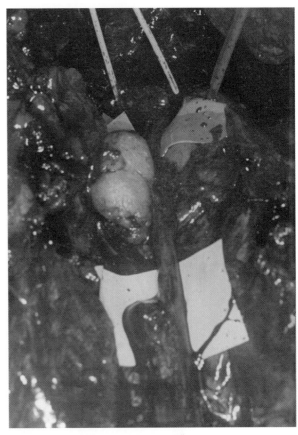

Fig. 13.32 The severely damaged common peroneal component resected.

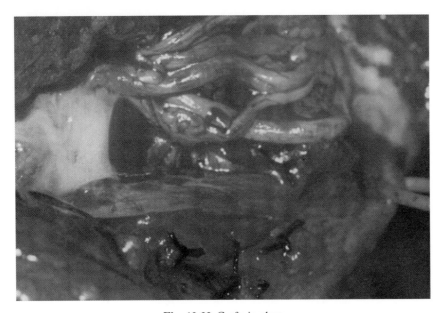

Fig. 13.33 Grafts in place.

Figs 13.34 and 13.35 Case 2 (described in text).

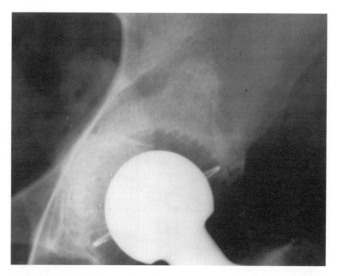

Fig. 13.34 Radiograph after operation shows cement intruding into the sciatic notch.

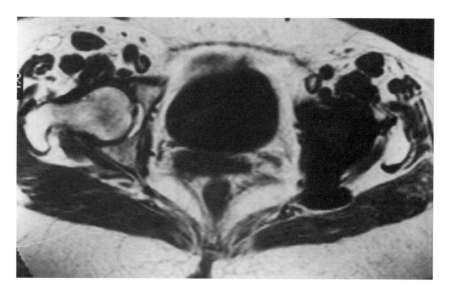

Fig. 13.35 Magnetic resonance image shows the relation of the cement to the notch and sciatic nerve. (Investigation by magnetic resonance imaging done at the instance of Mr Gordon Bannister.)

Table 13.1 Nerve damage associated with arthroplasty of the hip primary or secondary arthroplasty

Nerve injured	Primary arthroplasty	"Revision"
Sciatic	31	6
Femoral	6	4
Sciatic and femoral	6	1

Table 13.2 Nerve damage associated with arthroplasty of the hip: mechanism of injury demonstrated at exploration

Mechanism of injury	No. of nerves
Direct	
Cement burn	2
Cut	3
Included in suture	4
Retractor	8
Indirect	
Ischaemia (rupture of femoral vessels)	1
Extraneural bleeding	7
Intraneural bleeding	3
Traction/compression	26

Table 13.3 Damage to nerves about the hip: operation other than arthroplasty

Nerve injured	No. of nerves	Operation
Direct injury		
Obturator (extrapelvic)	3	
Obturator (intrapelvic)	3	Removal of tumour
Sciatic	3	Femoral nailing or nail removal
Femoral	6	Node biopsy (2) Arterial (2) Tumour (1) CDH (1)
Indirect injury		
Sciatic	6	Injection
Femoral	12	Injection (3) Catheterisation (9)
Ischaemic femoral neuropathy after aortofemoral bypass	1	

Table 13.4 Nerve damage associated with arthroplasty of the hip: results of operation

Operation type	No. of nerves
Early operation	
Drainage of hematoma	5
Removal of suture	3
Release of intraneural haematoma	1
Removal of cement	1
Late operation	
Removal of cement	1
Removal of suture	1
Exploration and neurolysis	42★

★ One aneurysm; two cut nerves.

indicated the likelihood of particular vulnerability in cases of severe dysplasia. In an interesting further note, Jacobs and Buxton (1990) recorded an increased incidence of a positive Trendelenburg test after arthroplasty of the hip by the lateral and transtrochanteric routes. The inferior gluteal nerve seems to be less vulnerable, though we have seen this nerve damaged with the sciatic during arthroplasty of the hip. Although the damage to the larger nerve was recognised within a week of operation, that to the inferior gluteal was not appreciated until the patient was seen by an independent examiner 2 years later.

It is, regrettably, the case that lesions of the sciatic nerve during hip arthroplasty are too often dismissed as "foot drop" and are not subjected to the investigation that they require. Such failure of recognition is particularly common in the case of associated lesions of the gluteal nerves. Although patients are required to rise from their beds and walk the day after operation, surgeons seem unwilling in the early stages to do more than inspect the foot and leg, without examining the function of the muscles of the thigh and buttock.

We are glad here to be able to narrate an instance of early recognition and prompt action by a surgeon who was so unfortunate as to cut the sciatic nerve during insertion of a medullary nail for fixation of the fragments of a broken femur. The case was that of a 19-year-old girl, 5 feet 4 inches in height and weighing 7 stone, who sustained a closed fracture through the middle of the right femur. Operation was undertaken 9 days after injury; during clearance with the scissors of soft tissues overlying the upper end of the femur, the muscles of the calf were seen to twitch. The exposure was extended, and it was found that the sciatic nerve had been cut. It was repaired then and there with sutures of 6/0 prolene. A month later the operator and one of us explored the site of the lesion: the suture line was intact, and bundles were seen to run within a few millimetres of it. When the patient was seen 2 years later there was remarkably good recovery of motor power and sensibility in the distribution of both components of the damaged nerve. This surgeon not only recognised instantly the fact of damage, but also proceeded at once to repair, and later sought advice from one with particular experience in the field. Although we regret the original mistake, for its effect on the patient and surgeon, we commend the prompt recognition and action that avoided serious continuing disability.

Cutaneous sensory nerves

Among the most disastrous consequences of iatropathic lesions of peripheral nerves are those of damage to nerves so small that few would believe that it could cause so much trouble. The nerves particularly concerned are the terminal branch of the radial nerve, the medial cutaneous nerve of forearm, the palmar cutaneous branch of the median nerve, the digital nerves, the supraclavicular nerves and the saphenous nerve. The first is damaged during operations for ganglion of the wrist or for de Quervain tenovaginitis; the second, during operations at the elbow; the third, during operation for decompression of the median nerve; the fourth during operation for Dupuytren's disease; the fifth, during operations on the thoracic outlet and brachial plexus; and the last during operations for arthroscopy of the knee and varicose veins. The last operation sometimes claims the sural nerve as a victim. Our experience of the distribution of these lesions is shown in Table 13.5. In most cases probably, the nerves are cut; sometimes they are ligated and then cut. In some patients such damage causes the development of a chronic painful state, with spontaneous or induced pain, hyper-aesthesia and hyperalgesia, and even with allodynia and hyperpathia. We have seen a limb amputated for persistent pain after damage to the superficial radial nerve at the wrist. In that case the persistent refusal of the defendants to accept a reasonable proposal for early settlement was undoubtedly a factor in prolonging and magnifying the patient's complaints. These painful states are not usually dependent on sympathetic activity. They are resistant to all methods of treatment; in fact, the piling of treatment on treatment in the "pain clinic" usually makes them worse. The cause is probably both central and peripheral: alteration of the central mechanism of analysis and modification of impulses; and peripheral alteration of incoming impulses by loss of the normal pattern of cutaneous innervation. Axonal sprouting from adjacent cutaneous nerves may cause further confusion of the pattern of innervation.

"There is no cure for this disease" (Belloc 1940): the only reasonable course is to avoid damage to cutaneous nerves by careful operating. If such a nerve is divided, the only treatment with any prospect of success is the restoration of neural continuity by direct suture or by insertion of a freeze–thawed muscle graft (Gattuso et al 1988, Glasby 1990). It is perverse to propose to treat the sequelae of damage to one cutaneous nerve by damaging another by taking it as a graft.

Table 13.5 Operations for damage to nerves of cutaneous sensibility

Nerve	No. of nerves
Neck and upper limb	
Supraclavicular	7
Medial cutaneous of forearm	11
Superficial radial	65
Palmar	38
Dorsal branch of ulnar	6
Total	127
Lower limb	
Lateral cutaneous of thigh	5
Saphenous	11
Sural	10
Plantar	9
Terminal branches common peroneal	7
Total	42

THE CRANIAL NERVES

Apart from the spinal accessory – itself hardly a cranial nerve – the nerve most often injured is the seventh (facial), damage to which causes grave disfigurement and dysfunction through the paralysis of the muscles of one side of the face. It is vulnerable in the cranial cavity, in the petrous temporal bone and in the face, in the last particularly because of its association with the parotid gland. In any of these sites some degree of damage may be inevitable because of difficulties imposed by the disease process and by restriction of space. Maran (1994) lists the circumstances in which damage to the facial nerve could be considered to be negligent. Hobsley (1994) says wise words about informed consent to parotidectomy for a lump. These words are in fact applicable to other situations in which a nerve is likely to be at risk in a prolonged operation.

We have seen the facial nerve of a woman in her thirties irretrievably damaged during an operation for the removal of what was thought to be a mixed parotid tumour but which was in fact a schwannoma of a facial nerve. In this case, unfortunately, a breakdown in the system operated by the Health Authority delayed repair for so long that reconstruction only was practicable. Doubtless, few surgeons nowadays embark on operation on the parotid gland without apparatus for magnification and for identifying by stimulation the facial nerve and its branches. When, often enough inevitably, the main nerve is cut, the indication is surely for instant repair by suture or by graft (Jacobs & Dean 1992). Since it is likely that much of the proprioceptive input from the facial muscles returns in branches of the fifth (trigeminal) nerve (Baumel 1974), early and accurate grafting of the facial nerve should give good results. Samii (1980) shows some excellent results of grafting.

The lingual branch of the fifth (trigeminal) nerve, involved as is the facial nerve with a salivary gland, is at risk during operations on the submandibular gland and on its duct. It is at risk too in operations for removal of the third lower molar tooth. Robinson (1994) reveals that the incidence of such damage in the UK (11–22%) compares poorly with that in the USA and in most of the rest of Europe (0.7%). He attributes this high incidence to the British practice of obtaining access by raising and retracting a lingual mucoperiosteal flap. Robinson concludes with a sentence applicable throughout this field: "It seems likely that, in the future, the threat of medical negligence will hang over not only the surgeon who caused the initial injury, but also the one who fails to refer the patient to an appropriate centre for nerve repair". What can be done in such centres is narrated by LaBanc and Gregg (1992), who report an overall success rate of 76.2% after microsurgical repair of the trigeminal nerve. Interestingly enough, an entrapment syndrome involving the lingual nerve has been described following the removal of the third lower molar (Ho & Lloyd 1987). The nerve was found to be compressed by a spicule of bone, the result, no doubt, of the operation for removal. The tenth (vagus) and twelfth (hypoglossal) nerves are at risk in many operations on the neck, and in particular operations on the carotid vessels (Vertu et al 1977, Hertzer et al 1980) and in the uppermost part of the cervical spine (Bonney 1991). In the last, the superior laryngeal nerve and its external laryngeal branch are quite easily damaged by traction. The consequent temporary loss of the action of the crico-thyroid muscle can cause trouble to singers.

The branch of the vagus nerve most famously vulnerable at operation is of course the recurrent laryngeal. Operations on the thyroid gland provide most of the injuries, but the nerve is at risk too in extensive operations on the lower cervical spine and the cervicothoracic junction. We are indebted to Professor A. G. D. Maran for guidance in this field and for the perception that the control of the muscles of the larynx is a complex matter; possibly too complex for adequate selective reinnervation after repair by suture or by graft. Professor Maran's help allows us to point to the work of Bigenzahn et al (1991) on the results of neurolysis or primary repair of the recurrent laryngeal nerve, and to that of Miyauchi et al (1993) on the results of repair. The latter concluded that "not only simple neuropathy of the recurrent nerve but also free grafting, vagus–recurrent nerve suture or ansa cervicalis–recurrent suture are effective in patients with peripheral and unilateral recurrent nerve paralysis". Professor Maran himself, writing in 1994 (Maran 1994) inclined to the view that "grafting of the recurrent laryngeal nerve was not as successful as grafting the facial nerve", and that "medialising" the paralysed cord was preferable to operation on the nerve.

A VIEW OF THE LEGAL ASPECTS

The occurrence after operation of a lesion of a peripheral nerve must create the presumption that there has been want of care, though that may not necessarily be the case. The factors to be considered are the depth of the lesion, the mechanism of the injury, the difficulty of the operation and the condition for which it was undertaken, and the speed with which the lesion is recognised, diagnosed and treated. In the case of primary arthroplasty of the hip, cutting the sciatic nerve plainly indicates a lack of care, whereas the occurrence of a transient lesion of the nerve just as plainly does not. On the other hand, serious damage to the sciatic nerve may truly be unavoidable in a secondary or tertiary operation of extreme difficulty, with the anatomy obscured and structures distorted by scarring. In such a case, failure to monitor function during operation could even now be taken to indicate lack of care. It is pretty certain that 5 years from now such a view will be taken.

Failure of recognition is only rarely forgivable; failure to diagnose and act appropriately is, in our view, never forgivable: it is this failure that may cause the patient to lose the best chance of recovery. Regrettably, it is this failure that seems to be the most common; it is on this failure that the "risk managers" must chiefly work.

FAILURE TO RECOGNISE ACUTE INJURY

Many factors make it difficult for the clinician to recognise nerve injury at an early stage, in the accident department, when and where it should be recognised. The patient may be drunk or mentally deranged or under the influence of drugs. He or she is certain to be distressed by the fact of injury and perhaps by the sight of blood. The patient may be a child, upset by the injury and frightened by the often appalling aspect of the modern accident department. There may be associated injuries sufficiently severe and painful to distract attention from the site of nerve injury. When a fracture or dislocation is associated with nerve injury, the pain of the former and the impairment of function may be attributed solely to the former injury. The examining medical officer may not be at his or her best in the early hours of the morning. A nurse in charge of "triage" may be as unfamiliar as any medical officer with the clinical aspects of peripheral nerve injury. Lastly, it is possible that in the first few hours after a clean severance of a nerve with a sharp instrument, sensibility may be preserved. Altogether, the circumstances are likely to be inimical to careful neurological examination. McAllister et al (1996), in their epidemiological study of 813 patients with 1111 nerve injuries, found that divisions of 93 nerves in 83 patients (8.3% of nerves; 10.2% of patients) "were treated other than by primary repair or elective secondary repair, due to delayed referral from accident and emergency departments, resulting from missed or uncertain diagnosis at presentation or otherwise unaccounted delay in the initial referral". Ten per cent is a lot. Accident officers and triage nurses must be made aware that when there is a wound across the line of a main nerve, the digits of the affected limb must be felt. If the digits in the area of supply of the nerve are warm and dry, the nerve has been cut and it must be so assumed unless and until exploration proves otherwise.

An illustrative case A woman of 56 living in a large town fell and injured her right shoulder. Because the accident department of the hospital in her town had been closed, she was taken by ambulance to that of the hospital in a large adjoining town. There she was seen, told that she was suffering from a "frozen shoulder", given two aspirin tablets and sent home. The same evening she was aware of progressive paralysis of and loss of sensibility in the limb. The next day she went 4 miles by taxicab to the accident department in which she had originally been seen. The advice given on the first day was repeated; two more aspirins were given. Recourse was had the next day to the general practitioner, he indicated that he could not override the advice given by the hospital medical officer. One month later, on her own initiative, the patient saw an orthopaedic surgeon, who instantly recognised that there was anterior dislocation of the shoulder with a deep lesion of the posterior and medial cords of the brachial plexus.

This case encapsulates for us the principal causes of clinical error and negligence: failure of knowledge, failure to observe and *failure to use common sense*. The medical officer should certainly have been able to recognise anterior dislocation of the shoulder in a woman of average build. He or she should, even without the benefit of knowledge, have realised that an elderly woman would not be at the trouble and expense of travelling 8 miles by taxicab for advice unless something serious was amiss. Sadly, although knowledge can be imparted and the need to observe can be stressed, it may be hard to impart common sense to those who have undergone a "medical education".

RADIATION NEUROPATHY

Contemporaneous interest in this subject indicated to us the need to examine it in some detail. Rather than accord it a separate chapter, we have chosen to discuss it in this section.

As a footnote to the article by Fallet et al (1967) indicates, our interest in the field of radiation neuropathy, and in particular in that of neuropathy after treatment of breast cancer, goes back at least 30 years. It is remarkable that Seddon (1975g) had little to say on this subject, though he narrated an interesting and tragic case of bilateral median neuropathy after radiotherapy for warts on the back of the wrists. We have experienced much difficulty in this field. First, we have up to recent times found it difficult to convince some radiotherapists of the reality of the condition; indeed, this discretion has often hindered disclosure of details of dosage and duration of treatment when we have been seeking a cause for the affection of particular patients by radiation neuropathy. Next, we have found it difficult to understand why one patient treated for breast cancer should develop radiation neuropathy whereas another, treated in an apparently similar manner, should not. Thirdly, the fact that so great an interval – in our experience, ranging up to 24 years – can separate treatment from onset of symptoms is an important obstacle to investigation. Hospital Authorities and Trusts are commonly averse to spending money on the storage and retrieval of records, and policies of routine destruction after (say) 6 years are common. A further element of uncertainty is introduced by the common difficulty of distinguishing between local recurrence and radiation neuropathy. Lastly, there is constant uncertainty about the role of intervention in radiation neuropathy: we have found it virtually impossible to come to any conclusion about its value except as a method for distinguishing between recurrence and neuropathy.

The most common site for radiation neuropathy is the brachial plexus of the adult woman, because of the frequency of breast cancer, the frequency with which radiotherapy is used and the position of the plexus in the field. We are of course aware of the occurrence of this lesion in the sacral plexus after pelvic irradiation, but our experience of this is limited to two cases.

The situation of the clinician directing radiotherapy is one of peculiar difficulty. On the one hand, the dose of radiation must be enough to destroy tumour cells; while, on the other hand, it should not be enough nor so directed as to cause serious damage to normal tissues, and in particular to nerves. The handicap of the long latency between treatment and the appearance of symptoms adds to the difficulties.

EFFECT OF X-RAYS ON PERIPHERAL NERVES

Cavanagh (1968a) investigated the effects of radiation on the sciatic nerves of rats. He found that "the capacity of cells in peripheral nerve to proliferate in response to nerve crush is seriously impaired if the limb has been previously X-irradiated with 1900 rads (19 Gy). No difference in this effect has been found whether the irradiation was done 3 weeks or 9 months before nerve crush". In the previous year, Cavanagh (1968b) had found significant nuclear abnormalities in the Schwann cells of rat sciatic nerve after exposure to as little as 200 rads (2 Gy).

RADIATION NEUROPATHY OR METASTASIS?

Stoll and Andrews (1966), working in Melbourne, began their account of "radiation-induced peripheral neuropathy" with the statement: "It has been thought that adult nervous tissues show a remarkable degree of resistance to injury by X-rays." They then went on to report a high incidence of neuropathy in patients receiving 63 Gy by megavoltage radiation over 25–28 days, after radical operation. Their criteria for the diagnosis of radiation neuropathy were later criticised by Thomas and Colby (1972), principally on the grounds that the distinction between neuropathy and metastatic plexopathy was imperfect. Mumenthaler (1964), reporting eight cases, based his differentiation either on the results of exploratory operation or on the presence of symptoms of neuropathy for 2–9 years without evidence of local recurrence or remote metastasis. In 1967, Maruyama et al in Minneapolis started their account of an unusual late complication of radiotherapy with the words "Peripheral neuropathy as a late consequence of radiation is generally considered rare." This patient, a woman aged 23 at the time of treatment, developed neuropathy 18 years after first being treated for Hodgkin's disease of the cervical lymph nodes. The experience of Maruyama et al was shared by Burns (1978), who described the cases of three women in whom symptoms of neuropathy began, respectively, 18, 12 and 17 years after radiation for breast cancer. Radical mastectomy had been done in all three cases. Burns recalled the findings of Lampert and Davis (1964) concerning "early" and "late" delayed reactions of the central nervous system to radiation.

Castaigne et al (1969) drew attention away from radiation neuropathy to neuropathy from secondary deposit, mentioning the remarkable case of a woman in whom the symptoms of "metastatic neuropathy" began as long as 26 years after treatment of a primary breast cancer. Indeed, in our own observation of a case of secondary deposit from breast cancer in the nerves of the cauda equina, symptoms began 10 years after treatment of the primary tumour. One of the introductory remarks by these authors bears repeating: "*La littérature concernant ces deux éventualités (envalissement des nerfs, ou souffrance consécutive à la radiothérapie) n'est pas très abondante. Il est évident que les observations d'envalissement cancéreux ne sont pas habituellement publiées parce qu'elles sont considérées comme trop classiques.*"

The debate about the differentiation of radiation from "metastatic" neuropathy was continued by Steiner et al (1971) and by Thomas and Colby (1972). Both sets of workers came to the view expressed by the latter workers: "A good deal stands to be gained from surgical exploration of the brachial plexus in any case in which diagnosis is uncertain". Both agreed that a long interval between primary treatment and the onset of symptoms of neuropathy was no certain indicator of damage by irradiation. Match (1974), however, reporting 15 cases of radiation neuropathy, thought that the condition might be "more common than is currently realised".

Kogelnik (1977) concluded that "the development of peripheral neuropathies of cranial nerve and of the brachial plexus following curative doses of irradiation is closely related with the total dose applied, the number and size of individual doses per fraction, and the overall time". He went on, "In the pathogenesis of peripheral neuropathy a combined effect of different factors seems likely".

Kori et al (1981), examining 100 patients with "plexopathy", were able to essay a clinical distinction which had been adumbrated by previous workers. In "metastatic" neuropathy, pain, affection of the lower part of the plexus, and Bernard–Horner syndrome were more common than in radiation neuropathy. These impressions were later confirmed by Lederman and Wilbourn's (1984) findings of fasciculation in radiation neuropathy as the "most useful diagnostic criteria". Roth et al (1988) also showed the value of the physiological finding of myokymic discharges as an indicator of radiation neuropathy, and indicated a connection with conduction block. In 1989, Harper et al were able to confirm the more common finding of myokymic discharges in radiation than in "metastatic" neuropathy. Myokymia is defined (De Lisa et al 1994) as

"a continuous quivering and undulation of surface and overlying skin ... associated with spontaneous, repetitive discharge of motor unit potentials". Myokymic discharges are motor unit action potentials that fire repetitively and may be associated with clinical myokymia. Hoàng et al (1986), describing three cases of metastatic neuropathy and one of bilateral radiation neuropathy of the plexus, found computed tomography unhelpful in differentiating "between tumour and radiation neuritis". Harper et al's (1989) findings with computed tomography were also rather disappointing, though in the previous year Cooke and colleagues presented evidence to show the role of that method of examination in distinguishing metastatic disease from "radiation fibrosis" (Cooke et al 1988). The role of magnetic resonance imaging in making this distinction has been explored in the last 10 years. Glazer et al (1985) found that radiation fibrosis, like muscle, "usually remained low on signal intensity on T2-weighted images, while tumours demonstrated higher signal intensity". However, a relatively high signal density on T2-weighted images was not specific for tumour recurrence. Castagno and Shuman (1987) examined 47 patients suspected of having tumour involvement of the brachial plexus, and concluded that "MR may have substantial clinical utility in evaluating patients with suspected brachial plexus tumours, particularly in patients with suggestive neurologic signs and symptoms." Ebner et al (1988) used magnetic resonance imaging for differentiating fibrosis from recurrent tumour in the female pelvis: in 11 of 12 cases of recurrence, they found that magnetic resonance imaging showed tumour as an area of increased signal density. Rapaport et al (1988) correlated findings on magnetic resonance imaging with pathological findings and appearances on computed tomography: magnetic resonance imaging was found to be more accurate than computed tomography. Posniak et al (1993) found that "the accuracy of magnetic resonance imaging in differentiating metastatic disease from radiation changes is unclear because both hypointensive and hyperintensive lesions on T2-weighted images have been described in radiation fibrosis. Biopsy may be required to make a definitive diagnosis." Similarly, Thyayagarajan et al (1995) found the presence of an increased T2-weighted signal ambivalent, and relied particularly on the finding of a mass as a predictor of tumour. As Harper et al (1989) had done before, they noted the frequent finding of myokymia in radiation neuropathy.

INCIDENCE OF RADIATION NEUROPATHY

Barr and Kissin (1987) found that 6 of 250 patients treated by local excision and irradiation at the Royal Marsden Hospital in the period 1980–1983 developed radiation neuropathy over periods of 4 to 24 months. Total doses of 51 Gy in fractions of 3.4 Gy were given. The authors considered the condition to be dose-dependent and related to the size of individual fractions. Cooke et al (1988), reviewing the results reported by Stoll and Andrews (1966), Kori et al (1981) and Pierquin and Huart (1985), found that the incidence of significant neurological disability after radiation ranged from 0% to 73%. Surely some mistake! In order properly to assess the incidence of radiation neuropathy Cooke et al (1988) analysed the cases of all patients treated by radiation after operation over a period of 30 months. Ten of the 459 patients treated developed lesions of the brachial plexus: a figure close to that of Barr and Kissin (1987). Again, the incidence was higher in the 336 patients treated with a large dose per fraction than in the 126 treated with a small fraction size.

Olsen et al (1990) suggested that the addition of chemotherapy to radiotherapy increased the incidence of neuropathy; they also indicated the predominant (56%) affection of the entire plexus. This Danish team (Olsen et al 1993), in a very important study, later examined 161 recurrence-free breast cancer patients for radiation plexopathy after a median follow-up period of 50 months (range 13–99 months) 5% and 9% of patients receiving radiotherapy had, respectively, disabling and mild radiation plexopathy. Neuropathy was more common in patients receiving cytotoxic therapy ($P = 0.04$) and in younger patients ($P = 0.04$). They concluded that fractions of 2 Gy or less were advisable. A year later, Falk (1994) concluded rather pessimistically: "axillary radiotherapy can also provide equivalent levels of long term control in the clinically node-negative axilla, but the chronic disabling symptom of brachial plexopathy is documented at all radiation doses that can sterilise microscopic disease, irrespective of the radiotherapy technique".

Two very important steps were taken in 1994 by the Royal College of Radiologists (London), partly under the stimulus of a group action taken by a number of women who had received radiotherapy and believed that they had suffered as a consequence (Radiation Action Group Exposure). An independent review by Drs Thelma Bates and R. G. B. Evans was commissioned; a committee chaired by Dr Jane Maher reviewed the "management of adverse effects following radiotherapy". Bates and Evans' (1995) most important findings were perhaps:

- the association of neuropathy with movement of the patient between the treatment of the chest wall and the treatment of the lymph nodes
- the very high incidence of neuropathy in patients receiving "high dose" treatment coupled with moderate movement during treatment.

Maher's (1995) contribution is a wide-ranging study of the nature, diagnosis, natural course, and response to treatment of radiation neuropathy of the brachial plexus. Spittle (1995) performed a valuable service in bringing these reports to the notice of a wider audience.

PATHOLOGY AND NATURAL COURSE

The lesion is typically sclerotic; depending on occlusion of small vessels (Spiess 1972), but the large vessels are of course also involved in the process that tends to sclerosis of all irradiated tissues (Fig. 13.36). Gerard et al (1989) narrate the case of the rather sudden onset of neuropathy in a woman treated by irradiation and radical mastectomy 22 years previously. Arteriography showed a segmental occlusion of the subclavian artery. Similar arterial lesions have been reported by Butler et al (1980) and Barros D'Sa (1992a).

To the primarily neural lesion of vasculitis with damage to both axon and myelin sheath is added the external one of compression by sclerotic tissues such as the pectoralis minor and subclavius muscles. Merle et al (1988) liken these to "syndromes canalaires créés par la nécrose du petit pectoral et du sous-clavier," and we cannot improve on that.

In our experience of more than 70 cases, the natural course of this disorder is almost always towards steady deterioration. The initial symptom is usually that of paraesthesiae in the fingers; it is at this stage that a diagnosis of "carpal tunnel syndrome" or "cervical radiculopathy" is commonly made. Less commonly, muscle weakness is the initial symptom, and even less commonly the patient presents with pain. The condition progresses to severe alteration of sensibility and motor paralysis; sometimes pain develops or progresses to become constant and severe. Salner et al (1981) reported spontaneous remission in eight cases of radiation neuropathy; in five of these there was complete resolution of all symptoms. The experience of Killer and Hess (1990) was, however, similar to ours; in all their cases the condition progressed without remission.

Little has been said about another, even more dangerous, consequence of radiotherapy: the development of sarcoma in the irradiated nervous tissue. Our experience of this condition is narrated in Chapter 14.

RADIATION NEUROPATHY IN THE LOWER LIMB OF THE MALE

In a wide-ranging paper, Bowen et al (1996) consider the cases of six men who received radiotherapy to the groin and para-aortic glands (T10 to L4) for testicular malignancies, and who later developed neuropathy. The mean dose was 45.5 Gy; the latencies ranged from 3 to 25 years; and the affection was predominantly motor, but in two cases it was initially monomelic. The course of the condition was regularly one of slow but relentless deterioration. Myokymia was noted in three patients; the sural nerve action potential was obtained in five. Magnetic resonance imaging with gadolinium showed linear and focal enhancement of the lumbosacral roots within the spinal canal in two of three cases. Pathological examination of the conus and cauda equina was possible in one case: this

Figs 13.36 and 13.37 Radiation neuropathy.

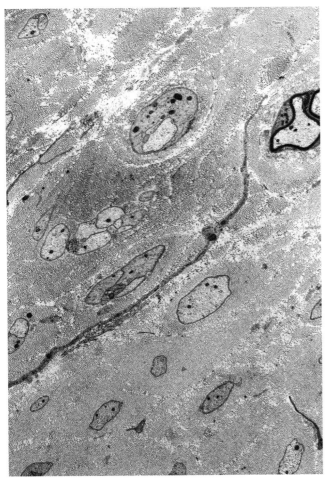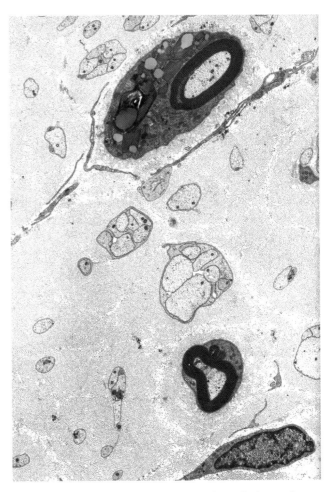

Fig. 13.36 Electron microphotographs of specimens from biopsy of the lateral trunk of the brachial plexus taken 2½ years after radiotherapy for cancer of the breast. Note the extensive collagenisation, the loss of axons and myelin, and the macrophage clearing debris. × 4125.

showed a "vasculopathy of the proximal spinal roots, with preservation of motor neuronal cell bodies and spinal cord architecture". The authors conclude that the affection is a radiculopathy rather than a neuronopathy.

This important paper offers no new insight on the possibilities of treatment, though the role of anticoagulants is briefly mentioned. It does, however, offer good clear evidence about pathology and differential diagnosis, and suggests possibilities for avoidance.

TREATMENT

Mondrup et al (1990), reporting from Denmark, stated bleakly: "Because the treatment of brachial plexopathy is unsuccessful, prevention is warranted". Opinion is certainly divided. For years we recommended and practised

exploration, biopsy, external neurolysis and occasionally epineurotomy, for confirmation of diagnosis and in the hope of giving relief. This attitude was certainly shared by the Geneva workers (Fallet et al 1967) and, with reservations, by Steiner et al (1971). So far as we are aware, the suggestion made by von Albert and Mackert (1970) from observations in seven cases of radiation neuropathy, that treatment with Actihaemyl, an albumen-free extract of blood, produced a rapid clinical and electromyographic improvement, has not received later confirmation.

In 1963, Kiricuta in Romania drew attention to the use of a pedicled omental flap for treatment of radionecrosis of the chest wall and of chronic oedema of the upper limb, and for reconstruction of the breast. Uhlschmid and Clodius (1978) followed the suggestion by free transplantation of the omentum with microvascular anastomosis, combined with external neurolysis, for radiation neuropathy of the plexus. They concluded, modestly enough, after reviewing the seven patients treated: *"Als wesentlicher Erfolg muss jedoch die sofortige und anhaltende Schmerzfreiheit aller Patienten angesehen werden"*. That is certainly right, even though the effect on neuropathy was probably, at the best to halt it. Later, Narakas (1984b) reported the results of operative treatment for radiation-induced and metastatic brachial plexopathy in 45 cases, 15 having an omentoplasty. Narakas thought that omentoplasty was most likely to succeed if used early; he achieved a "functional result" in only 20% of cases.

Le Quang (1989) attempted to answer the questions: (a) Should we operate on radiation plexitis: (b) If so, when? (c) What operation? The answers arising from an extensive experience were: (a) yes, whenever possible; (b) at the earliest possible time; and (c) selective neurolysis completed by a pedicled omentoplasty. Le Quang stated clearly the limitations of operation. Much weight should be given to those careful conclusions, based as they are on a careful observation and wide practical experience.

Our experience with omentoplasty was discouraging. In one of our two cases a 50-year-old woman began getting symptoms of neuropathy 10 years after mastectomy and radiotherapy. Symptoms progressed, and severe, unremitting pain was added. The plexus was explored and decompressed both above and below the clavicle, and, in order to remove any possible obstruction at the thoracic outlet, the first rib was removed. Biopsies were taken: there was no suggestion of metastasis, but there was severe sclerosis of all tissues, particularly of the scalenus anterior, the subclavius and the pectoralis minor. A free omental graft was taken and its main vessels were anastomosed to convenient vessels (Mr Angus Jamieson). There was good perfusion of the graft, which was wrapped around the plexus. Progress after operation was uncomplicated, but pain persisted and there was no regression of the neurological affection.

In contrast, outstandingly good results were achieved in two cases in which a pedicled graft of the latissimus dorsi muscle was used. These operations were done in collaboration with Professor Roy Sanders.

Case report 1. A woman with a family history of ankylosing spondylitis and diabetes mellitus underwent at the age of 35 a local excision of the left breast for carcinoma. An axillary lymph node was taken for examination: it showed no evidence of infiltration. Operation was followed by radiotherapy (60 Gy in 30 fractions). Symptoms of neuropathy principally affecting the medial cord of the plexus began 11 months later and progressed to pain, motor weakness and sensory change. Fifteen months after the primary operation the plexus was explored above and below the clavicle. There was no evidence of recurrence of tumour, but there was considerable fibrosis around the plexus. External neurolysis by release of the scalenus

anterior, subclavius and pectoralis minor was done. It is possible that after some months there was improvement in function of the hand.

Three and a half years after the primary operation there was a pathological fracture through the left clavicle, the site of radiation necrosis. Failure of the fragments to unite led to a partial excision, done at another hospital. The condition of the left upper limb continued to deteriorate and pain continued to increase until, in 1995, 8$\frac{1}{2}$ years after the primary operation, it was decided to attempt further neurolysis, coupled with cover by a pedicled graft of the latissimus dorsi muscle. The related vessels had not been affected by radiotherapy.

At operation a band of scar connecting the clavicular fragments was found to be compressing the plexus; in addition, the lateral clavicular fragment was found to be indenting the upper trunk. The scar tissue was removed and the clavicular fragments were mobilised and an enveloping mass of scar tissue was removed. Some further removal of clavicle was done. Then a pedicled graft of latissimus dorsi was taken and transferred to lie between the plexus and the residual clavicular fragments. No evidence of recurrent tumour was found.

After this operation there was marked relief of pain; it seems too, that motor function may be improving.

Case report 2. A man born in 1972 was treated at the ages of 3, 6 and 8 years for "lesions" of the left pectoral region later thought to be those of malignant fibrous histiocytoma. In 1992 a recurrent tumour was widely excised and the site was irradiated (60 Gy in 18 fractions over 6 weeks). Symptoms of radiation neuropathy began soon after treatment and progressed until at 6 months there was serious pain with deep affection of motor and sensory function. There was serious damage to the skin over the clavicle. Electrophysiological examination showed severe affection of the medial and posterior cords: in particular, there were frequent fibrillations and positive sharp waves in the left first dorsal interosseous muscle.

At operation in 1994, 2 years after radiotherapy, an extensive neurolysis of the plexus was done, with division of the scaleni, pectoralis minor and clavicular head of pectoralis major. Stimulation of roots and recording from cords showed potentials of diminished amplitude and velocity (medial cord 25 m/s, posterior cord 10 m/s). Professor Sanders then elevated and placed a pedicled musculocutaneous flap of latissimus dorsi and overlying skin to replace the burnt skin and to surround the plexus. There was early relief of pain; 2 years after operation there was good recovery of motor and sensory function (Fig. 13.37).

These two cases show the benefits to be obtained from extensive neurolysis and revascularisation by healthy living tissue. Perhaps the pedicled muscular or musculocutaneous flap provides revascularisation superior to that provided by the omental graft?

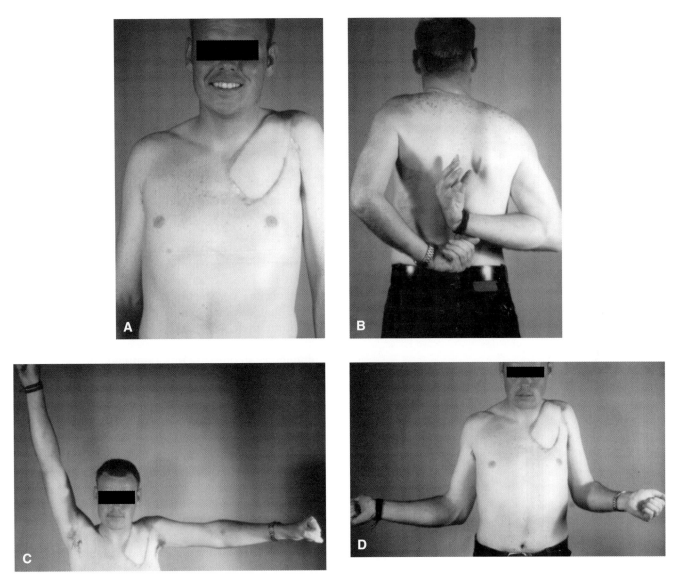

Fig. 13.37 Case 2 (described in the text). The patient 2 years after operation. (a) Appearance of the patient and flap. (b–d) Function at the shoulder.

Results of operation

Experience with 54 traced patients who underwent operation for radiation neuropathy suggests that the likelihood of true relief of pain and regression of the neurological abnormality is low (five patients). Twenty-four patients obtained relief of pain and stabilisation of the neurological state; twenty-five obtained no relief. Sex distribution and diagnoses are shown in Table 13.6. Recurrence of carcinoma was confirmed in three cases; remarkably, there was substantial relief of pain in two of these. Operation on the plexus in these cases is not free of danger: in one, necrosis of the artery led to amputation; in another there was thrombosis of the subclavian artery; in one there was delayed

healing with necrosis of part of the clavicle; and one patient died from cerebrovascular accident 3 months after operation. In one undoubted case of radiation neuropathy there was spontaneous remission over a period of 10 years. We are, albeit reluctantly, obliged to state that the place of operation in the treatment of radiation neuropathy remains uncertain. There are, probably, three indications for operation:

- establishment of diagnosis, and in particular the diagnosis of a radiation-induced malignant tumour of the peripheral nerve sheath
- severe and persistent pain
- rapid progressive loss of function.

Table 13.6 Sex distribution and diagnoses in radiation neuropathy

	No. of patients
Operation	
Total	55
Women	
Total	50
Carcinoma of the breast	45
Lymphoma	3
Carcinoma of the thyroid	1
Skin malignancy	1
Men	
Total	5
Lymphoma	3
Malignant fibrous histiocytoma*	2
Operations	
"Decompression"	46
Pedicled latissimus dorsi	5
Free latissimus dorsi	2
Omental transfer	2
Outcome of operation	
Relief of pain with neurological improvement	5
Relief of pain with stabilisation of neurological state	24
Transient or no relief	26
Recurrence of cancer confirmed	3
Complications	
Amputation (arterial necrosis)	1
Thrombosis of the subclavian artery	1
Delayed healing with necrosis of clavicle	1
Death (cardiovascular accident 3 months after operation)	1
No operation	
Total	7
Women	7
Lumbosacral (pelvic Ca.)	1
Ca. breast (very severe radiation effects)	5
Ca. breast: spontaneous remission (10-year observation)	1

*One received neutron therapy, and later had amputation.

The place of operation in the first seems to us to be undeniable. As to the second, it seems to us there is a worthwhile chance of relieving pain in most cases. As to loss of function, we think there is a worthwhile chance of, at least, arresting deterioration in most cases. Anything more is a bonus. We are aware that Bainbridge (1996) takes a more sanguine view; we can only hope that he is right.

RISK MANAGEMENT

No figures are available for the incidence of peripheral nerve damage during medical and surgical procedures, but the impression sustained by those working in this field is dismal. Evidently, there are lessons to be learned: about warning; about the position of nerves; about the vulnerability of nerves; about the symptoms and signs and diagnosis of nerve injury; and about the need for early and effective treatment. There are lessons to be learned, too, about procedures in the places where treatment is given, about recording and about proper communication with patients and their doctors.

Warning: In advising treatment, and in particular in advising operation, the clinician must be aware of the balance of advantage against risk, and should attempt to convey to the patient his or her assessment of that balance. This is not easy: if medicine were easy there would be little need for doctors; none for consultants. The final decision is, evidently, for the patient, but the clinician should not shrink from giving a clear indication of his or her view.

The surgeon should not think that because he or she carries that title it is necessary in every case to propose operation; more often, the task is rather to dissuade a patient from such a course. It has often seemed to us, examining the papers in cases of alleged medical negligence, that some claimants at least seem very eager to submit themselves to medical examination and treatment. The records of such patients *before the critical event* are voluminous: in one case they ran to 600 pages. A clinician seeing such a record and a correspondingly large general practitioner record could well conclude that it would be unwise to recommend operation of election to such a patient unless there were the strongest possible indications. One might speculate that some patients secretly relish the risk inherent in all medical and surgical procedures, and continue to tempt fate until, inevitably, a mistake is made and a penalty is claimed. Certainly, all clinicians should make themselves as familiar as possible with past medical history before recommending operation to any patient. Probably, examination of the medical records of patients taking suit for alleged medical negligence would provide a fruitful field of study for the medical defence organisations and for any unified body that may later be formed to examine such claims in the National Health Service.

ANATOMY AND VULNERABILITY

The decline of teaching of topographical anatomy has certainly produced a number of surgeons whose grasp of the location of nerves is defective. A similar lack of knowledge of the function and the vulnerability of peripheral nerves also seems to prevail. The common use during anaesthesia of agents blocking transmission at the neuromuscular junction has removed the warning sign of motor response to stimulation of a nerve. Those in charge of the education of clinicians may have to recognise that would-be surgeons will have to learn more about the position and function of nerves, about the need to handle them tenderly, about the simplicity and effectiveness of intraoperative stimulation and monitoring, and above all about the need to treat living tissues as if they were alive, which of course they are. It may be too, that in cases in which a special risk to nerves is perceived before operation, it will increasingly be necessary to rely on intraoperative monitoring of function, as indicated by Kennedy et al (1991) for arthroplasty of the hip.

Recognition and action

Surgeons must learn to treat seriously a patient's complaint of pain and loss of function after operation; to discard any habit of facile optimism; to investigate the site, nature, extent and depth of any lesion; and to act decisively. Above all, the diagnosis of "neurapraxia" should never be made unless 6 days after injury electrical stimulation of the injured nerve or nerves distal to the level of lesion produces a normal motor response. If there is a wound over the main nerve and there is a lesion of that nerve, the first possibility is that a nerve has been cut. If someone has been around that nerve with a knife in his or her hand, the possibility becomes a clear certainty.

PROCEDURES AND ATTITUDES

In "day case" operating in particular, the patient should not be sent home without being seen by a clinician of adequate experience, or without a record of the procedure and findings to take to his or her own doctor. General practitioners should discard the belief, real or assumed, that all hospital practitioners are all-wise and all-knowing. When evidence mounts to show that a diagnosis made in hospital is incorrect, the practitioner should be prepared to question it, and to ask the clinician who made it to think again or to ask someone else. All clinicians should bear in mind the fact that patients who complain generally have something to complain about. The expansion of knowledge and the growth of specialisation, whose effects have deliberately been intensified by the operations of lawyers and the law, have created new dangers for patients. Some clinicians may have forgotten that disease does not come neatly labelled as, for instance, "medical", "surgical", "orthopaedic" or "neurological", but as a patient with symptoms and signs which have to be construed. Pain in the neck may indicate myocardial ischaemia; pain in the lower limb may indicate aortoiliac disease; "cardiac" pain may indicate acute compression of nerves and vessels at the thoracic outlet. The clinician should not permit fear of legal process to deter him or her from, at least, thinking outside his or her speciality. It is agreeable to recall that, quite recently, in an aircraft at cruising altitude, a British Professor of Orthopaedic Surgery triumphantly ventured outside his speciality to save the life of a young woman with a tension pneumothorax.

Vincent and Clements (1995) summarised well the aims of risk management: "reduction of harm to patients; improvement in the quality of patient care; reduction of harm to the organisation; safeguarding the assets of the organisation (finance; reputation; staff morale); continuity of care for the injured patient; swift compensation for the justified claimant". They might perhaps have added reform of the system or policy that led to the error, and recording and dissemination for the benefit of others. We have outlined steps to be taken in this particular field with regard to the first two aims and the penultimate aim. The extent to which the other aims can be achieved depends on a degree of cooperation between clinicians, managers and lawyers which is, with the present constraints, unlikely to be realised. The clinician's dependence on reputation, the manager's dependence on financial success, the lawyer's dependence on success in adversarial process and the cumbersome processes of investigation and of law all militate against the injured person's chance of obtaining satisfaction either by adequate explanation or by adequate compensation. They act too against the organisation itself: the financial constraints operative in the National Health Service lead the managers of the organisation to take courses opposed to reform; opposed too to the aim of early compromise.

Two consecutive cases tell the story. In each, the ulnar nerve of a woman in work was damaged through clinical negligence; in each, the plaintiff made plain her willingness to settle for admission of liability and a small sum by way of compensation. Both Trusts concerned opposed the claims, and 5 years after the events the cases came to court. In both cases the plaintiffs were awarded £1500 by way of damages; in both the defendant Trusts incurred in addition their own and the plaintiff's costs for 4-day hearings. This folly and misjudgment cost them and their patients many thousands of pounds; they cost the plaintiffs 5 years of strain and a 4-day ordeal in court. The lawyers came off best. On the other hand, it has to be said that some claimants, regrettably but predictably, seek either from the start or after an initial rebuff from the defendant, to magnify the effects of their injuries on their work and daily life. Such an event is hardly likely to be avoided in an adversarial process in which all parties are seeking to justify their actions or to make them appear in the best possible light. It is an extremely likely event in a society which was said by a prominent politician not to exist. However that may be, it is certainly the unpleasant duty of lawyers and medical experts advising the court in such a case to probe obviously exaggerated claims, if necessary by covert surveillance. Modern techniques permit surveillance without the knowledge of the person under observation, and claimants should if necessary be made aware of this.

14. The peripheral nervous system and neoplastic disease

Classification of modes of affection: carcinomatous neuropathy; infiltration; pressure, distortion or infiltration from without; nerve tumours derived from non-neural elements; nerve tumours derived from neural elements. Recent advances in tissue culture, electron microscopy, immunohistochemistry, genetic analysis, imaging and operative techniques. Neurofibromatosis: classification, clinical features, treatment. Tumours of cranial, spinal and peripheral nerves. Schwannoma: clinical features, microscopic appearances and treatment. Solitary neurofibroma: clinical features; malignant change. Malignant peripheral nerve sheath tumours: clinical and other features; options for treatment. Deep musculoaponeurotic fibromatosis and other tumours.

The peripheral nervous system is affected in the following ways in neoplastic disease:

1. In neuropathy secondary to malignant disease elsewhere (usually in the lung).
2. By infiltration with disseminated malignant disease, in particular from cancer of the breast.
3. By pressure, infiltration or distortion from benign or malignant tumours arising from related structures.
4. By tumours arising within the nerve from non-neural elements.
5. By tumours arising within the nerve from neural elements; such tumours my be isolated or may form part of a generalised affection. They may be benign or primarily malignant. Benign tumours may undergo malignant transformation.

NEUROPATHY SECONDARY TO MALIGNANT DISEASE

The pathological changes in nonmetastatic carcinomatous neuropathy were described by Denny Brown (1948); other workers have described similar changes (Croft et al 1965, Dyck 1966, Croft & Wilkinson 1969). There are changes in the peripheral nerves. These changes affect nerve cells and nerve fibres. Recent studies (Anderson et al 1988) suggest a common basis in the formation of autoantibodies. McLeod (1993a) concludes that clinical neuropathy is apparent in 5% of patients with cancer, and that defects are detectable in 12% of patients by quantitative sensory testing. Neurophysiological investigation reveals abnormality in between 30% and 40%. A sensorimotor neuropathy is the most common pattern, characterised by axonal death affecting all types of fibres. The sensory neuropathy is particularly crippling. Symptoms may precede manifestation of the primary tumour by up to 15 months, and include numbness, dysaesthesia and paraesthesia commencing distally and advancing proximally. There is aching pain, and ataxia and orthostatic hypotension are common findings.

Similar "paraneoplastic" neuropathies are seen in lymphoma, leukaemias and Hodgkin's disease. McLeod (1993b) says that clinical evidence of involvement of the central nervous system is found in 10–25% of patients with leukaemia, from paraneoplastic neuropathy, bleeding or direct invasion.

INFILTRATION BY DISSEMINATED MALIGNANT DISEASE

Infiltration of the brachial plexus occurs in cases of dissemination of carcinoma of the breast. In rare cases, the cauda equina is similarly involved. We have seen only one instance of this event; years after mastectomy a woman reattended complaining of back pain. There was no evidence of bony metastases; myelography showed patchy, small defects of the contrast medium in the lumbar sac. At laminectomy, the cauda equina was found to be diffusely infiltrated by small foci of malignant disease. Haematogenous metastases from carcinoma of the colon and lung to posterior root ganglia have been reported (Johnson 1977). McLeod (1993b) writes that "direct infiltration of roots and peripheral nerves is not uncommon in lymphoma, particularly in non-Hodgkin's types". Axonal degeneration is accompanied by segmental demyelination.

INFILTRATION, PRESSURE AND DISTORTION BY ADJACENT MALIGNANT AND BENIGN TUMOURS

The most proximal part of the brachial plexus may be infiltrated by tumours of the apex of the lung; the more distal part may, rarely, be invaded by the spread of cancer of the breast. The lumbosacral plexus may be invaded

335

by the malignant tumours of the pelvic organs. Donaghy (1993) says that locally invasive colorectal carcinoma is the most common cause of neoplastic (lumbosacral) plexus lesion. Wetzel et al (1963) indicate that the initial pain may resemble that of prolapse of an intervertebral disc; Suber and Massey (1979) relate a presentation simulating meralgia paraesthetica. Clearly, the possibility of such a presentation must always be borne in mind. The spinal column is commonly involved by metastatic disease, causing compression of the spinal roots or of the cord. Christian Thomas et al (1992) discuss indications for and the techniques of operation in a series of 76 patients. Their patients ranged in age from 29 to 75 years. In 28 cases the primary tumour was of the breast. Vascular metastases from the kidney or thyroid were treated by spinal angiography and selective embolisation before operation on the spine. Pain in the upper limb or within the dermatome of the affected spinal nerve was the most common presentation in their 17 cervical cases. Compression of the cauda equina or the cord was the presenting feature in most of the 59 cases of thoracolumbar metastases. Compression in the cervical canal was usually posterior and operation involved posterior decompression with internal fixation. Compression in the thoracolumbar spine was usually anterior and this was treated by vertebrectomy, with bone graft or prosthesis and internal fixation. There were six early deaths. Relief, or improvement in pain followed in all cases. Before operation 27% of patients were able to walk; 85% walked afterwards. Bladder control returned in 27 of 35 patients presenting with incontinence or retention. The mean survival time of the 47 who died was 32 weeks, while of the 29 still alive it was 20 months. These workers point out that deep irradiation is useful in the relief of pain, but less so in improving function.

The more distal peripheral nerves are less commonly involved in direct spread of malignant disease than are their plexus of origin because of the relative infrequency of peripheral tumour. Benign tumours such as osteoma, chondroma, lipoma and others distort peripheral nerves, but less often interfere with conduction, unless they are placed so as to distort the nerve in a natural canal or tunnel. Thus, many cases of "tarsal tunnel syndrome" or of compression within the canal of Guyon are due to the presence of a benign tumour in the tunnel adjacent to the nerve. Infiltration of the paravertebral chain is of course well known in cases of cancer of the apex of the lungs, with the production of a Bernard–Horner syndrome (Olsen 1993).

PERIPHERAL NERVE TUMOURS

As Kehoe et al (1995) point out in their review of 104 cases, tumours arising from peripheral nerves cause difficulties in classification, clinical diagnosis and treatment.

Unnecessary resection of a major nerve trunk or trunks is seen far too often in operations for benign nerve tumours. In neurofibromatosis nice judgement is necessary in deciding which tumours must be removed and which can be left alone; involvement of other systems in this disease can be more significant than the presenting lump within a nerve. Patients need advice about the risks of malignant transformation within a benign tumour and about the risks of inheritance. Malignant tumours of nerves have a bad prognosis and the indications for excision, compartmentectomy and amputation are not clear.

The earlier literature is extensive and important, but it betrays uncertainty about the cell of origin, leading to widely different systems of classification. Dodge and Craig (1957) and Das Gupta et al (1969) made no distinction between the schwannoma and the neurofibroma. Geschickter (1935) and Stewart and Copeland (1931) considered malignant nerve tumours to be among the most common of sarcomas, although Stout (1937) stipulated the diagnostic significance of origin from a nerve trunk or neurofibroma. Earlier material was reconsidered by D'Agostino et al (1963) who reviewed 104 cases of malignant tumours seen at the Mayo Clinic. They reclassified 10 as benign schwannomas, and corrected the diagnosis to synovial sarcoma, rhabdomyosarcoma and leiomyosarcoma in others, leaving a total of 45 malignant nerve tumours. The pleomorphism of malignant nerve tumours continues to cause differing views. Enzinger and Weiss (1988) prefer the term "malignant schwannoma". Lapiere and Maheut (1986) retain malignant schwannoma, malignant neurofibroma, and fibrosarcoma in their classification. Harkin and Reed (1969) preferred "peripheral nerve sheath tumours" (MPNST) in their beautifully illustrated atlas, and this is now the most widely used designation. We follow the classification set out in Table 14.1.

Recent advances

There have been substantial advances in the understanding of peripheral nerve tumours in the last 25 years allowing a more rational approach in diagnosis, in clinical definition and in treatment.

1. Bunge et al (1989) have proved that the perineurial cells arise from fibroblasts, and have thus put an end to decades of controversy. Purified cultures of Schwann cells, of sensory neurons, and of fibroblasts were selectively labelled with a recombinant retrovirus, the gene product of which, β-galactoside, was found only in the infected cells. The perineurial cells were labelled only when the fibroblasts were infected. This confirms the observation made by Thomas and Jones (1967) that perineurial cells assumed the morphological features of fibroblasts. This important observation goes some way to explain the complex forms of tumour within neurofibromatosis, with

Table 14.1 Classification of peripheral nerve tumours

Benign	Malignant
Nerve sheath tumours	
Schwannoma (neurilemmoma)	Malignant peripheral nerve sheath tumour (malignant schwannoma, neurofibrosarcoma, nerve sheath fibrosarcoma)
Solitary neurofibroma	Malignant neurofibroma
Plexiform neurofibroma (diagnostic of NF1)	Primitive neuroectodermal tumour (PNET) (includes neuroepithelioma, extraosseous Ewings, PNET of bone, Askin tumour)
Lipoma, fibrolipoma, angioma, "Perineurioma"	Non-neural sarcomas arising in nerve trunks
Neural tumours	
Ganglioneuroma	Ganglioneuroblastoma, neuroblastoma

NFI, neurofibromatosis 1; PNET, peripheral neuroectodermal tumour.

differing contributions from Schwann cells, from perineurial cells and from fibroblasts. Definition of a true perineurial neoplasm, the perineurioma, is more controversial. Lusk et al (1987), in an impressive review of 57 tumours of the brachial plexus commented that "it is our contention that the epineurial fibrocyte, a more embryological primitive cell gives rise to the more 'invasive' neurofibroma and that the Schwann cell which seems to be a more highly differentiated perineurial cell gives rise to the comparatively more 'benign' schwannoma".

2. Electron microscopy has established beyond any doubt that the Schwannoma is formed by Schwann cells. The ultrastructural characteristics of benign peripheral nerve sheath tumours are summarised by Henderson et al (1986). Three of these are particularly useful in distinguishing between the schwannoma, the neurofibroma and the perineurioma. In the schwannoma, cell processes are long and interleaving, with infolding reminiscent of mesaxons (Fig. 14.1). Intercellular junctions are rare, the external lamina is continuous in single or multiple layers.

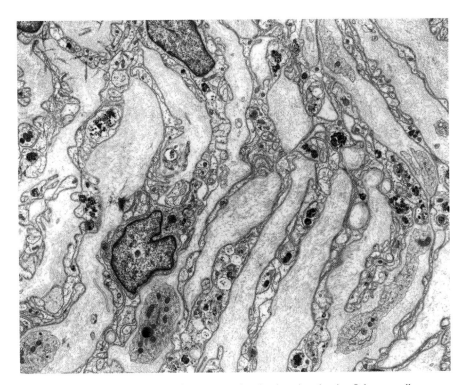

Fig. 14.1 Electron micrograph of a benign schwannoma, showing long interleaving Schwann cell processes. × 2250.

In the neurofibroma, cell processes are irregular and have the features of fibroblasts. Intercellular junctions are rare, the external lamina is usually absent. Cells of a perineurioma exhibit long thin processes, but without infoldings; intercellular junctions are frequent; and the external lamina is discontinuous, but may become concentrated along one side of the cell. Erlandson and Woodruff (1982) described the electron microscopic appearances of 23 schwannomas, 10 neurofibromas and 10 malignant peripheral nerve sheath tumours (MPNSTs). The solitary schwannomas were composed of differentiated Schwann cells. In six of the neurofibromas the cells were indistinguishable from those of normal perineurium. In the MPNSTs they found poorly differentiated cells with occasional intermediate forms between Schwann, perineurial and fibroblast-like cells.

3. With regard to the immunocytochemistry, tumour cells of different origin possess different antigens that can be demonstrated by polyclonal or monoclonal antibodies. Those of neural origin possess specific antigens termed "neural markers". This technique, now widely used by pathologists, is replacing electron microscopy as an adjunct to light microscopy in diagnosis. Urich (1993), in his review of the pathology of peripheral nerve tumours, outlines the usefulness of immunocytochemistry. The Schwann cell exhibits the S-100 protein, the LEU-7 membrane antigen and vimentin. Glial fibrillary acidic protein (GFAP) is found in Schwann cells supporting unmyelinated nerve fibres. The perineurial cell is S-100 negative, but expresses the epithelial membrane antigen EMA. Fibroblasts express vimentin and fibronectin.

The strong expression of S-100 by Schwann cells is particularly important in distinguishing between the large schwannomas of the retroperitoneum and soft tissue sarcomas, notably leiomyosarcoma or rhabdomyosarcoma.

On occasion they still are confused, with serious results for the patient when large portions of the lumbosacral plexus are unnecessarily resected. Weiss et al (1983) studied S-100 in the cells of benign and malignant tumours, confirming that the benign Schwannomas contained numerous immunoreactive cells. They found many such cells throughout neurofibromas too. S-100 positive cells were found in only half of malignant tumours. Wick et al (1987) studied 62 cases of MPNST using three neural markers: S-100 protein, myelin based protein and LEU 7. Staining was positive for at least one of these three in two-thirds of cases, there was coexpression of antigens in one-third. Rose et al (1992) reported on a case of MPNST with rhabdomyoblastic and glandular differentiation; it showed co-staining for desmin and S-100 in rhabdomyoblasts and for S-100 and cytokeratin in epithelioid cells. They suggested that divergent differentiation might be reflected in antigen coexpression at an individual cellular level. Peltonen et al (1988) reported on cellular differentiation in neurofibromatosis. Cells that stained only peripherally for S-100 were regarded as neoplastic perineurial cells, and immunostaining displayed distinct structures with epithelial, endothelial or smooth muscle differentiation within benign tumours (Fig. 14.2; A&B see also Plate section).

4. Understanding of round cell tumours of bone has been enhanced by combining the above technique with others that are yet more refined. Triche and Cavazzana (1988) collect evidence suggesting that Ewing's tumour, the Askin tumour of the chest wall, the primitive neurectodermal of bone and neuroepithelioma are variations from a common neural origin, and that they are distinct from neuroblastoma. Immunoreactivity is enormously improved in frozen section or tumour imprints, and this allows the use of monoclonal antibody typing. Short-term culture of

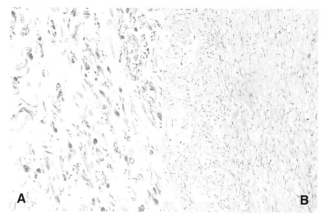

Fig. 14.2 a and b S-100 positive staining of Schwann cells in an intact fascicle within a plexiform neurofibroma; the myelinated nerve fibres are demonstrated by solochrome cyanin. A × 400, B × 160. (See also Plate section.) (Courtesy of Dr Jean Pringle.)

tumour cells allows cytogenetic and molecular genetic analysis, and is also useful in diagnosis as neural tumours frequently demonstrate spontaneous differentiation with neural features in vitro. Other sarcomas of bone, cartilage or the lymphatic system never show such differentiation. They argue that these four tumours are a range of peripheral neural tumours of common origin, with Ewing's sarcoma as the extreme undifferentiated member of the group, and overt peripheral neuroepithelioma as the most differentiated. The single most important piece of evidence for this is the observation that cells of Ewing's sarcoma have a characteristic reciprocal translocation of the long arms of chromosomes 11 and 21. This has been found in Askin tumour, peripheral neuroepithelioma, and extraosseous Ewing's tumour. It has not been found in neuroblastoma. These writers comment that "this cytogenetic data has been the single most compelling to date to implicate a common histogenesis for this group of tumours".

5. The widespread use of computed tomography (CT) with contrast enhancement and the introduction of magnetic resonance imaging (MRI) have considerably improved definition of the nature and extent of tumours, particularly of those within the body cavities, adjacent to or within the spinal column. The morbidity of digital subtraction angiography (DSA) is much less than that of intra-arterial catheterisation, and this facilitates the demonstration of the relation of larger tumours to vessels within the posterior triangle of the neck and within the pelvis.

6. There have been improvements in techniques of taking and interpreting biopsy. In the expert hands of those working in specialist tumour units, needle biopsy, frozen section and air-dried touch (imprint) preparations can reach very high levels of diagnostic accuracy in musculoskeletal lesions, as shown by Stoker et al (1991) and Pringle (1996) – but these are experts.

7. Notable advances in operative technique have been made. These rest on improvements in anaesthesia that allow the control and maintenance of circulation and ventilation during extensive and time-consuming procedures. These advances include new methods of exposure, notably the transclavicular approach to the cervicodorsal column developed by Bonney (Birch et al 1990), the transoral transclival approach to the uppermost segment of the cervical spinal cord of Crockard and Bradford (1985) and the extreme lateral approach to the upper part of the cervical spine described by Sen and Sekhar (1990) and Kratimenos and Crockard (1993). Regular use of the operating microscope diminishes the hazard of damage to conducting tissue and is particularly valuable in tumours of spinal nerves or within the spinal canal. Lessons have been learned from sometimes catastrophic instability of the spinal column following extensive and destructive laminectomy, now replaced by appropriate anterior or anterolateral approaches combined with adequate primary stabilisation of the spine with bone graft and internal fixation.

NEUROFIBROMATOSIS

Although this condition is associated with the name of von Recklinghausen, in 1849 Smith provided a very full clinical and pathological description. He described the progress in a 35-year-old man followed for over 3 years. On his last admission there were two large tumours, one in the neck and one in the thigh, which "exceeded in magnitude the size of the head of the patient". The patient's general health had greatly deteriorated before admission and he died the following day. At necropsy Smith found a total of 800 tumours, 150 in the right lumbar plexus and its branches, and similar numbers in the sciatic and brachial plexus. The tumours "presented as striking uniformity, within their external characters and their internal structures; their form was oval or oblong; their colour, a yellowish white; they were solid, and each was surrounded by a capsule, which was continuous with the neurolemma; their surface was smooth; their long axis corresponded with the direction of the nerve on which they exist, and they were movable only from side to side. Their section exhibited an exceedingly dense, close texture, of a whitish colour, and a somewhat glistening aspect, presenting a uniform degree of solidity and remarkable for the total absence of vascularity". Different patterns of the disease have been recognised for many years, described as central (affecting the neuraxis) peripheral, (von Recklinghausen's disease) and atypical. In the last 20 years the incidence, patterns of inheritance, and natural history have been defined in careful population studies. Cytogenetic studies have established underlying chromosomal abnormalities for the two major types. A study of Riccardi's (1990) excellent and comprehensive review is recommended (Table 14.2).

NF2 or central neurofibromatosis: bilateral acoustic neurofibromatosis

This is rare, with an incidence of 0.1 per 100 000. It is characterised by tumours within the central nervous system. The plexiform neurofibroma is rare, and cognitive defects and skeletal or vascular dysplasia exceptionally so. Inheritance is autosomal dominant and the gene locus is in the distal long arm of chromosome 22 (Seizinger et al 1986). New mutations are responsible for up to two-thirds of cases.

Patients with NF2 present with symptoms of a brain tumour, usually an acoustic neuroma or meningioma, or with compression of the spinal cord by paraspinal or intradural tumour. The tumours may become overt, or progress, during pregnancy.

Tumours of the acoustic nerve are the most common of cranial nerve tumours, forming 94% of King's personal series of 500 such tumours (1993). He describes the value of MRI imaging in diagnosis, and explains the substantial

Table 14.2 Diagnostic criteria for NF1 and NF2

NF1	NF2
1. Six or more café au lait macules over 5 mm in greatest diameter in prepubertal individuals and over 15 mm in greatest diameter in postpubertal individuals	1. Bilateral eighth cranial nerve masses seen with appropriate imaging techniques (e.g. CT or MRI)
2. Two or more neurofibromas of any type, *or* one plexiform neurofibroma	*or*
3. Freckling in the axilla or inguinal region	2. A first-degree relative with NF2 and either: (a) Unilateral eighth nerve mass
4. Optic gliomas	*or*
5. Two or more Lisch nodules (iris hamartoma)	(b) Two of the following: (i) Neurofibroma (ii) Meningioma (iii) Glioma (iv) Schwannoma (v) Juvenile posterior subcapsular lenticular opacity
6. A distinctive osseous lesion, such as sphenoid dysplasia or thinning of long bone cortex, with or without pseudarthrosis	
7. A first-degree relative (parent, sibling or offspring) with NF1 by the above criteria	

improvement in mortality and morbidity following operation by better methods of exposure, the use of the operating microscope, and the referral of these patients to centres equipped to diagnose and to treat them. Wright and Bradford (1995) review the matter.

NF1, von Recklinghausen's disease, peripheral neurofibromatosis

Inheritance in NF1 is also autosomal dominant, the gene locus being in the proximal long arm of chromosome 17. It is much more common than NF2, with a frequency of about 1 in 3000 to 4000 persons. Huson et al (1989a) identified 69 families with 135 affected members, a prevalence of 1 in 4950 in a population study from south-east Wales. Of the 135 cases, 41 were thought to be new mutations. We have removed benign tumours from 39 patients with NF1 and have operated on 11 malignant tumours (Table 14.3). Only one-half of our patients knew of their condition, and the complications of the disease for themselves and their families were known by only a few. The surgeon may be the first to make the diagnosis, and should work closely with a clinical geneticist so that the patient and family are adequately advised and supported. Support groups such as LINK in the UK have produced excellent fact sheets on NF1 and NF2, and patients have been much helped by contact with such groups.

Table 14.3 Benign tumours in NF1: 39 cases

Age (years)	0–9	10–19	20–29	30–39	40–49	50–59	60–69	≥70
No. of cases	2	6	10	9	4	4	4	0

14 male; 25 female

Location	No. of cases	Location	No. of cases
Upper limb		**Lower limb**	
Cranial nerves	2	Lumbosacral plexus	3
Supraclavicular brachial plexus	10	Sciatic nerve	5
Infraclavicular brachial plexus	4	Leg:	
Arm:		Tibial nerve	2
Ulnar	1	Cutaneous nerve	1
Forearm:		Common peroneal nerve	3
Median nerve	2		
Ulnar nerve	1		
Cutaneous nerve	1		
Posterior interosseous	1		
Hand:			
Cutaneous nerve	3		

1. The table describes the site of tumours *removed*. The abnormality was generalised. Dumb-bell tumours were noted in 15 patients. Histological diagnosis of the removed tumours: schwannoma, 18; solitary neurofibroma, 16; plexiform neurofibroma, 17.
2. All three tumours were seen in most patients.
3. Hypertrophy of limb or digit has been seen in a further nine cases of known neurofibromatosis.

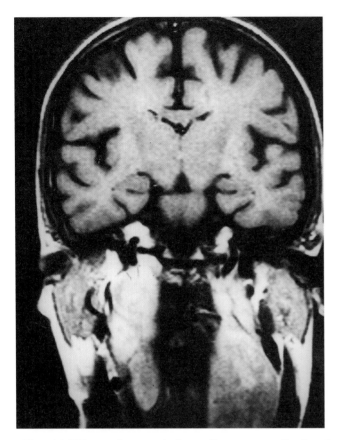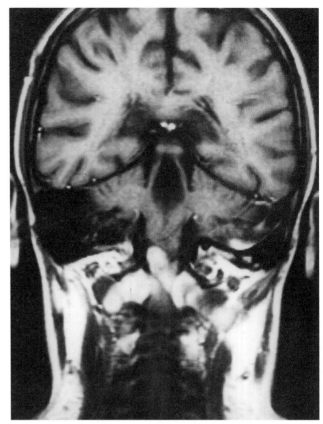

Fig. 14.3 NF1: massive paraspinal neurofibromata extending into the spinal canal and compressing the trachea. (Mr Alan Crockard's case)

NF1 is a disorder of the central and peripheral nervous systems, the skeleton and the vessels. It is a progressive condition and there are four major causes of premature death:

- massive plexiform neurofibroma in the mediastinum involving the airways
- astrocytoma of the optic chiasma, brain or cerebellum
- cervicoparaspinal neurofibroma (Fig. 14.3)
- malignant peripheral nerve sheath tumours (MPNSTs) (Fig. 14.4; see also Plate section).

The chief causes of morbidity include: plexiform neurofibroma, gigantism of a limb, intracranial astrocytomas, congenital glaucoma, tibial pseudoarthrosis and spinal deformity, renovascular hypertension, seizures, and speech defects and learning disabilities (Fig. 14.5; see also Plate section). Huson et al (1989b) defined four categories of complications of NF1. Intellectual handicap occurred in one-third of their patients; complications developing in childhood causing life-long morbidity in 8.5%; a treatable complication developing which can develop at any age in 15.7%; and a malignant or central nervous system tumour in 4.4–5.2%. Sorenson et al (1986) followed a nationwide cohort of 212 affected patients in Denmark for 42 years.

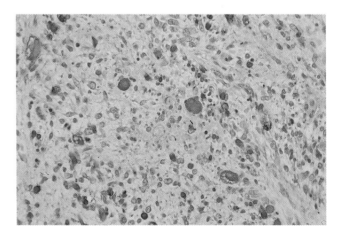

Fig. 14.4 MPNST in a patient with NF1, arising from the brachial plexus. A proportion of the tumour cells are expressing myoglobin, in particular, larger cells (triton tumour). × 400. (See also Plate section.) (Courtesy of Dr Kim Suvarna)

They found 21 malignant tumours of the central nervous system, 6 of the peripheral nervous system and 57 nonneurogenic malignant tumours. There were three cases of phaeochromocytoma. It is now possible to give a reasonable estimate of the risk of MPNST in a patient

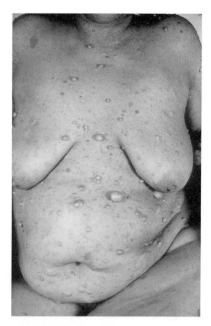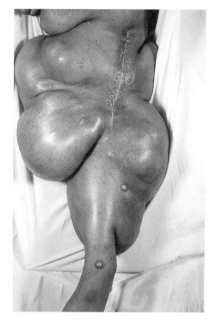

Fig. 14.5 (Left) A 48-year-old woman with NF1. (Right) Deformity of the lower limb in this case. (See also Plate section.)

with NF1. These tumours occur in about 3% of such patients: they are very rare in the first decade, presenting in adolescence or early adult life. They are characterised by pain, increase in size of pre-existing neurofibroma and loss of neural function.

Urich (1993) described the pathological features of tumours in both forms of neurofibromatosis. Virtually all the acoustic neuromas are schwannomas. The plexiform neurofibroma is diagnostic of NF1 and he describes it as "a monstrous caricature of a normal nerve with hyperplasia of all its components, albeit in various degrees". Microscopically the endoneurium is expanded by a loose myxomatous matrix, the fascicles are consistently enlarged and the perineurium may also be hypertrophic. Although the Schwann cell is important in all types of neurofibroma, perineurial cells and fibroblasts also contribute. Peltonen et al (1988) studied the cells of cutaneous tumours from nine patients with NF1. They found that Schwann-like cells, which were S-100 positive, formed 60–80% of the total cell population, but they also described a wide range of cellular differentiation into perineurial, epithelial, endothelial and smooth muscle types. This may explain the perplexing array of cell types seen in MPNSTs.

Localised forms of neurofibromatosis

Ricardi (1990) has argued for the recognition of a number of other types of the condition. Two of these are of particular interest to surgeons concerned with peripheral nerves. Segmental neurofibromatosis, involving one limb or even a dermatome, is rare and usually sporadic. Gigantism of one or several digits is another variant, and is associated with a fibrolipoma of median nerve.

The spine in neurofibromatosis

Kyphoscoliosis is a common complication of neurofibromatosis. Its incidence in patients with the disease is estimated at 3%, rising to 40% in publications discussing scoliosis. Calvert et al (1985) studied 52 patients with scoliosis and neurofibromatosis over the course of 30 years. Two spinal deformities were characteristic. Dystrophic changes were found in 47 of their cases; scoliosis and kyphosis progressed rapidly, especially before the age of 10 years. The prognosis was related to the extent of dystrophic changes. The most severe progression occurred in three patients with severe anterior scalloping of the apical vertebra. They strongly advised myelography as a prerequisite before any operative treatment of the spine. Curtis et al (1969) described eight cases of neurofibromatosis with paraplegia and reviewed 32 previously reported cases. In four of their cases the paraplegia was caused by vertebral deformity and instability, and in four more the cause was nerve tumour. Verbiest (1988) described seven cases with severe compromise of the spinal cord from disorganisation of the spinal column. Intradural extramedullary tumours were noted in six of these. He emphasised the danger of laminectomy, which precipitated instability and paraparesis in three of his cases. The results from extensive decompression

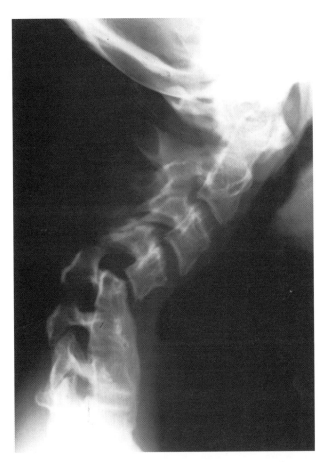

Fig. 14.6 The cervical spine in neurofibromatosis. Tetraparesis followed extensive laminectomy and incomplete anterior stabilisation in this 17-year-old boy. (Mr T Morley's case). Neurological recovery was good after a period of halo-traction. Mr Tim Morley then successfully stabilised the spine by long anterior fusion.

with stabilisation by long bone grafts, if necessary supplemented by posterior fusion, were impressive. There was one early death: that of a patient presenting with quadriplegia who developed pneumonia after operation (Fig. 14.6).

TUMOURS OF CRANIAL NERVES

The third to the twelfth cranial nerves are invested by Schwann cells close to their origin from the brainstem, and so are potential sites for tumours derived from neural elements. Such tumours are, however, rare except in the case of the eighth (auditory) nerve. King (1993) refers to 20 reports of Schwannomas of the third, fourth and 6th cranial nerves; he found four schwannomas involving the trigeminal nerve in his personal series of 500 cranial nerve tumours. Samii et al (1995) treated 27 cases of schwannoma arising from the 5th (trigeminal) nerve, an incidence of 1% of 2600 intracranial tumours, and 3% of 810 intracranial schwannomas. Tumours of the facial nerve are more common, Lipkin et al describing 248 reported cases in 1987. Roos et al (1958), Gibson and Hora (1970) and Conley and Janecka (1973) also described cases. The last authors commented on the difficulty of distinguishing tumours arising in the extraosseous part of the nerve from "mixed parotid tumours". Nine of their 23 tumours affected the nerve in its course in the petrous temporal bone. A group of tumours of more general interest are those involving the ninth, tenth and eleventh nerves at the jugular foramen. The clinical features accord with the site of the tumour, and three types have been described. In the first the tumour is almost entirely within the cranial cavity and presents rather like an acoustic neuroma with deafness, vertigo, ataxia or raised intracranial pressure. In the second, the lesion is within the bone channel, in the third it is extracranial. Patients with tumours of the second and third types come with "jugular foramen syndrome": hoarseness, swallowing difficulty and weakness of the shoulder. In the second type deafness may also be a feature.

TUMOURS OF SPINAL NERVES

In 1899, Victor Horsley successfully removed a spinal tumour in a man with a 3-year history of pain who, by the time of operation had become paraplegic with urinary retention and faecal incontinence. The patient made a complete recovery. It is still common in such cases to read of a prolonged interval between onset of symptoms and diagnosis. Gautier-Smith (1967) described 115 spinal nerve tumours, which he termed "neurofibromas". The length of history ranged from 20 months (cervical) to 4 years (lumbar), and most patients had signs of cord compression at preoperative examination. Salah et al (1975) reported 47 cases of intradural extramedullary neurinomas. Evidence of spinal cord compression was apparent in all but 11 of these, 3 patients presenting with clinical cord transection, and a further 19 with marked paraparesis. In earlier large series the schwannoma was not distinguished from the neurofibroma; the term "neurinoma" being preferred. The schwannoma is the most common: Nittner (1976) reviewed papers describing a total of over 4800 spinal cord tumours and found that the "neurinoma" was most common (23%); it was followed by meningioma (22%), then glioma and sarcoma (20%), and ependymoma (2.6%). The incidence of metastasis was 6.6%. There is no predilection for either sex, 60% occur between the ages of 30 and 60 years, and the incidence is estimated at between 0.3% and 1% per 100 000 by Alter (1975). The tumours usually lie dorsally within the spinal canal, behind the denticulate ligament; they are rarely intramedullary. About 20% are dumb-bell tumours with extradural or paravertebral extension, a feature shared by ganglioneuromas and also by plexiform neurofibromas arising outside the vertebral foramen (Figs 14.7 to 14.10; see also Plate section).

The predominant symptom is pain and it is the earliest and most common complaint. Although this may be experienced at the site of lesion in the spine (suboccipital pain is particularly important in diagnosis of a meningioma of the foramen magnum) it is not commonly felt within the dermatome of the affected nerve. Pain is described as deep seated; it is resistant to non-narcotic analgesics, and is often worse at night or when the patient is lying flat. The limb of the affected dermatome or dermatomes may feel swollen. Pain within the dermatome, exacerbated by posture, sneezing or straining, is a particular feature of tumours within the lumbar canal. In one of our cases of schwannoma in the lowest part of the lumbar sac, a particular clinical feature was marked hyperaesthesia of the skin over the sacrum. In another, hyperaesthesia of the skin of the outer aspect of the thigh, worsened by coughing, pointed to a tumour of L3 in a patient with NF1. These root symptoms are followed by evidence of progressive spinal cord compression. Signs of cord compression were apparent in four-fifths of Gautier–Smith's patients with tumours in the spinal and dorsal canal; more than one half had sphincter disturbance. The most common error was to ascribe symptoms to osteoarthritis or to prolapsed disc; as King (1993) points out, a tumour of a spinal nerve or the cauda equina is the cause in 2–4% of patients presenting with back pain and sciatica. As the tumour is considerably higher than a disc producing equivalent symptoms, the risk of error in diagnosis is high unless adequate myelography or MRI is used. Such findings are a salutary warning to those who advocate investigation of a presumed disc lesion by clinical evidence alone or by CT scanning confined to the presumed level of lesion. Vasquez-Burquero et al (1994) describe cervical Schwannoma presenting as spinal subdural haematoma. Viard et al (1989) point out the risks of spinal deformity after operations to remove dumb-bell tumours in children, as well as the hazard of malignant transformation in NF1. Sharma et al (1989) relate the case of malignant dumb-bell tumour presenting with tetraparesis. Two of our malignant tumours presented in this way.

Radiological abnormality is found in about one-half of cases, most commonly in the cervical region. Enlargement of the foramina indicates dumb-bell tumour; other changes include erosion of the dorsal surface of the body, erosion of the pedicle, widening of the interpedicular space and a paravertebral soft tissue mass. Until quite recently, myelography with a water-soluble medium was the basis of diagnosis; supplementing this with CT scanning provided more information about the relation of the tumour to the spinal cord and also the extension of the soft tissue mass. The investigation of choice, now, is MRI.

Treatment

The chief problem in treatment is the difficulty in gaining safe access to the tumour without compromising the spinal cord or causing instability of the column. This is a particular problem for those tumours within the uppermost part of the spinal canal, for those lying ventral to the denticulate ligament and for those with large extraspinal extensions. King (1993) points out that laminectomy is usually a straightforward operation for tumours placed dorsally, but excludes this approach for the ventral lesions as "virtually no retraction of the spinal cord is permissible if a good result is to be obtained". He recommends an anterolateral approach in the dorsal spine, removing the articular facets and the pedicle on the side of the tumour. Fusion is necessary if the whole of the facet is removed in the cervical or lumbar spine. Crockard and Bradford (1985) developed the transoral, transclival route to remove a schwannoma lying anterior to the craniovertebral junction. Their patient, who presented with a severe tetraparesis, made a full recovery. Kocher (1911) developed the transmandibular approach to the retropharynx for sepsis, and this was extended by Hall et al (1977) in a case of tetraparesis from spinal deformity. The transclavicular approach (Birch et al 1990) was developed to gain access to tumours of the spinal column extending from C7 to T2, and this exposure is particularly valuable in the treatment of tumours involving the lower roots of the brachial plexus with extension adjacent to it or within the canal. Abernathey et al (1986) described successful treatment of 13 cases of giant sacral schwannoma. In all these patients a benign schwannoma had eroded through the anterior sacrum and extended into the retrorectal space. These were excised, usually by anterior abdominal approach or by a posterior retrorectal transacral exposure. They attempted to preserve the first three sacral nerves and the pudendal nerves, finding that unilateral section of the third root could be performed without severe significant neurological deficit. More than this invariably led to bladder and bowel dysfunction. Preservation of the conducting elements within the involved nerve should always be attempted, but Kim et al (1989) described 31 patients where a spinal nerve from C5 to T1 or from L3 to S1 was excised. Only seven of these patients developed detectable motor or sensory deficit postoperatively. Fifteen of their patients had large dumb-bell tumours; in six more the tumour was probably a plexiform neurofibroma.

Case report. A 22-year-old man presented with a 3-month history of pain, weakness, hypersensitivity and anaesthesia about the right shoulder girdle and arm. Electromyography confirmed denervation of muscles innervated by C4, C5 and C6. A diagnosis of neuralgic amyotrophy was made. He was referred to the Royal National Orthopaedic Hospital 14 months later for

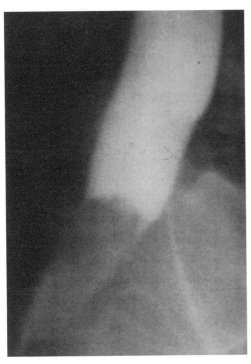

Fig. 14.7 Myelograph showing an intradural extramedullary schwannoma. The patient presented with back pain.

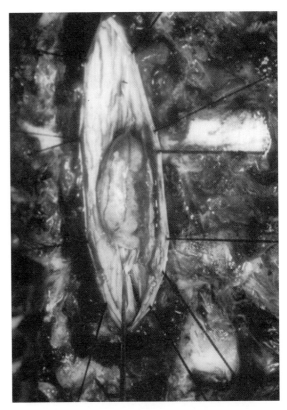

Fig. 14.8 Meningioma within the thoracic spinal canal.

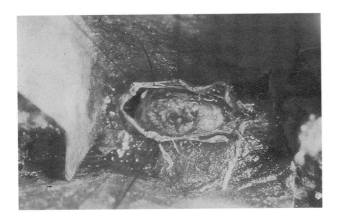

Fig. 14.9 Intradural extramedullary schwannoma exposed at operation. The patient presented with back pain. (See also Plate section.)

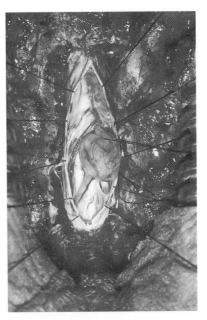

Fig. 14.10 Intradural extramedullary neurofibroma exposed at operation. The patient presented with back pain and paraparesis. (See also Plate section.)

confirmation of this diagnosis, at which time evidence of cord compression was all too plain, with a sensory level at T3, marked upper motor neurone signs, but with no sphincter dysfunction. A clinical diagnosis of intradural extramedullary tumour was confirmed radiologically.

The tumour was approached first by laminectomy of C4 to C6, allowing the intradural extramedullary component to be excised (Mr R. Bradford). Six weeks later the remainder was excised by anterolateral approach, and the spine stabilised with bone graft and plate (Fig. 14.11).

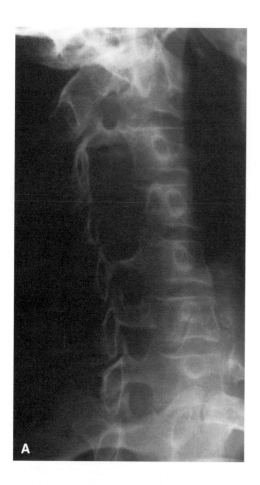

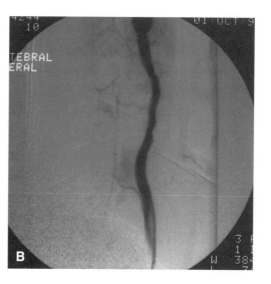

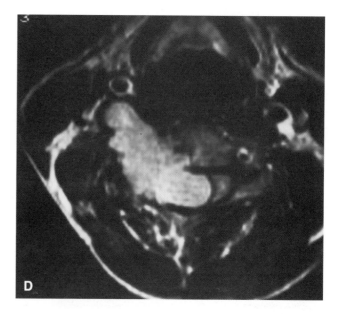

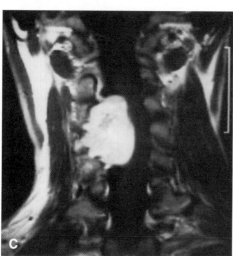

Fig. 14.11 Dumb-bell tumour (Schwannoma) in the cervical region. Plain radiograph (upper left) shows erosion of pedicles and enlargement of the foramina. Digital subtraction angiography (upper right) shows distortion of the vertebral artery. Magnetic resonance imaging (below, right and left) shows the extent of the tumour at levels C2/3 and C3/4.

THE SOLITARY BENIGN SCHWANNOMA (NEURILEMMOMA, NEURINOMA)

The characteristics of this most common of all peripheral nerve tumours are clearly defined. Brooks (1984), Enzinger and Weiss (1988), and Seddon (1975) analysed large series showing equal distribution between the sexes, with peak incidence between the third and the sixth decades. The most common site is the head and the neck, including the brachial plexus and spinal nerves, followed by the upper and lower limbs. Deep seated tumours in the posterior mediastinum and the lumbosacral spinal nerves and plexus can grow to an impressive size. Henigan et al (1992) described a 46-year-old man who presented with a short history of vomiting and left flank pain. A retroperitoneal mass was palpable per rectum. Neither open biopsy nor biopsy guided by ultrasound contributed to the diagnosis. The tumour was excised; it was found to be closely related to the sacral nerve root. A foot drop improved over the following 3 months. Histological examination confirmed a schwannoma, with areas of necrosis, calcification and ossification, which are to be expected in such a large "ancient" tumour. Whiston et al (1995) described a

massive retroperitoneal schwannoma causing anaemia by forming a fistula with the stomach. Schwannoma within the psoas caused back pain for 15 years before diagnosis in the case described by Downey et al (1989). Schwannomas have been described in bone (Fawcett & Dahlin 1967) (Fig. 14.12), skeletal muscle and viscera, and they are also found within the spinal cord.

One patient sent to us for review exemplifies the difficulties surrounding the large abdominal tumour. A 43-year-old woman presented with a 3-year history of intermittent abdominal symptoms; a mass was palpable. MRI showed a large tumour in the retroperitoneum, extending from L1 to the sacrum. A diagnosis of soft tissue sarcoma was made on the basis of needle biopsy, and the mass was excised, including a segment of the lumbosacral plexus L4, L5 and S1. Chemo- and radiotherapy followed, complicated by massive pulmonary embolism.

We reviewed the histological material: the diagnosis was revised to benign schwannoma. The patient now has profound weakness of the abductors and extensors of the hip, paralysis of the dorsiflexors of the ankle and foot, and weakness of the quadriceps and other muscles of the lower limb. She is able to walk 50 yards with two sticks.

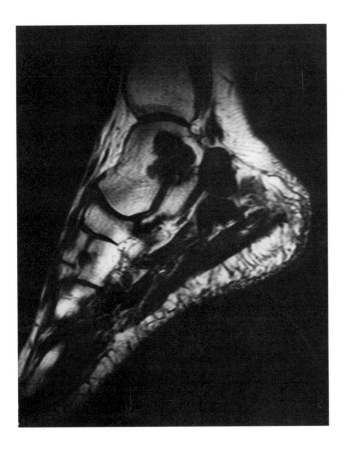
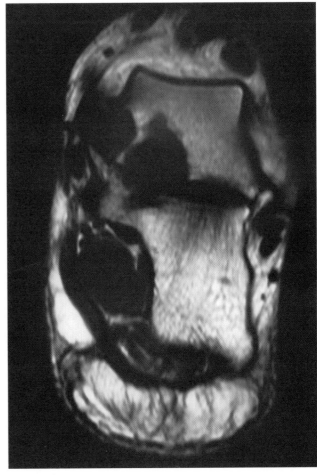

Fig. 14.12 Multiple schwannomas in the foot (left) and ankle (right).

Clinical features

The most frequent presentation is a swelling which is painful to pressure. Progressive neurological deficit occurs only when the tumour arises in a confined space, as in intradural extramedullary extension, or when it is deep to the clavicle. Diagnosis in the limbs is straightforward. The lump is mobile from side to side but not in the vertical axis of the limb. Percussion induces painful paraesthesia in the territory of the nerve of origin, similar to the Tinel sign. This finding is the single most useful sign in the diagnosis of schwannoma. At times the Schwannoma causes severe pain, particularly when it arises in the sole of the foot or in the buttock and is exposed to pressure on walking or sitting. Brooks (1984c) described a case of a 14-cm long schwannoma in the median nerve of an 18-year-old girl in whom pain was so intense that resection of the nerve was necessary. In 15 of our patients multiple schwannomas were noted in the same nerve or in different parts of the body. In none of these was there any evidence of neurofibromatosis. Purcell and Dixon (1989) and Rongioletto et al (1989) described three cases of multiple plexiform cutaneous schwannomas in patients with tumours of the central nervous system, but one of these patients had bilateral acoustic neuromata suggesting a diagnosis of NF2. Schwannoma is a common tumour in neurofibromatosis.

Pathology

The epineurium forms a capsule about the tumour which forms an eccentric oval swelling, usually less than 3 cm in diameter with nerve bundles stretched over it. It may be multinodular or plexiform infiltrating the nerve of origin, so that enucleation is impossible. Enzinger and Weiss (1988) described 5% of schwannomas behaving in this fashion. Larger tumours within the body cavities in the buttock or axilla develop cysts and show degenerative changes of haemorrhage, calcification and hyalinisation. The appearance of the epineurial vessels coursing over the capsule of the tumour is quite characteristic; they are engorged and tortuous. The cut surface is yellowish, and in larger tumours is cystic and may be blood stained (Fig. 14.13). Rarely, the tumour is semifluid, of the consistency of toothpaste, and appears to infiltrate between nerve bundles.

Microscopic appearance

The characteristic histological features are well reviewed by Enzinger and Weiss (1988) and Harkin and Reed (1969). The diagnostic feature is the organisation of Schwann cells either into areas of compact bundles (Antoni-A tissue) or a less orderly arrangement of spindle or oval cells in a loose matrix (Antoni-B tissue). There may be an abrupt change from one to the other. Palisading or compact parallel rows of cells forming Verocay bodies are features of Antoni-A tissue (Fig. 14.14; see also Plate

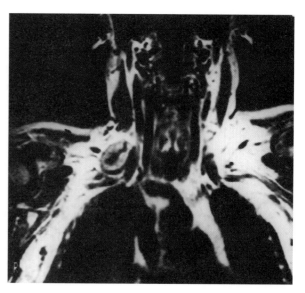

Fig. 14.13 MRI of a schwannoma of the upper trunk of the brachial plexus, with cystic change.

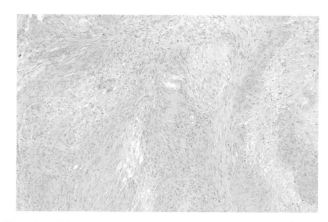

Fig. 14.14 Schwannoma, showing Antoni A and B tissue, palisading and Verocay bodies. Haematoxylin and eosin, × 250. (See also Plate section.) (Courtesy of Dr Jean Pringle.)

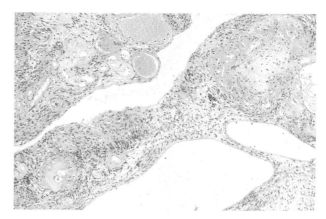

Fig. 14.15 Ancient changes in schwannoma. There is hyalinisation of the walls of the small blood vessels, haemorrhage, haemosiderin pigment and cystic change. Haematoxylin and eosin, × 250. (See also Plate section.) (Courtesy of Dr Jean Pringle.)

section). In larger tumours nuclei may appear hyperchromatic, large, and multilobed (ancient schwannoma) (Fig. 14.15; see also Plate section). A diagnosis of malignancy may be made on the basis of these findings, as it may also be for those schwannomas formed exclusively from Antoni-A tumours (the "cellular" variety). Errors are prevented by considering the nature of the tumour as a whole, and by supplementing examination with electron microscopy and immunohistochemistry. Schwannomas, particularly cellular areas, strongly express the S-100 protein, and this is particularly useful in distinguishing the large retroperitoneal tumours from soft tissue sarcomas such as leiomyosarcomas. Electron microscopy shows Schwann cells forming stacks and layers of long cytoplasmic extensions surrounded by basement membrane. Nerve fibres are sometimes seen in looser Antoni-B tissues.

Treatment

The schwannoma can be removed from its nerve of origin without loss of function in that nerve. In cases in which the tumour is centrally placed in the nerve, the appearances on first exposure can be daunting. The inexperienced operator may think that he or she is dealing with an invasive tumour, and may go on to resect the tumour-bearing segment of the nerve. In cases in which the tumour is peripherally placed, the danger is reduced. On the other hand, the appearances of the tumour in such cases may suggest a diagnosis of "ganglion". The inexperienced operator may proceed on the assumption without recognising the intimate connection with the peripheral nerve. Thus, part of or all the nerve may be damaged during removal of a "ganglion".

With the help of the loupe or microscope, in a bloodless field where possible, the operator should make a longitudinal incision in the epineurium over the most prominent part of the tumour (Figs 14.16 to 14.18). In nearly all cases it will be possible to develop a plane of cleavage between the tumour and the nerve bundles and to remove the tumour whole, without disturbance of conducting tissue. Sometimes a small bundle may have to be divided to permit removal. The occluding cuff is then removed

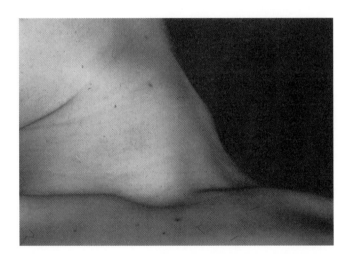

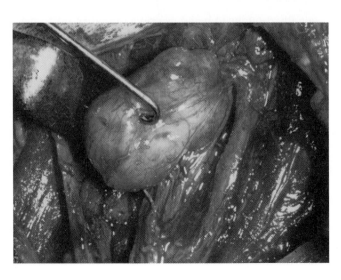

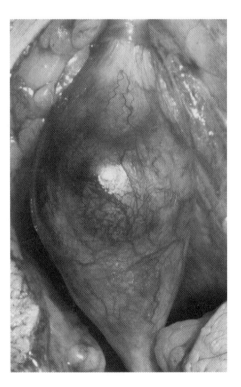

Fig. 14.16 Schwannoma of upper trunk of the left brachial plexus. Appearance before operation (top left): note swelling in left side of neck. The tumour exposed at operation (top right). Note the central position, with uniform expansion of the nerve. The tumour during enucleation (below). There was no neurological deficit after operation.

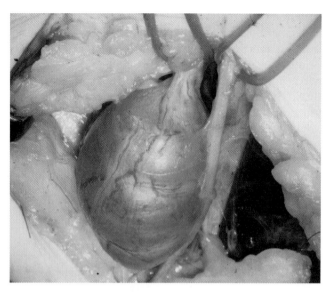

Fig. 14.17 A schwannoma of the radial nerve.

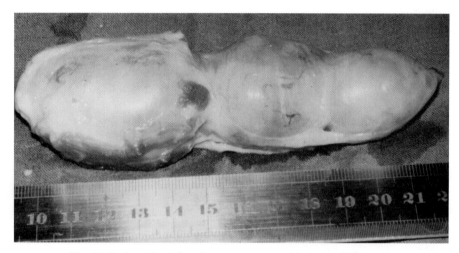

Fig. 14.18 A multinodular schwannoma removed from the tibial nerve.

and bleeding is checked with the bipolar diathermy in all parts of the wound. We have seen 119 patients; in 20 of these, unnecessary and severe neurological deficit followed resection of an unrecognised schwannoma, and partial injury to a major nerve trunk was noted in 18 others (Tables 14.4 and 14.5).

MALIGNANT TRANSFORMATION

This is exceptionally rare, if indeed it occurs at all (Birch 1993a). Carstens and Schroedt (1969) found a small area of cells within a benign schwannoma which appeared malignant on light-microscopic examination. This is not a persuasive case. Urich (1993) writes: "As a rule, the solitary malignant schwannoma arises, de novo, not in pre-existing benign schwannomas". In one of our cases,

originally thought to be an example of malignant transformation from a previously benign schwannoma, later review of the original material showed that the tumour had been malignant all along.

Case report. A 31-year-old Indian man had noted a lump in the right posterior triangle for about 6 months. At operation this was seen to arise from the upper trunk of the brachial plexus, and the surgeon excised the lump together with the upper trunk. The initial diagnosis was of a benign schwannoma, and 6 weeks later the upper trunk was repaired by nerve graft. No tumour was seen in any of the material excised at this operation. The patient regained function at the shoulder and at the elbow over the course of the next 2 years, but he came again at 40 months with a large and painful swelling above and below the clavicle. Elbow flexion had been lost. MPNST

Table 14.4 Solitary benign schwannoma: 119 cases

Age (years)	≤20	≤30	≤40	≤50	≤60	≤70	>70
No. of cases	5	15	38	30	22	5	4

43 male; 74 female

Location	No. of cases	Location	No. of cases
Upper limb		**Lower limb**	
Cranial nerves	2	Lumbosacral plexus:	7
Sympathetic chain		Femoral	3
Supraclavicular brachial plexus	26	Sciatic	5
Infraclavicular brachial plexus	11	Buttock and thigh:	
Arm:		Common peroneal nerve	3
Median nerve	6	Tibial nerve	3
Ulnar nerve	8		
Radial nerve	8	Foot:	
Cutaneous nerve	3	Tibial nerve	6
Forearm:		Cutaneous nerve	1
Median nerve	7		
Ulnar nerve	6	Total	28
Radial nerve	2		
Cutaneous nerve	3		
Hand:			
Median nerve	3		
Ulnar nerve	3		
Cutaneous nerve	3		

Table 14.5 Multiple benign schwannomas: 15 cases

Patient No.	Age (years)	Sex	Origin	No. of tumours	Treatment
1	27	F	Median nerve, forearm	4	Excised
2	31	F	Median nerve, forearm Brachial plexus Cutaneous nerve of thigh	Infiltrative	Could not be excised Excised Excised
3	33	M	Ulnar nerve, upper limb	6 (from elbow to hand)	Excised
4	63	M	Common peroneal nerve	Massive tumour	27 cm of nerve excised
5	43	M	Median nerve, forearm Ulnar nerve, forearm Tibial nerve, leg		Excised Excised Excised
6	48	M	Median nerve, forearm Tibial nerve, leg		Excised Excised
7	54	F	Sciatic, thigh	5	Excised
8	50	F	Common peroneal nerve Sural nerve Ulnar nerve, elbow		Excised Excised Excised
9	38	F	Tibial nerve, ankle and foot	6 (extending into bone)	Excised
10	36	F	Common peroneal nerve, knee	3	Excised
11	66	M	Median nerve, axilla and arm	3	Excised
12	50	M	Brachial plexus (upper trunk) Common peroneal nerve Cutaneous nerve	5	Excised
13	30	M	Median nerve, hand Sural nerve	2	Excised
14	58	F	Median nerve, forearm	5	Excised
15	41	M	Sciatic nerve, thigh Tibial nerve, leg	5	Excised

was confirmed by excision biopsy. The patient is alive and free of disease 5 years after forequarter amputation. This man did not have neurofibromatosis; there was no history of previous irradiation. It appears that the tumour arose from the graft, presumably from seedlings from the original tumour. Whilst the histological appearance of the first and last specimen were very different, review of the original material suggested that the tumour was, in fact, malignant from the outset.

SOLITARY NEUROFIBROMA

The prevalence of solitary neurofibroma varies according to the view of the author on the differences between schwannoma and neurofibroma. Despite this, the typical neurofibroma arising in a major nerve trunk is easily recognisable. Enzinger and Weiss (1988) pointed out that neurofibromas occur in younger patients, that cutaneous nerves are most commonly involved and that degenerative changes are unusual. Neurofibromas do not possess a true capsule, and staining for S-100 protein is less intense and less uniform than in the schwannoma (Fig. 14.19; see also Plate section).

The tumours appear uniformly grey-white and translucent, and in consistency they are rubbery and fibrous. The dilated and tortuous epineurial vessels so characteristic of the schwannoma are absent. Light microscopy shows interlacing bundles of elongated cells, with wavy dark staining nuclei interspersed with strands of collagen. Enneking (1983) describes some findings helpful in diagnosis: "a large avascular nonreactive oval fusiform mass in intimate proximity to a displaced vascular bundle is highly suggestive of neurofibroma". A second feature is multiple

Fig. 14.19 Solitary benign neurofibroma. The matrix is fibrillary and there are comma-shaped nuclei. Haematoxylin and eosin, × 250 and × 960 (Inset). (See also Plate section.) (Courtesy of Dr Jean Pringle.)

nodules within the mass. There are three chief reasons why neurofibromas are clinically significant. First, they may grow to a very large size causing pressure on adjacent structures; they may also extend along a spinal nerve into the spinal canal (Fig. 14.20). Hu and Lu (1993) describe a case of tumour forming one-quarter of the patient's body weight. Next, the neurofibroma of a *trunk* nerve is not separable from nerve bundles, which become intimately involved within it. Enucleation is not possible. Finally, there is a slight but definite risk of malignant transformation, which has been estimated at just under 1%. We have found that the large peripheral neurofibromas arose from slender nerves adjacent to the brachial plexus or major nerve trunks, and their removal was relatively straightforward, causing little loss of function. In four of the

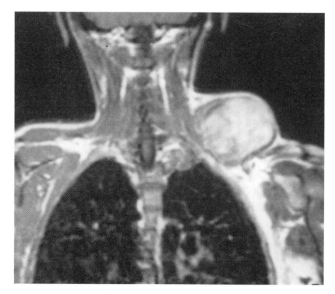

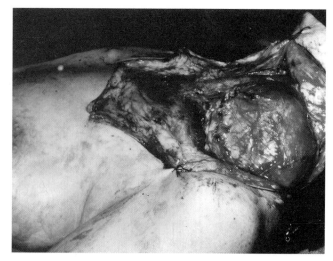

Fig. 14.20 Massive solitary benign neurofibroma. After removal of the tumour by the transclavicular approach, pain was relieved and there was no neurological deficit.

dumb-bell tumours conduction in the spinal nerve had been lost before operation, so that removal did not add to neural deficit. In other tumours arising within the cervical spinal nerves, the greater part of the tumour was removed, preserving displaced nerve bundles. Painful recurrence indicates malignant transformation, and an example of this is described below.

Case report. A 34-year-old man presented with a palpable lump in the posterior triangle which had been present for at least 12 months. It had increased in size and was causing pain. There was no clinical evidence of neurofibromatosis nor any suggestive family history. The tumour appeared to arise from the first rib, with no extension into the spinal canal. At operation, the tumour ($10 \times 8 \times 8$ cm)

arose from the first rib, distorting and stretching the whole of the plexus and accessory nerve and the subclavian artery, indenting the pleura, but not involving it, and merging into the scalene muscle. The tumour and rib were removed, together with the affected soft tissues (Fig. 14.21). The pathological diagnosis was benign neurofibroma with foci of myxoid degeneration. There was no evidence of malignancy, no hypercellularity and very scanty mitoses, but there was extension into the medullary cavity of the first rib.

Eight years later, a routine radiograph of chest showed two nodules in the upper and lower lobe of the left lung. Upper lobectomy was done; histological appearances were identical with those of the first tumour. Four years later,

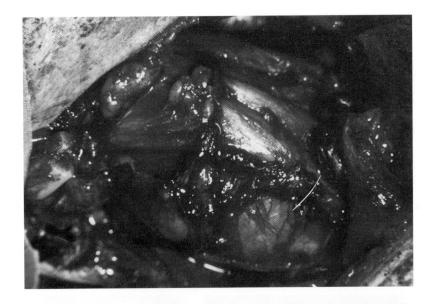

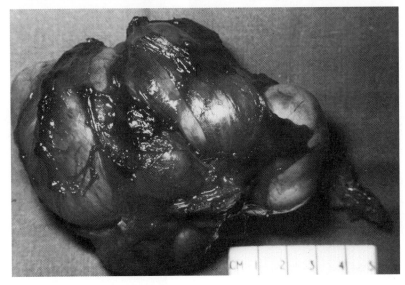

Fig. 14.21 Large solitary neurofibroma arising from the first rib. The tumour exposed and removed at the first operation.

the patient re-presented with a further mass in the left posterior triangle of the neck with increasing pain and weakness in the left upper limbs. MRI showed massive recurrence. The tumour was incompletely removed and in this specimen there were pleomorphism and small areas of multinucleated tumour cells, but the mitotic rate remained low at less than 1 per 10 high powered field (hpf). A course of radiotherapy was completed. A further partial excision of tumour from the left chest wall was performed 2 years later: histological appearances now were frankly malignant, with loosely arranged spindle and round or oval cells, nucleur pleomorphism and a mitotic index of 1 per 10 hpf. Sixteen years after the original presentation, extensive metastases in the abdomen and chest were evident. Chemotherapy was given (Fig. 14.22).

The clinical behaviour of this tumour, invading the first rib and scalenus anterior, suggests that it was malignant from the outset. The slow but inexorable progression in this case is reminiscent of the behaviour of some other soft tissue sarcomas, and reminds us that neurofibromas are always potentially malignant. Findings in six other cases are summarised in Table 14.6. These were massive tumours extending the length of between three and six vertebrae (Fig. 14.23). The transclavicular approach, sometimes supplemented by removal of the first rib, provided adequate access in all. The neurological deficit after excision was trivial in five cases; it was significant in case 2 (paralysis of glenohumeral muscles) and in case 4 (paralysis of long flexor muscles and small muscles of the hand).

OTHER BENIGN TUMOURS OR TUMOUR-LIKE CONDITIONS

ENCAPSULATED LIPOMAS

Encapsulated lipomas are rare. The diagnosis is usually made at operation, when the tumour can usually be enucleated without damage to connective tissues (Morley 1964, Watson Jones 1964). Rather different is *fatty infiltration or lipofibromatous hamartoma* (Johnson & Bonfiglio 1969). Brunelli (1964), Yeoman (1964) and Pulvertaft

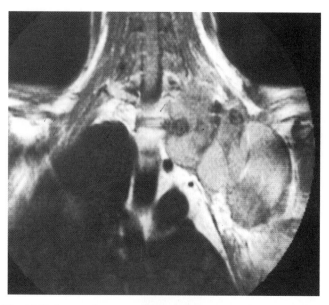

Fig. 14.22 Large solitary neurofibroma. Malignant change. The final recurrence 14 years later.

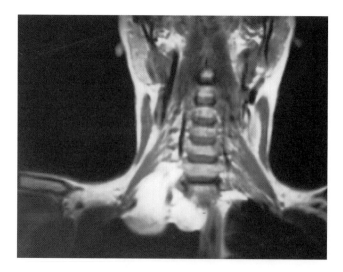
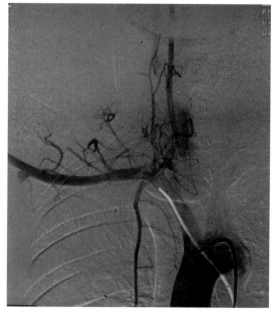

Fig. 14.23 Malignant solitary neurofibroma arising from the cervical sympathetic chain. There is an abnormal vascular pattern on DSA (right).

Table 14.6 Solitary malignant neurofibromas of the brachial plexus

Patient No.	Sex	Age (years)	Origin	Operations	Histological	Course diagnosis
1	F	36	C8. Extending from C6 to T2 bodies	Two previous excision biopsies. Excision lower trunk, first rib	Benign neurofibroma	DXT. Disease free at 3 years
2	F	71	C5, C6. Extending from C4 to T2 bodies	Previous partial excision. Excision of C5 and C6, of tumour, of first rib. Graft of C5 and C6. Tumour infiltrating scalenus muscle	Malignant neurofibroma	DXT. Disease quiescent at 2 years
3	F	38	Sympathetic chain extending from C6 to T3 bodies	Excision of tumour extending from C6 to T3, of sympathetic chain, of first and second ribs	Benign neurofibroma	Recurrence in vertebral body C7 at 18 months. Further excision and bone graft planned
4	F	36	C7 involving C7, C8, T1. Extending from C6 to T4 bodies	20-year history, four previous excision biopsies. C7, C8, T1 with first and second ribs excised	Benign neurofibroma	Disease free at 18 months
5	F	70	C5–C6. Extending into scalene muscle, transverse process C6	Excision	Benign neurofibroma	Disease free at 3 years
6	F	51	C6 extending from C4 to C7 bodies	10-year history, two previous excision biopsies. C6 root with tumour excised	Benign neurofibroma	Disease free at 4 years

(1964) described instances of this condition involving the median nerve. We have seen 20 cases. The median nerve was involved in 18 cases, the ulnar nerve in 2. The presenting sign is a fluctuant, tender swelling extending from above the wrist into the palm of the hand. At operation the nerve is found entering a large yellowish fatty tumour, and individual nerve bundles are so closely involved that removal of the tumour is impossible without resection of the nerve, which is not justified. Previous biopsy caused persisting pain and disturbance in sensation in seven of these patients. The ulnar nerve was resected in one case. MRI shows the carpal tunnel largely occupied by fibrofatty tumour, with hypertrophy of the nerve bundles. The pathological features include overgrowth of epineurium, perineurium and endoneurium. Electron microscopy confirms a greatly thickened perineurium with much collagen.

HAEMANGIOMA

Haemangioma within a nerve is very rare, presenting in adolescence or early adult life as a diffuse soft swelling with minimal interference of function. Since it cannot be removed without damage to conducting tissue, Seddon's (1975) advice to do no more than ligate the vessel connected with the affected part of the nerve is wise. The venae comitantes of nerves in the lower limb may be varicose, a malformation that perhaps should be more widely known than it is: we have seen cases of accidental injury to the common peroneal nerve during operations for varicose vein when, unknown to the surgeon, the stripper passed within the sural nerve to the common peroneal.

INTRANEURAL GANGLION

Intraneural ganglion is best known in the common peroneal nerve (Brooks 1952, Gurdjian et al 1965), but it also occurs in the median nerve and ulnar nerves at the wrist, and also in the sciatic nerve. It is most troublesome when it affects the common peroneal nerve, where it may interfere with conduction. The surgeon should resist the temptation to excise the nerve, or to do anything more than decompress it.

LOCAL HYPERTROPHIC NEUROPATHY: GIANT NERVES

Concentric Schwann cell proliferation, the onion-bulb formation, is a striking and characteristic feature in a number of chronic demyelinating neuropathies exhibiting enlargement of nerves. It is a feature of hereditary motor and sensory neuropathies of types 1 and 2 (including Charcot Marie tooth disease and Déjérine–Sottas disease). It may also be found in chronic progressive inflammatory polyneuropathies which are not inherited. It may be so confined to the brachial plexus or to a trunk nerve as to justify the term "local" or "focal" hypertrophic neuropathy. In an important review carried out by Thomas and colleagues, evidence is presented in nine cases. We have seen 10 "giant nerves". Leprosy is an important differential diagnosis in countries where that disease is prevalent.

DEEP MUSCULOAPONEUROTIC FIBROMATOSIS (EXTRA-ABDOMINAL FIBROMATOSIS, EXTRA-ABDOMINAL DESMOID)

Though microscopically benign, this condition demonstrates an alarming tendency to infiltrate and recur. Enzinger and Weiss (1988) described 360 cases. The tumour arose in the neck, shoulder and upper arm in 35%, and from the back of the chest wall in a further 17.2%. The buttock, thigh and knee accounted for a further 25.6%. Although the tumour is usually confined to muscle and to overlying aponeurosis or fascia, on occasion it arises from a nerve trunk or from the axillary sheath, so that the neurovascular bundle becomes deeply embedded in it. The lesion is poorly circumscribed and infiltrates surrounding tissue. The microscopic appearance is uniform, of masses of elongated spindle-shaped cells embedded within collagen without atypical or hyperchromatic nuclei. Paradoxically, the extensive infiltrative nature of the tumour is not characteristic of the smaller fibrosarcomas. In 16 of our patients, nerves were so closely involved that operations were necessary. In two cases, the tumour arose from the nerve trunks, along the musculocutaneous in one, and the common peroneal in the other. These patients presented with pain, swelling, disturbance of sensation and weakness, features suggesting to us that these were MPNSTs. The nerves were resected, and the functional deficit mitigated by appropriate musculotendinous transfer. There has been no recurrence. In 14 other cases the tumour arose from the axillary sheath and the neurovascular bundle was deeply embedded within it. These cases were exceptionally difficult to treat: only incomplete resection was possible, preserving the major nerve trunks with excision and repair by graft of the axillary vein and artery in three cases. Early recurrence in one patient was treated by radiotherapy. In another case a large tumour arose from the upper humerus or from structures near it, and enwrapped the radial nerve. The upper humerus and the tumour were resected together with the radial nerve, the tumour mass was stripped to the bone and the autoclaved humerus was reinserted to form an arthrodesis of the shoulder. Later, appropriate tendon transfer was done to restore extension of the wrist and fingers. Wide excision is the correct action for this condition; amputation should be avoided. Irradiation carries with it the risk of later development of a malignant tumour (Table 14.7; Figs 14.24 to 14.27).

Table 14.7 Other benign tumours or tumour-like conditions: 70 cases

Tumour type	No. of cases	Nerves affected	Sex
Intraneural ganglion	12	1 tibial, 7 common peroneal, 2 ulnar, 2 sciatic	10 M, 2 F
Angioma	5	1 tibial nerve (foot), 2 median, 2 ulnar (forearm and hand)	1 M, 4 F
Lipoma	6	1 posterior interosseous, 1 ulnar (elbow), 1 brachial plexus (middle trunk), 2 ulnar (hand), 1 radial (arm)	4 M, 2 F
Amyloid	1	1 radial (arm)	1 F
"Hypertrophic neuropathy"	10	3 brachial plexus, 2 ulnar, 2 sciatic, 2 median, 2 radial	4 M, 6 F
Aponeurotic fibromatosis (extra-abdominal desmoid)	16	14 brachial plexus, 1 common peroneal, 1 musculocutaneous	2 M, 14 F
Lipofibrohamartoma	20	18 median (forearm and wrist), 2 ulnar	6 M, 14 F

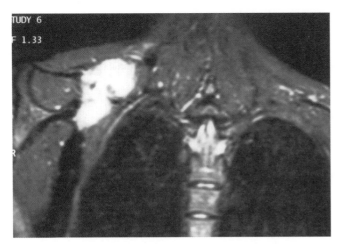

Fig. 14.24 MRI of aponeurotic fibromatosis involving the brachial plexus, showing the extension characteristic of the condition.

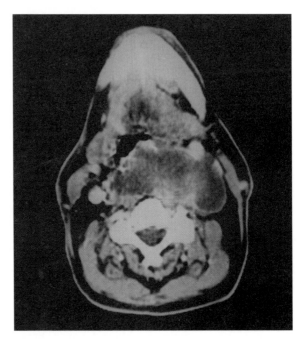

Fig. 14.26 Massive aponeurotic fibromatosis extending from C2 to D3, causing asphyxia. The tumour was removed through an extended transclavicular approach.

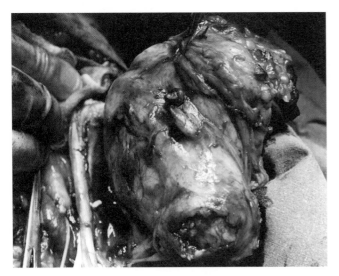

Fig. 14.25 Aponeurotic fibromatosis enveloping the axillary brachial plexus.

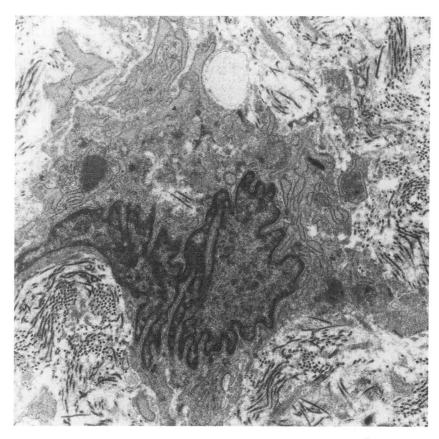

Fig. 14.27 Electron micrograph showing fibroblasts. × 10 650. (Prepared by Mr Stephen Gschmeissner.)

MALIGNANT TUMOURS

Malignant tumours of nerves are among the most terrible of soft tissue tumours. Increased understanding of their origin and improved methods of diagnosis have not altered their prognosis. There are three groups. The most danger-ous are those arising in patients with neurofibromatosis, and these account for one-third of the total. The patients are younger, the peak decade for incidence being 20–30 years. There is a tendency for tumours to arise more centrally, and the prognosis is very much worse than it is for the solitary malignancies. The long-term population study from Sorenson et al (1986) and the recent detailed analysis of 120 cases from the Mayo Clinic (Ducatman et al 1986) suggest that MPNST will develop in between 3% and 5% of patients with NF1. This compares with an incidence of the general population in the Mayo Clinic of 0.001% (Table 14.8; Figs 14.28 and 14.29).

The next identifiable group are those tumours arising years after irradiation. Sordillo et al (1981) identified 14 such cases from a total of 165 malignant tumours, and Ducatman et al (1983, 1986) reported on 12 malignant tumours developing in previously irradiated sites at a mean interval of 15.6 years from treatment. We have encountered three probable postirradiation tumours. Some features of

Table 14.8 Five-year survival or disease-free intervals in MPNST

Study	No. of cases	% survival
Solitary		
Das Gupta & Brasfield (1970)	184	49.4 (disease free)
Ducatman et al (1986)	58	53
Sordillo et al 1981	100	47
Neurofibromatosis		
Ghosh et al (1973)	30	30
Ducatman et al (1986)	62	16
Sordillo et al (1981)	65	23

one case are outlined in Chapter 13. In the case of a 63-year-old man who presented with massive swelling deep to and below the clavicle, full mantle radiotherapy had been used for Hodgkin's disease 15 years previously. When we saw him the history and physical signs admitted only one possible diagnosis, that of MPNST. Two biopsies had already been performed, one by needle and one at open operation; both of these were incorrectly reported as benign. The tumour arose from the medial cord.

Figs 14.28 and 14.29 MPNST in NFI. A man of 48 with a large, rapidly growing tumour in the right brachial plexus.

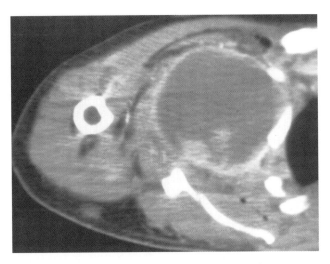

Fig. 14.28 CT scan shows large tumour. The homogenecity of the tumour image suggests a high mitotic rate.

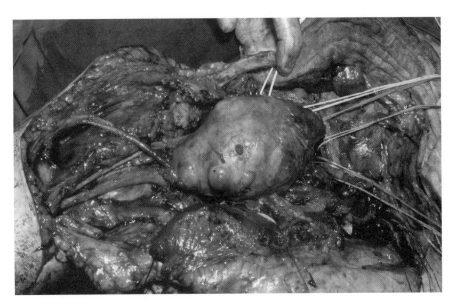

Fig. 14.29 The tumour exposed at the primary operation, after division of the clavicle.

Frozen sections revealed tumour in the eighth cervical nerve root, 15 cm proximal to the main mass. Forequarter amputation had been considered, but had to be abandoned because the chance of cure had already passed due to dissemination of the tumour throughout the field.

The solitary MPNST is somewhat less dangerous. The peak incidence is in the fourth, fifth and sixth decades, and the tumour tends to arise more peripherally. There is no significant difference between the sexes. The head, neck and upper limb are the most common sites, accounting for over 40% of tumours; the lower limb is the site of approximately one-third, and the remainder are found within the trunk, usually arising from spinal nerves and in close relation of the spinal column.

Difficulties in treating tumours of the plexus are well set out in two excellent series, which include over 50 cases (Lusk et al 1987, Sedel et al 1989). The prognosis is very bad. Forequarter amputation is advised for most cases, but this is impracticable in those in which tumour extends to the spinal column or spinal canal. Intradural extramedullary extension occurred in five of our cases of MPNST and in two of the PNET. Two further papers emphasised the serious nature of over 70 cases in the lower limb and sciatic nerve (Lapiere and Maheut 1986, Hruban et al 1990). These workers showed that large tumour size and high mitotic rate led to a particularly poor outcome. The general condition of the patient was always affected, and weight loss and anaemia were usual.

Clinical features

The cardinal clinical feature of MPNST is pain. This is usually attended by clear evidence of impairment of nerve conduction. A tender and enlarging mass is found in all but the most deeply located tumours. Errors in diagnosis are not uncommon; there are numerous references to unnecessary laminectomy or excision of a cervical rib before a correct diagnosis of tumour was made. Nerve conduction studies are not useful. CT and MRI are always valuable in showing the extent of tumour and in distinguishing between benign and malignant tumours. Myelography has a place in defining intradural extramedullary extension, and is extremely good for this when combined with CT scan. Clinical features and findings at operation are more important in diagnosis of MPNST than are histological characteristics, most of all in the so-called low-grade malignant neurofibromata. Detection of metastases, notably in the lungs, has obvious implications for the planned treatment (Figs 14.30 and 14.31).

One of our cases exemplifies the significance of pain. A 48-year-old man complained of intense pain in the foot. Diagnosis was not made for over 2 years, when an impression of fullness in the heel prompted biopsy. An infiltrative lesion was displayed in the heel pad and this was shown to be a malignant schwannoma. The patient remains well and disease free 11 years after below-knee amputation. Professor John Sharrard has kindly provided us with details of a case which exemplifies the behaviour of some of these tumours during pregnancy. His patient, a young woman, presented with MPNST in the median nerve at the elbow. The tumour was widely excised and the patient chose to adopt children, but at the age of 25 years she became pregnant. A recurrence at the original site was noted soon after the birth of her baby. The tumour was removed. The histological appearances were similar to those of the original tumour. The patient remains well. Professor Robert Duthie has advised us of a similar case.

Biopsy

Two reasons lead us to agree with Seddon in discouraging biopsy. First, dissemination of the tumour into the field rules out prospects of cure by radical excision of the affected nerve; next, the biopsy may miss the malignant tumour altogether. Seddon stated: "because the proper treatment for a neurosarcoma should not be less than a radical excision, the biopsy should be of the whole specimen and of a considerable length of the nerve trunk on either side of it – provided it is possible to make the diagnosis of malignancy on the clinical evidence and on the appearances disclosed at operation. A history of increasing pain, of a fairly rapidly developing swelling, the finding of a hard lump in the line of a nerve strongly suggest a neurosarcoma". He goes on to say that the swelling, when exposed, can really be only one of three things, a schwannoma, a benign neurofibroma or MPNST. We have already seen that serious errors followed interpretation of biopsies of benign tumours. An incorrect diagnosis of a benign lesion was made in nine of our cases before they were referred to our unit, and in five this precluded adequate surgical excision because of dissemination about the biopsy site or because of the inexorable extension of the tumour. A note of caution is introduced by one of our own cases in which wide resection of the common peroneal nerve was made because of a confident clinical diagnosis of MPNST; this proved to be aponeurotic fibromatosis.

These strictures do not necessarily apply to experts in the technique of taking and interpreting needle biopsies. Stoker et al (1991) achieved an extremely high level of accuracy in 208 needle biopsies of musculocutaneous lesions.

Small tumours appear as fusiform swellings within the nerve trunk: they are hard, the nerve is surrounded by vascular adhesions, and oedema of adjacent tissues is a significant finding. In other, larger tumours, the diagnosis is all too plain. The tumour may have burst out of the epineurium, extending into muscle or bone. Larger tumours develop as multilobular masses, and there may be cystic changes, haemorrhage and, in the most malignant and rapidly growing tissue, there may be extensive areas of necrosis. Frozen section of the nerve stump may reveal extension of tumour within the perineurium at a considerable distance from the main trunk: in one of our cases tumour was seen at 20 cm proximal to the main mass.

Pathology

Detailed and beautifully illustrated accounts of the histological characteristics can be found in Harkin and Reed (1969), Enzinger and Weiss (1988) and Urich (1993). The most common histological appearance is reminiscent of fibrosarcoma, with masses of spindle-shaped cells organised into sweeping bundles or lamellae (Fig. 14.32; see also Plate section). Irregularity of the cells and a characteristic wavy or buckled appearance of the nuclei is often found. Metaplastic differentiation occurs in about 20% of tumours. Bone, cartilage and muscle are the most

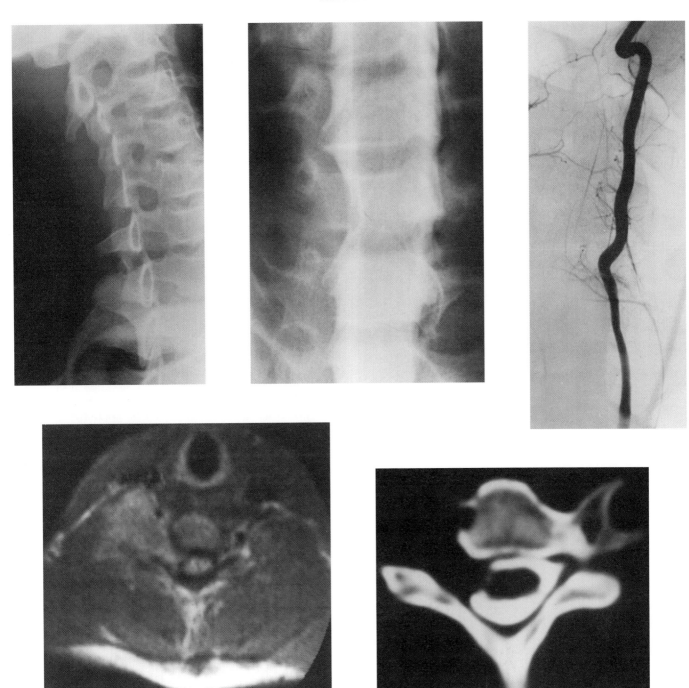

Fig. 14.30 Solitary MPNST arising at C7 level in an 18-year-old man. Radiograph (top left) shows foraminal enlargement. Myelograph (top middle) shows displacement of theca and obliteration of root pouch. Angiograph shows anterior displacement of the vertebral artery, with abnormal vessels. MRI (lower left) shows the extent of the tumour. CT scan (lower right) shows extent of bone destruction and invasion of the subarachnoid space.

common tissues seen; epithelioid differentiation into glandular or squamous tissue is less common. Woodruff et al (1973) described three new cases of rhabdomyosarcomatous change, the so-called triton tumour, and reviewed the seven previously published cases. They agreed with Masson and Martin (1938) in proposing that muscle is formed from malignant Schwann cells. Nine of their patients were dead within a year of diagnosis. A further nine cases were described by Brooks et al (1985).

Electron microscopic studies are rather disappointing, because so many tumours are undifferentiated. One-quarter of tumours show characteristic features of Schwann cells,

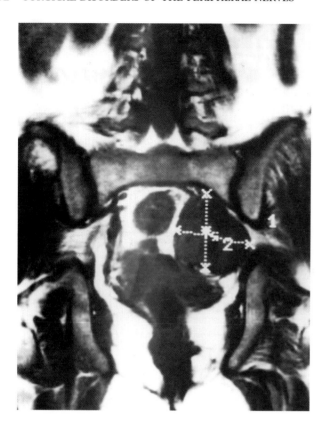

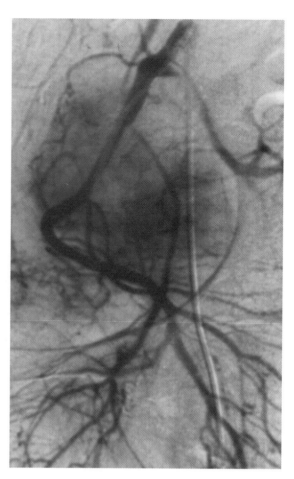

Fig. 14.31 Solitary MPNST of the sciatic nerve. MRI (left) shows situation and extent of tumour. Angiograph (right) shows the "tumour blush".

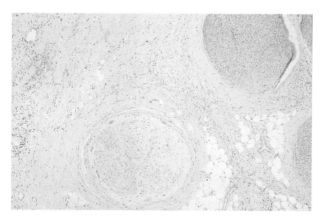

Fig. 14.32 MPNST in the medial cord of the brachial plexus in a patient with NF1. A biopsy of C8, 15 cm proximal to the main tumour mass, shows one bundle completely replaced by tumour and some degenerative changes in adjacent bundles. Haematoxylin and eosin, × 160. (See also Plate section.) (Courtesy of Dr Jean Pringle.)

and in about another quarter fibroblasts predominate. We have not found that the electron microscope is helpful in determining progress, although Verola et al (1985) did so in six cases of MPNST in NFI (Figs 14.33 to 14.35). Immunohistochemical studies are interesting, but may be confusing as nearly one-half of tumours do not stain for S-100 protein. Wick et al (1987) recommended examination for multiple neural markers, showing positive staining for the epithelial membrane antigen in the two epithelioid tumours and positive Desmin staining in the eight spindle cell tumours in their 62 cases (Figs 14.36 A&B, 14.37; see also Plate section).

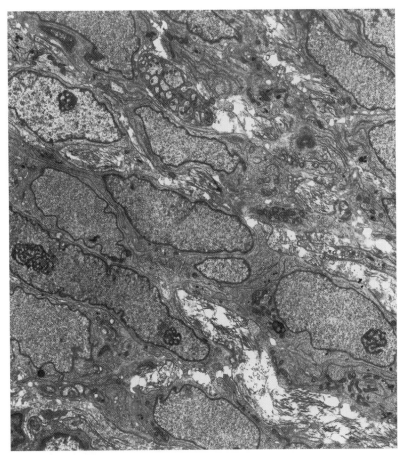

Fig. 14.33 Solitary MPNST of the radial nerve. The tumour is composed largely of Schwann-like cells. × 4500. (Prepared by Mr Stephen Gschmeissner.)

Treatment

This should be undertaken by a surgeon with experience of the treatment of tumours of peripheral nerves and of soft tissue sarcomas who is able to collaborate closely with an experienced pathologist with access to electron microscopic and immunostaining techniques. Adequate radiological facilities are essential. As we have seen in five of our cases, incorrect technique and interpretation of biopsy directly contributed towards a fatal outcome. Notwithstanding our reservation about biopsy in these tumours, there are occasions when correct tissue diagnosis must be obtained before subjecting the patient to loss of a major trunk nerve or ablation of the limb. We are indeed fortunate in the accuracy of interpretation of frozen sections granted us by Dr Jean Pringle and Dr Anne Sandison of the Royal National Orthopaedic Hospital.

Much of what is written about the staging of these tumours is confusing. The epineurium is the sheath within which the tumour starts. Once the epineurium is breached an excision of the nerve alone must be inadequate. An adequate excision of the trunk nerve is the correct treatment for tumour which is still confined in the epineurium, and frozen sections are essential to establish adequate clearance. In four of our cases we found it necessary to section the spinal nerve at the foramen to secure this. As Bolton et al (1989) point out, local recurrence after "limb sparing" operations is much more common on MPNST than it is in non-neural soft tissue sarcomas arising in the extremities.

Amputation is probably indicated when the epineurium has been breached, and, perhaps, in rapidly growing recurrence, although excision of the recurrence was adequate in Professor Sharrard's case and in our case 15. Lusk et al (1988) recommended forequarter amputation for MPNST arising within the brachial plexus. We agree that this is necessary with recurrence after apparently adequate excision or when there is such involvement of the plexus that no function can be preserved. It may be necessary for palliation even if it cannot cure.

The outcome of treatment in our 35 cases of true MPNST is bleak. Of the nine tumours in known NF1, six

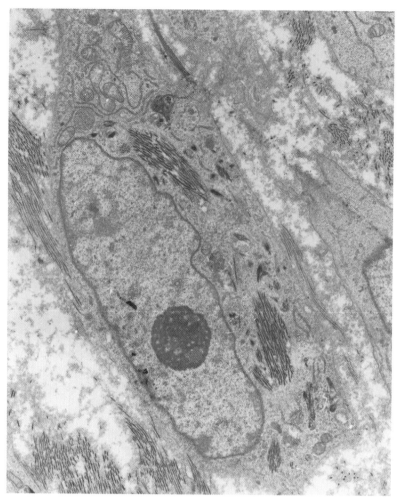

Fig. 14.34 Electron micrograph of a MPNST of the common peroneal nerve in NF1. Fibroblast-like cells predominate. × 5600. (Prepared by Professor F. Scaravelli.)

died within 2 years of treatment: one from a second intra-pelvic MPNST, one from disseminated intravascular coagulation (DIC) after operation. Two more patients still have disease at less than 12 months from operation (Tables 14.9, 14.10).

Of the 26 patients with solitary tumours, four died within 2 years and six are known to have disease. Nine appear free of disease at a minimum of 4 years from operation. Of those "cured", nine were treated by excision of the nerve, one by amputation of the limb and one by forequarter amputation.

Surgical ablation was impossible in six cases because of intradural extramedullary extension. Death was caused by invasion of great vessels, of the spinal canal or viscera in four cases, and in six more the threat of this remains. Death was caused by pulmonary and visceral metastases in three cases.

The outcome from non-neural sarcomas arising within peripheral nerve trunks is rather better, and is summarised in Table 14.11. These tumours were located more distally, and wide excision was possible in every case.

Our experience with primitive neurectodermal tumours is too small to be worthy of discussion. These tumours are radio- and chemosensitive, and case 3 remains apparently disease free 5 years after wide excision of the common peroneal nerve followed by intensive radio- and chemotherapy (Table 14.12; Figs 14.38 to 14.40). (Figs 14.41 A&B, 14.42 A&B; see also Plate section)

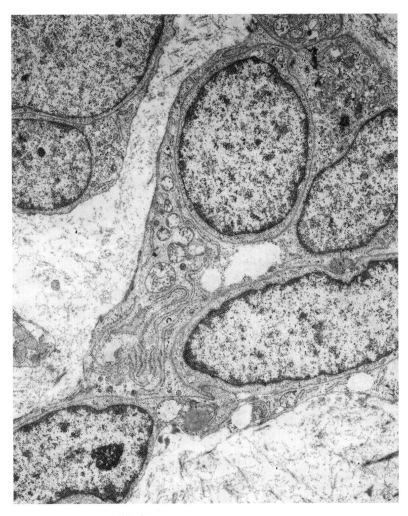

Fig. 14.35 Solitary MPNST of the brachial plexus. Some cells resemble those of Schwann, others resemble fibroblasts, and others are undifferentiated. × 7275. (Prepared by Mr Stephen Gschmeissner.)

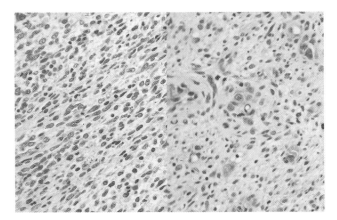

Fig. 14.36 MPNST. The tumour is densely cellular with moderate pleomorphism and high mitotic index. Haematoxylin and eosin, × 400. (See also Plate section.) (Courtesy of Dr Jean Pringle.)

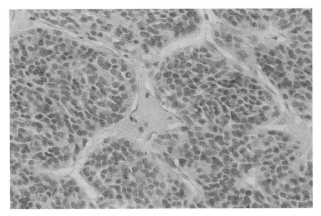

Fig. 14.37 Haemangiopericytoma of the common peroneal nerve showing the characteristic stag horn pattern of the vessels. Haematoxylin and eosin, × 400 (See also Plate section.) (Courtesy of Dr Jean Pringle.)

Table 14.9 MPNST in neurofibromatosis type 1: 9 cases

Patient No.	Age (years)	Sex	Origin	Operation	Histological diagnosis	Course
1	18	F	Posterior cord	Wide excision of posterior cord: margin 4 cm. Flexor to extensor tendon transfer.	Schwannoma	DXT. Disease free at 1 year
2	45	F	Upper and middle trunks	Partial excision	Muscle metaplasia	DXT. Disease present at 6 months
3	28	F	Sciatic nerve intra- and extrapelvic	Complete excision: margin 5 cm.	Schwannoma.	Died at 1 year
4	35	M	Medial cord and lower trunk	Excision lower trunk, medial cord 7 months later: forequarter amputation.	Glandular and epithelioid metaplasia	Death at 14 months from erosion of great vessels in neck
5	20	M	Tibial nerve	Wide excision	Fibroblastic tumour	DXT and chemotherapy. Death at 18 months from pulmonary metastases and local recurrence
6	20	M	Entire brachial plexus	Forequarter amputation	Schwannoma	DXT. Disease free at 2 years
7	14	F	Ulnar nerve (arm)	Wide excision	Schwannoma	DXT. Disease free at 2 years
8	35	F	C5	Decompression of spinal cord	Schwannoma	Tetraparesis improved. Disease present at 9 months
9	54	M	C8, T1	Wide excision. Vertebrectomy C7 and T1. Fusion	Neurofibroma	Death from DIC at 3 days

Case 8 was operated on with Mr R. Bradford FRCS.
Five from nine patients died within 2 years of diagnosis, and disease is present in at least two more.

Table 14.10 Solitary MPNST: 26 cases

Patient No.	Age (years)	Sex	Origin	Operation	Histological diagnosis	Course
1	65	F	Medial cord (postirradiation)	Wide excision	"Schwannoma"	Recurrence in chest wall at 15 months
2	18	M	Supraclavicular nerve	Wide excision	Bone metaplasia	Disease free at 1 year
3	60	F	Sciatic nerve in notch	Wide excision	Cartilage metaplasia	Disease free at 1 year
4	24	M	C5, extra- and intradural extramedullary	(a) Incomplete excision (b) Decompression of spinal cord	Schwannoma	Tetraparesis relieved: DXT. Disease present at 9 months
5	45	F	Sciatic nerve at notch	Wide excision	Schwannoma, multiple metaplasia	Recurrence in ilium at 3 years (removed)
6	20	M	Ulnar (forearm)	Wide excision	Schwannoma	Disease free at 6 months
7	66	F	Medial cord (postirradiation)	Wide excision	Schwannoma	Disease free at 6 months
8	56	M	Ulnar (arm)	Wide excision (recurrence). Forequarter amputation	Schwannoma, proximal intraneural extension for 20 cm	Disease free at 1 year
9	58	M	Medial cord (postirradiation)	Wide excision	Triton tumour, proximal intraneural extension 15 cm	DXT. Death at 18 months
10	18	M	C7 intradural extramedullary extension	Partial excision	Spindle cell tumour	DXT. Disease free at 4 years
11	30	M	Upper trunk	Excision and grafting (recurrence). Forequarter amputation	Schwannoma	Disease free at 1 year
12	41	M	Median nerve in axilla	Wide excision	Primitive mesenchymal tumour	Disease free at 7 years
13	33	F	Median at elbow	Wide excision (recurrence excised). Later amputation through shoulder	Schwannoma	Regional chemotherapy. DXT. Death at 3 years (pulmonary metastases)
14	55	M	Radial axilla	Wide excision	Schwannoma. Epithelial metaplasia	Disease free at 7 years
15	50	F	Posterior interosseous forearm	Wide excision (2 recurrences excised)	Schwannoma	Disease free at 5 years
16	69	M	Digital nerve finger	Ray amputation	Epithelioid schwannoma	Death at 1 year from pulmonary metastases
17	38	F	Median nerve hand	Incomplete excision	Schwannoma	DXT. Disease present at 1 year
18	51	M	T1	Incomplete excision	Triton tumour	DXT. Disease present at 9 months
19	62	M	Common peroneal nerve at knee	Wide excision	Schwannoma	Disease free at 5 years
20	50	F	Median nerve arm	Wide excision (recurrence at 4 years; excised)	Schwannoma	Disease free at 9 months
21	37	F	Lower trunk	Incomplete excision	Schwannoma	Disease present
22	55	M	Plantar nerve heel	Below knee amputation	Schwannoma	Disease free at 5 years
23	12	F	Ulnar nerve arm	Wide excision (of medial cord and lower trunk	Schwannoma (intraneural extension 12 cm)	Disease free at 4 years
24	30	M	Ulnar nerve axilla	Wide excision (of medial cord and lower trunk)	Glandular metaplasia (intraneural extension 10 cm)	Disease free at 10 years
25	28	F	Sciatic nerve thigh	Wide excision	Schwannoma. Muscle metaplasia	DXT. Disease free at 2 years
26	33	M	Median nerve forearm	Excision with graft	Schwannoma	Recurrence at 9 months

Cases 17, 18, and 21 seen in consultation. Cases 3 and 5 operated on with Mr T.W. Briggs FRCS, and case 12 with Professor A.O. Narakas.

Table 14.11 Sarcomas arising from nerves: 5 cases

Patient No.	Sex	Age (years)	Origin	Operation	Histological	Course
1	F	69	Ulnar nerve (arm)	Wide excision	Lymphoma	DXT. Disease free at 2 years
2	F	76	Ulnar nerve (axilla)	Wide excision	Liposarcoma	DXT. Death from septicaemia at 8 months
3	M	68	Musculocutaneous nerve	Wide excision	Liposarcoma	DXT. Disease free at 8 months
4	F	68	Common peroneal nerve (knee)	Wide excision	Haemangiopericytoma	DXT. Disease free at 9 months
5	F	70	Ulnar nerve (hand)	Wide excision, amputation little and ring and midrays	Haemangiopericytoma	DXT. Metastasis in skull at 2 years

Table 14.12 Primitive neurectodermal tumours: 4 cases

Patient No.	Age (years)	Sex	Origin	Operation	Histological diagnosis	Course
1	37	F	C7	Excision C7, middle trunk with vertebrectomy	Extraosseous Ewing's tumour	Chemotherapy. Disease present at 18 months
2 (NF1)	16	M	Sciatic nerve (thigh)	Wide excision	Neuroepithelioma	DXT, chemotherapy. Death at 18 months, pulmonary metastases
3 (NF1)	30	F	Common peroneal nerve (knee)	Wide excision	Neuroepithelioma	DXT, chemotherapy. Disease free at 5 years
4	19	F	Cervical sympathetic chain and lower trunk	Partial excision	Extraosseous Ewing's tumour	DXT. Chemotherapy. Death at 2 years, local recurrence, invasion mediastinum

Case 1 operated on with Mr A.O. Ransford FRCS. One patient in four may be considered cured.

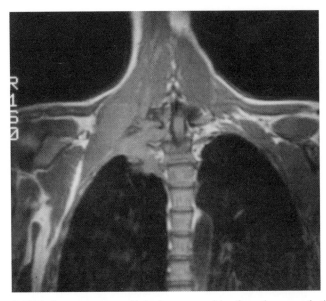

Fig. 14.38 MRI of an extraosseous Ewing's tumour arising from the sympathetic chain.

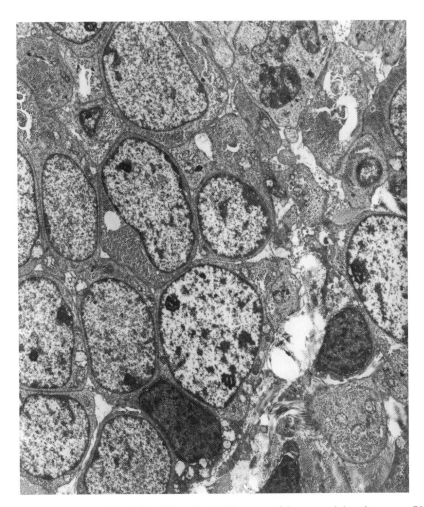

Fig. 14.39 The tumour consisted of undifferentiated cells, many of these containing glycogen. × 7000.

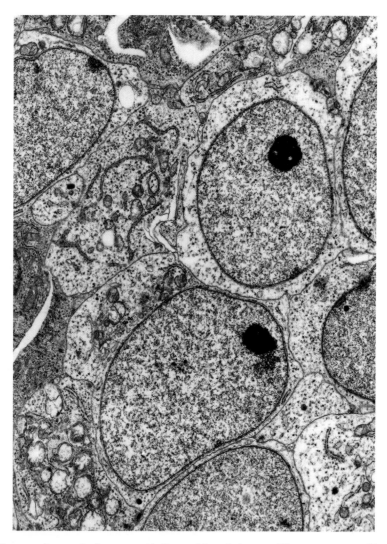

Fig. 14.40 Electron micrograph of a neuroepithelioma of the sciatic nerve. The tumour grew with great rapidity. The cells are undifferentiated, and the mitotic index is high. × 8075. (Prepared by Mr Stephen Gschmeissner.)

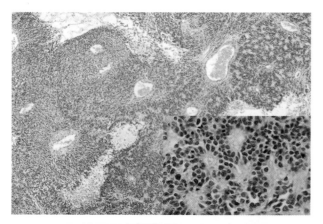

Fig. 14.41 Neuroepithelioma arising from the sciatic nerve in a 14-year-old boy with NF1. There is focal necrosis; viable tissue surrounding the blood vessels. There are areas of rosette formation. Haematoxylin and eosin, × 160 (left) and × 400 (right). (See also Plate section.) (Courtesy of Dr Jean Pringle.)

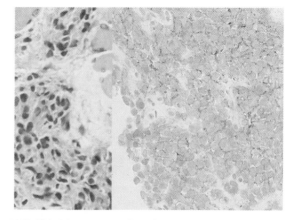

Fig. 14.42 Primitive neuroectodermal tumour arising from the median nerve. The tumour is infiltrating muscle and there is positive staining for MIC 2. Haematoxylin and eosin, left (inset) × 400 and right × 400. (See also Plate section.) (Courtesy of Dr Jean Pringle.)

TUMOURS OF THE SYMPATHETIC CHAIN

These tumours form a spectrum from the undifferentiated and malignant neuroblastoma to the fully differentiated and nonmetastasising ganglioneuroma. A full discussion of neuroblastoma is beyond the scope of this work, but there are certain features of particular interest and relevance. The neuroblastoma is the third most common childhood malignancy after leukaemia and brain tumour. One-quarter are evident at birth, and 50% have been detected by the age of 2 years (Enzinger & Weiss 1988). Eighty per cent have an abnormality on chromosome 1, which distinguishes them from primitive neurectodermal tumours (Brodeur et al 1980). The cells secrete neurotransmitters, over 80% of children showing elevated urinary levels of catecholamine and their derivatives, and there are occasional examples of tumours secreting acetylcholine. The N-MYC oncogene and its product are found in the cells; this is amplified in the more extensive and aggressive tumour (Slamon et al 1986). There are well-documented cases of maturation of neuroblastoma to ganglioneuroma (Cushing & Wolback 1927).

GANGLIONEUROMA

The ganglioneuroma is quite rare compared to other benign tumours, but it exceeds neuroblastoma along the sympathetic chain in the ratio of 3 : 1. Most are diagnosed over the age of 10 years. The posterior mediastinum and retroperitoneum are the most common sites. The tumour is circumscribed, with a fibrous capsule, grey or yellow in texture and sometimes walled, like a leiomyoma. Light microscopy shows bundles and fascicles of Schwann cells with scattered ganglion cells. Although Stout (1947) found no metastases in his series of 146 ganglioneuromas, there have been occasional reports of transformation into MPNST.

Patients with cathecholamine secreting tumour may present with systemic manifestations. Although contrast-enhanced axial CT is the most widely used technique for the localisation of phaeochromocytomas (Velchick et al 1989). Mukherjee et al (1996) describe the value of measuring noradrenaline and adrenaline levels by venous catheterisation in a case of secreting ganglioneuroma adjacent to a venal vein.

We have seen two cases of ganglioneuroma, neither were secreting tumours. The difficulties in their treatment are exemplified by one of them. A 9-year-old boy presented with a tender mass in the right side of the neck. A biopsy showed ganglioneuroma. The tumour extended from C3 to T3, indenting the apex of the right lung. There was little functional deficit; the mass did not extend into the spinal canal. There was no evidence that the tumour was secreting any abnormal substance. Operation was performed using the transclavicular approach, demonstrating a tumour 15 cm long, 10 cm deep and 7 cm wide, closely adherent to the internal jugular and subclavian veins, enveloping the vertebral artery. The mass was removed piecemeal. Recovery was uneventful and the patient remained well at 2.5 years.

for although wind up may induce central sensitisation, the latter, a more general phenomenon, can "be produced by the asynchronous activation of skin, joint or visceral afferents directly by chemical irritants, or as a consequence of inflammation, neither of which produces a detectable pattern of progressively increasing action potential discharge".

Munglani and Hunt (1995) persuasively argue that protein synthesis is a useful indicator of nociceptor activity in the dorsal horn. The protein Fos is synthesised under the control of a gene which is rapidly expressed in some dorsal horn neurones after peripheral noxious stimulation. Most Fos-positive neurones are found in laminae 1 and 2, with some in lamina 5. In the experiment, a rat sciatic nerve was loosely sutured, to provide a model of neuropathic pain; after this some neurones in laminae 3 and 4 became Fos positive.

CENTRAL PROJECTIONS

The central transmissions of nociceptive information from the dorsal horn is largely through the crossed spinothalamic tract in the ventrolateral quadrant of the cord. The cell bodies from which axons arise are found mainly in laminae 1, 4 and 5, with lesser contributions from 2 and 3 (Willis et al 1979). Axons may ascend up to two segmental levels before joining the tract that contains fibres conveying information about touch and temperature, so explaining the different levels of temperature, light touch and pinprick disturbance in Brown–Séquard syndrome and other cord lesions. The somatotopic arrangement within the tract is the basis of cordotomy for pain (Fig. 15.3). Some axons pass directly to synapse with neurones in the thalamus that lie in the nucleus ventralis posterolateralis (VPL). Lesions within the VPL cause loss of somatic sensation. Any pain relief is transient. Indeed, destruction of the VPL causes a state of continuous burning pain that is experienced mainly contralaterally, with exaggeration of autonomic and emotional responses. There is an orderly somatatopic arrangement of fibres entering the VPL, not only of nociceptors but also from the lemniscal system relaying touch and joint sensation (Poggio & Mountcastle 1963). It is tempting to see in this a possible basis for the ability to recognise the site, nature and volume of a painful event, but the VPL is certainly not the seat of pain. Stimulation of its neurones induces localised paraesthesia, and, rarely, evokes painful sensation (White & Sweet 1969). The anatomically precise link between the dorsal horn and the thalamus applies to only a proportion of the nociceptors within the spinothalamic tract, perhaps a minority. Many others enter a polysynaptic system which passes to the reticular formation, nuclei in the brainstem, the hypothalamus, and the medial and posterior group of thalamic nuclei. Bowsher (1976) thought that up to one-half of spinothalamic fibres never reached the thalamus

but ended in the reticular formation on both sides of the brainstem to synapse with cells in the nucleus gigantocellularis. Mehler et al (1960) proposed two components of the spinothalamic system: the neospinothalamic, of crossed fibres with a few synapses and an orderly somatotopic arrangement of terminals largely in the VPL; and the palaeospinothalamic of crossed and uncrossed fibres, polysynaptic, with much less somatotopic organisation, ultimately ending in the medial and posterior thalamus. Intraoperative stimulation in the course of ablative neurosurgical work provides data of considerable interest. Nashold et al (1969a) stimulated the periaqueductal grey matter deep to the superior colliculus of the midbrain in patients, evoking a diffuse centrally located pain which was associated with intense fear. There was a marked sympathetic response, an increase in heart rate and contralateral piloerection. More lateral stimulation evoked brighter or sharper pain felt on the contralateral side. Mark et al (1963) found considerable evidence to support a functional organisation for pain perception within the thalamus. Lesions of the medial thalamus relieved pain or at least the suffering from pain without disturbing sensation, whereas lesions in the VPL caused loss of sensation and did not relieve pain. Ishijma et al (1975) recorded from neurones in the central median thalamus during operations for chronic pain, finding that they had a very wide receptive field. Their stimulation evoked burning pain in a wide area of the body, and sometimes this was felt on both sides of the body. Lesions here caused no loss of sensibility. The central projections from the medial and posterior thalamus are far more widespread than from the VPL and include the limbic system.

Little is known of cerebral mechanisms. Direct stimulation of the human cerebral cortex rarely induces pain. Penfield and Boldrey (1937) reported their observations in 126 operations conducted under local anaesthetic. The cortex was stimulated on 364 occasions: in 11 of these, patients described pain, which was rarely severe. One recent study of interest (Flor et al 1995) followed 13 patients after amputation of the upper limb. Some of these had severe phantom-limb pain and five had no pain at all. Reorganisation of the cerebral cortex was measured by recording cortical magnetic fields in response to peripheral stimulation. These fields were most widespread in those with severe pain. There was a strong relationship between the amount of cortical reorganisation and the magnitude of phantom-limb pain; the authors suggest that such pain may be a consequence of plastic changes in the primary somatosensory cortex (Fig. 15.4; see also Plate section).

DESCENDING PATHWAYS: CONTROLS

Reynolds (1969) stimulated the central grey matter of the midbrain of the rat and induced such a degree of analgesia that the animals could be operated on without anaesthesia.

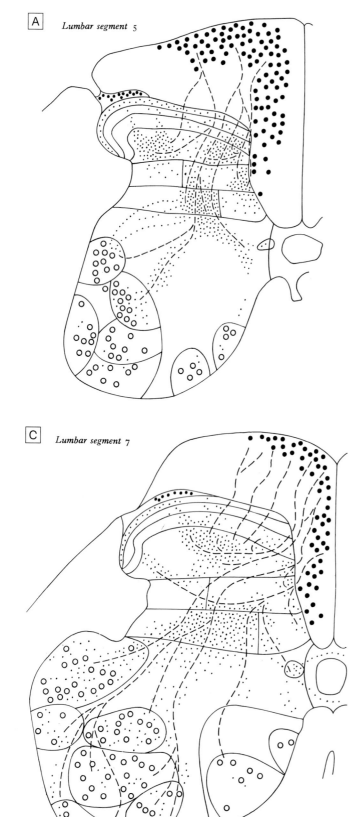

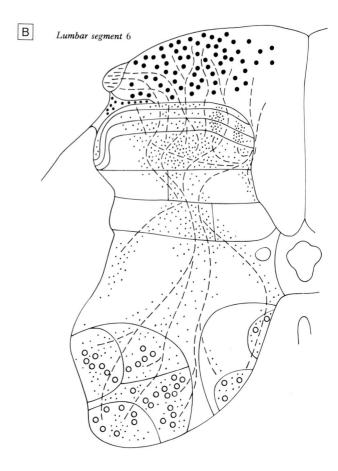

Fig. 15.3 The pattern of degeneration of nerve fibres and their terminals demonstrated with the Nauta–Laidlaw technique in the ipsilateral half of the spinal cord at various segmental levels, 5 days after surgical division of the sixth lumbar dorsal spinal nerve root of the cat. (A) The fifth lumbar segment; (B) the sixth lumbar segment; (C) the seventh lumbar segment. The large dots indicate degeneration of fibres in the dorsal funiculus; the smaller dots indicate degenerating fibres in the dorsolateral tract of Lissauer; the smallest dots indicate degenerating nerve terminals; dashed lines, degenerating fibres of passage; circles, neuronal somata of motor neurons. (From Sprague and Ha (1964), with the permission of the authors and Elsevier.)

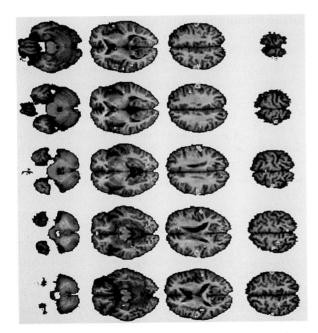

Fig. 15.4 Echo-planar functional magnetic resonance image using a 1.5 Tesla system showing the effects of repetitive stimulation of the left palm of a right-handed volunteer. The yellow areas indicate increased local oxygen concentration, a result of local increase in cerebral activity. There are several areas of activity; the bilateral anterior parietal activation probably represents somato-sensory cortex (by courtesy of Dr Jonathan Berman). Jonathan Berman permits us to refer to other findings as yet unpublished. In one patient with continuing pain, cerebral activity was seen in the midline, in the region of the cingulate cortex. In another case, in which pain disappeared with the return of muscular activity, cerebral activity was much less prominent in the cingulate cortex area. (See also Plate section.)

This analgesia was brought about by inhibition of nociceptor neurones in laminae 1 and 5: cell bodies able to do this are found in the diencephalic paraventricular region, the periaqueductal grey matter (PAG) and the raphe nuclei in the medulla. The pathway is not direct: PAG neurones relay in the raphe nucleus magnus projecting from there to the dorsal horn (Basbaum et al 1977a). The neurotransmitter released by the descending pathway from the raphe nucleus is the monoamine serotonin (5-HT) (Dahlstrom & Fuxe 1964). This serotonergic analgesic pathway was the first such descending control demonstrated. Substances that inhibit serotonin synthesis block the analgesic effect; if the serotonin precursor 5-hydroxy-tryptophan is given, analgesia increases. Morphine acts on it; it is blocked by naloxone. Other pathways using different transmitters have been described; one such tract passes from the locus caeruleus of the pons to the outer laminae of the dorsal horn. It is noradrenergic.

The demonstration of pathways producing analgesia similar to morphine led to the discovery of morphine binding sites throughout the central nervous system (Atweh & Kuhar 1977, Peri & Snyder 1979). Such receptors are found in particularly high concentrations within

the dorsal horn. The relevance of these in the inhibition of nociceptive neurones in the dorsal horn is indicated by the analgesia from intrathecal morphine. The demonstration of stimulation-induced analgesia in the experimental animal was soon followed by its demonstration in humans. Richardson and Akill (1977) relieved intractable pain in eight patients by stimulating the periventricular grey using implanted electrodes, and Adams (1976) eased perineal pain by stimulation close to the wall of the third ventricle. This effect was abolished by naloxone, which led Adams to suggest that the technique worked by provoking release of an endogenous opiate. One such was discovered in 1975 by Hughes, a peptide acting at morphine binding sites and antagonised by morphine antagonists. That inhibitory pathways descending from even higher levels within the central nervous system exist has been demonstrated by Tsubokawa et al (1993), who found encouraging results in the treatment of patients with thalamic pain from stimulation of the motor cortex. A more recent study of this technique used in two cases of central or thalamic pain following infarcts of the central nervous system attempted to correlate the electrophysiological and cerebral blood flow changes following stimulation at the precentral gyrus. Peyron et al (1995) followed two such patients. Pain was effectively relieved in one of them. They showed, with positron emission tomography, that stimulation increased blood flow in the thalamus, brainstem, cingulate gyrus and the orbitofrontal cortex. Stamford (1995) reviews the subject.

EVENTS AFTER NERVE INJURY

A tide of changes sweeps centripetally after wounding of a nerve; it can be described in the wound itself, in the proximal axon and dorsal root ganglion, in the dorsal horn and within the central nervous system.

Release of chemical agents

Many chemical agents are released by damaged tissue, blood vessels and by cut nerve fibres. They include cations, histamine, 5-HT, bradykinin, substance P, cytokines and purines. These induce spread of skin sensitivity from the damaged area to neighbouring skin. A zone of "primary hyperalgesia" extends to a "zone of secondary hyper-algesia", which reflects central changes of sensitisation or disinhibition, or both, of neurones in the dorsal horn. Lewis described this in 1936: "a profuse and widespread area of hyperalgesia appears in many normal subjects around the point of faradic stimulation or tiny crush of the skin. This hyperalgesia lasts for several or many hours and may be accompanied by a little smarting of the skin".

There is sensitisation of unmyelinated afferent fibres. Perhaps of greater significance are the changes that occur in the newly regenerating sprouts within the neuroma, and in particular their changing responsiveness to noradrenaline. Wall and Gutnick (1974a,b) studied events in neuromas made in the rat sciatic nerve. They found three major changes. First, the nerve fibres became spontaneously active, whereas in the normal state they are silent. This is the basis of spontaneous sensory symptoms, paraesthesiae and dysaesthesiae. Next, the fibres become sensitive to mechanical stimulation, an explanation for Tinel's sign. The spontaneous activity and the mechanical sensitivity were suppressed by stimulation of the intact nerve proximally, and by antidromic stimulation mimicking the action of transcutaneous nerve stimulation. This inhibition lasted for minutes or hours. Finally, the nerve sprouts become sensitive to noradrenaline. The time course of this sensitivity to injected adrenaline was confirmed by Scadding (1981) and Korenman and Devor (1981). Devor and Janig (1981) showed that stimulation of the sympathetic nerves to the limb released sufficient noradrenaline to excite the damaged sensory afferents. The firing of spontaneously active afferents from a neuroma of the rat sciatic nerve was increased by stimulation of lumbar sympathetic nerves, and also by intravenous injection of noradrenaline. Both these effects were blocked by phentolamine, an α-adrenergic antagonist. Korenman and Devor (1981) showed that, despite its powerful hypotensive effect, phentolamine did not affect the basal rate of spontaneous discharge from the neuroma, nor block the discharge caused by asphyxia. They also showed that adrenaline did not exert its effect simply by causing peripheral ischaemia.

Evidently, sprouting fibres within a neuroma become sensitive to locally released chemicals, to mechanical stimulation, and to a normal neurotransmitter. One more change, a structural one, is the development of new synapses between sprouting nerve fibres, ephapses, which permit the stimulation of one new fibre by an adjacent one (Seltzer and Devor 1979). These were described in the rat; they are rare in monkeys, and of doubtful relevance in man.

The sensitisation of distal receptors is not confined to the nerves. Akoev (1981) studied the sympathetic control of mechanoreceptors. Sympathetic fibres had been demonstrated adjacent to sensory receptors and muscle spindles for over 100 years and, until quite recently, their function was unknown. He concluded: "on the basis of available morphological and physiological data it seems reasonable to conclude that the autonomic efferent sympathetic nerve fibres probably do play a role of an effective feed back loop in regulation of the excitability in a variety of mechanoreceptors". It seems likely that this aspect of sympathetic function could contribute to allodynia.

Similar sensitisation has been observed within the proximal axon and also in the cells of the dorsal root ganglion. Some parent bodies of C-fibres become sensitive to circulating noradrenaline, develop spontaneous activity, and lose neuropeptides (Wall & Devor 1981).

Changes within the spinal cord

There are profound changes within the dorsal horn after injury to a peripheral nerve. Their nature is similar to those that occur peripherally, chiefly sensitisation, but to this is added loss of inhibition both from peripheral afferent and central descending pathways. Woolf (1995) has reviewed these events, and describes three mechanisms that bring about central sensitisation. First, the dorsal horn cells respond to an increase in C-fibre activity. There is a maintained state of central sensitisation from ectopic activity in the neuroma and dorsal root ganglion. Next, there is decreased inhibition because of loss of activity in A-β fibres, the input of which is diminished (Devor 1991). One aspect of failure of central descending inhibitory pathways has been displayed in the rat spinal cord by Besse et al (1990). Opioid receptors are most highly concentrated in the C-fibre terminal zone of lamina 1 and the substantia gelatinosa of the dorsal horn. Most of these receptors are presynaptic, on the afferent terminals. Cutting their afferent axons leads to degeneration of these terminals and loss of these opioid receptors. Third, there are new synapses within the spinal cord. Axonotomised A-β fibres sprout from deeper parts of the dorsal horn into laminae 1 and 2 (Woolf et al 1992), and new sympathetic fibres grow around large cells in the dorsal root ganglion (McLachlan et al 1993). It seems likely that sympathetic activity activates A-β neurones, providing an explanation for the role of the sympathetic system in A-β mediated pain.

These changes may permit an explanation for allodynia, the perception of normally nonpainful stimuli as pain. Lamotte et al (1992) recorded and stimulated single A-β fibres in human volunteers. The receptor field, which was usually a small area of skin, was defined by stimulation. Stimulation of the fibres evoked the usual innocuous response. Capsaicin, an agent which first stimulates and then blocks C-fibre activity, was injected. There followed a period when normally painless stimuli were perceived as painful ones. Afferent volleys passing through A-β fibres were interpreted as pain. It seems that hyperalgesia and allodynia after partial injury to a peripheral nerve is the central misinterpretation of normal inputs, and this occurs because of central sensitisation. The neurophysiological change that permits this is the summation of slow synaptic potentials from small-diameter axons, which depolarise neurones in the dorsal horn, in part by opening the NMDA receptors. There is wind up of action potential discharge in these spinal neurones, but there is also a prolonged increase in the excitability of their membranes.

Evidently, urgent steps should be taken to reverse the cause of these peripheral and central states of excitation and disinhibition, but some changes are irreversible. Chief amongst these is the death of neurones following axonotomy. Dyck et al (1984) studied the spinal cords of patients who had undergone amputation of lower limbs some years previously. They found that peripheral fibres were narrower, with shorter internodes, and they demonstrated a dramatic drop in the population of neurones in the anterior horn. Sendtner et al (1990) showed that a neurotrophic agent, ciliary neurotrophic factor, given exogenously, prevented cell death within the rat facial nucleus after section of the nerve.

Anand (1995) has assembled evidence showing that the first neurotrophin ever described, nerve growth factor (NGF), is involved in the maintenance of pain. NGF is a protein normally produced by such tissues as skin, blood vessels and bladder. It is taken up by sympathetic and small sensory fibres via a high-affinity receptor Tyrosine kinase receptor A (trkA) and transported to the cell bodies. It is essential for their development and survival. The first case of absence of NGF was described in 1991 by Anand et al. The patient presented with severe postural hypotension, and investigation confirmed autonomic failure. The sensory neuropeptides NGF and substance P were undetectable. There was no sensory axon reflex. Capsaicin injection was not painful. The threshold to heat pain was elevated, but the patient did feel pin prick and sharp pain. Three other studies in human neuropathies have been presented that show a possible role for NGF in the maintenance of chronic neuropathic pain. The concentration of NGF is low in the skin of those with leprosy (Anand et al 1994a). It is increased in sunburnt skin, which is notoriously hyperalgesic. NGF is diminished in diabetic neuropathy, which is usually painless (Anand et al 1994b). In about 10% of diabetic patients the neuropathy is painful, and nerve biopsies in these cases show considerable sprouting of myelinated fibres (Brown et al 1976). NGF has been measured in biopsies of damaged human nerves. It is still produced by the target organs in denervated skin, unlike the situation in diabetic neuropathy, and it is suggested that there is a relative excess of the neurotrophin, which is encountered by fewer than normal regenerating nerve fibres. It is possible that the hyperalgesia and exquisite capsaicin sensitivity of the skin of patients in the early stages of recovery after nerve suture is explicable on this basis (Anand et al 1994c).

One remarkable finding from biopsies from young animals and from infants who had sustained birth lesions of the brachial plexus was that there was no qualitative difference in NGF concentration between the mature and immature animal. However, autotomy and severe pain are not apparent, either in the neonatal rat nor in the baby. This is striking evidence for plasticity or adaptation within the immature spinal cord (Anand 1992).

Central pain: the preganglionic injury of the brachial plexus

Evidently, wounds of the brachial plexus can be associated with true causalgia or other painful states just as can other lesions of other peripheral nerves. However, of all the pains associated with injury to peripheral nerves, it is the pain associated with traction lesions that is perhaps the most severe, the most persistent, and the most resistant to treatment. The clinical features and results of treatment will be described later, but it is now possible to ascribe some of the characteristics of traction or avulsion pain to anatomical and physiological change within the spinal cord.

The pain is usually immediate in onset. Typically it has two components. First there is the constant pain, which is usually felt in the insensate hand. This is described as crushing or boring, bursting or burning. Superimposed on this are lightning-like shooting pains, which course down the whole of the limb. These last a few seconds, they may occur up to 30 or 40 times in every hour, and are exceptionally severe in intensity. It is usually the case that patients will report the distribution of these pains within the territory of avulsed nerves. The shooting pain is not experienced in those parts of the limb that have not been denervated.

Pain after traction lesion of the brachial plexus is usually worse in cold weather, if the patient is otherwise ill, or when the patient is stressed or depressed. Engagement of the mind in work, hobbies or conversation usually eases the pain.

Of some relevance here perhaps, is the observation made by Bonney and Jamieson in 1978 that in a human cord observed 24 hours after avulsion of the roots of the brachial plexus, the level of separation was in fact about 1 mm proud of the surface of the cord (Bonney & Jamieson 1979). Later histological studies confirm that in many cases of preganglionic injury the line of separation is within the peripheral nerve, through or distal to the transitional zone. The lesion is akin to rhizotomy. In more extreme cases, however, the rootlets are torn from within the spinal cord, and the fragments of this are seen attached to those rootlets when they are exposed within the posterior triangle of the neck. This is true avulsion. A partial Brown–Séquard syndrome is detectable in at least 10% of patients with deep preganglionic injury of the brachial plexus. Probably these are true avulsion injuries. Bonney (1973) thought of the pain as arising in the spinal cord as a result of damage and later gliosis in the substantia gelatinosa, and this has been confirmed in the lumbar spinal cord of the cat after dorsal rhizotomy or avulsion (Ovelmen-Levitt et al 1984). Consistent pathological changes were noted after avulsion, and included damage to the medial portion of Lissauers' tract, and gliosis within the substantia gelatinosa. Extracellular microelectrode recording from neurones within the deep laminae of the dorsal horn showed differences between the rhizotomy and avulsion model. The receptive fields extended more widely after rhizotomy. Spontaneous activity from recorded neurones were seen in both preparations, but the pattern was different, with more regular firing being seen in the chronically avulsed cells.

Ovelmen-Levitt et al (1982) found a different pattern of depletion of neuropeptides within the damaged dorsal horn after rhizotomy or avulsion.

The intradural rupture or rhizotomy is, in effect, an injury of the peripheral nerve; an avulsion is an injury of the central nervous system. In an experimental study of rat spinal nerves, Bristol and Fraher (1989) found that most myelinated fibres within the ventral roots ruptured at the transition zone junction. Hoffmann et al (1993a) described electron microscopic changes in the spinal cord at different intervals after avulsion of a cervical ventral root in the cat. There was progressive degeneration of motor axons between the ventral horn cell and the surface of the cord. There was an increase in population in glial cells. In the first few weeks there was evidence of proximal motor axons entering a phase of regeneration by forming "terminal clubs", an observation made earlier by Cajal (1928). By 3 months these nascent regenerating terminal clubs had disappeared.

An extreme example of the anatomical damage following avulsion is the rare complication of post-traumatic syrinx. Taylor (1962) and Richter and Schachenmayr (1984) provided evidence of cyst formation in the region of the posterior horn and intermediolateral (Lissauer's) tract long after avulsion. Taylor indeed produced instant and lasting relief of pain by excision of the cyst. The severe traction lesion of the brachial plexus brings about loss of all afferent input, disruption of the descending central inhibitory pathways, and damage to both dorsal and ventral horns. The neurophysiological sequelae of de-afferentation were described by Loeser and Ward (1967) and Anderson et al (1977), who showed that experimental deafferentation produced spontaneous firing in lamina. 1 and 5 of the posterior horn – the sites of relay of the nociceptor fibres. This spontaneous firing began a few days after the lesion, and gradually increased to reach a maximum at about 1 month. Two varieties of activity were observed: a continuous barrage, and superimposed paroxysmal bursts of high-frequency firing. Microelectrode recordings made from the deafferented cords of human subjects show paroxysmal discharges that coincided with the occurrence of painful flexor spasms. Albé-Fessard and Lombard (1983) showed experimentally that spontaneous firing found in the posterior horn after experimental section of the roots was gradually transmitted more rostrally. Some months after injury impulses could be detected in the thalamus. If transcutaneous stimulation was applied before and immediately after the lesion was inflicted, spontaneous firing could be reduced considerably. Rinaldi et al (1991) recorded electrical activity from single cells in the thalamus of 10 patients with chronic pain associated with deafferentation. One of their patients suffered a traction injury of the brachial plexus; lesions of peripheral nerves accounted for seven others, in two cases pain followed cerebral infarction or spinal cord injury.

They confirmed spontaneous activity in neurones in the VPL, but also showed, for the first time in humans, hyperactivity within the medial thalamus. They commented: "the findings of a dual representation of neuronal hyperactivity in the lateral and medial thalamus is perhaps not surprising in view of the fact that these are the two primary thalamic targets for the pain related relays from the spinal cord, carried by the neo spino thalamic and palaeo-spinothalamic systems".

With the present paucity of light or electron microscopic evidence about the state of the human cord and of its posterior horn in particular after "avulsion" it is still difficult to define the cause or to determine why some should have pain, why some should lose it and why some should have no pain at all. It may be that the occurrence of pain indicates true avulsion – that is, avulsion of material from the substance of the cord. In contrast, simple separation of the level of the transitional zone might not give rise to pain: on the other hand, the knowledge of spontaneous firing of neurones in the substantia gelatinosa and of the inhibitory impulses in the posterior columns makes attractive the theory of "deafferentation pain". Further observations on human subjects are required.

THE SYMPATHETIC NERVOUS SYSTEM AND PAIN

The sympathetic nervous system has been implicated in the onset and maintenance of many neuropathic pain states, so much that the terms *sympathetically maintained*, and *sympathetically independent*, pain have been used extensively in the literature of the last 10 years. Before introducing a classification of pain states that we find useful, it might now be useful to review some evidence. The endings of the sympathetic efferent fibres secrete noradrenaline. This increases the sensitivity of mechanoreceptors (or diminishes their threshold to stimulation), and it increases spontaneous activity in demyelinated or newly regenerating nerve fibres and in some neurones in the dorsal root ganglion. Probably there is a similar secondary effect on neurones in the dorsal horn. The net effect of this spontaneous activity is to increase the sensitivity of cells in the deeper laminae of the dorsal horn. These central changes may underly allodynia and hyperpathia.

There *may* be ambiguity about the phrase "sympathetic blockade": different people use the term "sympathetic block" indiscriminately for guanethidine infusion or injection of local anaesthetic into sympathetic ganglia, just as some people mean a "chemical sympathectomy" when they say "sympathectomy". We define our use of these terms as follows:

- Chemical blockade: regional infusion of guanethidine or equivalent agent; or systemic infusion of phentolamine or equivalent agent

- Ganglionic or stellate sympathetic block: injection of local anaesthetic into the ganglionic chain
- Sympathectomy: ganglionectomy or coagulation under vision
- Chemical sympathectomy: the injection of a destructive agent into sympathetic ganglia.

The placebo effect introduces further ambiguity in the interpretation of the effects of these interventions. Sympathectomy is perhaps the only true test of whether sympathectomy will succeed. Ganglionic block and stellate block are bound to have a true or false "placebo effect" – from systemic absorption, from the cuff, from spread of local anaesthetic or from the experience of having a needle stuck into the front of one's neck. It is not possible to control all these factors, and even a false guanethidine injection could produce a result from the tourniquet, or ganglionic block with saline could produce an effect from the act of injection. It is necessary, perhaps, to say what we mean by successful sympathetic block. It is the relief of pain together with the production of vaso-dilatation and anhidrosis in the painful limb.

The role of the sympathetic nerves has been recognised by surgeons for many years, from experience in treating causalgia from war wounds. Leriche (1916) relieved such pain by periarterial sympathectomy. Spurling (1930) relieved causalgia from a bullet wound of the brachial plexus by sympathetic ganglionectomy, a technique used by Adson and Brown (1929) for the treatment of "Raynaud's disease". The Special Committee of the Medical Research Council (MRC) defined causalgia in 1920:

- it is spontaneous
- it is hot or burning, intense and diffuse
- it is brought on by light, normally nonpainful stimulation of limb
- it often leads to great psychological distress.

The Second World War led to a closer definition of causalgia and establishment of its successful treatment by sympathectomy. Barnes, writing in the MRC Special Report No. 282 (1954), reserved the diagnosis of causalgia for pain after injury to a trunk nerve with the following characteristics:

- the pain is severe, spontaneous and persistent
- there is usually a burning quality
- the pain extends beyond the territory of the involved nerve
- the pain is invariably aggravated by physical and emotional stimuli.

Walters (1959) defined it as "tender, painful syndrome in the hands or feet which follows injury to the larger peripheral nerves. The part with the damaged sensory innervation develops intense, burning pains spontaneously. Burning pain is also evoked by surface stimuli, heat, dryness, noise, excitement, emotion or even the thought of being touched".

In his series of 48 cases, Barnes (1953) found that in the upper limb there was always a partial lesion of the lower trunk or the medial cord of the brachial plexus or of the median nerve. All these nerves have a large cutaneous sensory component. In the lower limb there was always a partial lesion of the medial part of the sciatic or tibial nerves. In all but two cases the lesion lay proximal to the knee or elbow. Without exception the cause was bomb or shell splinters or high-velocity missile. Twenty-seven of 31 complete sympathetic blocks brought complete relief, and in four more there was partial relief. There was one failure. Barnes elegantly disposed of the idea of sympathetic afferents by low spinal blocks in two cases, the somatic afferents for the lower limb were blocked but not the sympathetic outflow from ganglia L1 and L2. Pain was relieved in these two patients. He further found that pre-ganglionic sympathectomy was more reliable than post-ganglionic.

Richards (1967) reviewed data drawn from the Second World War on the centenary of the original publication of Weir Mitchell, Moorehouse and Keane. There were 377 cases of causalgia from 9781 peripheral nerve injuries, an incidence of 3.9%. In 83% the median or tibial or trunks of origin were damaged, and in most cases the damage was partial. In 88% the injury lay proximal to the knee or the elbow. Multiple nerve injuries were common. Vasomotor disturbance was usually seen, the part often being warmer. Most patients found relief by keeping the part wet. The onset was within 24 hours in over 50%, and within 7 days in over 80%. He made a significant observation: "It was a common experience of those working in nerve injury centres during World War Two to meet patients who gave a good history of causalgic pain which had subsided before the patient reached the centre." We have had similar experience with patients with incomplete injuries to the brachial plexus or sciatic nerves wounded during operation or diagnostic intervention. Sympathectomy was followed by excellent or good results in 89% of cases; the operation was successful even when performed years after injury, as in prisoners of war. Here is causalgia, uncommon rather than rare, a most severe neuropathic pain following swiftly on a partial injury of the lower trunk of the brachial plexus, the median or ulnar nerves, or the sciatic or tibial nerves. There is hyperpathia. Relief follows adequate sympathetic block, sympathectomy removes the pain, leaving the residual symptoms from the nerve injury itself (Fig. 15.5). Bonney (1973) and Sweet and Poletti (1985) stipulate that sympathetic block is diagnostic. The latter writers state: "if a successful sympathetic block does not stop or greatly lessen the pain it is, by definition of the term for many of us, not causalgia". Omer and Thomas (1972) described their experience with 77 cases of causalgia from the war in Vietnam. In 41 the nerves were injured in the

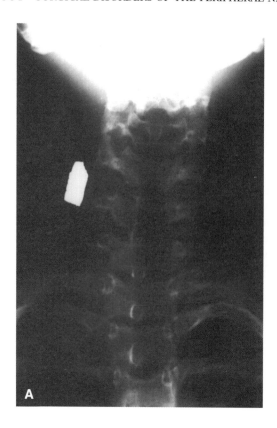

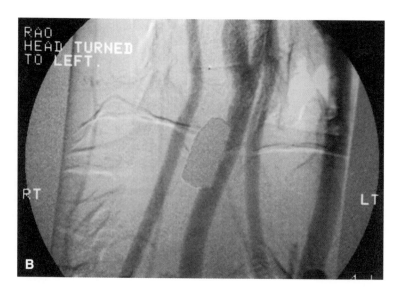

Fig. 15.5 Causalgia. The bullet had sectioned the seventh cervical nerve. Relief by sympathectomy and grafting of the nerve. (A) Radiograph shows bullet close to the cervical spine. (B) Angiograph shows the bullet's relation to the right carotid and vertebral arteries.

lower limb. The lesion was proximal to the knee or elbow in 61 cases, and in 16 it was distal. Onset of pain was immediate in 38 cases, and it had developed in 30 more by 3 weeks from injury. The initial treatment in these cases was by infusion of local anaesthetic close to the damaged nerve. If this was unsuccessful, central sympathetic blockade was introduced. These methods secured pain relief in 47% of cases. Surgical sympathectomy was reserved for the 41 cases where pain persisted, and it was successful in 34.

Sweet and Poletti (1985) reviewed published data on sympathectomy. In the upper limb the preganglionic operation is more effective than the postganglionic one, and it has the merit of avoiding a Bernard–Horner syndrome. The sympathectomy must be complete, and a number of cases are described where completion of sympathetic denervation at a second operation relieved the pain. Relief is lasting in most cases, but vigorous treatment is necessary to overcome disuse atrophy and deformity.

Search for the cause of this pain has stimulated many ideas. Ischaemia or blood flow abnormality were first in this field. In about one-quarter of published series there is an associated injury to the adjacent great artery. In some of our own cases causalgia appeared to be related to false aneurysm or arteriovenous fistula (see Chapter 8 for a description of these cases).

Artificial synapses between efferent sympathetic fibres and afferent somatic fibres were proposed by Doupe et al (1944) and Barnes (1954a). Nathan (1947) first supported

this in a study which proved that the pain was not caused by vascular stasis, vasodilation or vasoconstriction, or indeed by afferent sympathetic impulses. In his later work with Loh (1978), Nathan abandoned this view because pain is relieved not only by sympathectomy but also by guanethidine infusions distal to the lesion (Hannington-Kiff 1974). Guanethedine displaces noradrenaline at adrenergic nerve endings. Its repeated administration in high doses, in rats, may actually destroy them (Burnstock et al 1971). The idea of abnormal sensitivity to noradrenaline was produced, and its place in causalgia was described by Torebjörk and Hallin (1979a,b) in a series of observations in patients cured of causalgia by sympathectomy, and in one further patient whose pain later recurred. In the patient with recurrence of pain, intracutaneous injection of noradrenaline lowered the threshold to heat and cold stimuli, producing very severe pain. This was blocked by topical local anaesthesia. Microneurography showed abnormal activity in both A- and C-fibres. In patients whose pain was relieved by sympathectomy there was a remarkable reduction in pain thresholds to cold and mechanical stimuli after intracutaneous injection of noradrenaline. When a suprasystolic cuff was applied to the limb, sensitivity disappeared with the abolition of touch and cold sensation from ischaemia.

Schott (1994) has raised again the question of conveyance of pain impulses in "visceral afferent" fibres. He returns to Langley's (1903) concept of a single sensory system, which comprises afferents that travel within both somatic and autonomic nerves. He includes "visceral afferents," that is, those fibres conveying impulses from peripheral structures, especially blood vessels, as well as those conveying impulses from the cervicothoracic and abdominal viscera. Schott cites in particular the observation by Walker and Nulson (1948) that stimulation of the upper thoracic part of the sympathetic chain produced pain in the arm and the hand in the 3 patients of 10 whose sympathectomy was done for causalgia. These observers attached electrodes to the chain and led the connection out of the wound so that stimulation could be done after the effects of anaesthesia had worn off. Schott cites too the painful state that often enough arises after sympathectomy, and after lumbar sympathectomy in particular. After a wide-ranging, indeed exhaustive, examination of the evidence, he proposes that "damage to previously normal visceral afferents can generate pain but perhaps also cause allodynia", and that "visceral afferents are usually clinically silent, and generally only subserve pain when damaged". Schott's arguments are, at least, persuasive. It is perhaps unfortunate that with today's supposedly higher ethical standards and certainly stricter controls on the activities of surgeons, proceedings such as those of Walker and Nulson (1948) would, in this country, be received with so much disfavour as to oblige the observers to cease the practice of medicine. Kramis et al (1996) pursue the possible role for visceral afferents further. They discuss postsympathectomy pain, and they say that the syndrome occurs in 30–50% of cases. It is rare after sympathectomy for nonpainful states and the pain is different in its nature and in its distribution from that which provoked the operation. They suggest that postsympathetic neuralgia is a deafferentation and reafferentation complex. Paraspinal somatic and visceral afferent fibres are cut and many of the cell bodies of these fibres die, leading to a state of central deafferentation. A state of deafferentation hyperexcitability is now superimposed on the persistent sensitisation of central spinal nociceptor neurones by the painful condition that existed before the sympathectomy. These important and interesting observations need not necessarily surprise us. After all, the pain from a damaged somatic nerve is usually only temporarily relieved by proximal section of that trunk. The cell bodies of sympathetic fibres are no more immune to effects of permanent axonotomy than are somatic neurones; as Lisney (1989), Ygge (1989) and Melville et al (1989) have shown, a significant proportion of the neurones of C-fibre afferents die after axonotomy. One of us saw frequent cases of pain after sympathectomy for such nonpainful states as the circulatory disturbance of poliomyelitis. Anand (1986), who studied the matter closely, pointed out that postsympathectomy pain was usually transient, and continued to the border zone of the sympathectomised skin.

"Reflex sympathetic dystrophy"

The net of sympathetic involvement has been thrown far wider by the term "reflex sympathetic dystrophy", which embraces numerous others, among them being Sudek's atrophy, minor causalgia and sympathetic algodystrophy. This is very different from causalgia in that partial injury to a major nerve is not seen. The "diagnosis", if such a term is appropriate, is usually made when there has been no wounding of a nerve at all. A particularly significant study was that by Loh and Nathan (1978) in 45 patients with chronic neuropathic pain in the face, trunk and the upper and lower limbs. Peripheral nerves were damaged by partial section, compression, amputation or herpes zoster in 23. Lasting relief of pain followed sympathetic block in 11. There was success in some cases where the lesion lay within the central nervous system. Nathan and Loh emphasised the significance of hyperpathia in which blocks were likely to succeed and which were likely to fail in its absence. Clinical evidence of disturbance of the sympathetic function was not an indication for success or failure.

They proposed that these pain states were brought about by abnormal firing of peripheral nerve fibres – in particular the mechanoreceptors – which alter the behaviour of neurones in the substantia gelatinosa and lamina 5, either by diminishing their inhibition, by facilitating their activity, or by both. "Thus, stopping the emission of the normal sympathetic transmitter stops the firing of peripheral nerve fibres and that stops the abnormal function within the central nervous system. The abnormal state is kept going by mechanoreceptors and the large afferent fibres. The sympathetic outflow is acting on these fibres or receptors to cause the input to the spinal cord which causes a state of disinhibition or facilitation spreading from the original site of input."

This idea was extended by Roberts (1986) who suggested the term *sympathetically maintained pain* (SMP) for conditions responding to sympathetic block, to include causalgia and reflex sympathetic dystrophy. This term could be extended to conditions without nerve injury or dystrophic tissues. In order to define the neural mechanisms of this pain he elaborated an hypothesis that depended on two assumptions:

- that a high rate of firing in multireceptive neurones in the cord results in painful sensations
- that nociceptor responses associated with trauma can produce long-term sensitisation of such neurones.

Activity in low-threshold myelinated fibres from mechanoreceptors resulted from sympathetic efferent activity on the receptors or, when there had been nerve injury, on the neuroma. Removal of the efferent activity would relieve pain. The concept of sympathetically independent pain was later introduced for those conditions that did not respond to sympathetic block. Wahren et al (1991) went further in this matter. They studied patients with chronic pain after nerve injury, measuring the changes in various modalities of sensation before and after treatment with regional guanethidine blocks. They found, in the patients whose pain was relieved by the blocks, that the sensory impairment and allodynia were reduced, whereas in those who did not benefit from the block there was no such improvement. Roberts' work has indicated an abnormal central sensitisation as "the crucial element": it follows that "the emphasis in the acute phase should be to prevent or minimise the sensitisation of spinal neurones by reducing the nociceptor input"; or in other words, to treat the patent with a degree of urgency.

This proposal has the advantages of simplicity, and it provides a rational explanation for many of the clinical features of causalgia and reflex sympathetic dystrophy and their response to treatment. It has had considerable influence, but evidence from some recent studies is contradictory. Treede et al (1992) investigated sensory and vasomotor effects following diagnostic sympathetic ganglion blocks in 24 patients suffering from chronic pain. Overt lesions of peripheral nerves were noted in seven. Pain relief was significant in nine patients, four of whom had peripheral nerve injuries. This relief did not correlate with the extent of change in skin temperature or blood flow, and in some it preceded cutaneous vasodilation. In those patients with pain relief even vigorous stimulation of the skin did not "rekindle" hyperalgesia. The authors concluded that: cutaneous hyperalgesia could rapidly be reversed by a sympathetic block, even when it was of long-standing; that there was no clear correlation between pain relief and the extent of sympathetic blockade; and that maintained nociceptor activity must contribute to central sensitisation. Some of these conclusions were confirmed by Dellemijn et al (1994), who studied 24 patients with presumed sympathetic mediated pain in the upper limb. None of these had identified peripheral nerve injuries. They found no clear relation between the clinical features and the response to the block, nor did they find close correlation between pain relief and the degree of the sympathetic block. Pain relief followed stellate ganglion block more frequently than it did phentolamine infusion. Spread of local anaesthetic to the somatic fibres within the brachial plexus is a likely explanation for this. Unease about a simple classification of pain states arising from diverse injuries is heightened by two recently published long-term studies of patients with sympathetic mediated pain. Torebjörk et al (1995) examined the effect of topical application of noradrenaline into the sensitive skin of 25 patients whose neuropathic pain had been relieved by sympathetic block. Pain and hyperalgesia was aggravated in only seven. Differential nerve blocks using a supra-systolic cuff suggested that noradrenaline induced ongoing pain and heat algesia through C-fibres and that cold evoked and touch pain passed through myelinated afferents. Twelve patients were followed for a minimum of 12 years; of these, nine had responded favourably to sympathetic block at their first presentation. When they were seen later, only three of these showed a similar response. Some with earlier noradrenaline hypersensitivity had lost it at the later study. A similar change from initial favourable response to sympathetic block to no response was noted by Wahren et al (1995), who followed seven patients with neuropathic pain in the hand from nerve injuries in the arm over an interval of 10 years. Five had responded to the first block, but when last seen only three did so.

Thomas and Ochoa (1993) urged caution in accepting an explanation of pain state apparently so simple and attractive. They pointed out that the disorders labelled as causalgia-reflex sympathetic dystrophy might be no more than a group of symptoms provoked by a wide range of causes, each demanding accurate diagnosis and treatment: "This classification apparently carries pathophysiological connotation in that it endorses or rejects a role for the sympathetic system in maintaining the pain. The term has been understandably welcomed by anaesthesiologists who are handed the privilege and responsibility of issuing a pathophysiological diagnosis that may condemn neurological patients to multiple diagnostic therapeutic blocks or to sympathectomy. While sympathetic events might well influence the abnormal sensory physiology in some of these patients, it is not scientifically rigorous to assume that the sympathetic nervous system has a pathogenic role in determining pain, on the weaknesses of the subjective response of a patient to a ritualistic medical intervention." To this severe caution is added the suggestion of Verdugo and Ochoa (1994) that pain relief in the absence of successful sympathetic block is in fact a placebo effect. Bonney (1973) suggested this some years ago, adding that, unfortunately, relief after successful block might also be a placebo effect!

Perhaps inevitably, dissatisfaction with the terms reflex sympathetic dystrophy and sympathetically maintained and sympathetically independent pain has led to a new classification proposed by Stanton Hicks et al (1995) and adopted by the International Association for the Study of Pain (IASP). These writers state, that "SMP can be associated with a number of disease and a positive response to a sympathetic block should neither be a factor in the nomenclature of the disease nor define the disease". New terms are proposed to replace the older ones of causalgia and reflex sympathetic dystrophy. They are:

- *Complex regional pain syndrome (CRPS) type 1 (reflex sympathetic dystrophy)*. The diagnostic criteria that must be satisfied include:

  – an initiating noxious event
  – spontaneous pain or allodynia, not necessarily

limited to the territory of a single peripheral nerve and disproportionate to the inciting event
- evidence at some time of vasomotor or sudomotor abnormality in the region of the pain.
- *CRPS type 2 (causalgia)*. The diagnostic criteria include:

  - the syndrome develops after a nerve injury
  - spontaneous pain or allodynia occurs not necessarily limited to the territory of the injured nerve
  - there has at some time been a vaso- or sudomotor abnormality.

The presence of other pathological states which would account for the pain and loss of function excludes the diagnosis.

Some of us have been concerned for a long time by the tendency to lump all patients with painful, swollen hands or feet within the "diagnosis" reflex sympathetic dystrophy, so consigning them to a pain clinic. We believe that the diagnosis is made far too often in fracture clinics. Many cases of pain, swelling and stiffness after a fracture or soft tissue injury are a reflection of inadequate treatment. However, we think that the IASP taxonomy is a retrograde step. It does not help us in any way towards analysis of the different states of pain that may follow injuries to peripheral nerves. The characteristics of causalgia are so clearly defined that it serves no useful purpose to abandon the use of the term. It does not seem rational entirely to discard all the evidence that has been assembled demonstrating the role of the sympathetic nerves on mechanoreceptors, on damaged or regenerating nerve fibres, or their parent neurones. Nor does it seem rational entirely to discard the evidence that has been assembled concerning the role of visceral afferents.

THE GATE THEORY

In 1965, Melzack and Wall proposed a theory of pain mechanisms which provoked a great deal of critical interest. Wall restated the theory in 1978 and again in 1983, embracing criticisms about the role of the substantia gelatinosa, the extent of presynaptic inhibition on nociceptor afferents in the dorsal horn, and the known fact of stimulus specificity of nerve fibres. It has been summarised in Wall (1978) (Fig. 15.6):

1. *Information about the presence of injury is transmitted to the central nervous system by peripheral nerves. Certain small diameter fibres (a-δ and C) respond only to injury, while others with lower thresholds increase their discharge frequency if the stimulus reaches noxious levels.*
2. *Cells in the spinal cord or the fifth nerve nucleus which are excited by these injury signals are also facilitated or inhibited by other nerve fibres which carry information about innocuous events.*

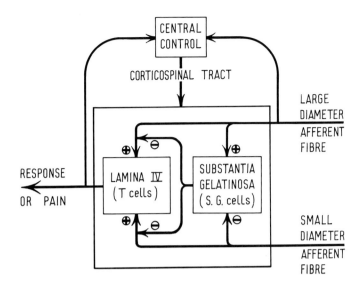

Fig. 15.6 The sensory "gate" mechanism as originally proposed by R. Melzack and P.D. Wall for the modus operandi of the dorsal laminae of grey matter of the spinal cord. See text for a discussion of the effects of an imbalance in the sensory inflow along the large and small diameter afferent fibres. (From an illustration in Melzack and Wall (1965), with permission of the authors and publishers.) (See also Plate section.)

3. *Descending control systems originating in the brain modulate the excitability of the cells which transmit information about injury*

Therefore the brain receives messages about injury by way of a gate control system which is influenced by:
1) injury signals; 2) other types of afferent impulse and 3) descending controls.

It is remarkable how many of the assumptions implicit in the gate theory have been proven since it was first proposed. Central descending inhibitory pathways exist, and presynaptic inhibitions of afferent fibres within the dorsal horn has been shown. Disinhibition of neurones within the dorsal horn following interruption of peripheral afferents is established. Their facilitation by increased input of nociceptors either from their terminals in sensitive skin or from regenerating sprouts within the neuroma has been demonstrated. There is experimental and clinical evidence which supports the notion that A-β mechanoreceptors do inhibit spontaneous activity within small fibres and diminish the sensitisation of central neurones.

Some success has followed the application of the principles underlying the gate theory in the treatment of patients. Two examples are particularly impressive. First is the successful application of transcutaneous nerve stimulation or implanted electrodes in the treatment of pain following some peripheral nerve lesions. Next is the dramatic improvement in pain that we have seen in many patients with severe traction lesions of the brachial plexus coincident with the return of muscular function. In most of these cases relief of pain preceded any significant cutaneous reinnervation.

It must be admitted that many aspects of neuropathic pain cannot be understood within the framework of the gate theory. The instantaneous onset of pain in some cases of causalgia or of traction lesion is one such difficulty. Indeed the pain of avulsion injury is more consistent with smashing the gate than lifting it. However, there is one central tenet that has been a source of constant encouragement for those treating patients with severe neuropathic pain. It is that the initial cause of the disturbance from injury to a peripheral nerve should be put right; and flowing from this that reasonable attempts must be made to restore afferent impulses to the spinal cord.

CLASSIFICATION

Injury to peripheral nerves is not always accompanied or followed by pain; most cases of complete division are painless. On the other hand, incomplete lesions are, from time to time, followed by or accompanied by pain of varying duration and severity. We have classed pain after nerve injury as follows:

1. *Causalgia* (CRPS type 2).
2. *Reflex sympathetic dystrophy* (CRPS type 1).
3. *Post-traumatic neuralgia*, which can be divided between that following major injury to a major nerve trunk and that following injury to a nerve of cutaneous sensation.
4. *Pain due to persistent compression, distortion or ischaemia.* We have called this pain neurostenalgia, (from στενος {stenos}, narrow, as in stenosis, added to νευρον {neuron} a nerve or tendon). It is agreeable that the verb στενω means to moan or groan, so that there is a dual reference to the idea of pain. This group undoubtedly contains many examples of Seddon's "irritative" lesions.
5. *Central pain.* This too can be divided between that following rupture of spinal nerves at the level of the transitional zone leading to pure deafferentation and that following avulsion of roots of a limb plexus from the spinal cord itself, a lesion which is truly an injury of the central nervous system.
6. *Pain maintained either deliberately or subconsciously by the patient* in response to a challenge such as the wish to obtain compensation, or resentment against a public body such as an insurance company, or other provocation.

CAUSALGIA

The clinical presentation of this, the most severe of neuropathic pain, is characteristic. There is a partial wound of the lower roots of the brachial plexus, or median and ulnar nerves, or proximal sciatic or tibial nerves. There is burning pain. There is obvious disturbance of skin colour and temperature and of sweating. Allodynia is intense: the patient cannot tolerate examination of the affected part. Often, the hand or foot is kept covered in moist wrappings. We have seen one patient who kept his foot in a bucket of water; another who wore an oversize waterproof glove which he kept filled with water. Pain is exacerbated by emotional stimuli. Analgesic drugs are rarely effective.

The following description is typical. One of our patients, a 23-year-old man, was shot in the arm by a bullet from a hand gun during a bank robbery. He was, in truth, an innocent bystander. He experienced immediate and intense searing pain in the arm, forearm, thumb, and index, middle and ring fingers. Nothing relieved this. We first saw him at 3 weeks. He was quiet, even withdrawn, answering questions in monosyllables. He had lost weight, and was exhausted from lack of sleep. The affected arm was held cradled against his body; he could not tolerate light touch or the pressure of contact from a sleeve. Light draught was intolerably painful. The hand itself was swollen, mottled with alternating red and blue discolouration. There was profuse sweating. The nails were coarse, the hair on the back of the hand had overgrown. This man found some relief from keeping the hand and forearm wrapped in a moist towel, onto which he frequently poured cool, but not cold, water (Fig. 15.7).

An injection of local anaesthetic into the cervical sympathetic chain brought relief within minutes, the relief coming seconds after his showing a Bernard–Horner sign, and a short while before vaso- and sudomotor paralysis

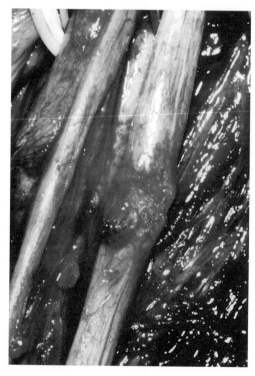

Fig. 15.7 The nerve lesion in causalgia. A 23-year-old, shot with hand gun in the axilla. The bullet partially severed the median nerve: the ulnar nerve was unscathed. Relief by sympathectomy.

appeared in the hand. Sympathectomy abolished burning pain and allodynia: this unmasked the deficit from the injury to the median nerve itself. This nerve was repaired by partial resection and grafting: two-thirds of it had been transected by the bullet. Pain relief was complete. At 3 years the patient noted only imperfect sensation in the thumb and index finger, but little else abnormal.

Notwithstanding uncertainties about the role of the sympathetic nervous system in pain states previously considered "sympathetically maintained" (see above), causalgia remains as clearly defined as the pain after pre-ganglionic injury of the brachial plexus. Diagnosis can be made from the history alone. There has been a wound to the proximal part of a limb. There has been partial damage to a major nerve trunk. There is spontaneous persistent pain, very often of a burning nature; pain is localised principally in the distribution of the nerve or nerves affected, but spreading beyond that distribution; pain is aggravated by physical and emotional stimuli; there is association of pain with hyperaesthesia and hyperalgesia of the skin in the distribution of the nerves affected; and there is association with disturbances of circulation and of sweating. Allodynia and hyperpathia are present. Some of our patients, with all these clinical features show variation in onset, course and response to treatment.

A 63-year-old woman sustained a deep incomplete sciatic neuropathy during operation for replacement of an osteoarthritic hip. The common peroneal division was worse affected. This was relatively painless for 3 weeks, when there was a sudden onset of intense burning pain in the leg and foot. This was followed, over the next 2 days, by discolouration of the skin, increased sweating and allodynia. Fresh deep vein thrombosis was excluded. Lumbar sympathetic block, with local anaesthetic, abolished the allodynia and sweating, but not the burning pain. The nerve was exposed 3 months later and there was a partial lesion at the level of the neck of the femur, where the nerve was tethered in a mass of scar tissue; there was intraneural fibrosis; some fascicles had been interrupted. An external neurolysis was done. A tissue catheter left in the wound permitted continuous infusion of local anaesthetic for several days. The burning pain disappeared. At 18 months pain relief was maintained. There was useful motor recovery.

In some other cases of ours, following gunshot injuries, it seemed as if causalgia became dominant with the development and expansion of false aneurysms or arteriovenous fistulae (see Chapter 8).

Spontaneous resolution of pain

Seddon noted this, and referred to Hirschmann's (1943) finding that remission occurred without treatment in one-half of cases. This seems to have occurred in 17 of our patients who sustained sciatic or femoral neuropathies during operations for hip arthroplasty, and in 18 others with wounds of the brachial plexus. These patients described severe burning pain, allodynia and vaso- and sudomotor disturbance which lasted several weeks to several months, but which resolved before we saw them.

Response to treatment

Information about the 26 cases we deem as suffering classical causalgia is set out in Tables 15.1 and 15.2. Missile injury, of one sort or another, was the cause in 21 cases. In nine, there was a major vascular injury. In 13 cases, operation was directed to the nerve lesion itself and to the associated vascular injury, and pain was relieved without recourse to sympathetic block or sympathectomy. It could be said that these patients did *not* have causalgia. It could be the case that our practice of infusing local anaesthetic about the nerves proximal to the lesion induced an element of sympathetic blockade.

Patients with causalgia should be treated urgently. The core of treatment is operative, directed towards diagnosis and rectification of the prime cause of the injured nerve and vessels. Sympathetic block is invaluable both in diagnosis and in treatment. Although the indications for formal sympathectomy seem less than before, a successful block does strengthen the case for operation.

The techniques of sympathetic block used are described below.

Sympathetic ganglionic block

The posterolateral approach formerly used has now fallen into desuetude, though it has been revived in a different form – that of providing an approach for electrocoagulation. It was certainly more difficult and more time-consuming than is the anterior approach, but it did give the opportunity for direct injection into the second and third thoracic ganglia.

With an anterior approach the object is to flood the stellate and upper thoracic ganglia with local anaesthetic introduced deep to the fascia over the anterior vertebral muscles. The patient is put into a semisedentary position and, under local anaesthetic, a needle is introduced above the sternoclavicular joint to pass posteriorly and slightly caudally between the carotid sheath and the laryngo-pharynx to touch the transverse process of the sixth cervical vertebra. It is best to do this with screening control so that the object can be the transverse process of the seventh vertebra, though in this case the risk of entering one of the vertebral vessels or puncturing the pleura is rather increased. However, the advantage is gained of a more direct injection into the ganglia concerned with the maintenance of the pain.

When the tip of the needle is in place, aspiration is done, in order to make as sure as possible that the point is

Table 15.1 Causalgia: response to direct treatment only

Age	Sex	Nerve level	Cause	Treatment	Outcome
18	F	Tibial – leg – posterior tibial aneurysm	Iatropathic (osteotomy)	Excision aneurysm (Prof. A Mansfield)	Pain relief. Nerve recovery
28	M	Medial cord	Rifle bullet	Graft medial cord	Pain relief. Little recovery
24	M	C5/C6/C7/C8	Rifle bullet	Graft C7/C8 Neurolysis C5/C6	Pain relief. Recovery C5/C6
49	M	Radial nerve – axilla	Rifle bullet	Graft radial nerve	Pain relief. Recovery
27	F	Median, ulnar, musculocutaneous nerves – axilla	Fragments	Graft of all three nerves	Pain relief. Recovery musculocutaneous median
37	M	C5/C6/C7	Shotgun	Graft C5/C6/C7	Pain relief. Recovery C5/C6
32	M	Median – axilla Arteriovenous fistula	Hand gun	Excision fistula. Graft median	Pain relief. Little recovery
21	M	C5 Arteriovenous fistula	Fragment	Embolisation fistula (Dr Al Khutoubi) Graft C5	Pain relief. Recovery
34	M	Lateral medial cords with axillary aneurysm	Rifle bullet	Excision aneurysm. Neurolysis	Pain relief. Recovery
34	M	Lateral medial cords axillary aneurysm	Hand gun	Excision aneurysm. Neurolysis	Pain relief. Recovery
16	M	Sciatic – buttock	Shotgun	Removal pellets	Pain relief. Recovery
21	F	Sciatic – thigh	Fragments	Removal fragments. Graft partial lesion	Pain relief. Recovery
31	M	Sciatic – thigh	Shotgun	Removal pellets	Pain relief. Recovery

Table 15.2 Causalgia: response to sympathetic block

Age	Sex	Nerve level	Cause	Response to sympathetic block	Response to sympathectomy	
23	M	Median – arm	Hand gun	Pain relief	Pain relief	
18	M	C7	Hand gun		Pain relief	
24	M	Medial cord	Shotgun	Pain relief	Pain relief	
31	M	Sciatic – thigh	Fragments	Pain relief	Pain relief	
34	M	Lateral cord – arteriovenous fistula	Shotgun	Pain relief	Pain relief	
43	M	Median – axilla – axillary artery rupture	Shotgun	Pain relief	Pain relief	
24	M	Upper and middle trunks. Retroclavicular subclavian aneurysm	Shotgun	Pain relief	Pain relief	
31	M	Median nerve, ulnar nerve – axilla	Fragment	No relief	Pain relief	
28	M	Sciatic – hip	Rifle bullet	Pain relief	Pain relief	
34	F	Median – arm Brachial aneurysm	Iatropathic	Pain relief		
55	F	Sciatic – hip	Cement burn	Partial relief	No relief	Partial relief from graft of tibial division
64	F	Sciatic – hip	Hip arthroplasty, retractor injury	Relief of allodynia		Neurolysis with tissue catheter. Relief of burning pain
68	F	Femoral – hip	Hip arthroplasty, crush injury	Relief lasting 5–7 days only	No relief	Neurolysis with tissue catheter. Transient relief

not in a vein or artery. Then, a measured amount of local anaesthetic (usually lignocaine or bupivacaine) is introduced. Ten millilitres should suffice: 0.5% or 1% in the case of lignocaine, and 0.25% in the case of bupivacaine. Very soon a Claude Bernard–Horner syndrome develops; later, the ipsilateral hand becomes warmer and ceases to sweat.

In a proportion of cases, pain and hyperalgesia diminish or disappear altogether, to return when the effects of the local anaesthetic have worn off. Such a reaction may indicate that the pain is sympathetically maintained, though it may almost as easily indicate a response to:

- having a long needle thrust into the front of the neck
- the local anaesthetic agent
- the bearing of the operator
- the preparation given by the operator to the patient
- the infiltration of the agent into the lower part of the brachial plexus
- all of the above factors.

It is always wise, before determining a course of action on the basis of the reaction to a single sympathetic block, to observe the effects of a similar injection with an inert agent. If the result of the true block is unequivocal, and if that of the "control" injection in the negative sense is unequivocal, adequate sympathectomy is very likely to give full and lasting relief. It is clear that if the effects of the block given as described are to be replicated exactly by operation, that operation must include removal of the stellate ganglion. If the production of a successful sympathetic block has no effect at all on the pain or hyperalgesia, it is very unlikely that sympathectomy will be lastingly effective. Carr and Todd (1991) describe a valuable extension of simple sympathetic block to continuous block. They introduced a catheter percutaneously by the anterior approach, and successfully relieved pain in 22 of 29 patients diagnosed as suffering from reflex sympathetic dystrophy following fractures or tunnel release, crush injury and other causes. This technique was first described by Linson et al (1983), who had been impressed by the results of continuous marcaine blocks of paravertebral sympathetic chain used in 100 cases by Betcher et al (1953).

Complications

To the hazard of entering a major vein or artery and of the associated risk of a large intravenous injection of lignocaine or bupivacaine are added those of production of pneumothorax and of infiltrating the brachial plexus. The former may be dangerous if the puncture of the lung stays open; the latter does no more than vitiate the result of the investigation. It is quite common for the recurrent laryngeal nerve to be affected temporarily by the local anaesthetic agent, but this is not of lasting significance. The hazard of entering the spinal canal can be avoided by the use of the screen, but anyone attempting this procedure in any case of traction injury to the brachial plexus must be aware that the needle may easily enter a pseudomeningocele (see Chapter 13).

Lumbar sympathetic block

Here, the anterior approach is not available. A posterolateral approach has to be used. A single needle may be used, on the principle of flooding the prevertebral space with local anaesthetic, but once one needle has been placed correctly, the introduction of others is easy. The patient lies on the side opposite to that of the pain. With control on the screen, the needle is advanced to touch the anterolateral aspect of the second lumbar vertebral body, and two others may then be placed at the third and the fourth levels. A small amount of contrast material may be introduced to confirm the correct placing, and a total of 20 ml of 1% lignocaine or 0.25% bupivacane is injected. "Successful" block is indicated by drying and warming of the skin of the ipsilateral foot. The first sign of vasomotor release is often dilation of the superficial veins.

The results and their interpretation are similar to those in the upper limb. It is fortunate in the case of the lumbar chain that the penalties attached to complete sympathetic denervation in the upper limb do not apply; all the lumbar ganglia can be removed on the one side without producing any unwanted effect. Also, the operation for sympathectomy is technically much easier than it is in the upper limb.

Complications

Accidental entry into the aorta or inferior vena cava may cause trouble from haematoma, but will rarely have any serious effect. It should be possible to avoid the kidney, and entry into the ureter seems to be very rare. Much more important complications are possible when neurolytic agents are used in order to produce "permanent" block: the chief of these is pain, produced either by action on sympathetic afferents or by injection of a somatic nerve. Rarely, but very seriously, a neurolytic agent introduced for the purpose of affecting the lumbar chain may affect the blood supply of the spinal cord and produce paraplegia.

Warning and preparation

The requirement to give adequate advice and warning and the requirement to avoid producing a "placebo effect" conflict in the case of diagnostic sympathetic block. For one thing, if the patient is told all that may occur and all that may go wrong, he or she may well, understandably, decline the investigation. Or, he or she may get the impression that the investigation proposed is purely therapeutic and so be inclined to lose pain and hyperalgesia. Or, the ghastly preparations for the deed may so daunt the patient that he or she will be inclined to say anything that will cut short the ordeal. In scarcely any other procedure is the need for tact and sympathy and empathy on the part of the operator and his or her assistants so great as it is in these procedures.

Guanethidine block

The present preferred method of guanethidine blockade is described. This procedure should be conducted in a room adequately equipped and staffed for resuscitation. A cuff is put round the affected limb well above the site of the pain, and is inflated to suprasystolic pressure. The pressure is maintained for 20 minutes. Once it has been inflated, guanethidine is injected into a vein as close as possible to the site of the pain. In the upper limb, 20 mg guanethidine in 20 ml saline is introduced; in the lower limb, 30 mg is given, with local anaesthetic to relieve the initial exacerbation of pain.

The pressure in the cuff is slowly released, while the patient's general condition is closely watched. There is often drowsiness. The local effect is one of flushing and warming. In a proportion of cases, pain and hyperalgesia will be relieved. Under these circumstances, the opportunity is taken to handle the previously sensitive limb and to require the patient to move and use it. Later, depending on the duration of the response, physiotherapy and occupational therapy are given.

The frequency of the blocks

In former days, we gave one block weekly in cases in which pain and hyperalgesia recurred after initial improvement. Now we give blocks on alternate days. We have indeed found that, even when the first block fails to produce improvement, repeated blocks may be effective. The present plan is to give six blocks on alternate days, in association with an intensive programme of rehabilitation, irrespective of the response to the first injection. If this regime is ineffective, we accept that the pain is not sympathetically maintained.

Hyperpathia

Much less satisfactory is the definition and treatment of patients whose pain has elements consistent with "sympathetic maintenance", or causalgia, following injury to nerves in the distal parts of the limbs. Girgis and Wynn Parry (1989) reported their experience with 78 such patients, treated for hyperpathia by serial guanethidine blockade. From 1979 to 1986 a total of 696 blocks were given. The total for each patient ranged from 4 to 39. All patients had transient relief of pain, presumably from ischaemia or cuff pressure. Thereafter there was, in successful blocks, pain relief lasting for some hours, an interval which tended to increase with further blocks. In other cases there was no relief at all. The nerves injured, and the causes of injury and the results of treatment, are set out in Table 15.3. An excellent result is reserved for complete abolition of pain. In 7 of 23 cases there was recurrence of pain at between 6 and 12 months from discharge, which required readmission and further treatment. Girgis and Wynn Parry emphasise the discipline of this treatment, which was given on an in-patient basis. Injections were given two or three times a week. Intensive physiotherapy was given with the aim of improving stiffness, swelling and skin sensitivity. Occupational therapy was used to enhance function, and to help patients learn techniques of adaptation whilst continuing to use the hand. Simple protective splints were, on occasion, useful. Three groups of patients did

Table 15.3 Effect of serial guanethidine blocks for hyperpathia (Wynn Parry and Gergis)

Site of lesion	Cause	No.	Total	Excellent	Partial relief	No relief
Median nerve at the wrist	Wound or fracture	12	25	9	10	6
	Iatropathic	13				
Palmar cutaneous nerve	Crush	20	21	8	11	2
	Iatropathic	1				
Ulnar nerve at the elbow	Tumour	1	12	2	0	10
	iatropathic	11				
Foot	Sprain	1	8	1	0	7
	Iatropathic	7				
Ulnar nerve at the wrist	Wounds	3	3	3	0	0
Knee	Wounds	2	3	0	3	0
	Iatropathic	1				
Superficial radial nerve at the wrist	Iatropathic	2	2	0	0	2
Postganglionic lesions of the brachial plexus	Traction	2	2	0	2	0
Post herpetic neuralgia	–	2	2	0	2	0

particularly badly: those with pain following operations to decompress or transpose the ulnar nerve at the elbow; those with iatropathic injury to the superficial radial nerve; and those with pain from damaged nerves of sensation to the foot. Our later experience confirms that those patients whose pain follows iatropathic injury to the ulnar nerve at the elbow and the superficial radial nerve at the wrist present quite exceptional difficulty in treatment.

REFLEX SYMPATHETIC DYSTROPHY

Reflex sympathetic dystrophy (RSD; CRPS type 1) is a strange disorder, which has at other times been called sympathetic algodystrophy, shoulder–hand syndrome and Sudek's atrophy, among other terms. There is usually an injury in which no major nerve trunk is damaged. This is followed by spontaneous pain, which spreads, and there is allodynia. There is vaso- and sudomotor disturbance, excess sweating, oedema, discolouration of skin and, later, changes in the nails and hair, with stiffness of the joints. The most common presentation to orthopaedic surgeons is after fractures or other injuries to the hand or foot, but the syndrome also presents after injuries or operations at the shoulder, elbow and knee. The initial stage is characteristic. The pain is diffuse and disturbs sleep. The hand is swollen and stiff. It is often wet and warm; it may be cold and blue. If untreated, fibrosis follows and the hand becomes a useless stiff appendage. We have seen cases where the pain and allodynia resolved spontaneously and we were faced with a very difficult problem of restoring function. Bonica (1990) described the progress of severe cases in three stages. First, the acute stage, is characterised by pain, oedema and warmth. The next stage, the dystrophic, is characterised by cold skin with trophic changes. Lastly, there is the atrophic stage, when the part is wasted and the joints fixed in deformity. We have seen patients coming to us in the last stage, and it is usual for them to describe a progression through the others. The atrophic stage represents the unrecognised or untreated case.

Trophic changes are interesting and significant, but indicate that earlier and more easily treated stages have passed. Nails become brittle and deformed, there is increased hair growth and the skin becomes atrophied and glossy. It is often dry and scaly. It is not unusual to see thickening of the palmar or plantar fascia reminiscent of Dupuytren's contracture.

In 1902, Sudek described periarticular osteoporosis but his radiological change is not seen in the acute phase. A three-phase bone scan detects diffuse uptake of tracer in periarticular tissues much earlier (Kozin et al 1981). Two recent reviews repay study. The first, from Baron et al (1996), described experience with 238 patients seen in Freiburg and Kiel. These writers found an age range from youth to old age, with a peak at 50 years, and a predominance of females over males. In all their cases there was some form of injury to a distal part of a limb, and this was most commonly a fracture, sprain or operation. The upper limb was involved more than the lower in a ratio of 2:1. Symptoms were apparently disproportionate to the cause, and they reflected disturbance of autonomic, sensory and motor function, which were not confined to the territory of one nerve. In all these patients there was spontaneous diffuse deep pain with allodynia and hyperpathia, which was often worst in the fingertips. Two groups of patients were recognised: warm patients and cold patients. There was measurable temperature difference between the injured and the noninjured sides. Similar differences in sweating and swelling were noted. Power was diminished in 90% of cases. Tremor was found in 50%, and there were trophic changes in 30%. Pain was made worse by activity and by environmental temperature change.

Low et al (1996) have studied over 500 cases. Patients ranged in age from 9 to 78 years; 67% were female. There had been a precipitating injury in 79%. Detailed measurements of skin blood flow, sweating and skin temperature were made in some of these patients. Detectable abnormality in skin blood flow was found in less than 50%; the incidence of alterations in skin temperature was higher. The sweat output at rest was measured (RSO) and a quantitative sudomotor axon reflex test (QSART) was developed. A prospective study of 102 patients led to a close definition of the diagnostic criteria and a prediction of response to sympathetic block. Clinical diagnosis rests on the presence of allodynia and swelling, with vasomotor abnormality supported by detectable unilateral changes in QSART, RSO and skin blood flow. Diagnosis is definite in the presence of allodynia to touch, pressure of movement and asymmetry of QSART or RSO. It is in these patients that sympathetic blockade has a high chance of success, and the best clinical indicators for successful sympathetic blockade included the presence of allodynia, severe pain and a duration of symptoms of less than 6 months. The term "complex regional pain syndrome" is preferable to "reflex sympathetic dystrophy", because it does not imply sympathetic dependence; however, it remains deeply unsatisfactory because of the suggestion that there is no nerve injury. In fact, there almost always is, either from compression or ischaemia of the trunk nerves, such as the median or tibial, from fracture haematoma, or direct injury to those nerves or to their terminal branches by displaced bone fragments, foreign bodies or wounds. We have seen many cases termed RSD where the trigger was an injury to the infrapatellar branch of the long saphenous nerve or to twigs of the medial cutaneous nerve of forearm or superficial radial nerve. Some of these cases are better considered as falling within the post-traumatic neuralgia group.

The great majority of cases in orthopaedic practice can be prevented by early treatment, and this calls for alertness in detection of the early stages of the syndrome. It is an error to label every painful, stiff and swollen hand presenting in a fracture clinic as RSD or CRPS type 1. More often these are examples of inadequate primary treatment. Some publications suggest Colles fracture is complicated by RSD in as many as 30% of cases. One might reasonably question the method of treatment used in these studies and contrast that with the rarity of RSD as a complication of Colles fractures treated by the regime proposed by Valentine Ellis and continued by John Crawford Adams, which was followed for a number of years in the fracture clinics at St Mary's Hospital. Adams emphasised that the fracture of the wrist must be well reduced and that it should be immobilised in a splint or slab, not a complete plaster, for the first week. The patient attended daily for the first 7 days after injury for rebandaging of the splint. This ensured that the splint was still holding the reduction as the swelling diminished. At every attendance the patient was taken through an exercise regime, to maintain a full range of movement of the shoulder, the elbow, and the fingers and thumb, with some vigour. In those patients with increasing pain or swelling more vigorous steps were taken. The key elements of Adams' policy include: accurate reduction, holding that reduction and, above all, early functional use, which prevents swelling.

We are forced to the conclusion that too many cases of this disorder are a reflection of lax medical care. In most early cases a cause will be found by those who look: the splint or bandage which is too tight; a limb improperly supported in a sling; a patient who is too frightened to keep the part elevated and in function. The surgeon should be alert for an underlying lesion of compression or irritation of a trunk nerve, either from swelling from a displaced bone fragment. The mainstay of treatment is use of the part.

POST-TRAUMATIC NEURALGIA

Post-traumatic neuralgia (PTN) is pain after nerve injury which is not sympathetically maintained. Writing of such patients, Seddon came to "an aspect of peripheral nerve injuries that is profoundly unsatisfactory: the painful syndromes lacking the distinctive features of causalgia". We are still there: even when the cases of central pain from traction injury to the brachial plexus and those of obvious continuing irritation are taken out, there remain patients with pain, hyperaesthesia, hyperalgesia, and even hyperpathia and allodynia that are resistant to all forms of treatment. The number and proportion of such cases is probably less than was found by Seddon: the introduction of sympathetic release by sympathetic guanethidine block (Hannington-Kiff 1977, 1979) brought into the "sympathetically maintained" group a number of patients who would in Seddon's day have been excluded.

PTN after injury to minor nerves (Table 15.4)

It is most common after injury to rather minor sensory (cutaneous) nerves, such as the superficial radial at the wrist, the medial cutaneous nerve of the forearm at the elbow, or the palmar branch of the median nerve at the wrist. Here too there is spontaneous pain with hyperalgesia and hyperaesthesia, even with allodynia and hyperpathia. However, the symptoms are not relieved by a sympathectomy; the condition is not "sympathetically maintained". Many have sought a cause: it was perhaps the work of Melzack and Wall (1965) and Wall (1978, 1985) in developing the gate theory of pain that did most to clarify matters, though it must be said that mechanism is still ill understood. The only method of treatment with

Table 15.4 Painful neuromas of cutaneous (sensory) nerves*

Nerve	Number	Neurolysis	Repair	Resection	Other
Upper limb					
Supraclavicular	5		2	3	
Medial cutaneous forearm	43	12	16	18	3
Superficial radial nerve	112	14	72	22	4
Palmar digital	183	18	128	23	14
Palmar median	11		1	5	5
Lateral cutaneous forearm	6	2	2	2	
Dorsal cutaneous ulnar	7	2	4	1	
Intercosto brachial	3		2	1	
Lower limb					
Lateral cutaneous thigh	4		1	3	
Sural	28	9	12	5	3
Long saphenous	14	2	4	8	
Infrapatellar terminal branches	14	7	5	2	
Plantar cutaneous	23	2	16	5	

* Operations have been performed in over 300 cases.

any hope of success is the restoration of a normal input of nonpainful impulses; this normally involves successful repair of the affected nerve or nerves. It is these cases that produce the most difficulty in treatment. It is a salutary reflection that many of these injuries were caused by surgeons and doctors in the course of treatment. In some patients the persistence of the symptoms may with certainty be related to the hope of securing compensation. The person whose livelihood has been removed by an injury is quite reasonably anxious to seek compensation from the person by whose fault that injury has been caused. The delays imposed on the process by insurance companies concerned for the interest of their shareholders or directors certainly confirm in many patients the determination to procure redress. The adversarial system used in British courts further increases the incentive to overstatement of the case: a litigant, who in a weak moment admits to even partial improvement, is likely to find him- or herself with very little at the end of the day.

We agree with Herndon and Hess (1991) that repair, if possible, is the best treatment. However, many forms of treatment have been described. They fall into one of four groups:

1. *The prevention of a neuroma.* Although ligation, or injection of sclerosants (Smith & Gomez 1970) have been shown to be successful, it is of course impossible to prevent nerve regeneration unless the parent neurone is dead. Langley and Anderson (1904) may have approached a state of inhibition of regeneration in their proposal to suture one nerve trunk to another. Kon and Bloen (1987) applied this to palmar digital nerves by suturing one to another, or, when the injury was unilateral, suturing the dorsal to palmar branches.

2. *Containment of neuroma.* The nerve end is secluded by epineurial flaps (Martini & Fromm 1989) or by silicone rubber caps (Swanson et al 1977). Good results are reported in about 80% of cases, but the abnormal neurophysiological activity within the neuroma is in no way altered.

3. *Translocation.* The nerve stump is passed into bone (Mass et al 1984), muscle (Laborde et al 1982, Dellon & MacKinnon 1986), or away from pressure-bearing skin (Herndon et al 1976). Reported results are good, and these techniques are useful when no repair is possible, as after amputations. However, the abnormal activity within the nerve persists.

4. *Repair.* This seems the most logical. A neuroma which is exquisitely tender to pressure or, by its tether onto scar tissue, is prone to traction, can cause disabling pain amenable to simple resection and relocation. However, when pain spreads beyond the territory of the nerve, with allodynia and even hyperpathia in adjacent skin, then the only possible way to rectify the situation is to restore volleys of afferent impulses from reinnervated skin, and so hope to reverse the changes described earlier in the dorsal horn; events predicted by the gate theory.

It is perhaps odd that transcutaneous stimulation is so rarely useful in these advanced cases, and that guanethidine infusion is only occasionally successful.

There are obstacles to repair, the most obvious being amputation, or an atrophied distal stump; there is too, the problem of injuring another nerve when the gap between healthy faces demands a graft.

We think that the idea of using the patient's own muscle as a graft is a most significant advance in treatment of these cases (Gattuso et al 1988, Glasby 1990). The freeze–thawed muscle graft (FTMG) provides a means of repairing nerves without damaging others. The technique is simple. The nerve stumps are prepared in the usual way. A segment of muscle, from an adjacent flexor carpi radialis or palmaris longus for example, is cut out, wrapped in aluminium foil, frozen in liquid nitrogen for 60 seconds, thawed in sterile water, cut to shape, and secured with sutures and fibrin clot glue.

Thomas et al (1994) described results in 50 cases of FTMG. Most of the patients had gone through prolonged courses of nonoperative treatment; some had previously undergone operations for repair or resection. Outcome was most successful for the repair of defects of 4 cm or less. Failures were usually seen when the gap was longer. Results seemed better in the upper limb than in the lower limb.

Occasionally a cutaneous neuroma goes unrecognised for years. The value of accurate diagnosis and of simple operation is exemplified by two of our patients whose treatment course included psychiatric referral. In both, the psychiatrist insisted that there must be some injury to a peripheral nerve!

Case report. A 34-year-old woman had severe pain in the left side of her face, neck, arm and chest for 8 years, after internal fixation of fracture of the clavicle. There was allodynia, but there was also a well-localised area of exquisite tenderness just above the scar of earlier incision. Movements of the neck brought on pain: the patient adopted a position of torticollis. At operation we displayed a neuroma of the supraclavicular nerve, 8 mm in diameter, which was tethered to the clavicle. The neuroma was excised and the stump was placed deep to the fat pad. Pain was abolished.

A second patient further illustrates the torment caused by tethering of a sensory neuroma.

Case report. A 43-year-old woman had a 7-year history of pain after laceration of her index finger. Any movement of the digit caused intolerable pain, and she kept all her fingers tightly flexed. The finger was amputated: there was a large digital neuroma stuck down to the scar over the proximal interphalangeal joint. Pain was relieved and useful function of the hand regained.

PTN after trunk nerve injury

Treatment of PTN following injury to nerves of cutaneous sensation remains unsatisfactory, and that following treatment for nonsympathetically maintained pain from injuries to trunk nerves even more so. We recognise some distinct groups.

The amputation neuroma

Prevention is the cure, and this is achieved by correct performance of the operation. Dederich (1963) described 560 cases of amputation of lower limbs using his myoplastic techniques. Many of these operations were revisions on painful stumps. His guiding principle was to restore normal physiological conditions within the stump, and pain-free function was achieved in nearly every case. His findings caused him to say: "in all cases stump pain, even those of causalgic character, have been eliminated. We attribute this to the attainment of normal muscular tension and we believe that many phantom sensations and pains are caused by cramped and retracted muscles". A painful amputation stump is, in all likelihood, a reflection of incorrect technique, an observation also made by London (1961) in his discussion of amputations in the hand.

The role of pre-emptive analgesia in preventing amputation pain has been described by Bach et al (1988), who reduced or eliminated phantom pain in patients enduring lower limb amputation for peripheral vascular disease by blockade of sympathetic outflow through epidural infusion before operation and continuing this for up to 72 hours. Wall (1988) commented that some experimental observations showed that the response to spinal cord neurones to intense stimuli could be prevented by these manoeuvres.

The pain of regeneration

It is usual for patients to experience dysaesthesia in the months or years after repair of the nerve, and some never progress beyond this. Most describe hyperalgesia, particularly to cold. However, crippling pain is rare after properly executed repair, and it is uncommon even after replantation of an amputated hand or forearm. Our own experience in treating these cases has been dismal. There were occasional cases of entrapment or tethering of the neuroma that have responded to neurolysis, but resection and regrafting of the previous repair when pain has been present for a year or more, as it usually has, fails with dismal regularity. It is unusual for these cases to respond to transcutaneous nerve stimulation or sympathetic blockade. A decisive course of sensory retraining and desensitisation sometimes does produce results, perhaps by a form of counter-irritation (Fig. 15.8).

A common feature of these cases is that the first nerve repair was not well performed and, in particular, there had been inadequate treatment of the associated soft tissues.

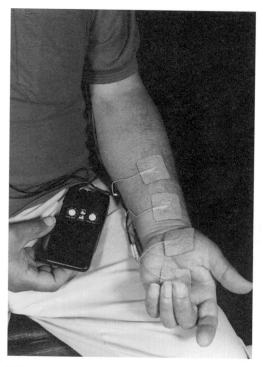

Fig. 15.8 Post-traumatic neuralgia in a 63-year-old man after damage to the median nerve. Relief was obtained, rather unexpectedly, by transcutaneous stimulation.

As we have indicated in the section on nerve repair, it does seem essential that tendons are secluded from the nerve, and repair of the synovium as a protective layer between these two structures is valuable.

Pain after operation for decompression of the median and ulnar nerves

This is a particularly unsatisfactory condition. Operation is necessary to establish diagnosis, and in the hope, often vain, that there is a remediable cause. We have already touched on the iatropathic lesion causing pain, such as damage to palmar cutaneous nerve or medial cutaneous nerve of forearm, or even to the trunk nerves themselves. Lax postoperative care, failure to insist on active movements, and failure to prevent swelling provoke reflex sympathetic dystrophy. Van der Molen (1996) has reviewed 22 of our cases of revision operations for ulnar neuropathy. The indication for our operation was pain. We found a number of obvious technical errors, chiefly relating to inadequate decompression, failure to remove causes of entrapment and redisplacement of the nerve, but the most common finding was of a nerve trunk tightly tethered in fibrous tissue. We could do no more than repeat the neurolysis, transferring the nerve to lie in unscarred fat and encourage early movement of the joints. An indwelling catheter, for infusion of local anaesthetic for 2–3 days was usually placed. Significant pain relief was achieved in 10 patients, the condition of 10 was unchanged, and 2 were made worse.

Pain from iatropathic lesion of the nerves at the hip

This growing problem warrants separate discussion. As we have seen, prompt attention to the cause of the lesion offers the best chance of pain relief. However, we found that in over half of our cases significant pain persisted, particularly when the nerve was re-explored late. Intraneural haematoma or traction from elongation of the limb seemed particularly serious causes of intractable pain.

It seems to us many of these nerves become embedded in scar so that gliding is blocked. Any movement of adjacent joints causes a local traction upon the afflicted nerve trunk. Lundborg (1988d) describes the connective tissues of a peripheral nerve as forming sliding interphase zones. The external layer, the adventitia, is loose and it acts as conjunctiva to the epineurium, which can slide considerable distances within it. In addition, the fascicles can slide against the deep layers of the epineurium. Millesi et al (1990) extend this idea and argue persuasively for the preservation of this gliding apparatus.

NEUROSTENALGIA

It is with a sense of relief that we turn now to this group of pain states, some of which fell into Seddon's category of irritative lesions, for they respond so well to surgical intervention. Patients in this group, together with those suffering from true causalgia, are the most rewarding to treat by operation. Chronic compression or distortion or chronic ischaemia of the nerve will produce pain: we all are, or should be, familiar with the history of the first Lord Nelson, who suffered constant "stump" pain after the amputation of his right upper limb through the arm. Years afterwards, the pain was suddenly relieved when the ligature round the median nerve came loose and was discharged through the wound. We see pain of this sort in the chronic ischaemia of diabetes or atherosclerosis, or traumatic obstruction of a main vessel or in "compartment syndrome", when raised pressure within a fascial compartment prevents adequate perfusion of structures. It is a constant pain; in chronic ischaemia of arterial disease, oddly enough, it seems to come on when the limb is warm in bed and is relieved when the limb is hung out of bed. The treatment of this variety of pain is, of course, the relief of the constriction or compression of ischaemia causing it. Of course, when there has been ischaemia for long enough, there are irreversible changes in the nerve or nerves affected.

In most cases the nerve trunk is intact, the lesion is neurapraxia, prolonged conduction block or, at worst, axonotmesis. The nerve is in some way irritated, tethered,

compressed or ischaemic, and treatment of the cause relieves the pain. We shall consider some examples.

Foreign body

Case report. An 11-year-old boy fell through a plate-glass window. There was torrential bleeding. His life and limb were saved by a master of vascular surgery. After operation a radial and ulnar palsy was noted, but in addition there was excruciating pain on attempted abduction of the shoulder and extension of the elbow. This alert surgeon recognised the cause and asked one of us to deal with it. As predicted, at re-exploration 5 days later, a suture which had been used to stem the haemorrhage had passed through the sheath of the ulnar nerve. We removed this. There was immediate relief of pain and rapid recovery of the nerve.

In a number of cases of gunshot wounds removal of pellets embedded in the nerve trunks brought similar gratifying results (see p. 139).

Much less acceptable is the encirclement or entrapment of a nerve by a suture in the course of an elective operation. One case report from the many we have treated will suffice.

Case report. A 43-year-old woman went through operation for ligation of the short saphenous vein. This was complicated by intense pain and foot drop. There were several striking features in this case, the pain was intense and it was related to the posture of the leg. The patient could find comfort only by lying immobile with the knee and ankle flexed. Any attempt at stretching of the leg brought on agonising pain. The nerve was re-explored at 7 days from the first operation, and we found the common peroneal nerve encircled by a suture, which had reduced its diameter to about one-half of normal. The epineurial vessels in the distal trunk were empty. The suture was removed and, with the microscope, it was confirmed that the epineurium had not been breached. The suture had been passed around the nerve, not through it. The distal epineurial vessels rapidly filled up after removal of this suture. This patient was free of pain on awakening, and recovery of the nerve lesion followed the pattern of an axonotmesis and was complete in 12 months.

Pressure from callus or bone spike or entrapment in a joint

A particularly dramatic example of this was Case 2 from Birch and St Clair Strange (1990). The patient suffered severe pain with peroneal palsy after successful treatment of a fracture of the pelvis. Nearly 3 years after the first operation the sciatic nerve was exposed at the notch. Its lateral part was narrowed to a translucent web by callus, and the latter was removed. Pain was abolished; the nerve made a wholly unexpected recovery over the next 3 weeks. Pain from entrapment in a joint or fracture line is a regular feature of this lesion, and abolition of the pain by removing that cause of entrapment is the rule.

Case report. An 8-year-old girl suffered a severely displaced supracondylar fracture which was fixed internally. There was great swelling. A complete ulnar and median palsy were recorded. She was in great pain, and this was the indication for re-exploration. The median nerve was found wrapped around a spike of bone, and the ulnar nerve tightly compressed in the cubital tunnel. The nerve trunks were released. There was relief of pain within hours and early recovery of both nerve trunks.

Case report. An 83-year-old woman suffered displaced fracture of the proximal part of the humerus and developed very severe pain which required opiates. This pain was resistant to all forms of block. We exposed the median nerve, found it impaled on a spike of bone, and released it. Pain relief was complete, but there was only limited recovery for the nerve trunk.

Vascular disorders

Some of these have already been described. There are two varieties. In the first an expanding haematoma or false aneurysm stretches or envelops the nerve, which stops working. Pain is severe, and at times presents the features of causalgia. Prompt treatment of the vascular problems has brought pain relief in nearly every case. Pain, in the conscious patient, is of course the cardinal sign of ischaemia of limbs or compartment syndrome. Some of this pain arises from the receptors in the dying muscle, but much of it arises from compression and ischaemia of the nerve trunks. Relief of pain is the indication that surgical decompression has been done in time and has been performed adequately. We have already seen that relief of pain with improvement in sensation is usual after late treatment of Volkmann's contracture.

CENTRAL PAIN IN BRACHIAL PLEXUS INJURY

In 1911, Frazier and Skillern set out to perform dorsal rhizotomy in a patient, a physician, with intractable pain from closed traction lesion of the brachial plexus. They exposed the cervical cord by laminectomy and found the anterior and posterior rootlet of C6, C7 and C8 absent: "the roots evidently had been torn completely from the cord". The patient's description of the pain was characteristic: "the pain is continuous, it does not stop a minute either day or night. It is either burning or compressing ... In addition, there is, every few minutes, a jerking sensation similar to that obtained by touching ... a Leyden jar. It is like a zig-zag made in the sky by a stroke of lightning. The upper part of the arm is mostly free of pain; the lower part from a little above the elbow to the tips of the fingers, never." It is all here. The pain is severe, there are two parts to it (one constant, the other intermittent), and it is worst in the hand and forearm. Later work has confirmed that this description is diagnostic of the avulsion lesion, and that the severity of the pain is related to the extent of lesion.

The natural history has been described. Bonney (1959) followed 25 patients for at least 2 years; pain was worst in those with no recovery. Seddon (1975) referred to Yeoman's studies. Yeoman found that severe pain persisted in 32 of 46 cases of complete paralysis, and in 22 of 44 who had regained spontaneous elbow flexion. Wynn Parry has made detailed studies in several large series which describe the characteristics, the time of onset, and the relation between extent of neural injury and the effect, for better or worse, of such factors as cold, illness, psychological state and occupation. In 1980, he reported on 122 cases of avulsion of at least one spinal nerve. Of these 112 had severe pain. Cold, worry or current illness deepened the pain. Distraction, by work, play or conversation considerably improved the pain in most cases. Pain remained severe at 3 years or more in 48 cases, while it had spontaneously abated in 28. Fifteen of those who obtained spontaneous improvement noted it within 12 months of injury, a further 11 between 12 and 36 months after injury. Wynn Parry (1989) later followed 404 patients with known avulsion lesions over periods of 3–35 years in order to clarify the natural history of the condition. In just over one-half, the patient's pain subsided over 3 years; in one-third the pain lasted for more than 3 years, but after that time was accepted and did not interfere with daily life. In 20%, however, severe pain persisted unchanged for many years and continued seriously to affect the lives of sufferers. In only 1% was there no pain at all. The first thoracic nerve was avulsed in every patient with severe pain persisting for more than 3 years: the whole plexus was also damaged in 48% of these.

Treatment by methods short of operation

Distraction

The first and best method is to create distraction, by appropriate rehabilitation designed to bring the patient back as soon as possible to work and recreation. We have had some success in this.

Transcutaneous stimulation

The second most valuable method is by transcutaneous stimulation. The basis of this is to increase input to the posterior column, and thereby to promote *inhibitory* impulses inhibiting rostral transmission of impulses from the dorsal horn. It will not do simply to give the patient a stimulator and tell him or her to get on with it. All our patients are admitted to the rehabilitation ward and a pain history is taken and a diary recorded. Various positions of the stimulator and variations of frequencies, duration and amplitude of pulse are tried. Patients are encouraged to wear the stimulator for many hours a day and for at least 2 weeks. The effect of use on daily activity, drug intake and subjective feelings are all recorded.

There seems to be no relation between the duration of symptoms and the effectiveness of the stimulator. An extreme case is that of the patient who had been in pain for some 50 years, whose pain was almost completely relieved by 2 days of treatment. There is no relation between the type of lesion and effectiveness. The particular advantage of transcutaneous stimulation is, of course, that it is noninvasive, simple, has no side-effects and is considerably cheaper than long-term treatment with drugs. Sindou and Keravel (1980) commented that nerve stimulation cannot work if the fibres of the dorsal columns are wholly degenerate; the technique can only work in postganglionic lesions or in cases where some of the fibres are preserved.

Drugs

The usual analgesics are virtually useless in avulsion pain. Very occasionally some relief is given by coproxamol or codeine derivatives. Controlled drugs such as morphine and the synthetic opiates have little effect on this pain, so it is, in our experience, rare to find addicts among these patients. On the other hand, Nashold and Ostdahl (1979), commenting on 17 patients with pain after avulsion of the plexus, noted that addiction to narcotics played "a major role" in nearly half their cases. Carbamazepine, phenytoin and sodium valproate, known for their use in controlling seizures in epilepsy, are worth trying in patients in whom shooting pains predominate. Carbamazepine is given in doses rising to a daily intake of 0.8–1.2 g. It has fewer side-effects than phenytoin, but drowsiness may limit its use. Eighteen of our patients obtained from its use relief sufficient to justify taking it regularly. Antidepressants have a central action on pain by their effect on the serotonin mechanism. Triptafen (amitriptyline and perphenazine) has proved the most useful. It is important to make sure that the patient should not, finding that he or she is being given an antidepressant, come to feel that the clinician feels that his or her pain is imaginary. The rationale for giving an antidepressant should, whenever possible, be explained.

Much the most successful drug for controlling plexus pain is cannabis. Many patients have told of relief by smoking this substance. In former days, of course, cannabis was regularly prescribed for the relief of pain. It is unfortunate that its mild hallucinogenic effect, at present inseparable from its analgesic action, prevents its regular use. It is unfortunate too that increasing misuse of the drug led Parliament to legislate against it. At present, of course, it has no *approved* medicinal use; it cannot be prescribed by doctors, except under licence from the Home Secretary, and its use is illegal in the UK.

Amputation and sympathectomy

It is hardly necessary to say that amputation of the affected limb has no part in the treatment of central pain: the origin of the pain is not in the affected limb. However, this is not to say that amputation has no place in rehabilitation, it certainly does. Fletcher (1981) found that 90% of his 80 patients, who were of course very carefully selected, used their prostheses and 63% found them particularly useful. Most of his patients were back at work; one working on the training ship *Sir Winston Churchill* used his prosthesis to climb rigging. We have found that amputations ease pain, but this is usually the dragging pain of the paralysed shoulder, not deafferentation pain. Although Taylor (1962) reported relief of pain by cervicothoracic sympathectomy in one case of avulsion of the plexus, our early experience firmly suggests otherwise. In those days, sympathectomy, which was done by the anterior route, was a matter of serious difficulty in the face of the extensive scarring in the region of the plexus. We are not aware of any evidence about the value of sympathectomy in such cases by the much easier method of the endoscopic operation.

Relief of pain by reinnervation of the limb

The relation between pain and recovery of function following operative repair remains obscure, but there is increasing evidence that repair by graft or by nerve transfer is indeed useful, and it seems increasingly to be the most important treatment of all. Narakas (1981b) and Bonnard and Narakas (1985) have reported to this effect. The pain of ruptures was eased in 90% of cases. Of patients with avulsions, 17% continued with disturbing pain at 3 years or more from neurotisation, compared with 25% among those who had not been operated on.

Berman, Taggant et al (1995, 1996) have gone further. In the first, 116 patients with root avulsions were studied prospectively over 12 years. The diagnosis was established at operation. In 34% of cases the whole plexus was avulsed, in the remainder there was a mixture of pre- and postganglionic injury. In all cases repair by nerve transfer and, where possible, graft had been performed. All patients experienced pain and this was graded as follows:

- *Severe*: continuous disturbance of daily life, of work, of study and of sleep (visual analogue scale (VAS 0–10) 9–10)
- *Significant*: able to sleep but cannot work or study, not enjoy hobbies (VAS 7–8)
- *Moderate*: able to work, but pain sometimes so severe the patient has to take time off (VAS 4–6)
- *Mild*: patient is aware of pain but leads a normal life (VAS 0–3).

All patients experienced pain, and in 88% this was described as severe at some time during their course. Pain began within 24 hours of the injury in 62%: the mean time to onset was 13 days (range 0–180 days); pain was at its most intense at, on average, 6 months from injury. Paroxysmal pain was never experienced in the absence of constant pain, and the intensity of the pain was closely related to the extent of deafferentation of the spinal cords. It was exceptionally severe in cases of avulsion of C4 to T1. No close relation between the depth of pain and the extent of associated multiple injuries was evident. A measurable decrease in pain was noted at a mean time of > 6 months after operation. In 34% of cases pain remained moderate or severe at 3 years or more from that operation. It seems reasonable to compare this study with that of Wynn Parry (1980). All the patients attended the same institution, the Royal National Orthopaedic Hospital. Those seen before 1980 did not have nerve transfers. All of those studied by Berman did.

In 1984 a young woman with proven avulsion of C5 and C6 and C7 had intercostal nerve transfer to the musculo-cutaneous and lateral root of the median nerves with the aim of regaining elbow flexion and some protective sensation within the territory of the hand. Nine months after operation she regained elbow flexion and told us that her pain had disappeared at the same time. This experience prompted us to use the operation for treatment of intractable pain. As Nagano et al (1989b) pointed out, useful motor recovery cannot be expected when the operation is performed more than 1 year after injury. In 1996, Berman, Chen et al described the outcome in 19 patients in whom intercostal nerve transfers were performed more than 1 year from injury with the sole purpose of pain relief. Seven of these patients had avulsion of five roots; six had avulsion of four roots; four had avulsion of three roots; and two had avulsion of two roots. In five patients a limited repair by graft was possible in addition to the intercostal transfer. T3, T4 and T5 were transferred to the lateral cord or its derivative branches in 9 cases, and to the medial cord or its branches in 10 cases. The choice of the recipient nerve was made on the basis of the location of the pain in the hand and the extent of recovery from either nerve graft or intact roots. The results are startling and unexpected: 16 of 19 patients reported significant relief of pain at an average of 8 months after intercostal transfer. Before operation 18 patients had severe pain and 1 had significant pain; in 10 cases pain dropped from severe to mild, and in 6 more it reduced from severe to moderate. The time between the intercostal nerve transfer and pain relief ranged from 3 days to 3 years, the average being 8 months.

Case report. A 42-year-old male Sikh suffered closed traction lesion to the right brachial plexus with a rupture of the subclavian artery and avulsion of C6, C7, C8 and T1. There was functional recovery from C5 into the shoulder and elbow flexor muscles. This patient had severe pain radiating into the ulnar three fingers of the hand, with additional shooting pain radiating from the shoulder to the hand, lasting for about 2 minutes and occurring between 30 and 40 times a day. Sleep was disturbed, he gained no lasting relief from analgesic tablets or from transcutaneous nerve stimulation. Two intercostal nerves were transferred to the ulnar nerve 43 months after injury. By 3 weeks he reported his pain much improved and his sleep undisturbed. Pain had dropped from 8 to 4 on the VAS scale, the shooting pains disappeared within the first week, and at 6 months from operation pain was insignificant.

Berman outlined possible explanations for these results. There are two types of preganglionic injury. There is, first, an intradural rupture of the rootlets and the peripheral segment at or distal to the transitional zone; in more severe cases there is avulsion from the cord itself. The more serious injury is associated with the partial Brown–Séquard syndrome. The constant pain probably arises from disinhibition of neurones within the substantia gelatinosa, which fire spontaneously (Loeser et al 1968). The convulsive pain, which may respond to such anti-convulsants as phenytoin or carbamazepine, arises from sudden outbursts of ectopic electrical activity in the damaged part of the dorsal horn.

Transfer of healthy intercostal nerves into the trunk nerves of the upper limb inhibits this abnormal electrical activity. The rationale for the use of intercostal nerve transfer for the relief of pain is that it restores the input from the damaged limb, from receptors in muscle or skin. Such an explanation is, of course, untenable in cases in which pain is modified before any reinnervation could have occurred, as happened in the case we reported here. Indeed, it could in any case be argued that the input was there all along, from receptors of the skin of the chest and intercostal muscles. Further proposals were made about the relief of pain:

1. It may depend on cortical inhibition initiated by the sight of activity in the formerly paralysed limb. It is well known that distraction regularly relieves pain during the period in which it operates.
2. It may be a purely nonspecific effect of operation, depending on the anaesthetic, the postoperative pain and the use of analgesics, or on suggestion alone. Against this view is the fact that the operations of former days often produced transient relief of pain; never permanent alleviation.
3. Relief may be produced by sectioning of functioning (but disconnected) axons of the posterior root system, impulses from which have in some way been reaching the central nervous system.

Berman's final study (1995) goes some way towards answering these questions. Fifteen patients with avulsion injuries were followed. All had repairs, by graft, and by intra- or extraplexus transfers. Pain was measured at direct interview using the McGill pain questionnaire and a verbal 10-point pain score (Melzack 1975). Power was measured by the MRC system; cutaneous sensation was assessed for light touch and prick. Return of C-fibre function into the skin was measured by capsaicin-induced axon reflex and of sympathetic sudomotor fibres by nicotine-induced sweating. Intradermal injection of capsaicin is painful in normal skin, and it is remarkable that these patients submitted to the investigation on at least two occasions! The 15 patients were followed for 18 months, and in five of them there was significant improvement of pain at the last examination. Berman found that this pain relief coincided with, or was preceded by a few days, by the return of muscle power. There was slight relation to return of light touch, but no improvement of C-fibre function was found over the 8-month period of study. The correlation between pain relief, measured by the McGill system, and the return of function was highly significant and there was no such relation in those patients with poor or no recovery. Berman comments: "this decrease in pain appears to accompany or slightly precede the first sign of recovery of function. As the capsaicin-induced flares did not show any signs of recovery at the time of the last follow up, the reduction in pain scores appears to be associated with returning large fibre function rather than A-δ or C-fibre function". This is an important observation, and suggests a different mechanism for pain relief from that following late intercostal transfer.

Case report. A 23-year-old woman sustained rupture of C5 and C6 with avulsion of C7, C8 and T1. Repair was performed 48 hours after the accident and, by combining graft with intra- and extraplexual transfer using the spinal accessory nerve and intercostal nerve, all the major trunks of the upper limb were, at least partially, innervated. She had severe pain, which reached its peak at about 3 months from injury. A marked improvement in her pain was recorded at 14 months from injury; this diminution occurred over the course of a few days. Two weeks later palpable activity was detected in deltoid, biceps and triceps. There was, by this time, no detectable change in cutaneous innervation, and there was no measurable change in the capsaicin-induced flare or the nicotine-induced axon reflex sweating.

This is all very encouraging, but there are, sadly, a number of patients in whom it is impossible to reinnervate the limb either by graft or by transfer. These are patients with complete avulsion in whom there is associated damage to the spinal cord, and who show the signs of partial Brown–Séquard syndrome. Their pain is truly central, it arises from damage to the central nervous system and it is both worse than and more intractable than deafferentation pain. We should now review the case for central interventions, either of destructive lesions in the spinal cord or implantation of central stimulators in the treatment of these patients.

Interventions on the spinal cord

The first serious attempts to relieve brachial plexus pain by operation arose from the identification of the cord as the site of origin of symptoms. The refinements of cordotomy introduced in this country by Lipton (1968) made that procedure far safer than it had formerly been. "Percutaneous" cordotomy became a standard treatment in cases of intractable pain in the terminal stages of malignant disease. It was tried in a few cases of plexus pain: the early results were good, but it soon became apparent that a procedure applicable in cases of terminal disease was inapplicable in the case of otherwise healthy young persons. There was recurrence of pain within a year. This disadvantage was additional to the theoretical one of intervening on the healthy side of a cord already damaged unilaterally.

With the increase of knowledge of inhibitor mechanisms, Shealy et al (1967) introduced posterior column stimulators in some cases. At that time, the advantages of this nondestructive method were widely canvassed. Later, fractures through movement of the implants and technical failure caused this method for a time to fall into disfavour. Recently, technical advances have again brought it to the fore. North et al (1991) promoted the idea of "multichannel" devices for the stimulation of the posterior columns; Watkins and Koeze (1993) gave an account of the present status of this method as used with the advantages of improved technology. Bennett and Tai (1994) found lasting and significant pain relief in their five cases of pain after traction lesions of the brachial plexus. These injuries had occurred between 5 and 16 years earlier. Electrodes were inserted under radiological control in the conscious patient, usually in the D6–D7 interspace and then advanced cranially to the lower cervical spinal cord. The stimulation pattern was adjusted according to the patient's experience (Fig. 15.9). Proposals for stimulating the natural production of enkephalins were canvassed by Richardson and Akill (1977). Using paraventricular electrodes they were able to locate the sites at which stimulation produced maximal secretion of these natural analgesics.

Sindou (1972) perfected an operation of selective posterior rhizotomy at the dorsal root entry zone (DREZ), by microsurgical technique, which rested on the topographical distribution of afferent fibres in the dorsal root injury zone. Small myelinated and unmyelinated fibres were found laterally, passing to the dorsal horn neurones; larger fibres, responsible for discriminative touch and proprioception concentrated medially, were found passing to the dorsal columns. Microsurgical lesion in the lateral part of DREZ achieves analgesia, and selective microcoagulation in the dorsal horn itself destroys hyperactive neurones responsible for deafferentation pain. The technique was extended for the treatment of plexus pain (Sindou and Daher 1988). The sum of experience with

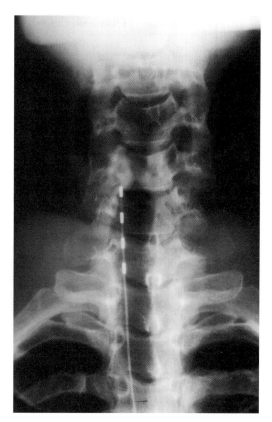
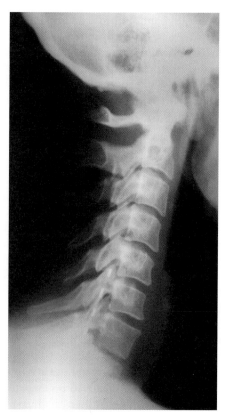

Fig. 15.9 A dorsal column stimulator lead in the cervical epidural space. The patient had suffered intractable pain for several years after brachial plexus injury. This was relieved. (Courtesy of Dr Michael Tai.)

this technique was reviewed by Sindou and Mertens (1993). A new proposal was made in 1979 by Nashold and Ostdahl. The former, with Friedman (Nashold & Friedman 1972), had previously studied the effect of posterior column stimulation and had become disenchanted with the results. They proposed coagulation of the "DREZ", on the basis that this procedure destroyed the part of the grey matter in which spontaneous firing was occurring – namely, the substantia gelatinosa. Radiofrequency coagulation was used, lesions being made at intervals along the intermediolateral suleus of the posterior aspect of the cord. Of 21 patients, 17 had suffered avulsion of the brachial plexus, and 1 has suffered avulsion of the upper limb. Good results were obtained in 13 cases but Nashold and Ostdahl note that in 11 cases there was some degree of residual weakness of the ipsilateral or, occasionally, both lower limbs. Since that time, Nashold (1981) has modified the duration of coagulation, amplitude of current and depth of penetration, with favourable effect on the incidence of long tract affection.

The principal objection to coagulation of the entry zone is that it inflicts another lesion on the damaged side of an already damaged cord. Thomas and Jones (1984) found evidence of subclinical affection of the posterior columns in 50% of their patients with avulsion of the brachial plexus

coming to operation for relief of pain. It is not uncommon in the acute case to find clinical evidence of affection of the ipsilateral corticospinal tract. There are serious potential complications: affection of the ipsilateral corticospinal tracts; damage to the ipsilateral posterior column; impotence; and unpleasant paraesthesiae. There is an incidence of failure of around 40%, and an unquantified evidence of late recurrence. Sometimes the recurrent pain is worse than that which went before. Thomas and Kitchen (1994) supply a long-term review of this operation. In 44 patients, at a minimum interval of 63 months from DREZ lesion for brachial plexus pain, 35 stated that there had been significant and lasting pain relief. Eight cases (18%) had persisting neurological deficit, which was usually mild.

It is plain that central operation of any sort, and entry zone coagulation in particular, should be reserved for patients who:

• have very severe and intractable pain persistently marring life
• have failed to respond to a full range of treatment short of operation
• have failed to show spontaneous improvement after 3 years, or have pain that has actually increased during this period

- have not experienced any relief after an otherwise successful neurotisation
- specifically require further treatment for persistent pain and understand well the drawbacks and hazards of central operation, particularly those of entry zone coagulation.

Patients addicted to controlled drugs are not suitable subjects for central operation.

CENTRAL PAIN

Déjérine and Roussy (1906) described the "thalamic syndrome" in patients with burning pain, dysaesthesiae and hyperpathia afflicting the side of the body opposite to the damaged thalamus, remarking that the motor deficit was often slight, and that the pain was resistant to conventional analgesics. Later, others described similar pain states after lesions other than in the thalamus (Head & Holmes 1911, Davison and Schick 1935, Garcin 1937, Retif et al 1967). Leijon et al (1989) proposed the term "central poststroke pain" (CPSP), but similar pain states are seen after other pathological states, or after injury to the spinal cord (Beric et al 1988). Mariano (1992) found that severe pain occurred in 18–63% of patients with spinal cord injuries. Hopkins and Rudge (1973) described seven patients with severe pain and allodynia in the chest and arms following hyperextension or flexion injury to the cervical spinal cord. They thought that the lesion was at the decussation of spinothalamic fibres in the cord. Cassinaris and Pagni (1969) and Pagni (1989) developed an important concept: that central pain was caused by lesions of the spinothalamicocortical pathways. Illis (1990) reviewed the subject, pointing out that "the definition of central pain is not, however, without some ambiguity". Davidoff and Roth (1991) and Boivie (1994) emphasised certain characteristic features of central pain: it is spontaneous, it is intermittent or continuous and there is allodynia.

We have seen two cases of severe pain after partial lesion of the spinal cord associated with traction lesions of the brachial plexus, which resolved with recovery of motor function.

Case report. A 28-year-old man suffered incomplete traction lesion of the brachial plexus, with avulsion of C7. Computed tomography with enhancement showed displacement of the spinal cord by haematoma at the level of lesion. There was clonus in both lower limbs; pin prick and temperature sensation were diminished, but not absent, from level T4. There was hyperhidrosis of both legs and feet. The patient had severe pain and, notably, allodynia in both lower limbs. This he relieved by keeping both feet in a bucket of cold water. Over the course of 6 weeks his neurological deficit improved spontaneously, and with it his pain.

Bowsher (1996) studied 156 patients with central pain after damage to the central nervous system, and recorded a number of very interesting observations. Allodynia was present in over 70% of cases, and was provoked by cutaneous, thermal or movement stimuli. Pain was experienced in an area smaller than the area of sensory impairment; it was most severe where sensory impairment was worst affected. Temperature and pin prick sensibility was much more impaired than was tactile sensibility. Bowsher said: "it is of very great interest that a substantial number of patients reported that their pain began as motor recovery took place"; the reverse of the usual course in patients with a brachial plexus lesion. Another difference between central pain and pain after brachial plexus lesion is the onset; this was immediate in only a minority of Bowsher's patients. He dismissed the idea that central pain is caused by abnormal discharges from "wide dynamic range" neurones in the spinal grey, and points out that two-thirds of his cases were improved by treatment with adrenergically active antidepressants, sometimes supplemented by Mexiletine, a membrane stabiliser, and that the sooner these are given the better. Bowsher concludes: "it seems, therefore, that the intensity of ongoing pain in these patients is proportional to the degree of deficit for pinprick and thermal (perhaps particularly cold) sensations, but it is influenced by the degree, or even the presence or absence of deficit for low threshold sub modalities ... The cortical disorder in central pain also seems to lie in the central processing of information coming from Aδ (cold and pinprick) rather than Aβ or C peripheral afferents." Other interesting observations from a study of 16 patients with spinal cord injury were made by Eide, Jorum and Stenehejm (1996), who compared somatosensory findings in painful denervated skin with those from nonpainful denervated skin as well as from normal skin. The threshold for thermal stimuli (spinothalamic tract) were significantly changed in denervated skin, but there was no significant difference between painful and nonpainful denervated skin. Furthermore, there was no significant difference in the threshold for touch, joint position sense, or two-point discrimination (dorsal column–medial lemniscus pathways) between painful and nonpainful denervated skin. Allodynia, and wind up pain, which these authors defined as pain caused by repeated pricking of the skin, was more common in painful than in nonpainful denervated skin. They concluded that: "central pain is not only dependent on the lesioning of either dorsal column–medial lemniscal pathways or spinothalamic pathways. The findings of abnormal evoked pain (allodynia and wind-up like pain) may be consistent with the experimental findings of hyperexcitability in nociceptive spinothalamic tract neurones that may be involved in the pathogenesis of central pain". We can only conclude that the pain from preganglionic injury to the brachial plexus arises from damage to both the peripheral and the central nervous system – and when the spinal cord is compromised, as it is in true avulsion, or by ischaemia or displacement by haematoma, then that pain takes on the characteristics, and difficulties, of central pain.

SUMMARY

Wall (1985) commented that the dualistic separation of physical from mental, which is one of the foundations of Western scientific thought, has been one of the factors responsible for confusion and error in analysis of pain. He sees this in the doctor's question about pain – "Is it real or is it in the mind?" – and in some ways he restates Aristotle: "pain is an agony of the soul". We hope that doctors treating patients with neuropathic pain will find our classification helpful and that they will recognise that appropriate surgical intervention is usually successful in true causalgia and in neurostenalgia. It is increasingly clear that reinnervation of the limb is important in relieving brachial plexus pain, but by how much remains uncertain because of the favourable natural history in some untreated patients. Success in these types of neuropathic pain works by modifying abnormal sympathetic activity, by removal of an irritative lesion and by restoring afferent impulses to the spinal cord. Operations on nerves have much less to offer in post-traumatic neuralgia, where our success, of about 50%, due to no more than a placebo effect. Such operations have scarcely anything at all to offer in the treatment of reflex sympathetic dystrophy (CRPS type 1), and for these patients a programme designed to modify their response to pain may help (we discuss this in Chapter 18).

Progress has been made, but a lot more is needed. It is always worth remembering that the history given by the patient, if followed carefully, will lead the doctor to the diagnosis of the cause in nearly every case.

16. Recovery of sensibility after nerve repair

Recovery of sensibility: the mechanism of sensation; regeneration and clinical quality of recovered sensibility; injury and regeneration; testing of sensibility; differential recovery of fibres of different sizes; assessment of function; re-education of sensibility; the value of re-education.

Recovery of sensibility after repair of a nerve in an adult is never perfect. That lack of perfection is no great matter for the patient when the proximal part of a limb is concerned, but in the hand in particular it imposes serious handicap. Such handicap is less serious in the case of the foot, though here too imperfect sensibility is often troublesome. The fact that recovery of sensibility after nerve repair is often very good in children must lead to the supposition that in their case the central apparatus for analysing incoming signals is much more plastic than it is in the adult. Thus, the child is able to reinterpret the altered signals produced by misdirection of regenerating fibres, leading to fibres reaching peripheral endings other than those proper to them. The generally superior results of repair of nerves with no cutaneous sensory component provide further evidence that misdirection of regenerating fibres is a main cause of failure.

In the case of the hand, recognition of objects is mediated through:

- cutaneous sensibility – static or dynamic
- sensibility in joints, tendons and muscles.

Static sensibility is shown in appreciation of temperature and of change in temperature, in pain, and in two-point discrimination. Dynamic sensibility is required for appreciation of texture and of shape. Deep sensibility is required in association with cutaneous sensibility for appreciation of consistency, shape and size. It arises from the receptors in ligaments, tendons and muscles, and joint capsules. The functional separation of superficial and deep sensibility can hardly ever be complete: it is not too surprising that correlation of histological evidence of regeneration of cutaneous nerves with clinical evidence of recovery is often imperfect. Thus, Jabaley et al (1976) attempted to correlate sensory function with evidence of cutaneous reinnervation after section and repair of the median nerve. They found that there was no such correlation. Indeed, in one case, after division and repair of the median and ulnar nerves, two-point discrimination was seriously defective in the thumb; yet blindfold identification of objects was regularly correct and the "pick-up"

test of Moberg (1958) was performed in 50 seconds. Histological examination of the skin of the index and the little fingers showed only an occasional nerve fibre and a few Meissner corpuscles. In contrast, a woman whose median nerve had been repaired by fascicular suture regained plentiful cutaneous innervation, but was unable to pick up objects because she could not feel them. On the other hand, Dellon and Munger (1983), using the partially denervated finger tips of three patients to correlate observations of sensibility with the presence of reinnervated sensory corpuscles as seen by light and electron microscopy, found that in all cases the reinnervated receptors identified were appropriate to provide the neurophysiological basis for the observed results of quality of sensibility.

The basis of stereognosis is a combination of stimuli from skin, tendons, muscles and joints relaying centrally, where comparison is made of memories of movements. The role of movement is vital: a blindfolded person cannot identify the nature of a material if it is simply placed on the finger. Identification is aided if the material is drawn across the finger tip. Recognition is, however, immediate if the subject is allowed to create temporal and spatial patterns by feeling the texture between the moving finger and thumb.

Cutaneous receptors

The question of the specificity of the various sensory nerve endings has been debated at least since von Frey's (1894, 1896) proposal of a correlation between modalities of cutaneous sensibility and the nature of the end-organ. As has been indicated in Chapter 3, the balance of evidence now favours von Frey's original view. The different receptors respond at different velocities: Merkel's discs and Ruffini endings adapt slowly and detect intensity and duration; Meissner's corpuscles and hair follicle receptors adapt with moderate rapidity to detect velocity; and Pacinian corpuscles, adapting rapidly, are detectors of acceleration (Iggo 1977, 1985). Mountcastle (1980) assigns to the specialised receptors a role as transducers responsible for amplification. He points out that in areas of skin subjected to sensory testing and later marked and excised, histological examination has shown only free nerve endings. No specialised mechanoreceptors transmitting through unmyelinated fibres have been identified; the same is so for nociceptors and for most thermoreceptors. All these receptors seem to be represented by fine branching unmyelinated nerve endings in the basal cell layers of the epidermis. The full range of quantitative sensibilities is represented by impulses transmitted in the Aα, Aβ, Aδ and C fibres. The highly organised encapsulated endings surrounding the terminals of myelinated mechano-receptor afferents condition the quantitative nature of the response. These rapidly adapting receptors are of two types. One, with densely packed overlapping fields, has sharply demarcated receptor fields of 1–10 mm.^{2} They are sensitive to brisk, light movements and respond to a velocity component of 30–40 Hz. The other type, with broader receptive fields, has a centrally located 2 cm of maximum sensitivity, with an optimum response rate of 200–300 Hz. These are the Pacinian corpuscles. Slowly adapting receptors have a threshold four times that of the rapidly adapting receptors.

Central analysis

Wall and Devor (1981) and others have shown that impulses entering the posterior horn of the grey matter are subject to modification by other entering impulses and by descending impulses. Thus (Wall and Sweet 1967) afferent impulses conveyed by large-diameter fibres can modify the transmission of nociceptive impulses reaching the posterior horn; this mechanism and central inhibition can greatly modify the perception of nociceptive input.

Further scope for modification and interpretation is provided at the periphery by the pattern of impulses propagated by a single cutaneous stimulus. A single stimulus falling on the skin activates the overlapping receptive fields of a number of different fibres. The activity provoked is maximal in the fibres stimulated at the centres of their fields, and minimal in those stimulated marginally. A pattern of impulses from a population of fibres is thus created, reflecting the size and shape of the stimulus. The localisation of a stimulus or the identification as such of a two-point stimulus, and the recognition of more complex spatial contours cannot be explained solely in terms of the activity of isolated neural lines; this is the function of the reciprocally arranged divergence and convergence at central relays and of the apparatus for central analysis.

The effect of injury and regeneration

The cutaneous end-organs atrophy after division of their supplying nerve. Dellon (1976) showed that in monkeys Meissner's corpuscles could be reinnervated after denervation for up to 9 months, but that they disappeared after a year's denervation. On the other hand, sensory function in skin grafts in which free endings only are present can be excellent. Cabaud et al (1982) cut and repaired the ulnar nerves of monkeys. He showed that "empty" sheaths in the distal stump had little, if any, part in redirecting regenerating axons. The new sprouts seemed to initiate production of their own endoneurial tubes. Not until the fibres reach the periphery do the chemotactic factors come into operation. It must follow that interpretation of impulses from a field so much altered must be done centrally.

Paul et al (1972) stimulated the paws of Macaque monkeys and mapped the cortical representation of the peripheral sensory receptors. They then divided and sutured the relevant nerve and again recorded from the cortex. They found marked alteration of the cortical representation of the peripheral sensory field. Scadding (1984) showed that, after suture, at least 40% of fibres failed to reach the periphery. Small-diameter C-fibres certainly regenerate more quickly than do large-diameter A-fibres, so that, certainly in the early stages of regeneration, there is every likelihood of an abnormal pattern of impulses reaching the central receptors.

It does not appear that similar attempts have been made to correlate the quality of recovered sensibility with evidence of reinnervation of muscle spindles. It was at one time thought that spindles were not affected by denervation, but more recent work has shown that this is not so. Myles and Glasby (1992) found that in denervated muscles the number of observable spindles declined markedly, but that in all groups in which repair had been undertaken the numbers of spindles were normal at 300 days. However, all reinnervated spindles showed morphological differences from healthy ones. They concluded that "nerve repair ... provides enough motor supply to reverse entirely the atrophy which follows denervation though it is unlikely that the reinnervation provides adequate specificity for the stretch reflex to operate in a physiological manner". Evidently, the limitations that apply to cutaneous reinnervation also apply to the reinnervation of muscle receptors.

TESTING OF SENSIBILITY

Sunderland (1991) reminds us that "in sensory perception many complex processes are involved. The ephemeral nature of the activity and the ever changing background to sensory perception make evaluation difficult". He went on to describe his system of sensory testing: (Table 16.1).

Two-point discrimination is valuable because it indicates the degree of reinnervation of slowly adapting receptors. It is subject to limitations. The patient easily gets confused; it is difficult or impossible to ensure that the same pressure is used throughout the test. Brand (1985) showed that even skilled clinicians used during the test pressures

Table 16.1 Modalities examined in sensory testing (Sunderland)

Factor
Time of recognition after stimulus
Localisation
Protective sensation
Pain
Pressure and position sense
Temperature sense
Identification of objects and textures
Effect of sensory defect on motor function
Subjective assessment of the effect of disability on the activities of daily life
Nerve conduction studies
Course of recovery assessed clinically and electrically

varying from 4 to 40 g per unit area. Such variability leads, of course, to error when results of different observers are compared. Bell and Burford (1982), using transducers and oscilloscopes, found that the difference between the pressure applied to one point and that applied to two easily exceeded the resolution threshold for normal sensitivity. They concluded that two-point discrimination had poor validity.

Refinements of the method were introduced by Greulich (1976) and by Mackinnon and Dellon (1985). These were based on the use of a ring with circumferential prongs set at varying intervals. Useful instruments had, of course, been developed previously by Mannerfeldt.

Dellon (1978) introduced the concept of *moving* two-point discrimination. The patient is asked to move his or her finger across a number of ridges separated by varying intervals. He or she then identifies the shortest interval appreciated, which is invariably less than that recorded by the static test. We think that this ingenious method is, to a certain extent, artificial: normal sensibility requires handling of an object between thumb and finger – a process that excites a far greater range of sensory receptors.

Conductance and resistance

Wilson (1985) and Smith and Mott (1986) developed tests which depended on the natural moisture of the skin, and the latter workers added a test of "sensory threshold". Wilson measured the resistance of the skin before and after repair of injuries to nerves. He showed a steady inverse relationship between resistance and sensibility in the acute cases. In cases in which the examination was done months after injury there was, inevitably, some lack of correlation, because of sweating determined by ingrowth of sudomotor fibres from neighbouring normally innervated skin, and by differential rates of growth of small and large fibres.

Smith and Mott (1986) used "sensory threshold" and "conductance". In the first technique, the smallest electrical stimulus to produce sensation is measured. In the latter, the ability of the skin to conduct direct electrical current is estimated. These workers were able to examine about 80% of all patients coming into Mount Vernon Hospital with nerve injuries. That amounted to 2342 clinical measurements in 374 patients over a period of 22 months. In some cases the results were "correlated with conventional EMG and conduction velocity". Smith and Mott concluded that these tests provided an "easily performed, objective measurement of nerve function". Disappointingly, Goldie et al (1992), reporting on the long-term results of repair of digital nerves, found no correlation between clinical results and conductance. Indeed, the difference of calibre between the fibres of the sympathetic system on the one hand, and those conducting fine cutaneous sensibility, on the other, suggests the possibility of such a finding. Indeed, one of us, years ago, found restoration of sweating to apparently insensitive skin after repair of a median nerve. It was, however, the work of Healy et al (1996) on the recovery of innervation after removal of the medial cutaneous nerve of the forearm that established the fact of recovery of sweating in insensitive skin. It may be that the chief value of such tests is in the investigation of patients in whom clinical examination is specially difficult and in the distinction between degenerative and nondegenerative lesions. The idea, or perhaps ideal, of a reliable objective measurement of sensibility remains attractive.

The results of electrodiagnosis using sensory conduction velocity have been disappointing. It is known (Ballantyne & Campbell 1973) that sensory conduction is markedly slowed for years after clinically satisfactory repair, and indeed is never fully recovered. A sensory action potential of reasonable amplitude with latency decreasing over time indicates a certain degree of reinnervation, but excellent function is sometimes compatible with gross abnormalities of sensory conduction. Thus, Birch and Raji (1991), studying the results of repair of the median and ulnar nerves, found that the best "neurophysiological" result after repair of the median nerve was obtained in a patient whose result was, on clinical grounds, considered poor because of hypersensitivity.

The MRC scale

The Medical Research Council (MRC) method of recording sensibility is shown in Table 16.2. This scheme offers a reasonable method for recording and measuring progress. As is the case with all such schemes it has obvious disadvantages, but no comprehensive method has yet been

Table 16.2 The MRC method of recording sensibility

Grade	Description
S0	No sensation
S1	Deep cutaneous pain in autonomous zone
S2	Some superficial pain and touch
S2+	Touch and pain sensation in autonomous zone with persistent overreaction
S3	As for S2+, without overreaction
S3+	Good localisation, with some two-point discrimination
S4	Normal sensibility

devised that does not have the overwhelming disadvantage of extreme complication.

Our methods

The modalities routinely tested are light touch, temperature, position sense, pain, two-point discrimination, localisation and pressure. Moberg's (1958) pick-up test is also used.

Light touch

A wisp of cotton wool is moved lightly across the area under test.

Temperature

Metal tubes are used: one contains ice, and the other contains water at 45°C. These are applied alternately to the area under test.

Position sense

All nearby joints other than the one being tested must be stabilised. The patient is first shown the directions in which the joint is to be moved. Then, with eyes closed, he or she is asked to indicate the direction in which the joint is being moved.

Pain

A scratch with a pin moving over an area of a few millimetres is adequate.

Two-point discrimination

This is done with the blunted points of a compass or the ends of a paper clip or with a special device. The patient is thus instructed: "I shall touch your finger now with one point; now with two. If you feel one, say 'one'; if you feel two, say 'two'; if you are in doubt, say 'one'." Then, with closed eyes, the patient attempts the distinction between one and two points.

Localisation

We have devised a chart in which the hand is divided into different numbered areas. The blindfold patient is asked to point to the point being touched, and this is recorded on the chart. Thus, if a touch on the tip of the index finger is felt as a touch on the base, the number of the former area is recorded on the latter area on the chart (Figs 16.1 to 16.3).

Pressure

The padded blunt end of a pencil is used to indent the skin only lightly. We also use von Frey hairs and the weighted pins (5 and 10 g) developed by Bowden.

Moberg's (1958) pick-up test

The patient is required to pick up a number of small objects, such as coins, safety pins and paper clips, and to put them as quickly as possible into a box. Each hand is tested separately. The patient then carries out the same task when blindfolded. All times are recorded. We found a high correlation between these times and the quality of two-point discrimination.

ASSESSMENT OF FUNCTION

Jones (1989) reviewed the various tests for assessment of function, and indicated that in most of these performance was measured in terms of speed. She suggests that methods are now needed to study how the hand executes tasks, and to quantify postures adopted, movements generated and forces exerted.

The pick-up test is, of course, a measurement of function as well as of sensibility. So is the assessment of ability to recognise objects, the importance of which we believe we were the first to recognise (Wynn Parry and Salter 1976, Wynn Parry 1981). The blindfolded patient is presented with a series of objects of different shape, texture and surface character and asked to distinguish them. The number correctly identified and the time taken are recorded. Later, common textures and small and large objects in daily use are presented for recognition.

It is best in functional testing to use simple tests appropriate to the patient's work and other interests and to compare function with that of the healthy hand.

RE-EDUCATION OF SENSIBILITY

Because the quality of recovery of sensibility in the adult depends so much on re-establishing the central analysis of input of new patterns, it should be possible to do much to aid recovery by retraining that central perception. We may have been the first to report on the methods and results of

Fig. 16.1 to 16.3 Localisation charts.

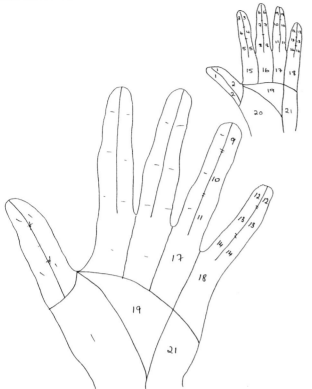

Fig. 16.1 Inability to localise 20 months after secondary suture of the median nerve.

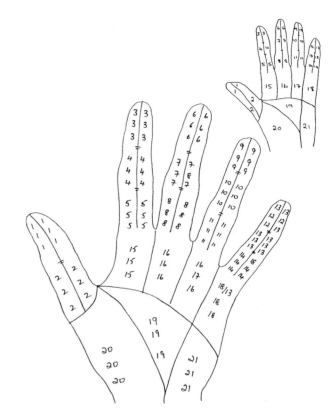

Fig. 16.2 Good ability to localise 15 months after primary suture of the median and ulnar nerves.

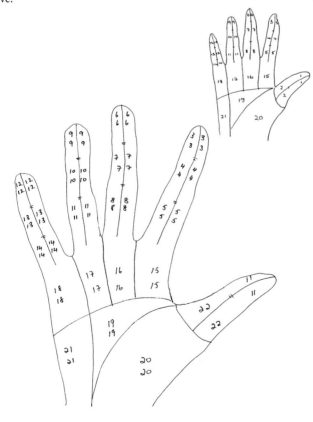

Fig. 16.3 Good ability to localise 2 years and again 40 months after primary suture of the ulnar nerve.

sensory retraining in adults (Wynn Parry & Salter 1976). Most workers in this field now accept that such retraining is an essential part of rehabilitation after nerve suture (Dellon 1981). Imai et al (1991) report that after sensory re-education 19 of 22 patients were able 2 years after nerve repair to recognise more than 9 of 12 small objects. Only 2 of 24 similar patients who did not receive sensory re-education were able to match this achievement. No patient who was not retrained achieved normal two-point discrimination; 15 of the 22 retrained patients achieved a moving two-point discrimination score equivalent to S3+. Imai and Tajima (1985) found that sensory re-education was very helpful in reducing paraesthesiae and improving function. They suggest that re-education is "of extreme value in returning practical use of the hand to the patient at a time when even our usual parameters of measurement may not suggest that the patient has this ability". Training, which is started as soon as the patient can recognise stimuli at the finger tips, aims to improve function by improvement of the qualities of localisation and of recognition. If the patient is distracted by paraesthesia or if allodynia makes testing unpleasant, an hour's transcutaneous stimulation is used before the session.

Localisation

The method described above (see p. 408) is used, the patient recognising error on the chart and attempting to correct it in further trials. With intensive training some patients can regain almost normal power of localisation after 3 or 4 weeks.

Recognition

The method described above (see p. 408) is used. First, the blindfolded patient attempts recognition of shapes. If unable to distinguish them, he or she is permitted to see and to feel, first with the healthy hand and later with the affected hand. The patient tries to relate the abnormal sensation to what is seen and what is felt by the healthy hand. Later, a similar process is followed with rough and smooth surfaces; after this, a variety of textures (sandpaper, wool, velvet, linen and so on) are presented. Finally, large and then small objects in daily use are presented, and the power of recognition is similarly trained. The choice of objects should relate to the patient's formerly usual activities: it is, for example, unlikely that one who has never lifted the bonnet of a car would recognise a spark plug. Textures most difficult to recognise are sheepskin, silk, plastic, wool and carpet. Those easiest to identify are sandpaper, leather, cotton wool, canvas and rubber. Objects most often misidentified are, in order of frequency, can opener, electric plug, safety pin, purse, spanner, small bottle, screw, hook, and nut and bolt. Those easiest to identify at first testing are, in order of frequency, nail brush, bulldog clip, pencil, matchbox, Yale key, cotton reel, tennis ball, ballpoint pen, scissors, marble and string. The treatment sessions last from 10 to 15 minutes; treatment is given four times a day. As soon as the patient understands the rationale, he or she can then practise at home with the help of a friend or partner. Variety is introduced by using sets of shapes and objects different from those in the training set (a "training effect" is easily produced). As an alternative, a variety of the lucky dip is used: objects are buried in a bowl of sand or bran and the patient is asked to find in this a named object. Alternatively, a cutout board can be presented to the blindfold patient, who is asked to select appropriate shapes to fit into the various cavities (Figs 16.4 to 16.9).

Figures 16.10 and 16.11 show representative examples of standards of ability to recognise and localise after primary suture of the median nerve. Sensory re-education

---

Figs 16.4 to 16.9 Sensory re-education.

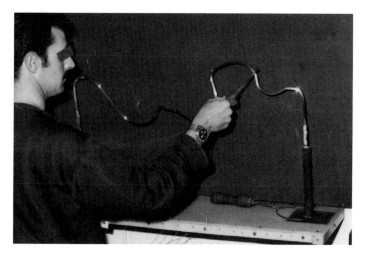

Fig. 16.4 Recognition and coordination. If the loop touches the metal, a buzzing noise is emitted.

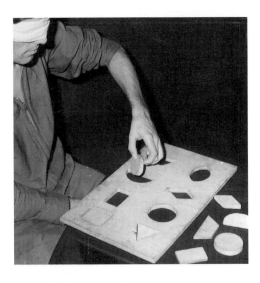

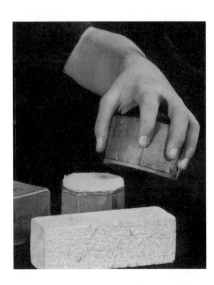

Fig. 16.5 Recognition of shape. Blindfolded fitting of shapes to the appropriate cavity.

Fig. 16.6 Recognition of shapes.

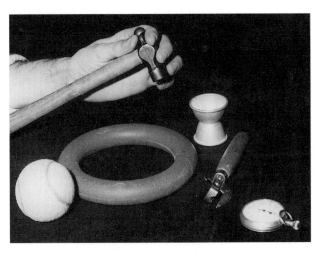

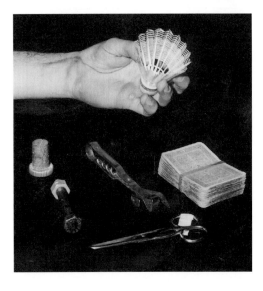

Fig. 16.7 Recognition of objects.

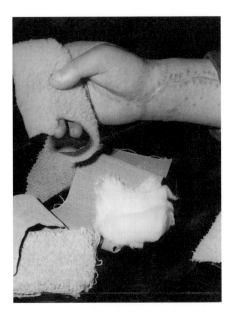

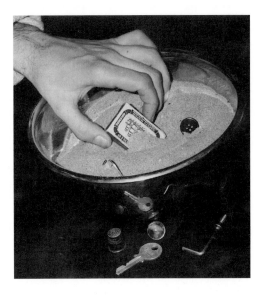

Fig. 16.8 Recognition of texture.

Fig. 16.9 Seeking a named object in the "lucky dip."

Figs 16.10 and 16.11 Measurement of ability to recognise and to localise.

DATE	11.8.86.						
	Interpretation	Time	Interpretation	Time	Interpretation	Time	
SHAPES – I section only							
Square	✓	4					
Oblong	✓	4					
Triangle	✓	2					
Diamond	Hexagon ✓	4					
Circle							
Oval							
Semi circle							
Moon							
AVERAGE TIME	4/4	·4					
COINS 50p + 2 others							
1p							
2p							
5p	✗1	10					
10p	✓	4					
50p	✓	2					
AVERAGE TIME	2/3	3					
TEXTURE – Test 6							
Sandpaper							
Formica							
Wood							
Rubber	✓	6					
Carpet	✓	7					
Leather	✓	5					
Velvet	✓	5					
Fur	✓	1					
Cotton wool							
Sheepskin							
Tissue							
Metal	✓	6					
AVERAGE TIME	6/6	5					

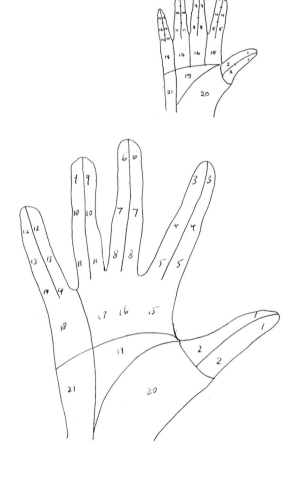

DATE	11.8.86.						
	Interpretation	Time	Interpretation	Time	Interpretation	Time	
OBJECTS							
SMALL							
Safety pin)	✓	9					
Paper clip) TEST 2	✓	4					
Nail)							
Screw)							
Nut							
Rubber)	✓	3					
Thimble)	✓	3					
Screw hook)							
Button) TEST 4	✓	7					
Yale key)	✓	2					
Ball of wool)							
Ball of string)							
AVERAGE	6/6	5					
LARGE							
Sink plug)	✓	3					
Cotton reel)							
Plug)	✓	5					
Bottle) TEST 3	✗	1·00					
Sellotape reel)							
Soap)							
Egg cup)							
Tea strainer)							
Pencil)	✓	4					
Fork)							
Metal comb)							
Ball point pen)							
Screwdriver) TEST 3	✓	2					
Teaspoon)							
Tooth brush)	✓	2					
Paint brush)							
Peg)							
AVERAGE	5/6	3					
LOCALISATION SCORE	35/35						
PROTECTIVE SENSATION	GOOD						

Fig. 16.10 Case 1: primary suture of the median nerve 5 years before testing. Both recognition and localisation are good.

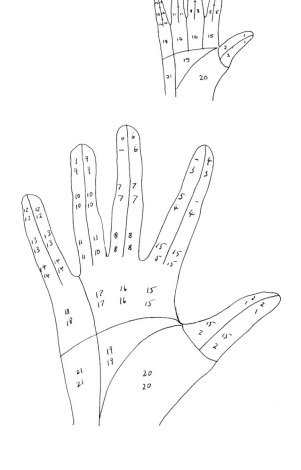

DATE	25.7.84		10.9.86			
	Interpretation	Time	Interpretation	Time	Interpretation	Time
SHAPES - I section only						
Square						
Oblong						
Triangle						
Diamond						
Circle	✓	07	✓	06		
Oval	Δ	21	Round	13		
Semi circle	✓	14	✓	13		
Moon	✓	24	X	12		
AVERAGE TIME	3/4	15	2/4	10		
COINS 50p + 2 others						
1p						
2p	5p	19	5p	33		
5p	1p	16				
10p			✓	18		
50p	10p	15	✓	25		
AVERAGE TIME	0/3	-	2/3	22		
TEXTURE - Test 6						
Sandpaper			✓	50		
Formica						
Wood	✓	10	✓	37		
Rubber	✓	07	✓	25		
Carpet	wood	30	foam	21		
Leather	plastic	07	cotton	13		
Velvet						
Fur			✓	11		
Cotton wool						
Sheepskin						
Tissue	✓	12				
Metal	✓	19	✓	23		
AVERAGE TIME	4/6	12	4/6	36		

DATE	25.7.84		10.9.86			
	Interpretation	Time	Interpretation	Time	Interpretation	Time
OBJECTS						
SMALL						
Safety pin)	1/2p	26	Key	54		
Paper clip) TEST 2			X	A90		
Nail)						
Screw)	✓	16				
Nut						
Rubber)	✓	21	Brick	16		
Thimble)	Plastic	34	small prece plate	1.00		
Screw hook)						
Button) TEST 4						
Yale key)	✓	09	✓			
Ball of wool)	✓	15	Soft ball	25		
Ball of string)						
AVERAGE	4/6	15	1/6	47		
LARGE						
Sink plug)			Beads	14		
Cotton reel)	Stopper (door)	15	X	15		
Plug)	✓	04	Metal	33		
Bottle) TEST 3						
Sellotape reel)						
Soap)	Plasticine	30				
Egg cup)						
Tea strainer)						
Pencil)			Pen	20		
Fork)						
Metal comb)						
Ball point pen)						
Screwdriver) TEST 3						
Teaspoon)						
Tooth brush)	✓	14	✓	18		
Paint brush)	Pen	05				
Peg)	plastic	41	tube	30		
AVERAGE						
LOCALISATION SCORE	2/6	09	1/6	18		
PROTECTIVE SENSATION	V POOR		V. POOR			

Fig. 16.11 Case 2: primary suture of the median nerve 7 and 33 months before testing. Both recognition and localisation are impaired; there is little change in the quality of the result in the 26 months intervening between the two tests.

was used in both cases. It will be seen that in the second case (Fig. 16.11) the result was worse than that in the first, and that there was little improvement during the second and third years after repair.

CONCLUSIONS

The results of peripheral nerve repair depend, inter alia, on the timing and technique of repair, on the quality of treatment after operation, and on the age, motivation, trainability, and qualifications of the patient (Jabaley et al 1976). Narakas (1985) indicated the following as being factors on which successful regeneration after nerve repair depended:

- survival of the neuron
- adequate sprouting and growth from the proximal stump
- establishment of proper synapses for atrophy of collateral sprouts and fibres
- maturation of the "neofibre"
- cerebral transduction.

Measurement of sensibility can indicate the success or otherwise of repair in effecting peripheral reinnervation, but the quality of reinnervation is not necessarily related to function. Thus for purposes of research both academic tests of sensory restoration and tests of function must be used.

17. Reconstruction

Definition. Limitations. History. Principles and practices. Correction of fixed deformity: Volkmann's contracture in upper and lower limbs. Active reconstruction by restoration of active movement: upper limb (scapulohumeral, glenohumeral, elbow and wrist joints; opposition of the thumb); lower limb (hip, knee, ankle and subtalar joints); transfer of vascularised bone and muscle. Results.

Am I God to kill or make alive, that this man doth send unto me to recover a man of his leprosy? (2 Kings 5:7)

We use the term "reconstruction" to signify operations, other than by nerve repair, designed to restore function. These include: the release or correction of fixed deformities; transfer of musculotendinous units to restore balance across joints; similar transfer to restore lost active movement; and, on occasion, arthrodesis. These are operations of palliation. Fixed deformity is a mark of failure of primary treatment, arthrodesis is an acknowledgement of failure to regain active movement, and, as Narakas (1987c) said, no musculotendinous transfer matches the outcome from good nerve regeneration. Throughout the world the most common indications for muscle transfer remain the infectious diseases poliomyelitis and leprosy. Our own experience is drawn largely from work with loss or disturbance of function from injury to the upper or lower motor neurones, or both (Table 17.1). Pulvertaft (1983) outlined a good classification of causes of paralysis (Table 17.2).

Table 17.1 Operations for reconstruction, 1977–1995

Operation type	No. of cases
Tetraplegia and cord lesions	12
Cerebral palsy, spasticity from head injury	64
Poliomyelitis	10
Brachial plexus lesions:	
Shoulder	110
Arm	315
Forearm and wrist	298
Hand	239
Total	962
Peripheral nerve lesions:	
Forearm and wrist	130
Hand	101
Thumb	181
Hip, knee, ankle and foot	181
Total	591*

*Including over 200 operations of release and 30 amputations.

Table 17.2 Causes of paralysis

I. Upper motor neuron disorders

A. Extrapyramidal tract lesions: ataxia, athetosis, chorea, rigidity, tremor and others, hysterical brachial palsy

B. Pyramidal tract lesions (examples on right)

1. Congenital	Cerebral agenesis
2. Trauma	Cerebral palsy; head injury
3. Vascular	Haemorrhage, thrombosis etc
4. Infection	Encephalitis; cerebral abscess
5. Neoplasm	Benign, malignant etc
6. Hamartoma	Haemangioma
7. Miscellaneous	Multiple sclerosis

II. Lower motor neuron disorders (examples on right)

A. Spinal cord and roots

1. Congenital	Craniovertebral anomalies
2. Trauma	Fracture dislocation; wounds
3. Vascular	Thrombosis anterior spinal artery
4. Infection	Poliomyelitis; herpes zoster
5. Neoplasm	
6. Hamartoma	
7. Metabolic	Subacute combined degeneration
8. Degenerative	Spondylosis
9. Miscellaneous	Motor neuron disease

B. Brachial plexus

1. Trauma	
2. Vascular	Subclavian aneurysm
3. Neoplasm	
4. Hamartoma	
5. Entrapment	Thoracic outlet syndrome
6. Miscellaneous	Radiation neuropathy

C. Peripheral nerves

1. Congenital	Hereditary sensorimotor neuropathy
2. Trauma	
3. Vascular	Postischaemic contracture
4. Infection	Leprosy is classified separately
5. Neoplasm	
6. Hamartoma	Haemangioma, fibrolipoma
7. Toxic	Peripheral neuropathy
8. Metabolic	Peripheral neuropathy
9. Entrapment	
10. Peripheral neuropathy	Infective: diphtheria, Guillain–Barré
	Toxic: drugs or poisons
	Metabolic: diabetes
	Deficiency: vitamin B complex
	Iatropathic

From Pulvertaft (1983).

The demands of these infectious diseases and of war wounds led to the definition of the principles underlying reconstructive work. Nicolodani (1880), Vulpius (1904), Codavilla (1899) and Lange (1900) laid the foundations in work largely directed to the treatment of the lower limb afflicted by poliomyelitis. Biesalski and Mayer (1916) and Jones (1921) developed operations for the injuries of war, particularly in the upper limb. It is to Robert Jones that credit is due for establishing specialised orthopaedic hospitals; to him also goes the accolade for defining the most important principles that should be followed in reconstruction. These include: the joints must be supple; the transferred muscle must be strong enough; the course of the transferred muscle and tendons should be direct; and the transplant should be attached with slight tension. These principles were developed by Starr (1922) in a large series of reconstructions for radial nerve palsy. Bunnell (1928) and Steindler (1939) defined technical considerations in reconstruction of the upper limb. Brand (1958) and Antia et al (1992) drew on their enormous experience of the treatment of leprosy. Huckstep (1975) crystallised his experience with poliomyelitis in an excellent monograph directed to those working in countries with much disease, and limited means. Zancolli (1979) presented detailed anatomical studies of the hand and forearm, and proposed logical explanations for the progression of certain types of deformity. Moberg (1976), and later with Lamb (1980), developed a functional classification of tetraplegia, which serves as a useful basis for reconstruction. The essays collected and edited by Lamb (1987) and by Tubiana (1993) are outstanding; the interested reader will learn a great deal from them.

REQUIREMENTS

Some of the prerequisites for success are as follows.

1. There must be a clearly defined loss of function which can be remedied only by transfer, the prognosis for neural function being known.
2. The patient is well motivated; even better, the patient defines what he or she needs from experience of work or from daily life. It is not for the surgeon to argue the case for operation; rather, it is for the patient to persuade the surgeon that there is indeed a justification for intervention. Operations for reconstruction in adult patients in process for compensation usually fail.
3. The treatment of continuing neuropathic pain takes precedence.
4. Ideally, there is useful sensation in the part, but this is by no means an absolute requirement; as Citron and Taylor (1987) showed from their study of transfers to improve hand function, sensation improves after the operation.

There are two essential requirements. First, fixed deformity must be overcome. Next, in dynamic deformity, the causal force must be realigned and/or so modified that the affected joints are rebalanced. This is of the utmost importance in the growing child or in the spastic deformities after head injury or cerebral palsy.

The muscle to be transferred should be dispensable: as our colleague Donal Brooks said "all transfers rob Peter to pay Paul". The price should not be too high. Only in exceptional circumstances would a surgeon transfer biceps to triceps for the sake of elbow extension. Transfer of the last remaining wrist flexor for the sake of wrist extension may lead to hyperextension of the wrist, so preventing extension of the digits.

The muscle should be of sufficient power when the indication for transfer is to restore movement against gravity: in restoring extension of knee or ankle, nothing less than Medical Research Council (MRC) grade 5 will do. Reinnervated muscles are predictably unreliable. They may be weak; there is often a degree of co-contraction after repairs of the brachial plexus; there is, in particular, deficiency of afferent function of proprioception and muscle spindle control, so that retraining is difficult or impossible.

The surgeon does need to know how to do the operation. It should be done cleanly and with kindness. Gentle handling of the tissues and meticulous haemostasis are as important in this as in any other operation.

The preferred plane of passage is through unscarred tissue, and preliminary operations to improve skin may be necessary. The plane is subcutaneous, in fatty areolar tissue. The only exception to this rule in our practice is in transfer of the tibialis posterior through the interosseous membrane for extension of the ankle. Brand (1987) used the term "drag" to sum up all those factors offering soft tissue resistance and friction to the transfer. He argued persuasively for preserving paratenon where possible, avoiding contact with naked bone or scarred fascia, and using a gentle tunnelling technique to provide an investing layer of living fat or loose areolar tissue. Compromise may be necessary; some muscles such as flexor carpi ulnaris, pronator teres and brachioradialis have lengthy attachments to periosteum or fascia, so that considerable dissection is necessary to mobilise them. Others, such as the tendons of flexor digitorum superficialis or extensor indicis, can be detached from their insertion and rerouted through small incisions with a minimum of dissection.

The muscle transferred can be asked to perform one function only. Although we have seen exceptions, on the whole it seems that three motors are necessary in radial palsy: one for wrist extension; one for extension of the metacarpophalangeal joints of the fingers and the interphalangeal joint of the thumb; and one for abduction of the thumb metacarpal. For a number of reasons we prefer tendon suture over other methods of insertion. First, because the weak muscle may recover; and, next, because union of tendon to tendon is stronger than that of tendon to bone. When a tendon is wound around another to create a pulley, neither should be scarified; the paratenon of both should always be respected.

The most important part of the operation is the splinting and postoperative care, and this is the sole responsibility of the surgeon. Swelling must be avoided and only those joints which require immobilisation should be so splinted (Fig. 17.1). Thereafter a balance is sought between risking the new attachment by premature or overvigorous force and too prolonged immobilisation leading to extensive scar formation. Protection of the transfer needs to be prolonged following such transfers as tibialis posterior for dorsiflexion of the ankle or hamstring transfer for knee extension, when some support is necessary for 3–6 months.

In the early stages of retraining it is often useful to introduce the muscle to its new function by mimicking the old: pectoralis major to serratus transfer is retrained by the patient strongly adducting the arm. This is a useful manoeuvre after elbow flexorplasty by transfer of pectoralis minor or latissimus dorsi. Transfers for wrist extension are first encouraged by clenching the hand. Some transfers are notoriously difficult to retrain; these include those for radial palsy and those for extension of the knee and of the ankle. In these, direct stimulation of muscle may prove necessary. Another group difficult to retrain are children under the age of 5 years. It is salutary to recall that these do badly after tendon grafting.

The tension of the transfer has long been a matter of debate. There are those operations in which posture is more important than power, as in placing the thumb into opposition or abduction. Overzealous transfer of brachio-radialis to flexor pollicis longus may lead to a thumb-in-palm deformity. Where transfers seek active power against

gravity, as at the ankle or wrist, then transfers are tight. As a rule of thumb, the joints should be at a neutral position or slightly into the desired posture when the transfer is completed. One of the advantages of performing these operations under regional anaesthesia is that the excursion of the transferred tendon can be demonstrated to the surgeon by the patient.

FIXED DEFORMITY

The chief causes of fixed deformity of such severity that active treatment is necessary include:

1. The unopposed action of muscles during growth (we have already seen the effects of muscle imbalance at the shoulder in obstetrical brachial plexus palsy (see Ch. 10); the effect on the posture of the foot after irreparable tibial or common peroneal lesion in the growing child is severe; and dislocation of the hip from unopposed action of the adductor muscles in cases of cerebral palsy or spina bifida is a shameful complication.
2. Next is the fixed deformity from postischaemic fibrosis of muscle. The importance of this is frequently underestimated; it is seen particularly involving the flexor muscles of forearm, the small muscles of hand and the deep flexor compartment of the leg.
3. Untreated pain is an important cause of fixed deformity, and in the upper limb may cause severe flexion deformity of the wrist with extension of the metacarpophalangeal joints and flexion of the proximal interphalangeal joints.
4. Lastly, it must be said that many cases of fixed deformity are a reflection of neglect of elementary principles in the treatment of paralysed limbs. Two of these are particularly common. They are the fixed extension deformity of the metacarpophalangeal joints of the hand, and the flexion deformity in the lower limb marring the function of hip, knee and ankle (Fig. 17.2).

We shall elaborate on two of these causes.

Children

Sharrard (1971) and Huckstep (1975) have described examples of preventable, crippling deformities following untreated poliomyelitis or cerebral palsy. Our own experience from peripheral nerve lesions is illustrated by some cases (Figs 17.3 to 17.5). These serve to illustrate the importance of *progression* of deformity in the growing hand and foot. Forward planning is needed, based on a clear understanding of the prognosis of the nerve lesion.

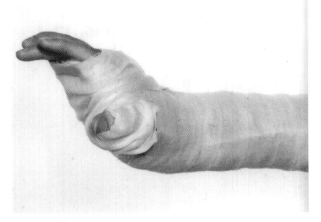

Fig. 17.1 Splint for flexor to extensor transfer. The distal interphalangeal joints are free.

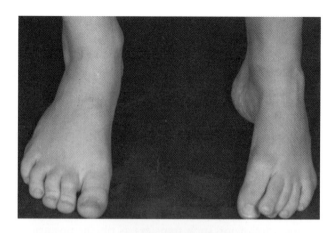

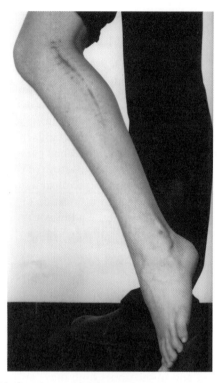

Fig. 17.2 Pain from iatropathic injury to the common peroneal nerve caused this flexion deformity of hip, knee, and ankle in a 17-year-old boy.

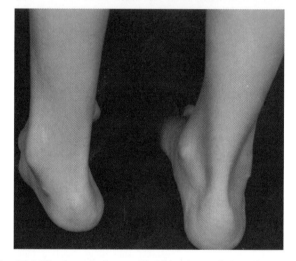

Fig. 17.4 The foot of a 6-year-old girl in whom a lesion of common peroneal nerve went unrecognised and untreated for 3 years.

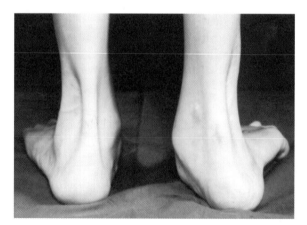

Fig. 17.3 The foot of a 17-year-old girl. Innominate osteotomy for hip dysplasia, performed at the age of 4 years, damaged the sciatic nerve.

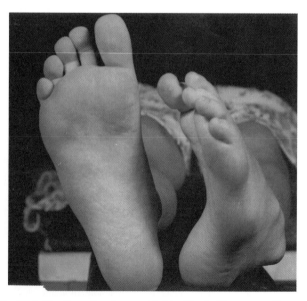

Fig. 17.5 The foot of an 8-year-old girl with plexiform neurofibroma of the lumbosacral plexus.

Postischaemic contracture: Volkmann's contracture

Volkmann (1881) described ischaemic contractures in the limbs from overtight bandages. Finochietto (1920) was probably the first surgeon to recognise the cause and effect on the hand of ischaemic contracture of the intrinsic muscles, and it was he who described a simple and valuable clinical test for the condition. When the finger is extended at the metacarpophalangeal joint the interosseous muscles are shortened and passive flexion of the proximal interphalangeal joint is possible. When the finger is flexed at the knuckle, passive flexion at the proximal interphalangeal joint is impossible (Fig. 17.6).

A number of important papers describe experience from the Second World War. Merle D'Aubigné and Postel (1956) considered Volkmann's contracture as falling into one of two types (with or without claw hand), an idea further developed by Zancolli (1979) who grouped ischaemic contractures of the upper limb under four headings:

- affliction confined to the flexor muscles of the forearm alone
- paralysis, but not contracture, of the small muscles of the hand in addition to the forearm problem
- contracture of both the forearm and the hand muscles
- paralysis and contracture of the small muscles in addition to the problem of the forearm.

Seddon (1956) thought of Volkmann's as a condition of progressive severity. First, there was diffuse ischaemia without infarct, with a good prognosis. Next, was the group with infarction of the flexor muscles of the forearm with or without a lesion of the median and ulnar nerves. Last, and worst, were cases of diffuse fibrosis with severe paralysis and deformity. We prefer Seddon's approach because it emphasises the physiological abnormality underlying the clinical lesion.

Our own experience is set out in Table 17.3. It is extremely important to distinguish between the paralysis

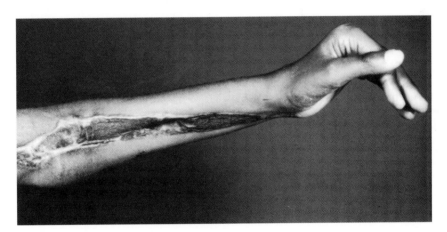

Fig. 17.6 Volkmann's ischaemic contracture of intrinsic muscles. The flexion deformity of wrist has been corrected by Scaglietti's muscle slide. The metacarpophalangeal joints are fixed in flexion; passive flexion of the proximal interphalangeal joints was impossible.

Table 17.3 Postischaemic contracture: cases requiring operative treatment, 1977–1995

Location of contracture	No. of limbs	Cause (No. of limbs)
Upper Limb		
Shoulder	3	Direct blow, coma, fracture
Arm	2	
Forearm	53	Fracture/dislocation of elbow, 38; other fracture, 15
Hand	23	Drug coma, 15; injection, 8
Total*	81	
Brachial plexus		
Forearm and hand	40	Arterial injury in all
Lower limb†		
Buttock and thigh	4	Direct crush or fracture, coma, 4
Leg	55	Arterial injury, 21; "compartment syndrome", 34
Total	59	

* Direct arterial injury in 36 cases.
† Direct arterial injury in 21 cases.

of the small muscles of hand or foot caused by degenerative lesion of nerves, whether from ischaemia, compression or both, from the less common problem of ischaemic contracture of those muscles (Fig. 17.7). In most of our cases of Volkmann's contracture in the upper limb there was some recovery into the small muscles of the hand. This led us to the view that prognosis is determined by the fate of the trunk nerves. Elaborate reconstructive work on an insensate hand is a waste of time. Nerves are a good deal more resistant to ischaemia than are muscles. It seemed, in many of our cases, that the lesion of the nerve was one more akin to compression than frank ischaemia. Our policy has been to determine the extent of lesion of the nerve. This demands operations of decompression to expose the nerves concerned, which are the median, the ulnar and the posterior tibial. In a number of such cases the outcome was remarkable: early relief of pain; and later improvement of sensation and vaso- and sudomotor function, and recovery of the small muscles, notably those innervated by the ulnar nerve. This may be a reflection of the fact that the ulnar neurovascular bundle runs in a discrete fascial compartment and is separate from the main body of the flexor muscles. The tibial nerve is similarly situated.

Parkes (1951) advocated musculotendinous transfer to restore function after ischaemic contracture. Seddon (1956) and Zancolli (1979) went further in their operations in which dead muscles were excised before appropriate reconstruction, either by tendon grafting or by transfer. We are a little more cautious, perhaps because the contracture in most of our cases is less severe. In any event we have found that total irreparable lesion of the ulnar nerve is rare. Furthermore, we believe that in the most severe cases the functioning muscle transfer is a better way forward than conventional tendon transfer. For these reasons it is our practice to determine the prognosis for the involved nerves before any attempt at reconstruction. Electromyography is useful; insertion of the concentric needle into an irretrievably fibrosed muscle is met with characteristic gritty resistance. There is scanty or no electrical activity.

We now describe four valuable operations in the treatment of fixed deformity. These have been indicated most often for: postischaemic fibrosis; severe spasticity from head injury or cerebral palsy; and for the treatment of joints contracted during severe pain states.

The equinovarus deformity of ankle and foot

A 34-year-old man (Fig. 17.8) presented with pain, degenerative lesion of the tibial nerve and deformity after fracture of the proximal tibia. The contracture involved not only the flexor muscles of the heel, but also the flexor muscles of the toes. The tibial neurovascular bundle was exposed through a posteromedial incision. The tibial artery was patent. The tendocalcaneus, and the tendons of tibialis posterior, flexor hallucis longus and flexor digitorum profundus were all lengthened widely, permitting the foot to come into a plantigrade posture. None of these muscles was completely infarcted. There was early relief of pain; functional plantar flexion of the heel and toes was evident at 1 year. Similar operations have been performed in 18 cases. The results have been worthwhile.

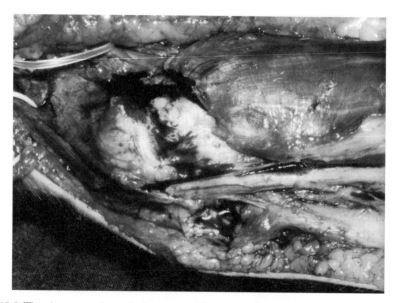

Fig. 17.7 The ulnar nerve shown in the course of flexor muscle slide. The nerve is narrowed where it passes into the infarcted muscle; there is obliteration of the longitudinal epineurial vessels. After decompression there was complete recovery of the nerve.

should be no swelling. The metacarpophalangeal joints are approached through linear incisions centred between the metacarpal heads. The extensor tendons are lifted up from the capsule which is then incised transversely. This may be all that is required; in more severe cases division of the collateral ligaments as described by the originator is necessary (Figs 17.10 to 17.12).

The joints are now flexed to 90° or more. There is a tendency for the extensor tendons to displace from their proper position, in which event a few fine absorbable sutures to the remnants of the capsule may prove necessary; the skin is closed and the position held with fine Kirschner wires passed from the dorsum of the head of the metacarpal into the proximal phalanx (Fig. 17.13). The hand is immobilised in two separate plaster of Paris splints. The wires are removed at between 2 and 3 weeks. The joints, however, are held in the position of flexion for a total of 6 weeks. Active and passive work is then started. It is mistake to use a transverse incision to expose the joints, for it may be impossible to close the skin without tension. Close supervision by the surgeon of the maintenance of the position and throughout the period of mobilisation is essential.

Release of contracted hand intrinsic muscles

This procedure (Littler 1949) is indicated when the metacarpophalangeal joint is free, but flexion of the proximal interphalangeal joint is impossible when the metacarpophalangeal joint is flexed. A dorsal linear midline incision over the proximal phalanx permits exposure of the intrinsic lateral band and the interosseous triangular laminae. These are excised. The hand is protected in a splint which holds the metacarpophalangeal joints in flexion; early active and passive flexion of the interphalangeal joints is encouraged. The operation is contraindicated when there

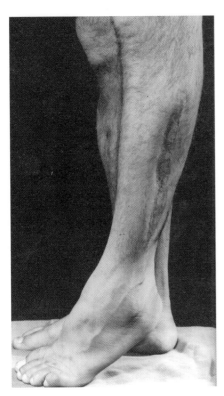

Fig. 17.8 Lateral view of left leg of a 34-year-old man three years after fibial fracture with ischaemic change in the flexor muscles. Note the scar of the fasciotomy and the equinovarous deformity of the foot.

Fixed extension at the metacarpophalangeal joints

This operation (Fig. 17.9) was described by Campbell Reid (1984). We have used it on 42 occasions, and have found it consistently reliable in restoring a reasonable passive range of movement in the metacarpophalangeal joints of the hand. It is important not to intervene too soon. The inflammatory phase must have settled; there

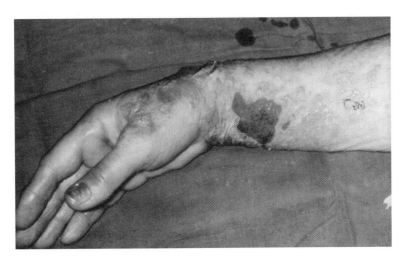

Fig. 17.9 A 63-year-old woman lay on her hand in a drug-induced coma for 18 hours. There was severe ischaemic contracture of the intrinsic muscles.

Figs 17.10 to 17.13 Metacarpophalangeal release.

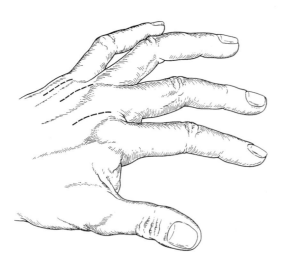

Fig. 17.10 The incisions.

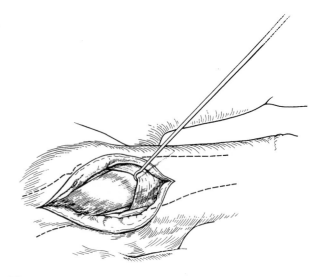

Fig. 17.11 Investing fascia released displaying the extensor tendon.

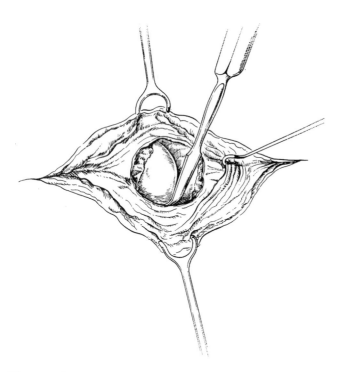

Fig. 17.12 Incision of capsule and of collateral ligaments after elevating extensor tendon.

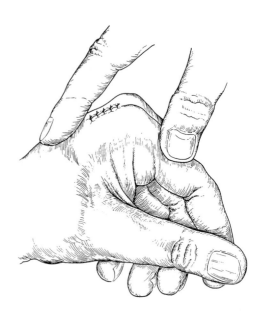

Fig. 17.13 Range of flexion of the joints which are now stabilised with fine Kirschner wires.

is fixed flexion deformity of the metacarpaphalangeal joints. In some cases the release must be proximal to the metacarpophalangeal joint and in severe cases an anterior approach permitting mobilisation of the volar plate may be necessary. We have only rarely encountered deformities of such severity (Fig. 17.14).

Adduction contracture of the thumb is common. Unless this is corrected (Fig. 17.15). all operations designed to restore active opposition of the thumb will fail. We favour the operation advised by Brooks (personal communication), who recommended a Z-plasty for the skin of the thumb web space combined with subperiosteal release, from their origin, of the first dorsal interosseous and adductor pollicus longus muscles. Rotation flaps or split skin grafts are sometimes needed.

Flexor muscle slide

Flexor muscle slide, by the technique of Brooks (1984a) is ascribed to Scaglietti. Operation is indicated where there is potential for function after partial recovery of long flexor muscles to at least Medical Research Council (MRC) grade 3 (Fig. 17.16). It is also useful in certain cases of spasticity following head injury or cerebral palsy.

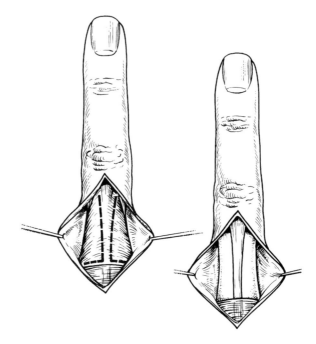

Fig. 17.14 Intrinsic release.

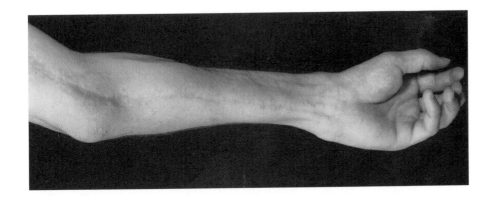

Fig. 17.15 Ischaemic contracture of the intrinsic muscles of the hand. A flexor muscle slide, performed years before, corrected the flexion deformity of the wrist and digits, but the thumb metacarpal remains adducted.

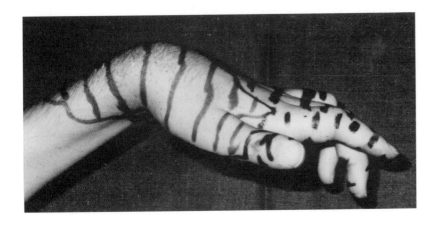

Fig. 17.16 Supracondylar fracture in an 8-year-old boy was complicated by ischaemic contracture of the flexor muscles of the forearm. The brachial artery was not damaged. The median, radial and ulnar nerves were afflicted by compression and by ischaemia. These recovered after decompression.

With a suprasystolic cuff in place an incision is made along the ulnar border of the forearm and lower arm from the wrist to above the elbow. The ulnar and median nerves are traced at the elbow, and the brachial artery is seen. The ulnar nerve is decompressed where it enters the cubital tunnel and dives deep to the flexor carpi ulnaris. The plane of dissection is from the ulnar border, starting distally, displaying the interosseous membrane. The flexor muscles are released from the ulna and radius. The anterior interosseous nerve and vessels are preserved. At the proximal end of the incision the ulnar nerve is transposed forward, whilst detaching the superficial flexor origin from the medial epicondyle of the humerus. The whole muscular mass displaces distally. Full correction of the deformity is achieved, but it is important to release the origin of flexor pollicus longus and flexor digitorum superficialis from their radial insertion by subperiosteal dissection; at times, detachment of pronator quadratus from the ulna is also necessary. After release of the cuff and haemostasis, the skin is closed and the forearm and hand are immobilised in a position of extension of wrist and digits. An indwelling catheter to permit the infusion of local anaesthetic, placed adjacent to the median and ulnar nerves in the arm, is useful to diminish postoperative pain. The splint is removed at 6 weeks, when a resting or night splint is reapplied in between periods of passive and active use of the wrist and of the digits (Figs 17.17 to 17.20).

This is an extremely valuable operation because it permits display of the artery and the nerve trunks, and preserves any vestigial muscular function. We think it preferable to excision of the flexor muscles, and far preferable to the operation of excision arthrodesis of the wrist joint. Excision of the infarcted flexor muscles is reserved for the most severe cases, as a prelude to musculotendinous or free muscle transfer.

SERIAL SPLINTING

Sister Evelyn Hunter RGN, Miss J. Laverty MCSP and Donal Brooks have developed, over a number of years, an extremely useful technique for the treatment of fixed deformities throughout the upper limb, notably for those at the elbow, the wrist and in the digits. Wynn Parry and his colleagues, first at RAF Chessington and later at the Royal National Orthopaedic Hospital, used similar techniques, achieving excellent results (Wynn Parry 1981). Carefully moulded plaster of Paris splints are applied and bandaged into position. After a few days the joints are stretched and new splints are fashioned. The technique demands a very high level of skill in the safe application of plaster of Paris splints, often onto insensitive and atrophic skin. However, it has successfully corrected many deformities of the upper limb without recourse to surgery, including the common and vexing deformity of flexion of the proximal interphalangeal joints. Seventy-nine cases of flexion deformity of proximal interphalangeal joints were treated. The mean deformity before treatment was 85°; after treatment this was reduced to 15°. The mean range of active movement achieved was in the range 15–110°. The duration of treatment ranged from 1 to 42 sessions; on average, six plaster changes were necessary; the time taken to achieve the result was 42 days (Figs 17.21 to 17.24).

METHODS OF ACTIVE RECONSTRUCTION

The priorities in reconstruction are (Moberg 1975), in order, restoration of:

- stability of the scapula
- rotation at the shoulder
- flexion at the elbow
- extension of the wrist
- perhaps most important of all, opposition or prehensile grip between the thumb and tips of the fingers, that is between the "eyes of the hand".

We think that, in the lower limb, the priorities are:

- a stable hip
- extension of the knee
- dorsiflexion of the ankle
- a balanced, supple, plantigrade foot.

THE UPPER LIMB

The shoulder girdle

There is a changing perception of the importance of this complex of joints from a better understanding of the great importance of the spinal accessory nerve and the nerve to the serratus anterior, and the relative contribution to function from the suprascapular nerve and rotator cuff. Bonnel (1989) estimated that no less than one-quarter of the fibres within the brachial plexus passed to the shoulder girdle. On the whole, muscle transfers to restore scapular and glenohumeral control in adults are disappointing. Comtet et al (1993) discussed control of the scapula, showing that the upper fibres of trapezius and the lower fibres of serratus are critical. They further showed that deltoid cannot elevate the shoulder unless the supra- and infraspinatus are innervated and not torn. Narakas (1993c) analysed shoulder function after different patterns of injury; he proposed measurement of the scapulo-humeral angle as a measure of abduction. This is least after damage to the suprascapular nerve or rotator cuff; it is equally poor when circumflex nerve palsy is associated with either of these.

In the following we outline some procedures that we have found useful when nerve repairs have failed.

Figs 17.17 to 17.19 Flexor muscle slide.

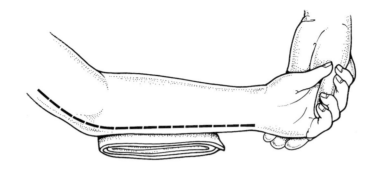

Fig. 17.17 The incision.

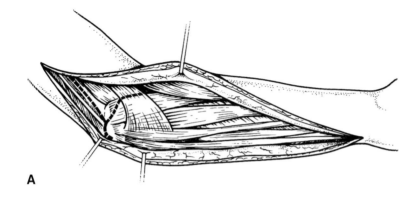

A

Fig. 17.18 (A) The flexor origin is defined. (B) Detachment of flexor muscles and transposition of the ulnar nerve.

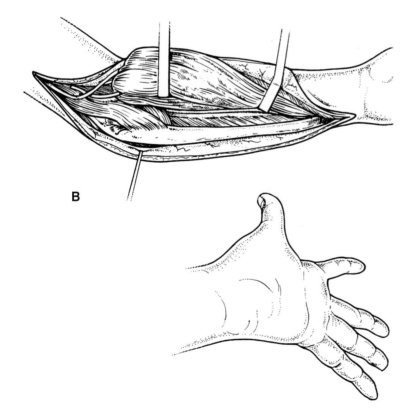

B

Fig. 17.19 The flexor muscle mass elevated from its origin, together with the ulnar, median and anterior interosseous nerves, with the radius, ulnar, and interosseous membrane behind. Full correction of the hand deformity should be obtained.

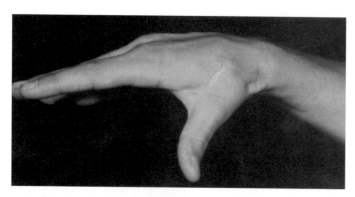
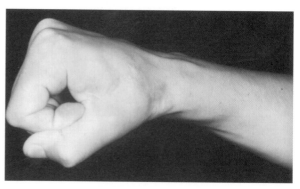

Fig. 17.20 A salutary tale. A 9-year-old boy sustained a fracture of the distal humerus, which was treated by complete above-elbow plaster of Paris splint. There was entrapment of the brachial artery and median nerve within the fracture. The ischaemic contracture of the forearm flexor muscles required a Scaglietti release; the contracture of the small muscles of the hand was corrected by a series of operations, including Littler's release and release of the deep origin of the adductor pollicis slide of the first dorsal interosseous and Z-plasty of the thumb web space. Neurological recovery was good. The hand shown at the age of 14 years.

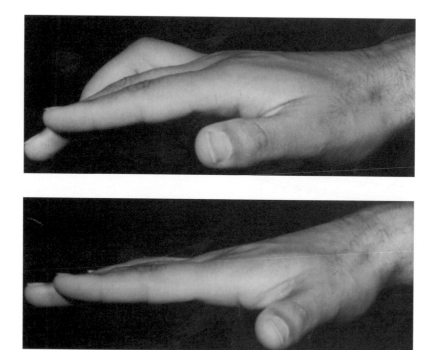

Fig. 17.21 Fixed flexion deformity of the proximal interphalangeal joint following fracture. A full range of movements was restored after three treatments with serial splinting.

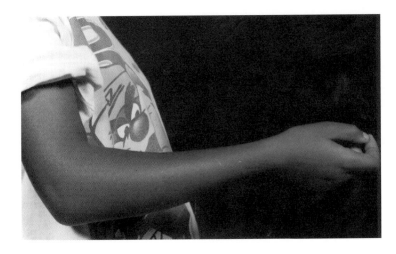

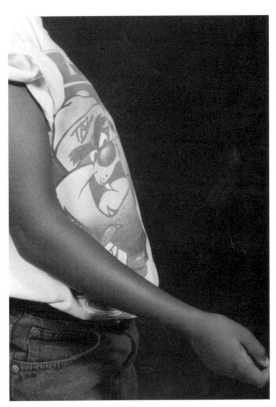

Fig. 17.22 A 10-year-old girl with 75° flexion deformity at the elbow from a birth lesion of the brachial plexus was treated four times with serial splinting. The deformity was reduced to 30°. Full flexion was maintained.

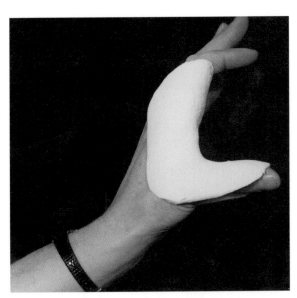

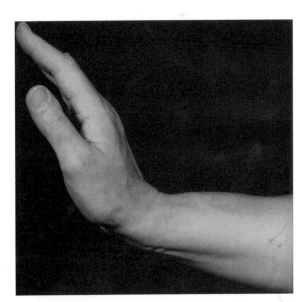

Fig. 17.23 The thumb web space splint used to treat stiffness after operations for Dupuytren's contracture in a 45-year-old woman.

Fig. 17.24 Restoration of active extension after six treatments with serial splinting in a 42-year-old woman presenting with a 70° flexion deformity of the wrist complicating a fracture of the forearm.

Transfer of the levator scapulae and rhomboids for paralysis of trapezius (Eden 1924, Lange 1951)

The patient is prone. Through an incision one finger's breadth medial to the vertebral margin of the scapula, the paralysed trapezius is detached to expose the levator scapulae and rhomboids. These are defined and mobilised, taking care for the dorsal scapular nerve. The muscles are detached with an osteoperiosteal flap, respecting the insertion of serratus. The rhomboids are advanced by about 3 cm deep to the infraspinatus and sutured to the scapula (Figs 17.25 and 17.26).

The second incision exposes the trapezius insertion to the spine of the scapula: the levator scapulae is brought into this wound by a tunnel deep to the trapezius and sutured to the outer margin of the spine. The supraspinatus muscle and suprascapular nerve must be protected. The trapezius and infraspinatus are securely reattached and the limb immobilised in a spica with the shoulder at 90° abduction for 6 weeks. Then, an abduction bolster is supplied. Passive and active movements of the glenohumeral joint are encouraged. At 9 weeks a broad arm sling is worn and gentle active elevation and protraction of the scapula is introduced.

Our results, from five cases, are at best moderate; these patients were in pain from the original injury to the accessory nerve; they had developed significant capsulitis of the shoulder. Bigliani et al (1985) found good results with pain relief in six of seven cases.

Transfer of the sternal portion of pectoralis major for paralysis of serratus anterior (Féry & Sommelet 1987)

This is a useful operation in the treatment of the irretrievably paralysed serratus anterior and it does seem to ease the pain from the unstable scapula more reliably than the operation described above for trapezius palsy. The patient is supine. The pectoralis major is exposed through a deltopectoral incision. The plane between the sternal and clavicular portion is defined and separated, respecting the medial pectoral neurovascular pedicle. The tendon of the sternal portions is the deepest of the three laminae and it is detached from the humerus. Now, through an incision in the midaxillary line, the scapula is exposed anterior to the thoracodorsal pedicle. The bone is brought into the wound by a stout suture. A capacious tunnel in the axillary fascia is prepared so that the sternal pectoralis major glides easily over pectoralis minor and ribs. It is sutured to the lower pole of the scapula. The arm is immobilised across the chest for 6 weeks (Figs 17.27 and 17.28). Passive and active abduction to about 40° with lateral rotation to neutral is then begun, and at 9 weeks from operation a more vigorous programme is followed with the aim of restoring full range of abduction and lateral rotation by 12 weeks. At 12 weeks vigorous resisted work can begin. Little is written about the outcome of this operation. Narakas (1993c) found some improvement in five cases after various muscle transfers for paralysis of serratus anterior. Seven from eight of our patients reported

Figs 17.25 and 17.26 Muscle transfer for trapezius paralysis.

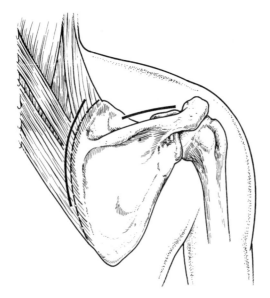

Fig. 17.25 The incisions.

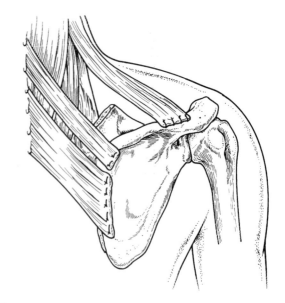

Fig. 17.26 The levator scapulae and rhomboid muscles reinserted.

Figs 17.27 and 17.28 Pectoralis major transfer for serratus palsy.

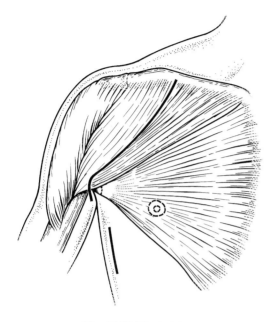

Fig. 17.27 The incisions.

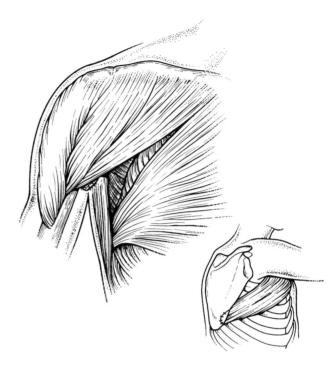

Fig. 17.28 The sternal head is inserted from the humerus, and sutured on to the inferior pole of the scapula.

improvement of function and some relief of pain at about 1 year from operation. In one patient the transferred tendon was torn from its new insertion following an injury; her symptoms recurred. Reattachment of the detached muscle was possible; there was improvement.

Transfer of the latissimus dorsi for lateral rotation of shoulder

This operation (L'Episcopo & Brooklyn 1939) is useful in shoulders which are supple and when there is some activity in the deltoid muscle. It does no more than give the patient a sense of stability if the shoulder is flail.

The patient is prone. The incision starts behind the acromion and follows the posterior border of the deltoid to curve forward into the axilla over the conjoined insertion of latissimus dorsi and teres major. It is extended inferiorly along the anterior margin of the latissimus dorsi. The latissimus dorsi tendon is defined, separated from the teres major, and released from the humerus. The muscle is mobilised and the thoracodorsal pedicle, which enters it anteriorly, is preserved.

The posterior border of the deltoid is elevated, permitting display of the tendon of infraspinatus. Splitting of the overlying fibres of deltoid permits display of supraspinatus tendon, and the latissimus dorsi is passed deep to the deltoid and interwoven in both of these tendons (Figs 17.29 and 17.30).

We no longer use a plaster of Paris spica for immobilisation, but prefer an abduction bolster. This is removed at 6 weeks and gentle active lateral rotation is encouraged. By 9 weeks unrestricted active lateral rotation is permitted. Unrestricted activities follow from 12 weeks. Ross and Birch (1993) reviewed 22 of our cases. Two-thirds of them found an improved sense of stability in the shoulder, one-half regained active lateral rotation, and none regained useful active abduction (Fig. 17.31).

Figs 17.29 and 17.30 Latissimus dorsi transfer rotator cuff.

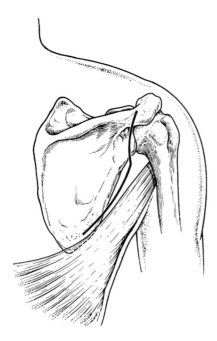

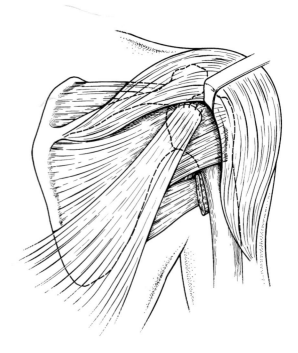

Fig. 17.29 The incision.

Fig. 17.30 The muscle inserted into the supra- and infraspinatus tendons.

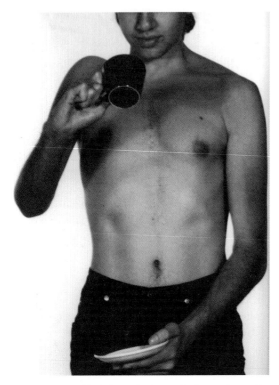

Fig. 17.31 Outcome of latissimus dorsi transfer in a patient with irreparable injury of C5 and C6. Elbow flexion was restored by Steindler flexorplasty.

Arthrodesis

Thoracoscapular arthrodesis. Fortunately, the indications for thoracoscapular arthrodesis are rare, for this operation is a trial for surgeon and patient alike. The largest experience is that of Copeland and Howard (1978), who used it with great success in the treatment of patients with scapulohumeral dystrophy. Copeland (1995c) describes the operation fully; further description is superfluous. We have used it in one case for combined palsy of the eleventh cranial nerve and the nerve to the serratus anterior (Fig. 17.32).

Glenohumeral arthrodesis. Glenohumeral arthrodesis is a time-honoured operation for the treatment of brachial plexus lesions; it has been given more importance than it deserves. It is an admission of failure for the treatment of the nerve lesion: it has the doubtful merit of according some stability to the rest of the limb by destroying the shoulder. However, there are occasions when a patient presents with such instability of the joint that arthrodesis is worthy of consideration as a method of transferring scapular function to the limb as a whole, and for the treatment of pain.

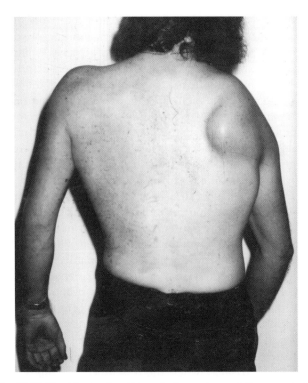

Fig. 17.32 Combined palsy of the spinal accessory and the nerve to the serratus anterior.

We agree to three indications:

- the flail shoulder causing pain because of subluxation
- the well-motivated patient who uses a prosthesis after amputation of the upper limb for complete, untreatable and irreversible paralysis
- the patient with C5/C6 or C5/C6/C7 palsy who has a useful hand, is in work, and needs a stable platform to use the hand.

The lengthy debate about the position of arthrodesis is answered simply by considering the purpose of operation – it is to enhance the function of the limb. The patient should retain or regain the grip function between the arm and the chest and should be able to bring the hand to the mouth. This gives us the desired position of 20–30° for abduction and a more or less similar angle for medial rotation and forward flexion. Copeland (1995c) uses a 10-hole pelvic reconstruction plate. Chammas et al (1995) prefer combined external and internal fixation: Nagano et al (1989a) choose external fixation alone, and theirs is a very large series. We have performed 52 arthrodeses. There was no case of sepsis; there was one failure of fusion, and one patient fractured the humerus in a subsequent fall (Figs 17.33 and 17.34).

The elbow

The number of operations described to restore elbow flexion indicates that none of them is particularly good. Alnot and colleagues (Alnot & Abols 1984, Alnot & Oberlin 1993, Alnot et al 1995) select certain transfers above others, finding the pectoralis minor, the triceps and proximal advancement of the flexor forearm muscles to be particularly useful. Sedel (personal communication) favoured pectoralis minor transfer; Narakas refined the technique of latissimus dorsi transfer.

Marshall et al (1988) reviewed 50 of our cases. Their findings are disturbing, for in less than one-half was there evidence of significant improvement of function. Five patients demonstrated a real increase in the active use of the damaged limb as a result of the operation. These cases were followed for, on average, 2–7 years. Latissimus dorsi proved the best of all transfers for range of elbow flexion, and for regaining supination. Triceps to biceps transfer achieved greatest improvement in power. Pectoralis major transfer was a disappointing operation.

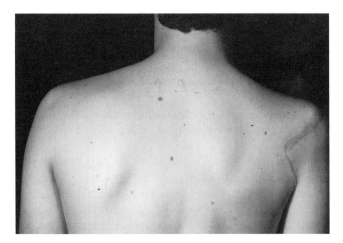
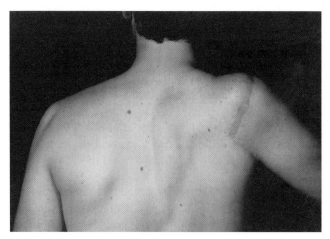

Fig. 17.33 Adduction after glenohumeral arthrodesis.

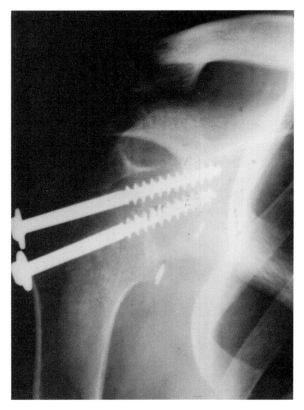

Fig. 17.34 The radiograph of the case shown in Figure 17.33.

Marshall and colleagues thought that 27 patients had a good result: elbow flexion of MRC grade 4 or better. Fourteen more had a fair result; elbow flexion MRC grade 4 with no useful shoulder stabilisation, or MRC grade 3 with shoulder stability. Eighteen patients could not lift any weight, the average was 1–2 kg. Those who achieved up to 8 kg or better had some biceps function, or had triceps to biceps transfer.

Pectoralis major transfer was described by Clark (1956) and by Brooks and Seddon (1959). They transferred the tendon into the long head of the biceps. Useful elbow flexion is the rule, but with a medial rotation posture. Dautry et al (1977) preferred transfer of virtually the whole muscle, inserting its tendon into the coracoid process and the muscle into the biceps tendon, a technique favoured by Bonney. There is, of course, loss of adduction power of the shoulder.

Pectoralis minor transfer (Lecouer 1967) is an elegant operation, and it is certainly useful in improving power of elbow flexion by at least one MRC grade. It is appropriate when elbow flexors have regained power to MRC grade 2 or 3, and it also enhances active supination.

Steindler (1918) proposed proximal advancement of the extensor origin of the forearm to the humerus, detaching a portion of bone and advancing this by up to 7 cm. Modifications of this operation have been widely practised.

Brooks elevated the flexor muscles and interwove them into the medial intermuscular septum, limiting proximal advancement to 3 cm. The operation achieves a limited range of flexion; it tends to increase pronation deformity, and I have had two cases of significant lesion of the ulnar nerve, from compression, in spite of exposing that nerve. The operation seems to have the same gain as pectoralis minor transfer, without the benefit of supination, and it should be reserved for cases in which elbow flexors reach power MRC grade 2 at least. Triceps transfer (Bunnell 1953, Carroll & Hill 1970) is undoubtedly effective, but costs most of all because of loss of active extension at elbow. The operation is indicated when there is co-contraction of the two muscles after repair of the brachial plexus if shoulder function is poor, but it should not be done when shoulder function is reasonable. Latissimus dorsi transfer (Schottstaedt et al 1955, Hovnanian 1956, Zancolli & Mitre 1973) is practised by a number of techniques. The best, and the most extensive, is to transfer the whole muscle with an overlying skin island, suturing the tendon to the coracoid or acromion, and the muscle to the biceps tendon. This is a considerable operation; it cannot be performed safely when there is much scarring within the axilla or when there has been previous damage to the axillary artery.

We suggest the following as guidance.

1. Some elbow flexion exists but it is weak; C7, C8 and T1 have recovered – pectoralis minor is the first choice; proximal advancement of the flexor muscles next.
2. The elbow flexors are completely paralysed; there is recovery through C7, C8 and T1 – bipolar transfer of latissimus dorsi with a skin island is the first choice; failing that pectoralis major transfers by the technique of Brooks and Seddon.
3. Co-contraction of triceps with biceps through lesions of C5, C6 and C7, with poor shoulder function – triceps to biceps transfer.

The operations

All of these are performed with the patient supine. Careful haemostasis and suction drainage are essential. In all the elbow is flexed at 90° for 6 weeks after operation, in a plaster of Paris splint. At 6 weeks the arm is put into a triangular sling and gentle active and passive flexion work is commenced. Active extension work is not permitted until 9 weeks have elapsed, when the arm can be set free from restraint.

Pectoralis minor transfer. The muscle is exposed through an incision inferior to the lower margin of pectoralis major, and is detached from its origin from the third to fifth ribs. The medial pectoral neurovascular bundle, which enters the superior margin of the muscle, is respected. Next, biceps muscle is exposed through an anterior incision in the upper arm and the biceps is drawn proximally by stay sutures. Pectoralis minor muscle is passed through a capacious tunnel in the axilla and sutured directly into biceps (Figs 17.35 to 17.37).

Proximal advancement of the flexor origin. The flexor origin is exposed through a posteromedial incision centred over the olecranon. The ulnar nerve is traced and the aponeurosis of the two heads of flexor carpi ulnaris is split. The flexor origin is dissected free from the medial epicondyle, the ulnar nerve is left in its normal position, and the ulnar origin of the flexor carpi ulnaris remains undisturbed. The muscle mass is advanced for 3–4 cm and interwoven into the medial intermuscular septum. If this is deficient, the flexor origin, with a piece of the medial epicondyle, must be fixed into the humerus with a screw and washer (Figs 17.38 to 17.41).

Figs 17.35 to 17.37 Pectoralis minor transfer.

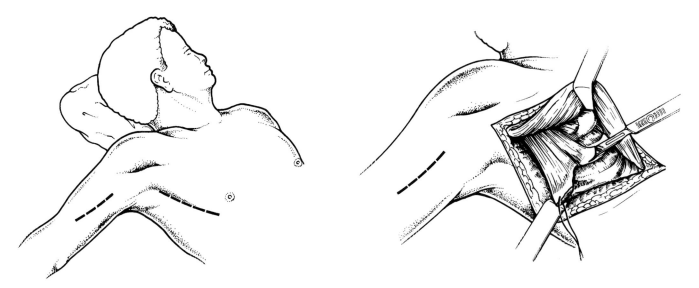

Fig. 17.35 The incisions.

Fig. 17.36 Elevation of the muscle.

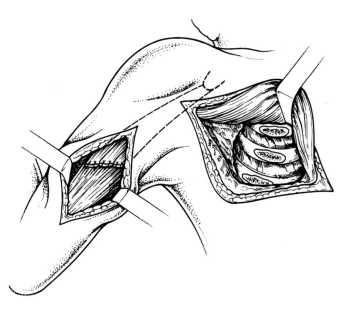

Fig. 17.37 The transferred muscle sutured directly onto the biceps belly.

Figs 17.38 to 17.41 Elbow flexorplasty.

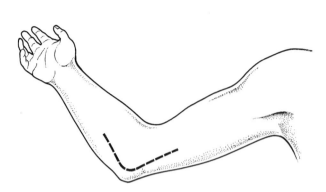

Fig. 17.38 The incision.

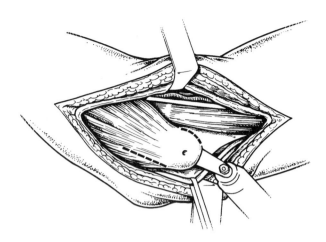

Fig. 17.39 Elevation of the flexor origin.

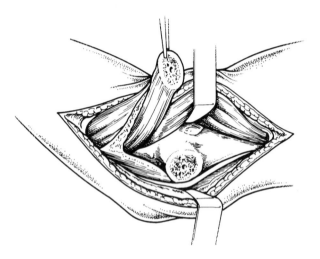

Fig. 17.40 Exposure of the anterior surface of the humerus. The ulnar nerve has been traced.

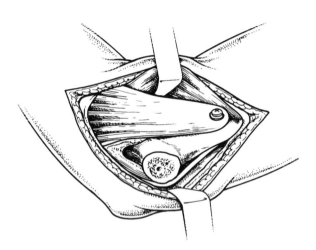

Fig. 17.41 Proximal advancement of the flexor muscles.

Pectoralis major transfer. The tendon of the muscle is exposed through a short anterior incision, it is detached and then interwoven into an interposed tendon, either the palmaris longus or a toe extensor, which is then passed subcutaneously to be sutured through biceps tendon exposed through a separate incision.

Triceps to biceps transfer. The muscle is exposed through a posterior midline incision. The ulnar and radial nerves are identified. It is not uncommon to find a motor branch passing from the ulnar nerve into the medial head of triceps. The muscle is detached with a strip of periosteum

from the olecranon and mobilised to the midportion of the arm. A wide subcutaneous tunnel is fashioned on the lateral aspect of the arm, and the transferred muscle is sutured around the biceps tendon (Fig 17.42 to 17.44).

Latissimus dorsi transfer. The first incision runs along the anterior margin of the muscle, designing a skin paddle 12 cm in length and 5–6 cm wide. The thoraco-dorsal pedicle is identified and mobilised proximally; the artery to serratus anterior requires ligation and division. The appropriate length of the muscle is measured to match the interval from the coracoid process to the elbow flexor

Figs 17.42 to 17.44 Triceps to biceps transfer.

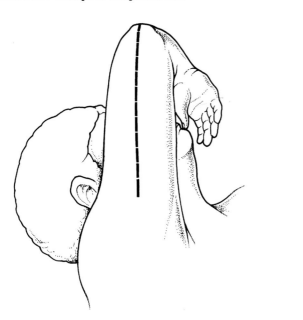

Fig. 17.42 The incision.

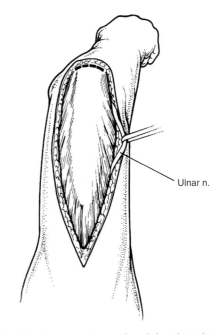

Ulnar n.

Fig. 17.43 The ulnar nerve is traced, and the triceps insertion defined.

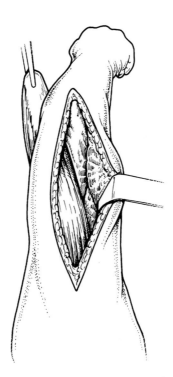

Fig. 17.44 The muscle is mobilised and passed subcutaneously about the lateral aspect of the arm.

crease, and it is then detached below and posteriorly. Next, the tendon is detached from its insertion and reinserted onto the coracoid. A lengthy incision, from the coracoid down the whole of the anterior aspect of the arm, is prepared and the muscle laid in this, suturing it to the biceps tendon distally and suturing the skin flap into position (Figs 17.45 to 17.48).

Elbow extension

Moberg (1975) emphasised the potential for valuable reconstruction in tetraplegics with sparing of C5 and C6. These are patients who have good control of the shoulder, flexion of the elbow and extension of the wrist, and, perhaps most important of all, good sensation in the thumb and the index and middle fingers. Moberg, together with Lamb (Moberg & Lamb 1980), clarified priorities in reconstruction, pointing out the benefit of active extension of the elbow and showing that this should take priority over tendon transfers within the hand. Lamb (1987b) describes in detail the operation of transfer of the posterior one-third of the deltoid to permit active extension of the elbow. We have followed his technique on three occasions. All three patients regained full active extension of the elbow against gravity, and one of them, who had a mild hyperextension posture of the elbow, was able to transfer from bed to chair. On two occasions we have used latissimus dorsi transfer for elbow extension in patients with injuries to the brachial plexus. The results were not impressive.

Figs 17.45 to 17.48 Latissimus dorsi transfer.

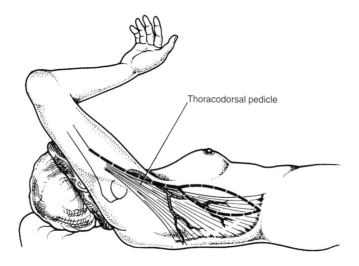

Fig. 17.45 The skin incision with skin paddle.

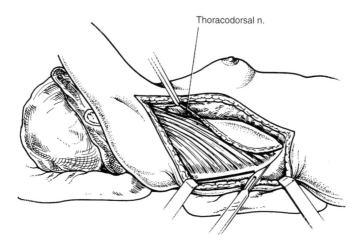

Fig. 17.46 The nerve and vessel to the latissimus dorsi are defined, and the muscle released from its origin.

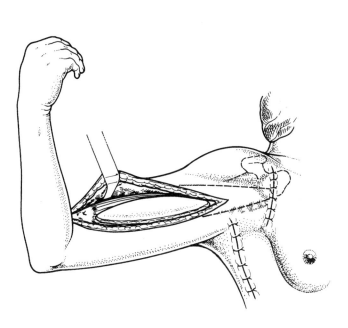

Fig. 17.47 Rerouting of the muscle with a skin paddle.

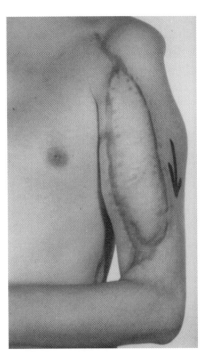

Fig. 17.48 Transfer in a 24-year-old man with a C5/C6 lesion. The range of elbow flexion was 0–130°; he was able to lift a weight of 2.5 kg.

The wrist and hand

Boyes (1960) recognised no less than 58 different operations to restore extension of wrist and of the digits. To Jones (1916) goes the credit for the idea of using pronator teres (PT) for wrist extension, and to Zachary (1946) that for recognising the importance of keeping at least one wrist flexor (Fig. 17.49). We condemn arthrodesis of the wrist, for this abolishes the function gained from the "tenodesis effect". The reader can demonstrate this quite simply by noting the posture of the fingers when their wrist is passively dorsiflexed and then permitted to drop

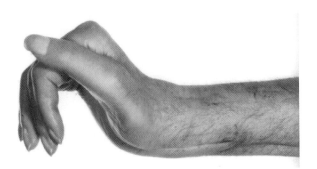

Fig. 17.49 Hyperextension deformity of the wrist after transfer of the sole remaining wrist flexor, flexor carpi radialis, in a patient with brachial plexus injury.

into palmar flexion. It is an operation of last resort. Napier (1955) showed that in full palmar flexion the power of grip is 25% of the best achieved when the wrist is extended. As Tubiana (1993b) points out, most wrists work in a position of semipronation, and there is a synergy between the radial wrist extensors (the extensor carpi radialis longus (ECRL) and extensor carpi radialis brevis (ECRB)) and the flexor carpi ulnaris (FCU). The extensor carpi ulnaris is the partner of the abductor pollicis longus (APL) and extensor pollicis longus (EPL). Merle d'Aubigné developed a technique similar to that used by British surgeons in which the PT was transferred to the wrist extensors, the FCU to the digital extensors, including the extensor pollicis longus and either the palmaris longus or one flexor digitorum superficialis to the APL and extensor pollicis brevis (EPB). He and Ramadier (1956) reviewed a series of these operations.

We favour a transfer of three muscles when there is complete paralysis of the forearm extensors. For wrist extension PT to ECRB is preferred; on occasion the brachioradialis or one of the wrist flexors will replace PT. Next, either the flexor carpi ulnaris or the flexor carpi radialis is transferred to extensor digitorum communis (EDC) and EPL. Last, a muscle must be transferred to the metacarpal of the thumb, in order to enhance its abduction and anteposition. The palmaris longus or one flexor digitorum superficialis (FDS) muscle, preferably that to the ring finger, is used for this. As a second string we use FDS for all the digital extensors, as proposed by Boyes and later modified by Brooks.

There are theoretical disadvantages in using FCU. It is the most powerful of the wrist flexors and it is responsible for powerful ulnar deviation, such as in holding a hammer (Fig. 17.50).

The operation

The patient lies supine. There are four incisions: the first in the middle of the anterior aspect of the forearm for display of pronator teres and the muscle belly of FCR; next, a short incision is made between the tendons of the PL and flexor carpi radialis (FCR); then, an incision is made on the dorsum proximal to the extensor retinaculum for display of the EDC and EPL tendons; and, finally, a short incision exposes the tendons of APL and EPB (Figs 17.51 and 17.52).

The pronator teres is detached from the radius, taking a strip of periosteum, and then interwoven into the tendon of ECRB. It may be passed either superficial or deep to BR, whichever seems easier. The tendon of FCR is cut at the wrist, and its muscle belly is withdrawn into the wound of the forearm and tunnelled subcutaneously to be interwoven into the tendons of EDC and EPL, which are held on stay sutures to permit a balance in tension. Lastly, the tendon of APL is sectioned at its junction with the muscle; traction on it indicates the extent of abduction of the thumb metacarpal. If this is limited, or if the metacarpophalangeal joint remains in flexion, then the tendon of EPB is similarly cut and the palmaris longus interwoven into these.

At 3 weeks this plaster is removed and a light supporting splint is applied, to be worn for a further 3 weeks, during which time active exercises are commenced. Passive stretching of the wrist or digits into flexion is forbidden for the first 6 weeks (Fig. 17.53).

If the flexor carpi ulnaris is chosen, an additional incision is required over the ulnar border of the forearm, and the muscle is released from its origin before subcutaneous passage to the dorsal forearm (Figs 17.54 and 17.55).

In cases of C5/C6/C7 lesion, pronator teres and the wrist flexors will be weak or paralysed and are not available. In these cases we use flexor digitorum superficialis (FDS). The tendons are identified through a short incision proximal to the carpal tunnel, drawn into the wound, and sectioned. These are mobilised proximally, separating those to the little and ring fingers from those to the middle and index fingers. The former group is passed through a subcutaneous tunnel around the ulna, and the latter passed similarly around the radial border, and interwoven through all four tendons of EDC and EPL. This operation does not achieve active extension of the wrist; rather there is a pulling upwards of the wrist from digital extension. It does not address the problem of control of the metacarpal of the thumb.

Dunnet et al (1995) reviewed 49 of our cases (22 for radial palsy, 27 for brachial plexus lesions). Forty-one were improved. There had been a subclavian or axillary arterial lesion in four of the eight failures. More than two-thirds of the patients reported impaired coordination and dexterity; over four-fifths cited loss of endurance. The average power of wrist extension was 22%, that of digital extension was 31% and power grip was 40% of normal. FCU was used in 14 cases and FCR in 12. Power grip was close to 50% with FCU; it was 35%, on average, with FCR. There was no difference in the range of ulnar and radial deviation irrespective of which wrist flexor was used. After all, it seems that FCU is the better of the two.

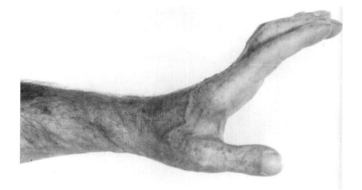
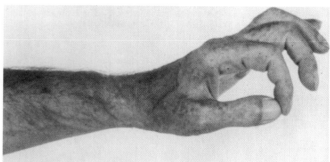

Fig. 17.50 A 51-year-old man with radial palsy. FCU, PT and PL transfer. This unusually good result is, in part, explained by unexpected recovery through the lesion of the nerve.

Figs 17.51 to 17.55 Flexor to extensor transfer.

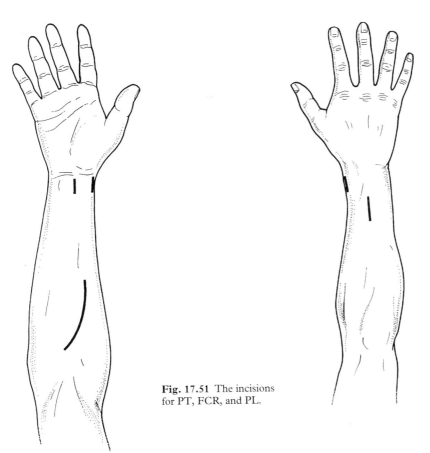

Fig. 17.51 The incisions for PT, FCR, and PL.

Fig. 17.52 The incisions to expose two extensor tendons to the thumb and fingers and the APL.

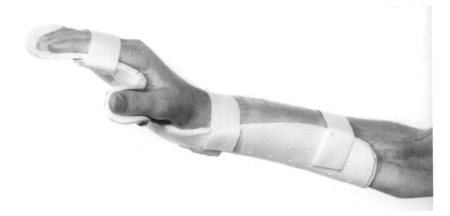

Fig. 17.53 The resting splint introduced at 3 weeks after flexor to extensor transfer.

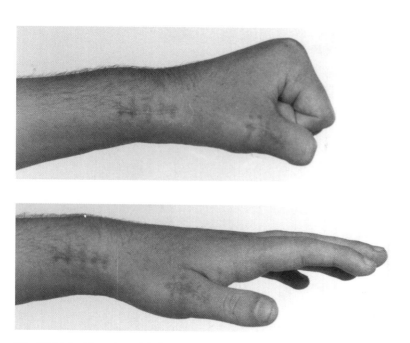

Fig. 17.54 In this patient with C5/C6/C7 lesion, no muscle was available for wrist extension. The flexor carpi ulnaris was transferred to extensors of the fingers and thumb and the palmaris longus to the extensor pollicis brevis.

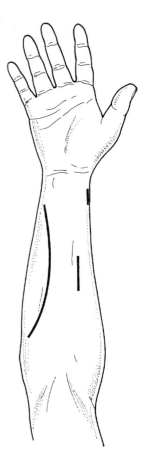

Fig. 17.55 The incisions for FCU, PT, and APL.

Paralysis of the flexor muscles of the forearm and the intrinsic muscles of the hand with preservation of the extensor muscles

This is a common problem in reconstruction, and there are significant differences between the different groups presenting in this situation. The tetraplegic, with sparing of C5 and C6, has no digital extension, but good sensation in the thumb and index and middle fingers. This pattern is similar to that following irreparable injury of C7, C8 and D1.

When the lower trunk or medial cord is afflicted there is preservation of digital extensors and of the pronator teres and flexor carpi radialis. The defect from a combined median and ulnar nerve lesion is a good deal worse, because in these patients sensation throughout the greater part of the hand is absent.

Judicious use of the available muscles can restore a useful grasp and, very much more importantly, restore prehensile grip between the thumb and sensate fingers. The key to success is active wrist extension: *extensor carpi radialis*

brevis must be preserved. Brachioradialis is useful for transfer, but only when the elbow is stable, for its action is dissipated in paralysis of triceps. When the biceps is paralysed it will, if transferred, be required to mediate two actions.

No two cases are the same, and each patient requires careful thought about the desired aim and, in particular, careful assessment of the power of the muscles available. Simple splints, modelled in different degrees of opposition or antepulsion, are useful to determine the best position for the thumb. If it seems that stabilisation of the joint is necessary, then this can be tried by passage of a Kirschner wire, allowing the patient to use the hand for a few days to test it out before proceeding to definitive arthrodesis.

Tetraplegia with C5/C6 sparing

The upper limb in such cases has as much in common with that seen in patients with preserved C5 and C6, but loss of the rest, after injuries to the brachial plexus. Those patients with intact 5th and 6th cervical nerves, as opposed to 5th and 6th spinal segments, often have some elbow extension, albeit weak, and some function in the flexor carpi radialis. We follow the programme developed by Lamb in these cases, acknowledging his insistence that some active extension of the elbow must be regained before brachioradialis is used (Lamb 1987b). ECRL is transferred anteriorly and interwoven into the flexor digitorum profundus tendons. FPL tendon is divided at its musculotendinus junction and buttonholed into the profundus tendon. Tension is important in this operation; the interphalangeal joint of the thumb must not be unduly flexed. With the wrist in neutral, the tips of the fingers should come to about 3 cm from the palm. With the wrist extended they come into the palm, and in that posture the tip of the thumb rests against the lateral border of the index finger. When the wrist is flexed, all digits extend fully (Brooks 1984a) (Figs 17.56 to 17.58).

High median palsy

The ECRL is used to restore power to the flexor digitorum profundus, the brachioradialis is available for the flexor pollicis longus and the extensor indicis is mobilised into the distal part of the forearm and then passed anteriorly to wind around the tendon of the flexor carpi radialis before insertion into the tendon of abductor pollicis brevis (Figs 17.59 to 17.61).

High ulnar palsy

Improving power of flexion of the little and ring fingers is a fairly straightforward matter; the tendons to these digits can be interwoven into the adjacent ones. Two problems remain. First is restoration of flexion of the metacarpophalangeal joints; next, improvement of control of the thumb. We have already seen that the one muscle consistently innervated by the median nerve in the hand is the

---

Figs 17.56 to 17.58 High median transfer.

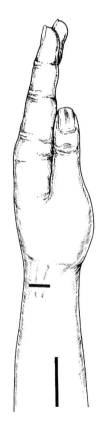 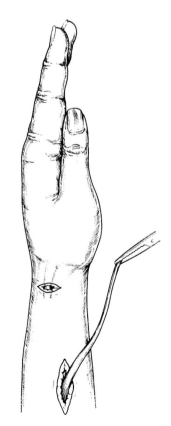 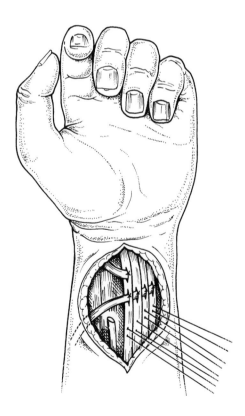

Fig. 17.56 The incisions.

Fig. 17.57 Elevation of the ECRL.

Fig. 17.58 The ECRL is passed through the FDP tendons; the FPL is buttonholed. Note the posture of the tips of the fingers and thumb.

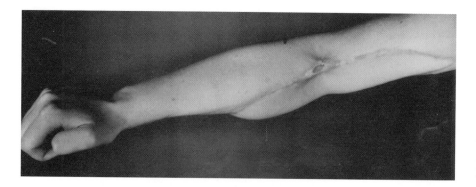

Fig. 17.59 A 28-year-old woman suffered a gunshot wound to the elbow, destroying the brachial artery and median nerve. The artery was repaired by reverse vein graft, and Professor Roy Sanders secured skin cover with a free latissimus myocutaneous flap. High median transfer was performed at 6 months.

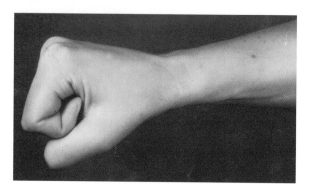

Fig. 17.60 The hand in flexion.

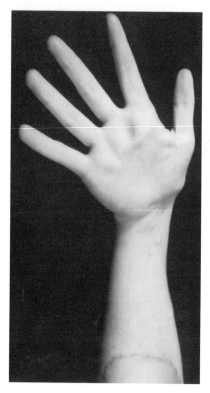

Fig. 17.61 The hand in extension.

abductor pollicis brevis, but that there is an overlap with the ulnar nerve in 50% of cases for the flexor pollicis brevis and opponens pollicis. The defect lies in the pinch grip between the thumb and the index fingers, because of paralysis of adductor pollicis (the most powerful of all the intrinsic muscles of the hand) and the first dorsal interosseous.

There are two useful ways of restoring active flexion of the metacarpophalangeal joints of the fingers. We like Brand's transfer, in which the extensor carpi radialis is detached, extended by tendon graft and divided into four slips, which are passed through the lumbrical canals, anterior to the deep transverse metacarpal ligament, to be inserted by interweaving suture into the interosseous hood. For the little, ring and middle fingers the tendon slip is passed on the radial side; for the index finger it is passed on the ulnar side. This transfer seems particularly suited to the supple, flexible hand (Figs 17.62 to 17.64). Zancolli's dynamic lasso procedure is more suitable for the strong, rather stiff hand (Zancolli 1957). In this operation metacarpophalangeal flexion is restored by cutting the tendons of the FDS and looping them through the flexor sheath.

We are then left with the thumb. The best operation that we have seen for restoration of pinch grip between the thumb and index finger is that developed by our colleague Mr David Evans FRCS (van der Molen & Evans 1996). The extensor indicis tendon is detached from its insertion, passed deep to the index metacarpal along the line of adductor pollicis and sutured into the insertion of that tendon. One slip of abductor pollicis longus is extended by a tendon graft to the insertion of the first dorsal interosseous muscle (Fig. 17.65).

Combined high ulnar and median paralysis

Reconstruction in these patients presents a difficult problem because there is so often poor sensation throughout the hand. The aims of operation include restoration of grasp between the thumb and the index finger. For this,

Figs 17.62 to 17.64 Transfer for intrinsic paralysis.

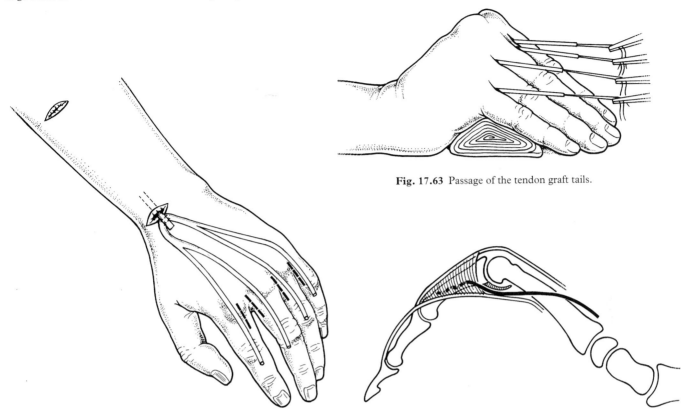

Fig. 17.63 Passage of the tendon graft tails.

Fig. 17.62 The ECRL is detached, mobilised and extended by a four-tailed tendon graft.

Fig. 17.64 The direction and method of insertion of the tails of the tendon graft.

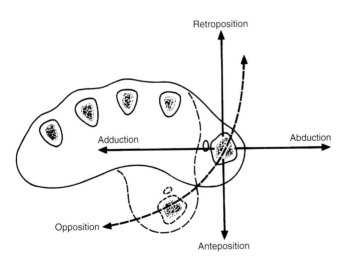

Fig. 17.65 Position of the thumb. (After Tubiana (1993a).)

both the ECRL and BR are available. It is always desirable to improve the posture of the thumb metacarpal, and the extensor indicis is useful for this.

The paralysed thumb

It is beyond our scope to discuss in detail the various techniques of restoring function into the hand. However, patients with lesions of the lower trunk, of C8 and T1, or some cases of hereditary sensorimotor neuropathy present real difficulties because of the complete paralysis of intrinsic and extensor muscles of the thumb, yet that digit retains worthwhile sensation. Bunnell (1938) stated two principles that are useful in considering such patients. The metacarpophalangeal joint of the thumb must be stable, and the thumb itself taken out from its position of supination. Arthrodesis of the metacarpophalangeal joint is sometimes indicated, particularly in cases where the passive range is limited. It may be worthwhile stabilising this joint and the interphalangeal joint of the thumb, using the silastic pegs developed by Nicolle. The position of the metacarpophalangeal joint should certainly not be more than 30° of flexion, preferably less: the interphalangeal joint should not be flexed to more than 15°. The surgeon then has muscles such as the brachioradialis or flexor carpi radialis available to restore extension and opposition of the thumb metacarpal, so that the carpometacarpal joint can be moved. Tubiana and McCullough (1984) and Tubiana (1993b) discuss the problem of the paralysed hand, and operations to relieve these problems, refreshingly: Merle et al (1993) consider the particularly perplexing problem of the hand in brachial plexus lesions.

THE LOWER LIMB

The extensive literature about reconstruction in the upper limb should not obscure the fact that the principles of all of this work arose from early attempts to treat the deformed lower limb. It may be that the decline of poliomyelitis in countries with large numbers of orthopaedic surgeons has something to do with this, but it is surprising that, whereas there are so many – perhaps too many – operations for reconstruction in the upper limb, there are possibly too few in the lower limb. We remain surprised to see the numbers of patients with paralytic deformities of the ankle and foot, the knee, and the hip for whom nothing has been proposed. Yet, nowhere else does skilfully performed appropriate intervention bring about such benefit. The ability to cross a road or go upstairs is an important function. We might reflect that one of the disadvantages of the welcome strength of the discipline of hand surgery is that it has turned away from its roots at a time when there is undoubted increase in nerve injuries of bad prognosis in the lower limb from road traffic accidents, missile wounds and, it must be said, from intraoperative damage to trunk nerves.

We shall discuss three aspects of lower limb deformity in adults. The first flaws from inadequacy of the abductors of the hip; the next from the extensors of the knee; and lastly those relating to the ankle and foot from partial lesions of the sciatic nerve.

The hip

Sharrard (1971) described transfer of the iliopsoas to secure location of the hip joint in children with spina bifida. The operation is an extensive one, but we have had occasion to use it in three young adults who had suffered iatropathic injury to the sciatic and gluteal nerves during the course of operations for hip dysplasia. All three experienced relief of pain, and described a sensation of improvement in gait, but in none could we demonstrate abduction of the hip against gravity, even at 1 year from the transfer.

The operation, which is a considerable one, is described at length in Sharrard's work. The elements of the operation include: detachment of the iliopsoas tendon with a piece of the lesser trochanter; mobilisation of this muscle, which is passed deep and lateral to the femoral nerve; transfer of the muscle mass through a large hole in the ilium; and then suture of the iliopsoas tendon through a tunnel fashioned in the greater trochanter of the hip. The hip must be protected in a spica for 12 weeks. After that, active weight bearing is encouraged, and in particular strengthening of hip flexion and hip abduction is taught.

The knee

It was common experience in times when poliomyelitis was common to see children and young adults walking quite well even though their quadriceps muscles were paralysed. Of course they did this by a form of adaptation, a trick movement, in which the tensor fascia lata was responsible for stabilisation of the knee. In many cases there was the added factor of a hyperextension deformity at the knee. It is, however, quite wrong to assume that an adult with a deep femoral nerve lesion can walk comfortably and without risk. In three of our cases of damage to the femoral nerve done during the course of operations for replacement of the hip, the lesion was brought to the attention of those concerned when the patients fell and damaged themselves, Ober (1933) and Herndon (1961) suggested transfer of muscles to restore active extension of the knee. Our technique is drawn from that proposed by Herndon (1961) and Clark (1956).

Anterior transfer of hamstrings for paralysis of knee extensors

There are two essential requirements. There must be no flexion deformity of the knee and the hamstring muscles must be of full power. As with other operations in the lower limb, the transferred muscles must work against gravity during weight bearing, and those innervated by nerves damaged in one way or another are always inadequate.

The patient lies supine. Two separate incisions are made over the biceps and semitendinosus tendons; it is advisable to trace the common peroneal nerve. The tendons are detached from their insertion and mobilised to the middle thigh, preserving the neurovascular pedicles. A large window is made in the lateral intermuscular septum for the passage of the biceps tendon; on the medial side the passage is subcutaneous, and the tendons are interwoven through the quadriceps tendon, through the retinaculum of the patella, and then sutured end to end beneath its lower pole. The tension of the transfer is such that when the lower limb is lifted from the operating table the knee drops into no more than 30° of flexion (Fig. 17.66). The limb is immobilised in a plaster of Paris cylinder for 6 weeks. The patient is encouraged to mimic quadriceps

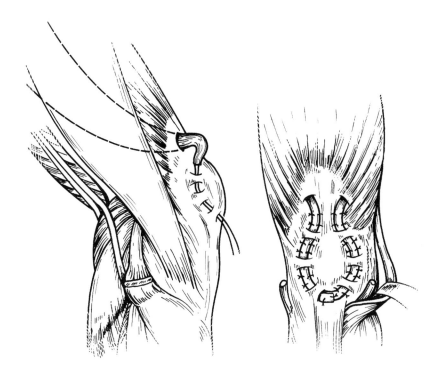

Fig. 17.66 Hamstring transfer for paralysis of the quadriceps muscle.

action during this time, but weight bearing is not permitted. At 6 weeks the plaster is removed, and a new splint applied holding the limb in full extension of the knee. This is retained for a further 6 weeks with periods of 1–2 hours in every day of active flexion to no more than 30° at the knee, with encouragement to active extension. This work is done with the patient standing; it should not be attempted against gravity. The process of retraining is helped by work in a swimming pool. At 3 months the resting splint is abandoned and the patient then goes into a simple knee splint which limits flexion to about 45°, and this should be retained for a further 3 months. By 6 months all restraints are cast aside.

We have performed this operation in six patients. Five regained active extension to the neutral position and were able to walk unencumbered and climb stairs without undue difficulty. In one patient the operation was a failure. The injury to the anterior compartment of the thigh had damaged the medial hamstrings also and only the biceps femoris was available for transfer. Schwartzman and Crego (1948) reviewed 134 cases. These patients had paralysis from poliomyelitis. They noted that transfer of biceps femoris alone resulted in a significant rate of lateral displacement of the patella. It seems that in adult patients, who do not have joint laxity, the risk of a hyperextension deformity when the semimembranosus is left undisturbed is minimal.

Foot and ankle: the dropped foot from common peroneal palsy

There have been two themes of treatment for this disorder. The first is by arthrodesis, triple arthrodesis or the more elegant operation of Lambrinudi (1927). *It is very important to remember that no arthrodesis should ever be performed in the growing limb unless the muscular imbalance provoking that deformity has been corrected.* Lambrinudi's operation is technically very difficult to do, and that is perhaps the reason why it seems to have fallen out of favour. When the operation was done in the young it was often followed by degenerative changes in the ankle. Seddon did this operation with mathematical precision: there was a significant failure rate. Those who did it less precisely but smashed the bone up more had a better success rate. Angus and Cowell (1986) followed a number of triple arthrodeses over an average period of 13 years. There were a large number of unsatisfactory results, with over half having persisting residual deformity, 22% with pseudoarthrosis and 25% of patients in continuing pain. Not all of these operations were performed for lesions of the common peroneal nerve. The idea of restoring active dorsiflexion comes from Ober (1933), who recommended forward transfer of the tibialis posterior muscle by a superficial route. Watkins et al (1954) reviewed 25 cases where Putti's idea of transferring the muscle through the interosseous membrane had been used, finding good results in

17 of 25 cases. Turner and Cooper (1972) and Lipscomb and Sanchez (1961) reported with guarded optimism. We have used this operation in 51 cases and follow a technique developed from that of Adams (1980), who advised suturing the transferred tibialis tendon to the peroneus tertius tendon rather than into bone. A prerequisite of this operation is that there is full passive dorsiflexion of the ankle. If there is any equinus deformity, subcutaneous elongation, through three separate stab incisions, of Achilles tendon is necessary.

The patient lies supine. The tendon of the tibialis posterior is exposed by a short transverse incision over the navicular bone. It is sectioned here. Next, the muscle belly is exposed through a posteromedial incision of about 8 cm. The tendon is drawn into this wound and the muscle mobilised from the interosseous membrane. Then an incision over the anterior aspect of the leg, lateral to the subcutaneous surface of the tibia, is made, retracting the tibialis anterior to expose the interosseous membrane, protecting the neurovascular bundle. A wide window is made in the interosseous membrane and, under direct vision, the muscle and tendon are passed through this. The tendon is now split into two parts. Now, an incision is made over the dorsum of the foot, midway between the tendons of tibialis anterior and peroneus tertius. The transferred tendon is passed deep to the retinaculum. One portion of it is sutured into the tibialis anterior tendon and the other into the peroneus tertius, if that is of good size. In a number of cases we have found the peroneus tertius to be deficient, and in these the peroneus brevis tendon is brought across the dorsum of the foot by dividing it at its musculotendinous junction in the lateral compartment of the leg, withdrawing this through a separate wound where the tendon passes into the sole of the foot and rerouting it across the dorsum of the foot. The tibialis posterior tendon forms a "Y", with equal tension applied to the medial and lateral borders of the foot. The tension of the transfer should be such that the foot is close to the neutral position and lies in neutral balance between inversion and eversion (Figs 17.67 and 17.68).

Figs 17.67 and 17.68 The transfer for common peroneal palsy.

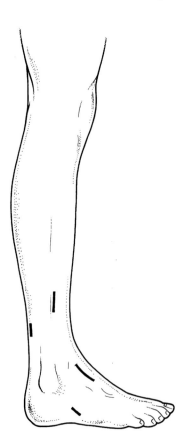

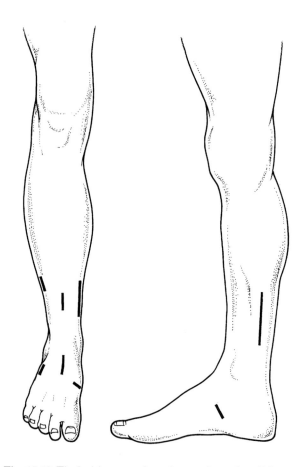

Fig. 17.67 The incisions seen from the lateral aspect.

Fig. 17.68 The incisions seen from the anterior and medial aspects.

The transfer is protected in a plaster of Paris below-knee splint for 6 weeks, during which time weight bearing is not allowed. At 6 weeks the splint is removed and the patient returns to the foot drop splint orthosis. Active exercises are started at this time but the transfer is protected for a total of 3 months.

One of us (G.B.) preferred passing the tendon of tibialis posterior through the base of the proximal tarsus, tying the sutures to a bar incorporated in the plaster.

Srinavasan et al (1968) described the two-tailed transfer of tibialis posterior for correction of drop foot in leprosy, and Richards (1989) reported on the outcome of 39 operations performed for leprosy. One tail of the transferred tendon was sutured to the extensor hallucis longus, and the other to the extensor digitorum longus and peroneus tertius. Richards recommends that the tendo-Achilles is lengthened whenever passive dorsiflexion is limited to less than 20°. He achieved active dorsiflexion to at least 10° in 17 cases. Soares (1996) transferred the tibialis posterior for foot drop deformity in 69 cases of leprosy, showing that passage of the muscle through the interosseous membrane is better than the circumtibial route. The transferred tendon is sutured into tibialis anterior and to the peroneal tendons. This is similar to the technique we favour.

The growing foot

The variety of progressive deformities seen in the growing foot is considerable and the surgeon should be alert to the need for a rebalancing operation to prevent fixed deformity of the skeleton. If this is permitted, then later bone correction by arthrodesis is unavoidable. Each case must be taken on its merit. It is as necessary to be on the watch for progressive deformity arising from transfer as it is to be on the look out for deformity produced by the initial lesion. Care to maintain a balance between eversion and inversion is essential. Calcaneus deformity is now uncommon, but we have seen cases of it in children with damage to the tibial division of the sciatic nerve and we have found the operation of posterior transfer of tibialis anterior (Herndon et al 1956) to be valuable. Once the prognosis of the nerve is known, and once it becomes apparent that a calcaneus deformity is developing, then the operation is indicated. We believe that it is important first to balance the forces of inversion and eversion before directing attention to the position of the heel.

The operation is a simple one. The tendon is divided from its insertion on the dorsum of the foot, drawn into an incision made over the lower part of the anterior aspect of the leg, and it is then passed through a window into the interosseous membrane to be interwoven into the calcaneus tendon. Tension should be such that the foot is drawn quite firmly into 30° of plantar flexion. The postoperative care is similar to that outlined for transfer of tibialis posterior (Fig. 17.69).

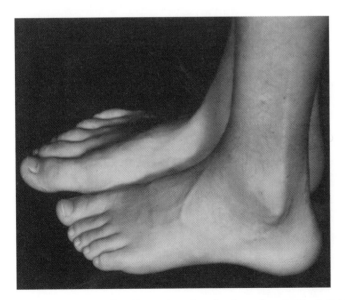
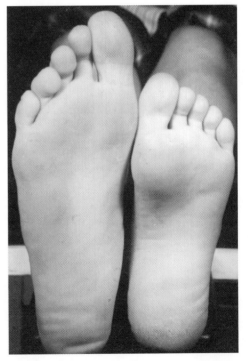

Fig. 17.69 A 5-year-old boy suffered laceration of popliteal vessels and of both divisions of the sciatic nerve at the knee. The vessels were repaired successfully. Recovery for the common peroneal division was good, but the repair of the tibial division failed. The posture of the foot is shown at age 10 years, 1 year after transfer of one-half of the peroneus brevis to the tibialis posterior and of the tibialis anterior to the Achilles tendon. Dorsiflexion was good through the long extensor tendons. Note the discrepancy in foot size.

VASCULARISED BONE AND MUSCLE TRANSFER

The development of free transfer of vascularised tissue is one of the greatest advances in the treatment of the severely damaged limb since the development of antibiotics and blood transfusion: it is, of course, the natural child of advances in vascular surgery. Some lessons and applications of what is now an enormous experience have been described in Chapters 7 and 8. The scope is so wide that we can do no more here than sketch the outlines of the application of these techniques. Two developments are particularly relevant in reconstruction. First is the free vascularised bone graft in the reconstruction of limbs. The free fibular graft was described by Taylor et al (1975). Other bone grafts were described later. Of interest to us is the occasional place for this operation in the upper limb: we touched on our experience in Birch (1987). Weiland and Russell-Moore (1988) reported 91 cases, 19 of these for severe injuries to the upper limb. Pho (1991) describes the technique. A precept of reconstructive work is stability of the skeleton, and what has become, in skillful hands, a standard and reliable operation should be remembered for the difficult case. Although improvements in understanding of fracture healing have led to increased use of bone transport, to such an extent that the technique is now rarely indicated in the lower limb, there is no doubt of its continuing validity in the upper limb (Fig. 17.70).

The next valuable technique is that of free functioning muscle transfer. The experimental foundation of this was laid by Tamai et al (1970). Harii et al (1976) performed the first free gracilis transfer for facial palsy. Surgeons in Shanghai did the first free muscle transfer for reconstruction of flexor muscles of forearm (Shanghai, 6th Peoples Hospital 1976). Ikuta et al (1976) described a number of cases in the treatment of Volkmann's contracture. Manktelow and McKee (1978) described their first two operations to restore active finger flexion. Both patients achieved good power grip, substantially better than that provided by conventional tendon transfer. The indications for and technique of operation are thoroughly reviewed by Manktelow (1988, 1993), who has a series of 98 cases. We have experience of the latissimus dorsi transfer for forearm flexor reconstruction in three cases. The latissimus dorsi was chosen because of our familiarity with it, but in fact gracilis and gastrocnemius probably provide a better range of movement. In our cases useful and powerful grip was

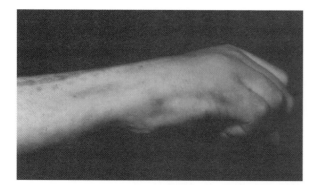

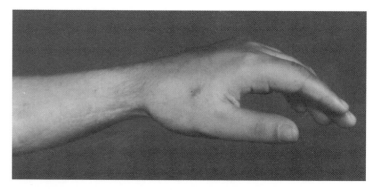

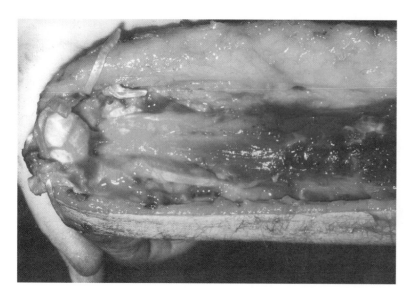

Fig. 17.70 Excision of the radius, ulna, and extensor compartment for extensive aponeurotic fibromatosis in a 9-year-old boy treated by free vascularised fibular graft and flexor to extensor transfer. The result at age 12 years.

restored, but range of digital flexion was deficient. We believe that free muscle transfer has a definite and valuable role in the treatment of the severely damaged upper limb, in which all the flexor muscles have been damaged by ischaemia or direct injury (Figs 17.71 and 17.72).

With our colleague Professor Roy Sanders, seven operations for transfer of latissimus dorsi have been done to restore active flexion of elbow in cases of brachial plexus lesion. Results are promising, but the paucity of potential motor donor nerves is a real difficulty. Akasaha et al

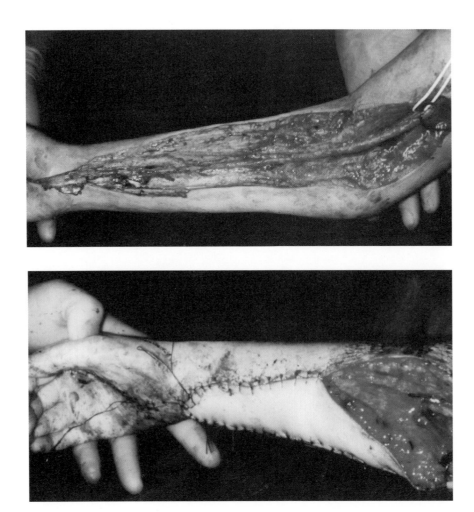

Fig. 17.71 A 31-year-old woman lay in a coma for 18 hours infarcting the whole of the flexor muscles of the forearm. The infarct was excised and replaced by free latissimus transfer. Useful power grip was gained, but the finger tips did not reach the palm.

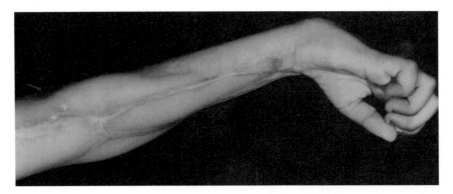

Fig. 17.72 A medial gastrocnemius free muscle transfer was used to restore flexor function in this 12-year-old boy with severe Volkmann's ischaemic contracture. There is full digital flexion, even with the wrist flexed. (Courtesy of Mr David Evans FRCS.)

(1991) described their experience with free muscle transfer in the restoration of elbow flexion and wrist extension for brachial plexus injury, a technique developed in 1978. By 1 year, 8 of 11 patients regained functional elbow flexion, and 9 of 17 regained useful wrist extension. These are impressive results. Through the good offices of Professor Akira Nagano, our colleagues have been kind enough to release to us unpublished data (1985) on a grand total of 111 cases: 76.9% of 26 cases of elbow flexorplasty regained useful function, and 56.7% of 81 cases of transfer for wrist extension recovered power to at least MRC grade 3. We have been disappointed by our failure to restore wrist extension in many cases of complete brachial plexus injury, and think that this work is strikingly good. Gilbert (1993) described two cases of muscle transfer for elbow flexion in obstetric brachial plexus palsy, in which a long nerve graft was passed from the opposite, undamaged arm, from one of the pectoral nerves across the chest. After an interval of 1 year a free gracilis muscle was inserted.

This technique has established itself as a useful one in serious cases where the conventional tendon transfers are inadequate. We think the operation is technically somewhat easier than free vascularised bone graft. The key to success lies in the selection of a suitable donor nerve, and a muscle of appropriate length and quality, adequate for the purpose.

18. Rehabilitation

Rehabilitation: history during war time; objectives (assessment, reduction of degree of disability; return to work; return to independent living and recreation). Methods of physical treatment: functional splinting; correction of deformity; abatement of pain. Return to work: modified; unmodified or wholly different; retraining; operation of Disability Discrimination Act. Adjustment to daily living. Organisation of rehabilitation services. Paralyses without demonstrable physical cause.

Rehabilitation is an important part of the treatment of patients recovering from serious illness or injury: it is particularly important in cases in which there has been serious damage to the central or peripheral nervous system. Experience gained from residential units for members of the armed services in Britain and in the USA during the war of 1939–1945 showed that an intensive programme of exercises and games and of occupational activities related to work or hobbies could, when combined with appropriate counselling, enable patients to return to duty in remarkably short times. Of 550 patients with tibial fractures, 95% returned to duty within 5 months of injury, and 90% of patients with femoral fractures returned within 8 months. Of course, these patients were, for the most part, previously fit and young men and women, and there was then no problem with unemployment. On the other hand, return to duty at that time often meant return to face the violence of the enemy. The enemies are different now; they are unemployment, the indifference of employers, the procedures of insurance companies, the erosion of good will and the deterioration of morale caused in part by the promulgation of the doctrine that "there is no such thing as society." The situation is different too: residential units in the country were appropriate for members of the armed services; such units are not suited to the requirements of civilian life. Service men and women were and are inured to being separated from their homes and families; most civilians still prefer to be with or near their homes and families, and so expect to be treated in a unit near home. The clientele is different: the members of the armed services were and are of necessity young fit men and women; in civilian practice patients of all ages and degrees of fitness come for treatment.

We are concerned here with the rehabilitation of patients who have suffered serious damage to the peripheral nervous system, and in particular those who have suffered serious damage to the brachial plexus.

The objects of rehabilitation are:

- the objective assessment of disability and the accurate measurement of the outcome of treatment

- the reduction of the degree of disability by physical and other therapy
- the return of the patient to his or her original work, to the original work modified or to suitable other work
- the restoration of the patient's ability to live in his or her own home, to enjoy recreation and social intercourse and to be independently mobile.

ASSESSMENT

Initial assessment: measurement of effect of treatment

The Medical Research Council (MRC) grading of motor power and sensibility remains an essential method for the objective measurement of those functions from the start to the finish of treatment. The assessment of motor function is extended by methods used to determine the stamina of muscles (Figs 18.1 to 18.3). The simplest method is to record with a stamina gauge or spring balance the length of time during which the subject can maintain the contraction as a standard percentage of his or her maximal strength. Or, repeated contractions are made at maximal strength and the number that can be made before amplitude falls to 50% of the original is recorded. A standard dynamometer or a sphygmomanometer with an aneroid or mercury gauge may be used. It is preferable to use a size of bulb to fit the size of hand. The function of the hand as a whole is well measured by Moberg's (1958) "pick-up" test; this involves both motor power and sensory appreciation. Other tests can be devised for assessment of the function of the upper limb as a whole, in grasping, reaching, handling and lifting (see Ch. 9). The lower limb is assessed by measurement of speed of walking, of duration of walking that can be sustained, of the length of stride and of the ability to walk up and down stairs.

"Trick" movements

Accuracy of assessment may be impaired by failure to recognise substitution of the action of a paralysed muscle

Figs 18.1 to 18.3 Measurement of grip and pinch.

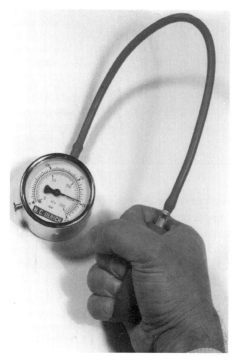

Fig. 18.1 "Median power grip" with use of thumb.

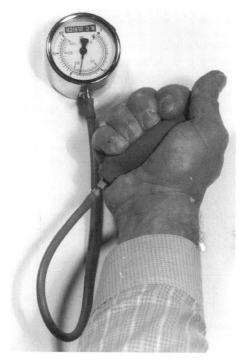

Fig. 18.2 "Ulnar power grip" with thumb excluded.

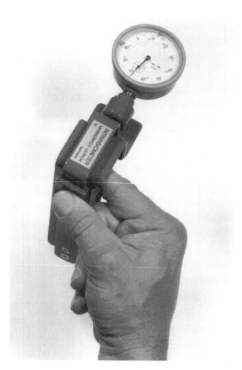

Fig. 18.3 Pinch grip (thumb to index finger).

by a "trick" movement. Such movements are, of course, useful for the patient in providing function when the primary movers are permanently paralysed. They may be produced by direct substitution, by an accessory insertion, by "tenodesis effect" or by rebound. Of course an anomalous nerve supply may leave active a muscle or muscles which would be expected to be paralysed.

Direct substitution. Most patients with paralysis of the deltoid muscle can, when the spinati and the rotator cuff are preserved, abduct the limb at the glenohumeral joint. Even the clavicular part of the pectoralis major and the long head of the triceps can effect abduction when the humerus is rotated laterally by the action of the infraspinatus. When the biceps brachii and the brachialis muscles are paralysed, the action of the brachioradialis alone often suffices to flex the elbow to power MRC grade 4. Of course, the power of gravity suffices to extend the elbow in the absence of the triceps. We have seen (see Ch. 6) how a kind of opposition of the thumb can be produced by action of the flexor brevis and abductor longus when the thenar muscles supplied by the median nerve are paralysed. Strong extension of the fingers can give an impression of an abducting action in the interossei, whilst strong flexion can give the appearance of adducting action.

Accessory insertion. The abductor and flexor breves pollicis have insertions to the extensor expansion, so that abduction of the thumb extends the interphalangeal joint, even when the extensor muscles are paralysed.

"Tenodesis" action. When the long flexors of the fingers are paralysed, extension of the wrist produces in them sufficient tension to cause flexion of the interphalangeal joints. It is this action that is exploited in the tenodesis of paralysed finger flexors to give a grip when the wrist is extended.

Rebound. When the antagonist to a paralysed muscle contracts strongly and relaxes quickly it may appear that there is a contraction of paralysed muscle. In paralysis of the common peroneal nerve the patient can mimic active extension of the toes by strong contraction and sudden relaxation of the flexors.

Regular assessment

Regular assessment is clearly necessary to:

- determine the effectiveness of treatment used
- to establish a point at which no further recovery can be expected.

The "sensory chart" reproduced in Figure 18.4 shows the extent of change in one case over 27 months. However, as Birch (1996) remarks in relation to patients with serious lesions of the brachial plexus: "early and accurate diagnosis is an essential first step towards achieving as normal an existence as is possible with the minimum of dependence". That early and accurate diagnosis depended and depends

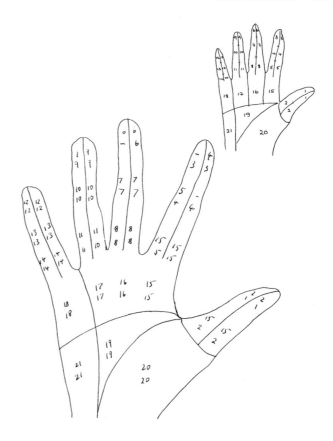

Fig. 18.4 Localisation chart showing ability in September 1986 compared with that in July 1984, in a case of primary suture of the median nerve in December 1983. Note particularly the improvement in the ability to localise in the thumb and index finger.

on early operation with recognition of the findings and, when possible, early repair. It is now possible in many cases of serious nerve injury to measure with some accuracy the likely end-state, to inform the patient accordingly and to plan ahead with his or her cooperation for return to work and ordinary life. This process, begun with diagnosis and repair, is continued soon after recovery from operation. Perhaps 6 weeks after operation the patient will be admitted for 1 or 2 weeks for a planned process of rehabilitation. Progress is monitored; if necessary, one or more further admissions for planned treatment may be arranged. In cases in which a patient is seen some months after injury and which contractures have developed and morale has deteriorated it may be necessary to admit for preliminary rehabilitation before operation.

TREATMENT

Treatment is by:

- physical therapy to muscles and joints
- correction of deformity by physical therapy and splinting
- relief or abatement of pain

- functional training, including the fitting of functional splints
- adjustment to daily living
- specific process for return to work.

PHYSICAL THERAPY

The aim during the stage of motor paralysis is to maintain a full range of passive movement of the joints the control of which is impaired. The patient and, if necessary, his or her carer is instructed in the appropriate manipulations so that they can be continued at home. It is particularly difficult to maintain a full range of movement of the meta-carpophalangeal and the glenohumeral joints. It is indeed remarkable how fixed extension deformity of the former and the medial rotation deformity of the latter develop in spite of what appears to be careful and continuing treatment. We have, however, no knowledge of the assiduity with which the exercise programmes are carried out by the patients in their homes. There must be a considerable tendency to neglect the paralysed limb, and to rely on the treatment given in the hospital. It is the business of a responsible clinician so far as possible to change such an attitude, and to impress upon the patient that the key to the avoidance or mitigation of permanent disability is in his or her own hands.

Spared muscle and recovering muscle are exercised; the patient is instructed about care for a limb to avoid accidental injury and the effects of disuse. The paralysed limb is especially sensitive to cold; patients may be tempted to warm an ice-cold limb by applying heat of a degree that would hardly be tolerated by a healthy limb. Anaesthesia of the skin allows exposure to such heat without the warning of pain; the disorder of vasomotor control certainly alters the reaction of the skin to such heat. Patients should be encouraged to protect the paralysed limb against external cold.

Once recovery of motor function begins, passive movements give way to active exercise. In the very early stages, gravity-assisted exercises on the plinth and exercises in a pool are best. Immersion in warm water assists weak muscles; in the later stages the water serves usefully as resistance. Bathers are familiar with the effort expended in walking and in trying to run in water. In these early stages techniques of proprioceptive neuromuscular facilitation are particularly useful. The cell bodies of the nerves supplying the weak muscles are subject to central inhibition; and activity in neighbouring healthy motor cells stimulates activity in those of a recovering nerve. Thus, a weak quadriceps muscle can better be stimulated by asking the patient to raise the lower limb with the ankle dorsiflexed than by requiring action by the quadriceps alone. Similarly, the action of the weak biceps brachii can be enhanced by requiring a combined movement of adduction flexion and medial rotation.

Once muscles are strong enough to move joints against gravity resistance can progressively be introduced: first, against the hand of the physiotherapist; later against springs and weights. Isokinetic machines represent an extension of this principle. "Cardiovascular training" – that is, exercises in the gymnasium and in the swimming pool – has been useful in restoring morale and in general fitness, especially in older patients. Pressure garments are useful for swollen and hyperaesthetic limbs.

"Biofeedback", in which the contraction of the muscle or an antagonist is visually recorded, is useful in the recovery phase, especially in cases of "co-contraction" of agonist and antagonist. Chronic pain and long-lasting disability are certain in some cases to produce depression. In such cases the advice of a clinical psychologist is likely to be helpful, but much of the burden of maintaining and improving morale must rest on those who are in daily contact with the patient.

In residential units, games and general exercise by walking, cycling and swimming can be added to the programme of rehabilitation. In the rehabilitation units of the Royal Air Force, blow, flip and bar football, beat the clock hand games and playing with weighted draughts amused service men and women and improved function of the hand. It is more difficult to introduce such competitive games in civilian environments: only extreme enthusiasm and commitment on the part of those in charge will bring success to this endeavour.

CORRECTION OF DEFORMITY

Deformity is corrected or lessened by passive stretching (Figs 18.5 and 18.6) and by serial plaster splinting. When there is a bad contracture, frequent treatment is necessary: to achieve that, a short period of in-patient care is advisable. The physiotherapist gently stretches the affected joint and applies a plaster in the position of correction. This treatment is repeated up to three times during the day. The splint is worn day and night. The duration of such intensive treatment is perhaps 1 week; after that, weekly treatments are given and the patient is instructed in passive stretching and application of the splint. The splints are dated and retained to serve as a measure of progress (Fig. 18.7). Cessation of progress when deformity has not adequately been corrected may be an indication for correction by operation. The achievement of a satisfactory state may be an indication for operation to preserve the correction (see Ch. 17 for other examples).

RELIEF OR ABATEMENT OF PAIN

Pain is particularly severe in cases of intradural injury of the brachial plexus, which may serve as a model for this discussion. The clinician and his or her colleagues are confronted with a serious problem of a young person – usually

Figs 18.5 and 18.6 Correction of deformity.

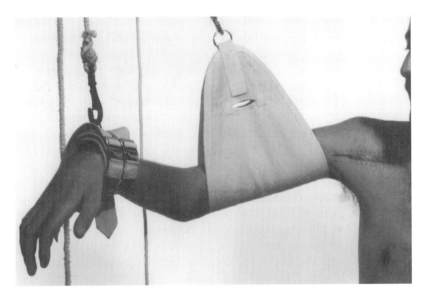

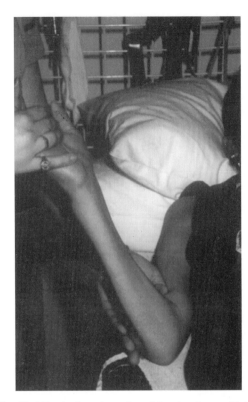

Fig. 18.5 Limb suspended in slings.

Fig. 18.6 Passive lateral rotation of the glenohumeral joint.

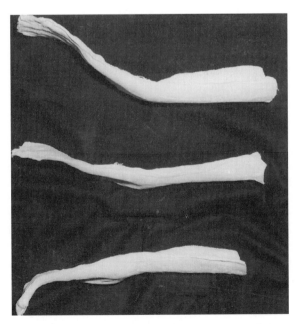

Fig. 18.7 Serial plasters for correction of deformity. A set of plasters showing progressive correction of flexion deformity of wrist.

a young man – with an upper limb wholly or almost wholly paralysed, often with severe continuing pain, often enough engaged before injury in unskilled or semiskilled manual work, and having few educational qualifications. The problem need not be so severe as it was in former days: early operation, early establishment of prognosis and early substitution by neurotisation can bring motivation and can lead, by restoration of activity at least, to early diminution of pain. If, as we hope, repair of intradural lesions becomes a practical proposition, the problem will be alleviated further. However, all this requires a great deal of work and organisation; for years yet there is likely to be a hard core of patients with useless limbs and chronic pain for a few of whom amputation offers a reasonable course. Ian Fletcher (1981) did a great deal for such patients with his work on the fitting of prostheses after amputations. He warned against amputation and the fitting of a prosthesis in patients with severe pain. His reasons were:

- disappointment felt by the patient, even after warning, because of the failure of amputation to relieve pain
- difficulty in using the prosthesis because of inhibition by pain.

Nevertheless, amputation and fitting of a prosthesis remains at treatment of last resort for patients with intradural injury of the plexus. Sometimes the functional results are remarkably good: Fletcher (1981) reproduces a photograph of a patient with a left below-elbow amputation and arthrodesis of the shoulder climbing rigging with the help of the prosthesis. So good an outcome must, however, be unusual. A more recent paper from Wilkinson et al (1993) discusses the indications for and timing of amputation.

Transcutaneous stimulation

Transcutaneous stimulation (TNS or TENS) was and is an offshoot of the proposal by Melzack and Wall (1965) of the "gate theory" of pain. It was argued, perhaps not quite logically, that the addition of a sensory input by another route would diminish the painful effect of "deafferentation"; in any case, it has for long been known that, irrespective of deafferentation, one massive painful input can dislodge another from conscious appreciation. Thus, apprehension in the waiting room can dull the appreciation of toothache, and the pain of a broken leg can "mask" the pain from an ipsilateral dislocation of the hip. In any case, transcutaneous stimulation has long progressed beyond the theoretical considerations to become an accepted and generally harmless adjuvant. Like other "harmless" treatments, it may of course lead indirectly to harm if it is used empirically for pain the cause of which has not been determined.

Miss P. Barsby gives us the following very useful information about the use of transcutaneous stimulation in neuropathic pain. She, with her colleagues, in the Physiotherapy Department of the Royal National Orthopaedic Hospital studied 281 in-patient episodes from January 1995 to the present. High-intensity, low-frequency stimulation was found to be preferable, in "bursts" or continuously for "stretching" pain; low-intensity, high-frequency stimulation, again in "bursts" or continuously, was preferable for "neuralgic" pains. Transcutaneous stimulation was not useful in the treatment of hyperaesthesia. About 80% of patients gained relief, but the results deteriorated after 3–6 months in more than half the patients. Acupuncture has been used over the past 4 years; it has been helpful in a few cases only.

The chronic pain programme

In 1984, Wynn Parry and Withrington describing their experience with 50 patients referred to our pain service with neuropathic pain. A total of 71 operations were performed by us for the purposes of establishing diagnosis and for relieving pain. In only one case was the operation successful in bringing about the relief of pain. Such patients form a hard core of those suffering from chronic pain, which prevents return to work and normal life. Their pain is resistant to all forms of treatment that have already been described, and these patients do cause despair amongst those trying to treat them. For some of these, pain management programmes do help: that is, carefully structured multidisciplinary programmes of rehabilitation which aim to modify behaviour so as to increase function, increase activity and relieve fear.

Many patients with severe pain retreat into themselves, cutting themselves off from family, friends and work. Fear of return to work, or of any painful activity leads to progressive dependence: learned abnormal behavioural patterns, including needless inactivity and display of suffering, become embedded. There may be an unconscious manipulation of the environment, with the patient at the centre of things, and a family dominated by the patient's pain behaviour. Fordyce (1981) studied 150 patients with chronic pain who were asked to record in a diary their perception of pain, their daily activities and their involvement in common activities. Fordyce found no clear correlation between the recorded level of perceived pain and the levels of activity. These methods do not set out to modify the pain experience: rather they seek to lessen the disability of chronic pain by increasing activity, diminishing medication, and diminishing dependence on doctors. Family involvement is important, so that a positive approach, of praise for achievements and of disregard for complaints of suffering, is established. The pattern of illness behaviour must not be reinforced.

In our hospital patients are admitted for progressive programmed exercises, relaxation, vocational assessment and retraining. Psychological counselling and adjustment of medication is a central theme. Many patients have been using a formidable list of analgesics and even narcotics, and it is important to wean them from their drugs. We have been surprised to see how often patients say they feel less tired and actually feel less pain once drugs have been withdrawn. A pain cocktail is used in which the active ingredients are successively reduced on a time-related, not demand, basis. The patient is told that medication is being reduced, but does not know the rate of attenuation or when the active ingredient has been entirely removed.

The approach is multidisciplinary. It is for the physician to explain in detail the nature of the patient's pain and why further intervention is inappropriate. This will involve explanation of theories of chronic pain, the risks of further operation and the severely deleterious long-term effects of passive and dependent lifestyle, taking increasing amounts of drugs and becoming ultimately a pain cripple. We emphasise that a single simple explanation of the cause of symptoms and prognosis is the single most valuable facet of this treatment programme. We have found that patients are usually much relieved when their pain is explained. Many patients with a paralysed yet painful arm have believed that they must be taking leave of their senses, particularly when they have been ill advised that pain is evidence of recovery or that it is "all in the mind". Understanding is the essential prelude to acceptance. We cannot overemphasise the value of a prolonged interview in which explanations are given and all questions answered. Empathy between the doctor and the patient is essential for the successful first faltering step of the long journey of rehabilitation.

Possibly, suitably qualified clinical psychologists should assume responsibility for the overall programme. Once that has been established no further medical or surgical intervention is appropriate. The patient is encouraged to take personal responsibility for coping with the effect of his or her pain. Continuing review by physicians leads the patient to believe there is still some further remedy, and this is one potent reason for yielding direction of the programme to the psychologist. *We emphasise again that no patient should be sent to a "pain" clinic or entered into a "pain" programme until an accurate diagnosis has been made.*

It may appear callous, but it is essential that no reference is made to pain. Only positive achievements are discussed, and continuing pain complaints are disregarded. Thus the behavioural pattern of pain complaining and inactivity and dependence becomes altered, progressively, to one of a positive attitude with increased activity. Behaviour is changed although the symptoms remain. An improvement in the response to symptoms permits progressive increase in function, greater social involvement and even return to work, although this last criterion cannot itself be a measure of success for there are many reasons why someone with a nerve injury cannot work, such as the severity of disability, levels of unemployment and age. If the clinical psychologist detects serious emotional problems or overt depression, then psychotherapists can make a most valuable contribution.

A typical pain management programme is conducted on an in-patient basis, within the rehabilitation unit. The patient comes in for 5 days, from Monday to Friday, and is expected to be independent. Physical exercise plays a major part, with swimming, group exercises, circuit training, and individual sessions for those with specific muscle weakness. Work skills and recreational pursuits are developed or relearned in the occupational therapy department to the level appropriate to the physical status and the patient's own interest and experience. Recreational outings on a small-group basis and group therapy are useful in encouraging reintegration into community life. Relaxation classes at the end of the day and counselling sessions help the patients to understand their pain and resolve any conflicts within the family, to regain self-control, and to take responsibility for their own care. Activities are monitored and on appropriate occasions recorded by video camera so that outcome measures can be regularly measured and results discussed with the patient and the team, so that all see progress is being made. Close liaison is kept at all times with the family and, where appropriate, the employer.

It is a constant source of pleasure, and often a surprise, to see how patients whose chronic pain has taken over their lives become cheerful, optimistic and positive human beings in such a relatively short time. Over the last 10 years we, with others (Fordyce), found that it is possible to merge the conventional rehabilitation programme and the behavioural programme so that the behavioural bias gradually takes prominence over active treatment for pain.

The constitution of the group is all important. Results may be significantly affected by one individual with an unyielding and morose sense of dependence or possessed of a determination to beat the system (Moore et al 1984). On the other hand, an enthusiastic individual can often "carry" some less well motivated members. The team leader has to be aware of these factors and be ready to take appropriate action. The work is demanding for all members of the multidisciplinary team, and regular frank discussions with agreed objectives are vital.

Certain techniques are common to all structured pain management programmes. We shall outline some of those that we think are particularly important.

1. The patient is persuaded that he or she is not helpless and that there is "life with pain".
2. The patient is encouraged to examine how pain is affecting daily life so that a problem-solving attitude is developed.
3. Factors that reinforce pain behaviour are identified and, where possible, modified. The spouse who treats the patient as an invalid protecting him or her from physical and emotional stress should gently be dissuaded from this attitude and encouraged rather to make the patient independent and be supported in disregarding complaints.
4. The patient is encouraged to keep a pain diary. In this way, he or she recognises that pain is not continuous, but that it may fluctuate, so permitting some activity.
5. Specific aims of a short-, medium- and long-term are set and scrupulously assessed.
6. The regular exercise programme is essential.
7. A planned reduction of medication is a sine qua non.
8. A full explanation of pain must be given and time allowed for the patient to voice all fears and anxieties, many of which are unreasonable. Some patients have extraordinary ideas about the nature of their pain and its possible effects on life expectancy, and they may be reluctant to open out these fears until they are actively encouraged to do so.
9. Patients are taught relaxation and controlled breathing exercises, which many find helpful in reducing spasms of pain.
10. Daily activities are increased regularly and monitored.
11. Some patients can learn self-hypnosis to reduce severity of pain – the help of psychologists and suitably qualified hypnotherapists should be sought.

Well-constructed programmes of behavioural therapy have a very real place in the treatment of chronic pain. Linton (1986) wrote a comprehensive review of published work on the subject. A statistically significant increase in activity and reduction of medication was found in no less than 30 studies.

George Omer (1987) wrote: "there are only two principles in the treatment of an established pain syndrome involving the upper extremity: to relieve the subjective pain experience and to institute active function of the involved extremity". He further commented that: "the best of functional activity occurs when the patient returns to daily work. Patients who continue functional activities will ultimately 'cure' themselves".

FUNCTIONAL TRAINING AND FUNCTIONAL SPLINTING

The restoration of function for return to unsupported daily life and to work can be helped by occupational therapy and by functional splinting. Therapy aims at reproducing the actions principally used in the patient's work. In a fully equipped rehabilitation unit appropriate facilities are available for stimulation of such activities. Functional splinting is particularly useful in disorders of the upper limb, but the simplest splints can greatly aid the patient with partial paralysis of the lower limb (Figs 18.8 to 18.14). Very simple splints aid function of the hand impaired by lesions of the ulnar and median nerves in simulating

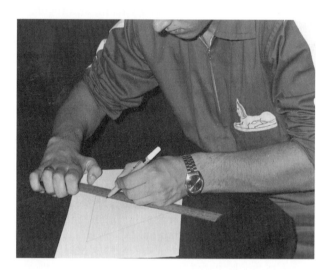
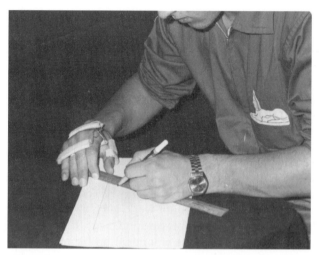

Fig. 18.8 Simple functional splinting. Writing with and without the now rarely used combined "knuckle duster" and opposition spring splints.

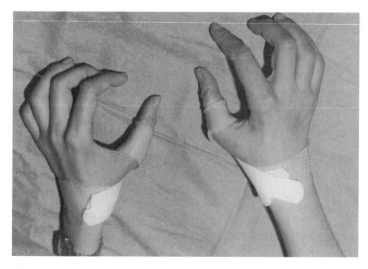

Fig. 18.9 The use of the new type of opposition splint in a patient with progressive neuropathy. (Courtesy of Sister Evelyn Hunter RGN.)

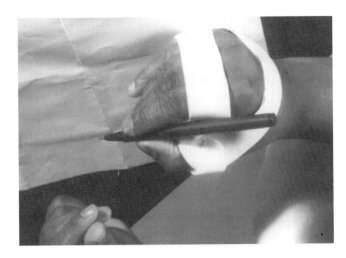

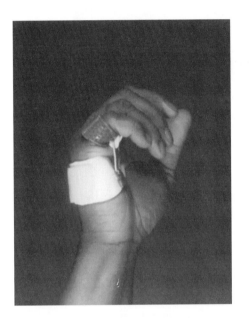

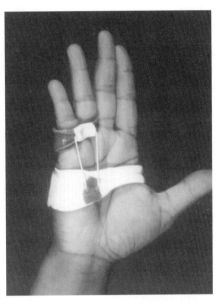

Fig. 18.10 The use of the combined "knuckle duster" and opposition splint in writing for a patient with a lesion of the median and ulnar nerves. (Courtesy of Miss Lydia Dean Dip, COT.)

Fig. 18.11 A "lively" splint conferring flexion of the metacarpophalangeal joints in cases of ulnar nerve damage. At rest, the joints are kept flexed; active extension is, however, possible. (Courtesy of Miss Lydia Dean Dip, COT.)

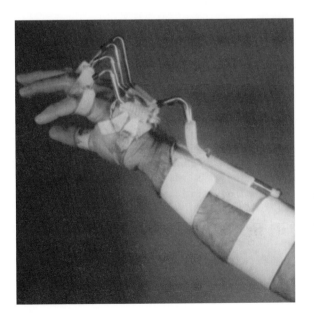

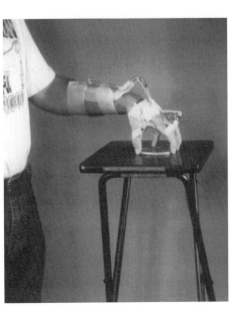

Fig. 18.12 A very elaborate splint for radial nerve palsy. Active extension for the wrist, fingers, and thumb is provided. The appearance of impracticability is belied by the fact that the patient found this splint extremely useful. (Courtesy of Miss Lydia Dean Dip. COT.)

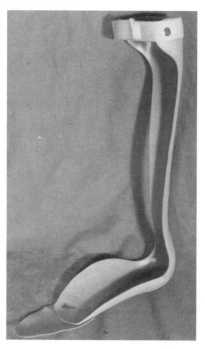

Fig. 18.13 Splints for the lower limb. Simple foot drop splint. (Courtesy of Miss Lydia Dean Dip, COT.)

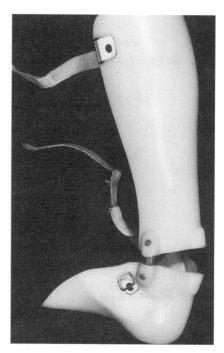

Fig. 18.14 An elaborate hinged, "springloaded" drop foot splint. (Courtesy of Miss Lydia Dean Dip, COT.)

opposition of the thumb and flexion of the metacarpo-phalangeal joints. More elaborate splinting is necessary in cases of severe damage to the brachial plexus. The *gauntlet splint* is useful when there is major and lasting loss of function in the forearm and hand. The *elbow lock splint* is useful in the absence of active control of the elbow. The *flail arm splint* is used when there is irreparable and irrecoverable damage to the whole plexus. The simplest of these is, of course, the elbow lock splint. The flail arm splint includes an elbow hinge and a wrist platform, to which can be attached various devices such a splint hook and a cable operated by the opposite shoulder (Figs 18.15 to 18.17). It is, in effect, an artificial limb over the paralysed limb. It consists of a shoulder supporting piece, an elbow ratchet which allows flexion in five different positions, and a forearm trough to which the appliances are fitted. The lower part of the splint is, in effect, the "gauntlet". It comes in three sizes. Adjustment by the orthotist and training by the occupational therapist takes about 10 days. During this time the therapist teaches the patient to cope with activities of daily life. In a long-term review of 200 patients fitted with these splints, Wynn Parry and Withrington (1984) found that 70% used them for work or recreation. The most useful devices are the tool holder, the split hook and the appliance for steadying a sheet of paper. Although "true success" is measured by continuing use of the splint, fitting and instruction are justified if:

- the temporary use of the splint carries the patient usefully through a period of recovery
- function conferred by temporary splintage gives sufficient function to distract patients from his or her pain
- temporary use gives the patient the motivation to start and continue rehabilitation.

In a later study, Wynn Parry et al (1987) were able to review 103 of 211 patients fitted with flail arm splints. Sixty-eight had continued to use these splints. It is probable that most of those failing to respond also failed to continue use of their splints.

Further important studies have been done at the Royal National Orthopaedic Hospital by Sarah Probert, Margaret Taggart and Manuella Schuette. Sarah Probert records that, since 1980, a data card has been completed for every patient fitted with one of these splints, and that the information on each card is, so far as is possible, kept up to date. Between 1987 and July 1996, 211 patients were fitted with brachial plexus splints; 103 responded to questionnaires. Sixty-eight of these patients indicated that they were wearing the splints. Thus, about one-third of patients supplied with splints used them. An earlier survey, of 446 patients fitted between 1980 and July 1996, showed that 205 responded to the questionnaire, and that 107 of these continued to use the splint: a "take-up" rate of perhaps one-quarter. The "take-up" rate was roughly the same for all three types of splint. Miss Probert points to the need for further examination of the design of these splints so that the failure rate may be reduced.

Margaret Taggart studied the cases of 324 patients who underwent operations for supraclavicular injury of the brachial plexus and were followed for at least 30 months. These were entered into the study between 1986 and 1993; all had a period of admission for rehabilitation. She examined five parameters of response to rehabilitation: usefulness of the admission; continued use of splints; value of transcutaneous nerve stimulation; return to work or study; and time off work. The results are shown in Tables 18.1 to 18.4. These are important figures, showing again the rather frequent failure of the splints in their present state; the general appreciation of a period of admission, and the rather high rate of return to work. Manuella Schuette reviews the use of flail arm splints between April 1995 and April 1996, and confirms the rather low rate of continued use (probably, 14 out of 35). We find it agreeable that one of our patients with brachial plexus lesion works in the orthotics unit at Stanmore; two more are studying orthotics.

Figs 18.15 to 18.17 Splints for extensive paralysis of the upper limb.

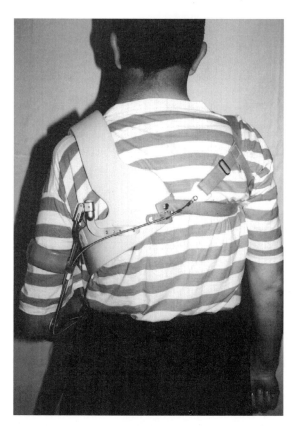

Fig. 18.15 Full flail arm splint with elbow lock and gauntlet.

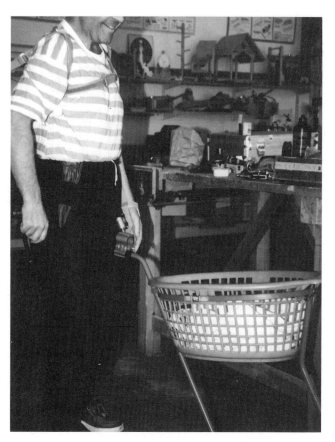

Fig. 18.16 Use with elbow extended.

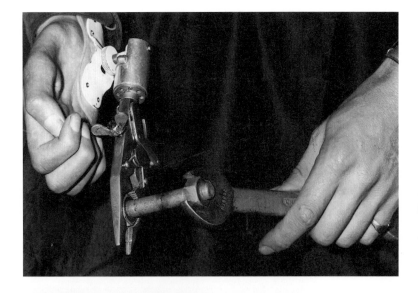

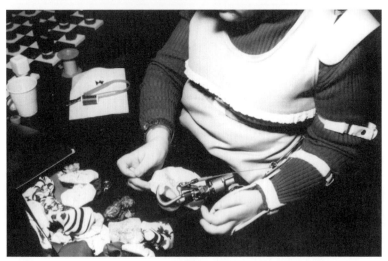

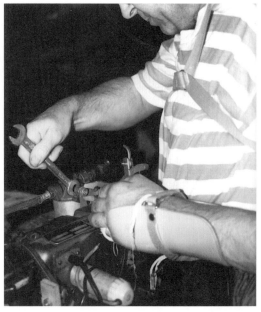

Fig. 18.17 Use of various attachments, including a split hook and pliers.

Table 18.1 Supraclavicular lesions of brachial plexus – usefulness of admission (patients' assessment): 324 cases

Assessment	No. of cases
Useful	301
Not useful	23
Benefits*	Mobilisation of limb
	Adaptation to disability
	Meeting others with same type of injury
	Enhancement of morale

*40% of all patients referred to all four of these benefits.

Table 18.2 Supraclavicular lesions of the brachial plexus – use of splint and TENS: 324 cases

	Yes	No
Splint used for more than 1 year*	87	195
TENS used for more than 1 year	48	
Never useful	168	

*Not fitted in 47 cases.
TENS, transcutaneous stimulation.

Table 18.3 Supraclavicular lesions of the brachial plexus – return to work or study: 324 cases

	No. of cases
Return to work or study	249
Did not return	75
Same occupation as before injury	54
Different occupation	195
Formal retraining	81

Table 18.4 Supraclavicular lesions of the brachial plexus – time off work: 201 cases

Time off work (months)	No. of cases
≤3	19
4–6	44
7–12	60
13–18	32
19–30	28
≥31	18
Total	201

Range: 1 week to 6 years.

RETURN TO WORK

Although Taggart's figures indicate that the rate of return to work after serious injury to the brachial plexus is encouragingly high, the findings that four out of five patients return to a different job indicates the importance of retraining and of systems of information about employment. Apart from physical disability, several factors militate against an early return to work. The patient may feel that, for a time, he or she has had enough and deserves a rest. If the question of compensation is raised, solicitors may well advise their client against early return to work, apprehending that the chief item in any sum awarded is likely to relate to loss of earnings. It must, however, be recalled that from any sum awarded for loss of earnings the Department of Social Security will deduct welfare payments made during the period of invalidity (a policy amended only very recently).

The attitude of employers to disabled applicants is often unhelpful: the 1990s ethos of a long day's work for the lowest acceptable pay is inimical to the employment of persons who may make special demands. However, recent changes in the medical criteria of unfitness for work may oblige many persons to resume work who otherwise would have been content to rely on social security payments. Formerly, employers of more than 20 persons were obliged to include a percentage of disabled people within their workforce. That obligation was widely disregarded; it was in fact virtually unenforceable. All that has been swept away by the Disability Discrimination Act of 1996.

Disability is defined as a physical or mental impairment that has a substantial and long-term adverse effect on a person's ability to carry out normal day to day activities. People who have a disability, and people who have had a disability but no longer have one, are covered by the Act. It is now unlawful for employers with 20 or more staff to discriminate against current or prospective employees with disability *because of reasons relating to this disability*. They may also have to make a reasonable adjustment if their employment arrangements or premises substantially disadvantage a disabled employee or a disabled applicant. Unlawful discrimination is defined; circumstances are defined in which less favourable treatment of a disabled person is justified. Those covered by the Act are named; and categories of exempt persons, such as those serving in the armed forces, are defined. One may speculate that, had these regulations been in force 200 years ago, the victor of the Nile, Copenhagen and Trafalgar would not have come as he did to his triumph and his death.

Evidently, the balance has decisively been altered: the employer is no longer obliged to include a proportion of disabled persons in the workforce; rather, it is for the disabled person refused a job to show that the refusal stemmed from discrimination because of his or her disability. Cox (1996) comments quite sharply that the guidance notes published to help interpretation of the provisions of the Act "signal a contentious time ahead for health professionals". He concludes: "it is in the area of employment that doctors, particularly occupational physicians, will be most involved. Their expertise must ensure that many of the Act's ambiguities and uncertainties are resolved with fairness to both disabled people and employers. It will require the wisdom of Solomon." Success in returning the patient to work depends on the capacity and motivation of the patient, on the efforts of those in charge of treatment, and on the availability of employment. At Job Centres, Disablement Resettlement Officers are available to advise on the possibilities of return to work. In 1969, Dr Derek Brewerton introduced at the Royal National Orthopaedic Hospital the concept and the practice of the *Hospital Employment Advisor*. We are very grateful to Mr Peter Cozens, the present holder of the post, for information about the advisor's functions, and also generally about the problems associated with return to work. Evidently, if there is no or only trifling residual disability, or if the patient is in the comfortable position of having easy access to transport and an assured job that is not physically demanding, there would be little difficulty. The Hospital Employment Advisor is available to help patients who, because of their disability, are likely to experience problems in returning to work. The patient is seen while he or she is in hospital. Problems can be discussed, and in favourable cases difficulties can be resolved before discharge. With the patient's permission the Advisor makes contact with the employer and discusses the job situation and any adjustments that will be required to accommodate the patient's disability. Best, of course, is return to the original work, but if that is not possible alternative employment with the same firm may be available. Since government grants of up to 80% of costs between £300 and £10 000 and 100% of costs over £10 000 are available for adaptation of premises or provision of special equipment, employers have an incentive to make suitable provision.

In cases in which permanent disability is, or is certain to be, so severe as to preclude a return to anything like the original work, the question of retraining may be raised. The Employment Advisor can arrange for such patients to be seen at one of the numerous Employment Assessment Centres. That may lead to a specialised training course, either locally or at one of the four residential training colleges maintained in Durham, Exeter, Leatherhead and Nottingham. The Employment Advisor can help too in the matter of transport and mobility: patients with serious disability of one upper limb are able to handle a car fitted with an automatic gearbox and adjustments for the steering wheel and handbrake. Modifications are available for the patient whose disability affects the lower limb (Cowal (Mobility Aids) Ltd, Holmer Green, Bucks; Reselco Engineering Ltd, Green Dragon Lane, Brentford, Middlesex).

ADJUSTMENT TO DAILY LIVING

For all patients with serious disability there has to be adjustment to make it possible to live at home with the greatest degree of independence. This is, of course, especially so for patients who are too old for retraining or who have retired from work. There are adjustments to the individual patient and there are adjustments to the home. The role of functional splinting has been considered. Often enough the patient's own ingenuity will suggest methods of reducing dependence.

At the Royal National Orthopaedic Hospital, Stanmore, the Graham Hill Unit provides facilities for patients suffering from progressive neurological disease, amputation, the effects of damage to the spinal cord, severe rheumatoid arthritis and the effects of serious damage to the peripheral nerves and the brachial plexus in particular. There are facilities for assessment and for treatment, including a flat equipped for most of the eventualities that may confront a disabled person, and a house built to the design of the local council. Patients can live in the house and discover many of the little problems likely to arise in daily living. They can then move to the flat and practise living with the appropriate aids.

There is, no doubt, a formidable case for the rehabilitation unit as a method of reducing permanent disability and invalidity, and for returning damaged patients to work and to active life. It is, no doubt, expensive: some time,

doubtless, costs will be calculated and will be balanced against those of merely paying incapacity benefit and disability allowance. It may be that further consideration will be given to regularising the payment for treatment and rehabilitation by insurance companies in cases in which disability flows from, for instance, road traffic accidents. At present, under the provision of the Road Traffic Act 1988, Hospital Authorities and Trusts can claim up to £2949 for in-patient treatment for injuries sustained in a road traffic accident. In theory the patient charged can then recover or try to recover the sum from insurers. It is doubtful whether the National Health Service benefits to any significant extent from this deeply unsatisfactory system. Even if, with the cooperation of insurance companies, the system were extended and improved and the collection of sums owed were regularised, the amount collected would hardly be more than a drop in the ocean. There are, according to Topliss (1993) 6 million disabled people in Britain, 69% of whom are aged over 60 years. The proportion of those with disability arising from road traffic accidents must be very small.

The break up of the National Hospital and Community Services into purchasers and providers with competing Trusts has hardly helped planning in general, or planning of rehabilitation facilities in particular. It is hardly possible for the management of district general hospital – even if such an entity still exists or is likely to continue in existence – to furnish a viable rehabilitation unit. Unfortunately, the important association of hospital and community services brought about by the "reforms" of 1974 were sundered by those of 1990. However, there is, as Barnes (1993) remarks "a case for the establishment of specialist rehabilitation centres each serving a population of around 3 000 000". In former days, that would have been the task of the Regional Health Authorities, but the removal of these bodies has left a void. It will, doubtless, be left to the initiative of clinicians and others working in special centres, district hospitals and community health services to preserve such specialist units as exist, and to formulate plans for a regional network of centres for the rehabilitation of the disabled patient with special needs. The palliative care of others will, as it does now, devolve on those working in the community medical services and on voluntary carers. Rehabilitation is difficult and demanding work: it is common to find that the success of a centre depends largely upon the enthusiasm and commitment of the person in charge. Unfortunately, there are scarcely enough such people to go round.

PARALYSIS NOT PHYSICALLY DETERMINED

Most clinicians have seen or will see at least one patient with a paralysis of a limb for which no physical cause can be assigned. The most likely cause is a "conversion" disorder or "conversion hysteria," in which resolution of some mental disorder is sought by converting it into a physical one. A few patients are actually malingering – consciously simulating a paralysis in order to claim compensation or to avoid some unpleasant task or experience. A very few are true exponents of the "Munchausen syndrome."

"Conversion hysteria"

Abse (1987) makes this definition: "In conversion hysteria there are dramatic somatic symptoms into which the patient's mental conflict is 'converted'". There may be gross paralytic, spasmodic, or convulsive motor disturbance or perversion of sensation. Oscar Wilde (1890) may have been near an understanding with: "That is one of the great secrets of life – to cure the soul by means of the senses and the senses by means of the soul". Tyrer (1989) noted that, although the typical case of conversion disorder was in most instances easy to identify, the diagnosis provided a fertile ground for clinical error. Although early descriptions of "conversion hysteria" "emphasise the equanimity of the patient in the face of a major handicap (the *belle indifférence* of Charcot), that feature is not now considered of prime importance in diagnosis". Indeed, patients with the very severe and doubtless physically determined pain of intradural injury of the brachial plexus seem to display a curious indifference to a pain described as constant and severe, with episodic exacerbations. Sunderland (1991b) dealt with "conversion hysteria" and noted certain features: area of sensory loss not corresponding to anatomical distribution; sensory defect not associated with loss of function; absence of trophic changes; and paralysis never an isolated nor predominant sign. None of these features is entirely constant, but that does not detract from the value of Sunderland's criteria as an initial guide.

Our experience has brought us into contact with patients with conversion disorders manifesting themselves in paralysis of the brachial plexus. The term "conversion paralysis" is perhaps the most appropriate for this condition. The narration of a typical case serves well as a description of the common clinical features.

Case report. A man was sent at the age of 22 for fitting of a functional splint for a complete lesion of the brachial plexus of the right (formerly dominant) upper limb. He was then living alone, running his own business as a window cleaner. He seemed perfectly well adjusted and, apart from the upper limb, perfectly fit. The patient's General Practitioner sent the medical record, which was enormously bulky and very informative. The patient, an only child, had been brought up by parents clearly obsessed with matters of health. Between the ages of 4 and 11 he had been seen intermittently by paediatricians for a variety of complaints, none of which was found to have a physical basis. At the age of 14 he developed a motor and

sensory paralysis of the right upper limb, which was investigated but never consistently treated. The patient left home at the age of 18, and never returned.

There was complete motor and sensory paralysis of the right upper limb, with marked wasting, brittle nails and other "trophic" changes. However, there was no history of unnoticed accidental injury of the limb. Electrophysiological examination (Dr Nicholas Murray) showed, in effect, normal responses. The patient was admitted and kept in for 6 weeks, during which the basis of his condition was explained to him, and regular treatment was given to encourage him to resume the use of the limb. The response of the "paralysed" muscles to electrical stimulation was shown, and the attempt was made to overcome resistance to voluntary activity. A functional splint was fitted. All that was obtained was some abduction of the shoulder and some flexion of the elbow. Even that small gain was lost in the weeks after this young man left hospital; he did not wear the "functional" splint and the paralysis returned in its full extent.

This case exemplifies the conversion paralysis in an extreme form. It is worth noting that there were undoubtedly trophic changes, though there was no history of unnoticed accidental injury. Over the years the patient had adjusted his life well to the disability: our intervention was, in the event, irrelevant. We have had slightly more success with other patients similarly affected, but the gain has never been commensurate with the effort expended.

The Munchausen syndrome

Richard Asher's (1951) description of this syndrome has not been bettered, though the picture of hospital mores drawn in his article now seems archaic. Thus: "it requires a bold casualty officer to refuse admission". Nowadays, decisions about admission have largely been removed from the control of the "casualty officers"; indeed, from clinicians in general. Other features of a bygone age, such as the "experienced front gate porter" are found, but the article remains the classic account of an extraordinary condition by an altogether exceptional clinician and thinker.

As Asher says, the person suffering from this condition resembles the famous Baron Munchausen in having or in affecting to have travelled widely; their stories, like those attributed to the Baron, are both dramatic and untruthful. The patient comes with apparently acute illness supported by a plausible, extensive and dramatic history. The last is largely made up of falsehoods; later, the patient is found to have attended a number of other hospitals and deceived many clinicians there. He or she nearly always discharges him- or herself against advice, after quarrelling violently with doctors and nurses. Asher goes on to list tell-tale signs, and names three well-known varieties of the syndrome: acute abdominal, haemorrhagic and neurological.

Our particular recollection, dating from the 1960s, is of a sturdily built man in his early thirties, who used to come with a complete motor and sensory paralysis of the right (dominant) upper limb, allegedly caused, in one version, by the fall of a heavy weight on the shoulder. There had been previous accidents: in particular, one sustained during service in the Royal Air Force, when the allegedly ruptured spleen had been removed. This man was admitted to St Mary's Hospital Paddington, referred from another hospital for investigation of a recent lesion of the brachial plexus. At the time, there was a rather convincing motor and sensory paralysis of the right upper limb, with much complaint of pain. The abdomen showed the large scar of the splenectomy, with other scars. It was perhaps fortunate that at that time the prime method of investigating lesions of the brachial plexus was by myelography: soon after that course was suggested, the patient slipped away. Investigation revealed previous visits to several other hospitals in the London area where similar dramas had been enacted. We continued to hear of this patient from various hospitals for several years afterwards. Evidently, his case combined the abdominal and neurological syndromes; as is so often the case, it was difficult to discover what advantage he sought from the deception.

Asher suggested as possible motives: the desire to be the centre of interest and attention; a grudge against hospitals and doctors that is satisfied by deceiving them; a desire for drugs; a desire to escape the attentions of the police; or a simple need for bread and lodging. Nowadays, of course, many more people than formerly harbour grudges against doctors and hospitals, just as many more seek refuge from the police and many more seek a bed for the night. On the other hand, in the UK today, controlled and prohibited drugs are readily available, at a price; attendance at hospital with symptoms and signs of serious disease no longer provides any guarantee of a bed for the night. Yet "Munchausen" patients are still seen and still cause unease and confusion (Kwan et al 1997). Asher commented on the remarkable tolerance of such patients to "the more brutish hospital measures": he could hardly have foreseen that 40 years later "brutish measures" would include keeping sick patients for up to 2 days on trolleys in accident departments. Even that prospect does not seem to have discouraged these patients.

Diagnosis is hard even for the most experienced clinician. Those who have learnt from harsh experience to distrust on sight the open faced, frank man or woman who looks his or her interlocutor straight in the eye and speaks openly, clearly and respectfully, will have less difficulty than will their more trustful colleagues. The "paralysis" can of course be shown by electrophysiological examination to be a fake; the sight of an abdomen looking like a battlefield is a sure giveaway. Nevertheless, the earnestness, clarity and frankness with which the patient initially expounds his or her condition constitute the first and most important warning sign. We are not aware that any clinician has successfully treated this condition.

Malingering

We think that when the patient with the "hysterical" paralysis of the brachial plexus is alone at home, his or her paralysis persists. On the other hand, when the malingerer is home alone or with his or her intimates, the paralysis disappears or reverts to its true physical extent. The object of deception is the natural one of wishing to gain a large sum in compensation or to avoid some tiresome or dangerous task. The latter is, of course, the common cause of malingering by persons in the armed services in wartime. It is hard, even for the shrewdest clinician armed with the most advanced technical aids, to penetrate the cloud of deception and come to a true assessment of motor power, sensibility, joint movement, degree of pain and level of function. Modern advances have come to the aid of clinicians and insurers: the video camera permits recording of a claimant's level of activity when he or she thinks him- or herself unnoticed. These are not agreeable pastures.

19. Electrodiagnosis

Shelagh J.M. Smith

Electrodiagnosis: Historical aspects. Techniques: nerve conduction studies; small fibre function; electromyography. Safety of investigations. Caution in interpretation of results. Pathophysiological correlates: conduction block axonotmesis, neurotmesis. Localisation of lesion. Variations in innervation. Entrapment neuropathies: median nerve; ulnar nerve; radial nerve; common peroneal; sciatic; femoral; uncommon entrapment syndromes. The brachial plexus; adult post-traumatic; obstetrical plexopathy; thoracic outlet syndrome; lumbosacral plexopathy. Radiculopathy. Generalised disorders.

The development of neurophysiological investigation has played a pivotal role in evaluation of disorders of the peripheral nervous system. Electrodiagnosis contributes in a number of ways to the investigation of neuromuscular disease, through its ability to localise lesions and to determine the severity of nerve injury and progress of recovery. Furthermore, electrodiagnostic procedures have advanced understanding of nerve pathophysiology. Nerve conduction studies and electromyography discriminate between disease occurring at different levels within the peripheral nervous system and should be considered as an extension of the clinical examination of nerve, muscle and the neuromuscular junction.

HISTORICAL ASPECTS

After the early physiological experimentation with electrical currents carried out during the 17th and early 18th centuries, Galvani in the 1780s came to recognise the relationship between electrical stimulation of a nerve and the contraction of its muscle. Subsequently, Valli observed that this effect was interrupted when the nerve was constricted. Duchenne showed that muscles could be stimulated percutaneously using localised currents at specific spots on the body, which were later identified as the motor points of muscles. Observation of the different effects of galvanic and faradic current on paralysed muscle allowed Erb to develop the use of electrical stimulation for electrodiagnosis and, subsequently, electrotherapy. Although these pioneering experiments established the role of electrodiagnosis, clinical applications were not exploited until after the Second World War. Advances in electronic engineering, many of which stemmed from applied military research, provided apparatus that could be used to study the peripheral nervous system in man (Gilliatt 1961). The first publication to describe altered nerve conduction in human disease was that of Hodes et al (1948), who reported that conduction velocity is slowed in regenerating nerve. Considerable advances occurred during the 1950s,

with the demonstration of delayed conduction of the median nerve in carpal tunnel syndrome by Simpson (1956) and the development of sensory nerve recording by Dawson in London using superimposition of photographic traces to record averaged potentials (Dawson & Scott 1949). Further work with Dawson's technique was carried out by Gilliatt and Sears at the Institute of Neurology in London, who applied it to the clinical study of nerve lesions (Gilliatt & Sears 1958), and P. K. Thomas, who described abnormalities of nerve conduction in ulnar neuropathies at the elbow and in the hand. An important contribution to the understanding of the basis of nerve conduction abnormalities was the experimental work by Lambert's group at the Mayo Clinic on diphtheritic neuropathy (Keaser & Lambert 1962), which identified segmental demyelination as the cause of slow conduction velocity. Developments in the investigation of electrical properties of muscle fibres, notably by Lord Adrian and colleagues in Cambridge in the 1920s (Adrian 1925), and later by Buchthal in Sweden during the 1940s and 1950s, led to the introduction of electromyography (EMG) into clinical practice. Buchthal's group went on to describe the characteristics of normal motor unit potentials, and the abnormalities seen on EMG in a wide range of myopathic and neurogenic disorders in man (Buchtal et al 1957).

In the years that have followed these fundamental clinical applications of nerve conduction studies and EMG, much progress has occurred in neurophysiological diagnosis. Techniques for studying a variety of peripheral and proximal nerves have been introduced, and the pathophysiological basis of nerve conduction abnormalities has been clarified through correlation between nerve conduction studies and morphological changes seen on nerve biopsy. Methods to evaluate previously inaccessible parts of the nervous system in man, including the central motor and sensory pathways and small myelinated and unmyelinated nerve fibres, have been developed to extend the diagnostic role of neurophysiological investigation.

ELECTRODIAGNOSTIC TECHNIQUES

Nerve conduction studies

Standard nerve conduction studies assess function and conduction in the large or fastest conducting nerve fibres. Compound action potentials can be measured in sensory, mixed nerve and motor fibres, using skin or surface electrodes both to stimulate supramaximally and to record the evoked response. In some situations, near-nerve needle electrode stimulation and recording is necessary, particularly if the nerve trunk is relatively inaccessible to surface study. The amplitude of the evoked response is measured to derive an estimate of the number of functioning axons that are contributing to the compound action potential. Responses from sensory and mixed nerves are small, with amplitudes in the order of microvolts, compared to those obtained from motor nerves, which produce compound muscle action potentials (CMAPs) of several millivolts. Hence, sensory action potential (SAP) recording depends on the technique of averaging of several responses to obtain measurable potentials. Nerve conduction velocity is obtained by stimulating a nerve trunk at two or more points, allowing the measurement of conduction in different segments of the nerve (Fig. 19.1).

Conduction velocity in proximal nerve is relatively difficult to measure by direct recording, although high voltage electrical stimulators have been developed for stimulation of the proximal segments of upper limb nerves. Additional techniques are available to estimate proximal nerve conduction. The most widely used method is the F response (Fisher 1992), so called because it was first recorded from a foot muscle. This is a late response evoked by peripheral nerve stimulation, whereby the action potential propagates antidromically to the anterior horn cells, which discharge to produce another axon potential, this being propagated orthodromically down the axon. The latency of F responses depends on nerve length and the distance between the point of nerve stimulation to the spinal cord (Fig. 19.2). In the arm, they have a latency of the order of 25–33 ms and in the leg the latency is 50–60 ms.

Another technique for assessment of proximal conduction is the H reflex, which includes Ia fibres in the afferent arc of the reflex. The latency of the H reflex may be used to provide a measure of conduction in these pathways (Fig. 19.3). H reflexes can be difficult to record in certain muscles, particularly those in the upper limb, and this limits their applicability. For a detailed description of nerve stimulation and recording techniques, the reader is directed to standard textbooks on this subject (DeLisa et al 1987, Kimura 1989, Brown & Bolton 1993).

The normal values for amplitude of nerve and muscle action potentials and conduction velocity vary from nerve to nerve, but, in general, nerves in the upper limbs conduct

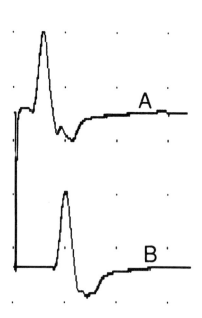

Fig. 19.1 Ulnar nerve motor study in a normal subject. CMAPs are evoked by stimulation at the wrist (A, amplitude 7.0 mV) and at the elbow (B, amplitude 7.0 mV). Motor conduction velocity between wrist and elbow is 59 m/s. (Recording setting: 10 ms per division; sensitivity 5 mV per division; filters 2 Hz–10 kHz.)

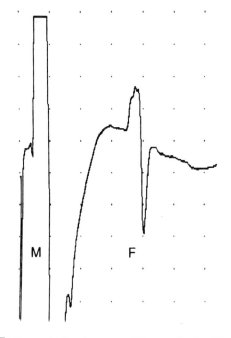

Fig. 19.2 F response in the ulnar nerve. The amplitude of the F response is small relative to the direct muscle response (M), as approximately 1–2% only of motoneurons contribute to the F response. Latency is 33–4 ms. (Subject's height 182 cm. Recording settings: 10 ms per division; sensitivity 100 μV per division; filters 2 Hz–10 kHz.)

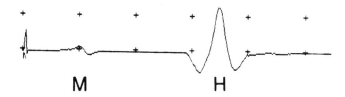

Fig. 19.3 H reflex recorded from soleus muscle. Low intensity, long duration stimulation of the posterior tibial nerve in the popliteal fossa evokes a very small direct muscle response from soleus (M) and an H reflex of latency 29 ms. (Recording settings: 10 ms per division; sensitivity 200 μV per division; filters 2 Hz–10 kHz.)

at faster velocities (50–70 m/s) than those in the lower limb (40–50 m/s), and there is a normal gradient of conduction velocity along the length of a nerve, such that the more peripheral segments conduct less rapidly than proximal parts. The reference range of normal values will differ between laboratories, and each should establish its own normative data. There are a number of biological variables that can affect nerve conduction, and these must be controlled for carefully. The most important variable in clinical practice is limb temperature. Skin temperature below 30°C will reduce nerve conduction velocity, increase the amplitude of nerve compound action potentials (possibly through longer duration opening of sodium channels in the nerve membrane), and enhance neuromuscular transmission (Denys 1991). Furthermore, fibrillations may disappear in a cool limb. Correction of limb temperature is, therefore, essential for diagnostic accuracy. Age is also an important factor (Hyllienmark et al 1995). In children below the age of 5 years, conduction velocities are approximately one-third to one-half those in older children and adults, which is in keeping with age-related myelination of peripheral nerves. In the elderly, amplitudes of sensory nerve potentials decline; sural nerve responses may be unrecordable using skin electrodes in normal subjects above the age of 65 years. The effect of height on normal nerve conduction has received relatively little attention until recently. Height may be a more important variable than age, although not all nerves show the same effect of height on conduction velocity. In the sural, tibial and peroneal nerves, conduction velocity is inversely correlated with height, whereas median nerve conduction velocity shows no relationship to height in normal subjects (Rivner et al 1990). One explanation for variation in conduction with height is axonal size, in that distal segments of longer axons have a smaller diameter and may also have less myelin and shorter internodal distances.

An important technical consideration for nerve conduction studies, particularly when used serially to evaluate progression of a neuropathy, is the inter- and intraexaminer variability. Chaudry et al (1991, 1994) showed that intraexaminer reliability is high, but that amplitudes of SAPs and CMAPs could vary considerably between different examiners. Conduction velocity measurement shows less interexaminer variability. Hence, longitudinal nerve conduction studies are best performed by the same examiner.

Assessment of small nerve fibre function

Standard nerve conduction studies assess function in large myelinated fibres, and therefore test only a minority of the fibres that constitute a peripheral nerve. Most of the fibres which constitute a peripheral nerve are of small diameter: A-δ or small myelinated fibres, and the C or unmyelinated fibres. Assessment of small nerve fibre function is a less straightforward matter than evaluation of large myelinated nerves, and the number of techniques that have been developed for investigation of small fibre neuropathies is testament to the difficulties. The compound nerve action potential evoked by electrical nerve stimulation can be resolved to yield later responses from slower conducting fibres, but this requires near-nerve needle recording and averaging of a thousand or more responses, making this method unsuitable for routine clinical practice (Buchthal et al 1984). Furthermore, activity of unmyelinated fibres is not detectable using this technique. Microneurography, whereby very fine needles are used to record from within individual axons of a nerve trunk, is also too invasive for routine use (Hallin et al 1982). Other methods for assessment of small fibre function include the axon reflex flare (Parkhouse & Le Quesne 1988), which depends on the integrity of nociceptive afferent nerves; cutaneous CO_2 laser evoked responses to measure peripheral and central pathways subserving pain; and the evaluation of thermal thresholds (Jamal et al 1987). Measurement of the thermal threshold for the sensation of cooling assesses small myelinated afferent pathways (A-δ fibres) and warming of the unmyelinated or C-fibre afferents (Fowler et al 1988). Indirect information about the integrity of small fibre afferent and afferent nerves may also be obtained by autonomic function tests.

Electromyography

The technique of EMG involves the recording of spontaneous activity and motor unit potentials in muscles (Daube 1991). It supplies important information about the characteristics of disease processes affecting motor units, and can distinguish between pathology of the lower motor neuron and muscle. The pattern or combination of muscle involvement on EMG is of considerable value in determining whether the pathological process involves the anterior horn cells, roots, plexus, a whole peripheral nerve or its branches. In conjunction with nerve conduction studies, EMG provides information on the duration of peripheral nerve injury and the likely prognosis.

EMG is recorded using needle electrodes inserted into the belly of a muscle with examination of the muscle at rest – for spontaneous potentials – and under voluntary contraction. In normal muscle, spontaneous activity should not be present, except in the regions of the motor end-plates ("motor end-plate noise") and immediately after the needle is inserted. There are a number of different types of abnormal spontaneous activity, but, in general, none is specific to a particular disease or pathological process. Thus, fibrillation potentials may be seen in denervated muscle, motor neuron diseases, and certain muscle disorders, such as polymyositis or endocrine myopathies. Fibrillation potentials and the related abnormal potentials, positive sharp waves, arise from abnormal single muscle fibres in which spontaneous depolarisation occurs. Fasiculations are spontaneous discharges of groups of muscle fibres innervated by the same axon or anterior horn cell, and are often visible through the skin, unlike fibrillations and positive sharp waves. Fasiculations can sometimes be seen as a benign phenomenon in normal subjects, but there is no definitive electrophysiological test that can reliably distinguish benign fasiculations from those which signify pathology. Whilst fasiculations are most often seen in chronic neurogenic disorders, such as neuropathy or anterior horn cell disease, they can occur in all neuromuscular diseases. Other types of nonspecific spontaneous activity include complex repetitive or pseudo-myotonic discharges, which are complexes of potentials with a relatively stable amplitude and frequency, found in neurogenic and some myopathic disorders. True myotonic discharges have variable frequency and amplitude; their sound has been likened to a dive bomber, but the noise of a motorbike engine is a better analogy. They occur in various myotonic muscle disorders, such as dystrophia myotonica and myotonia congenita (Thomsen's disease). Myokymic discharges consist of bursts of motor units discharging at regular intervals, and are seen quite commonly in radiation plexopathy and some chronic nerve entrapments (Fig. 19.4).

Motor unit potentials (MUPs) are assessed during voluntary contraction for their appearance, size, duration and firing pattern. In normal voluntary contraction, motor units increase their firing rates, up to 20 Hz, and larger motor units are recruited as the force of contraction increases. Any of these characteristics may be altered by disease processes. In neurogenic or neuropathic disorders, denervation causes a fallout or loss of motor units, resulting in reduced recruitment or interference patterns, and the firing rate of MUPs is increased (Fig. 19.5). Reinnervation can be identified by a change in the morphology of MUPs, which become polyphasic, of longer duration and, eventually, increased in size. These are features of reinnervation in a partial nerve lesion as a result of collateral sprouting from axons which are either unaffected or less affected by

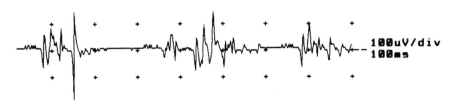

Fig. 19.4 Myokymic discharges in the biceps muscle of a 56-year-old woman who had received radiotherapy for breast carcinoma. Groups of motor unit potentials are seen firing in a rhythmic or repetitive fashion.

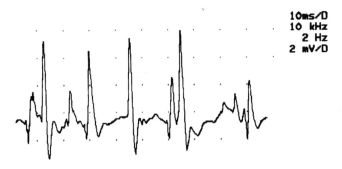

Fig. 19.5 Neurogenic EMG pattern. Motor unit recruitment is reduced, MUP morphology is complex or polyphasic, and firing rates and amplitude are increased.

Table 19.1 EMG findings in denervation and reinnervation

Denervation	Spontaneous activity (fibrillations, positive sharp waves in acute denervation; fasiculations and complex repetitive discharges in chronic denervation)
Reinnervation:	
Early	Normal motor units with increased duration because of late potentials (satellite fibres incorporated through collateral sprouting)
Ongoing	Moderate amplitude polyphasic motor units of long duration, unstable firing due to variable conduction along unmyelinated sprouts and low safety margin of neuromuscular transmission
Late	Large-amplitude polyphasic motor units with stable transmission

the disease process (Table 19.1). Nascent reinnervation through axonal regrowth results in MUPs with different characteristics; nascent units are of very low amplitude (typically less than 0.5 mV), unstable and often highly polyphasic.

The EMG features of myopathic disorders differ from those in neurogenic lesions. In myopathies individual muscle fibres are lost, resulting in small motor unit potentials (1–2 mV) that are polyphasic and of short duration. There is rapid recruitment of large numbers of these small MUPs, with relatively little voluntary effort ("crowded" interference pattern). Although it is usually a straightforward matter for an experienced electromyographer to distinguish between a neurogenic and myopathic disorder on EMG, difficulties may arise in very chronic neuromuscular disease, when there is some overlap in the changes in characteristics of motor units. Additional quantified EMG techniques (Yu & Murray 1984), such as macro-EMG, turns analysis and fibre density (which measures the number of fibres within a motor unit), may be helpful in these situations.

Safety of nerve conduction studies and EMG

Elecrodiagnostic tests are well tolerated and, being largely noninvasive, relatively safe. There is a theoretical risk of transmission of infectious diseases such as hepatitis B or C, and HIV, although there are no reports of cases occurring in clinical practice. Care should be taken with EMG in patients with coagulation disorders; there is an increased risk of bleeding if the prothrombin time is more than 2 or if the platelet count is less than $50\,000/cm^3$. Aspects of electrical safety are crucial, particularly in environments such as the operating theatre or intensive care unit, where attention must be paid to adequate grounding and electrical isolation of the patient from recording apparatus.

PATHOPHYSIOLOGICAL CORRELATES

The electrophysiological changes which occur with nerve pathology of various causes are relatively limited. There are three main pathological processes that affect peripheral nerves: axonal degeneration, segmental demyelination and neuronopathy or disease of the sensory and motor nerve cell bodies. General comments can be made about electrophysiological distinction between processes which primarily affect the axon and those which damage the Schwann cell or myelin sheath. In axonopathy, there is a reduction or loss of amplitude of nerve and compound muscle action potentials, with relatively little change in nerve conduction velocity, unless the axonal degeneration is of severe degree. Experimental data have shown that up to 30% reduction of conduction velocity may occur in axonal atrophy (Baba et al 1982), due probably to axonal shrinkage or secondary demyelination. Axonal degeneration will result in a reduction of the number of MUPs and the appearance of fibrillation potentials and other evidence of denervation on EMG. Demyelinating neuropathic processes have variable effects on the amplitude of compound action potentials and the characteristics of MUPs, the principal electrophysiological changes being a reduction in conduction velocity and the occurrence of conduction block (see p. 472). Formal criteria have been proposed for the diagnosis of demyelinating neuropathies, particularly those due to inflammatory processes, on the basis of conduction velocity, distal motor latency, F wave latency and CMAP amplitudes (Cornblath 1990; AAN AIDS Task Force 1991).

Nerve transection serves as a useful model of the neurophysiological changes that occur after nerve or axonal injury. Following section of a nerve, axons and their myelin sheaths begin to break down rapidly, as Wallerian degeneration takes place distal to the site of the lesion. Axons become inexcitable and neuromuscular transmission fails. Thus, there is no response to direct stimulation of the nerve distal to the lesion. However, some conduction may be maintained for a few days after the nerve injury, depending on the rate of Wallerian degeneration, which is determined in part by the length of the distal stump. The failure in conduction is evident on recording action potentials from sensory and muscle fibres, which show a progressive decline in amplitude. The reduction in CMAP size precedes that of sensory potentials. Chaudry and Cornblath (1992) have evaluated the sequential changes in nerve conduction studies in five subjects with acute nerve injury. The amplitude of CMAPs had fallen by 50% at 3–5 days after injury, and responses were absent by day 9. Sensory nerve action potentials were reduced in size by 50% at 1 week after injury and had disappeared by day 11. The rate at which the amplitude of both sensory and motor responses fell was greater in lesions with shorter distal stumps. In contrast to the amplitudes of compound nerve and muscle action potentials, there is relatively little acute effect on nerve conduction velocities, which may be maintained at near normal levels, whilst responses can still be evoked from sensory and motor nerves. Fibrillation potentials appear as muscles are denervated, but the timing of the appearance of denervation potentials depends on the distance between the site of the nerve lesion and the muscle. Thus there may be an interval of 10–40 days before fibrillations are seen, and these will be found in proximal muscles before they occur in distal muscles (Weddell et al 1944). Quantification of the amount of fibrillation potentials is not helpful in assessing the degree of axonal degeneration.

The process of regeneration or reinnervation begins at the same time as Wallerian degeneration is taking place. In partial or incomplete nerve lesions, reinnervation can occur quite rapidly, through collateral sprouting of surviving axons into areas of denervated muscle fibres. The collateral sprouts are initially thin and unmyelinated, and thus conduction in the terminal sprouts is variable and extremely slow, with rates of approximately 5 m/s (Feasby et al 1981). This results in unstable MUPs, in which neuromuscular transmission often fails. As the terminal axon sprouts become myelinated, conduction becomes more reliable and the threshold for stimulation is reduced. The conduction velocity in regenerated fibres improves to 80–100% of normal levels (Ballantyne & Campbell 1973). In more severe axonal degenerative lesions, reinnervation is dependent on axonal regrowth. The timing of appearance of nascent MUPs depends on the distance between the site of the lesion and muscle. The scope for clinical recovery in this type of reinnervation is determined by the efficiency with which the regenerated axons reach their target effector and receptor sites and the integrity of these structures. The reappearance of voluntary MUP activity signals that reinnervation is taking place, and EMG evidence of this usually precedes clinical evidence of recovery. However, the amount of MUP activity is not a quantitative measure of reinnervation; serial measurement of evoked responses or CMAPs provides the best guide to the degree of recovery in individual muscles. Furthermore, the finding of a few motor units showing reinnervation, even at an early stage after injury, does not imply that full recovery of the nerve will take place.

Conduction block

Conduction block refers to the phenomenon of failure of conduction in an intact axon or nerve fibre. As with degenerative lesions of nerves, the clinical manifestation or consequence of conduction block is weakness. There is, however, an important difference in that weakness due to conduction block is recoverable when the block is reversed, whereas recovery from axonal degeneration is less predictable and may be incomplete. Conduction block is a common feature of demyelinating neuropathies and compression neuropathies, such as the carpal tunnel syndrome, peroneal neuropathies at the knee and some ulnar neuropathies, particularly in the region of the cubital tunnel. It may occur transiently, as in the Saturday night palsy type of radial nerve entrapment, or last for several weeks or months (Trojaborg 1977). Conduction block which appears to persist for years is seen in some cases of chronic inflammatory demyelinating neuropathy. The pathophysiology of chronic conduction block is not well understood; it may be the consequence of intramyelin oedema or failure of remyelination.

The entity of paralysis in the setting of preserved electrical excitability of muscles has been recognised since the 19th century – Erb (1876) considered that motor nerves underwent a change in their molecular constitution which abolished their ability to conduct. Seddon (1943) was aware of the phenomenon of conduction block or neurapraxia when he devised his classification of nerve injury, although its morphological basis was not known at the time. It is now well established through experimental work on animal models of nerve compression (Ochoa et al 1972, Rudge et al 1974), and in man (Feasby et al 1985), that the pathological change which underlies conduction block is focal or paranodal demyelination. Demyelination limited to two or three nodes of Ranvier may be sufficient to result in failure of propagation of the nerve action potential. The susceptibility of individual nerve fibres to conduction block depends in part on the diameter of the axon, with large fibres being more affected than smaller axons, particularly those of 5 μm or less (Gilliatt 1980). However, the position of axons and fascicles within a nerve and thus their relation to a compressive agent such as underlying bony structures may also be an important factor in determining which nerve fibres show conduction block.

The electrophysiological changes which occur in conduction block differ from those in axonopathies. The CMAP is reduced in size, by at least 20–30% and often substantially more. Conduction velocity is relatively unaffected in the nerve segment below the site of the block, depending on the degree of involvement of faster conducting motor fibres, and there is typically no evidence of denervation on EMG. However, some fibrillations may sometimes be seen in nerve lesions where the primary pathological change is conduction block and focal demyelination, because an element of axonal degeneration will be present. The occurrence of some fibrillations in a focal compressive nerve lesion with conduction block is not necessarily an indication of a poorer prognosis (Gilliatt 1981). A direct relationship between the amount of reduction of the CMAP and the degree of conduction block cannot be assumed because of the effect of differential involvement of large and small fibres. Conduction block is more readily diagnosed in motor nerves than in sensory fibres, which is partly a consequence of the morphology and size of sensory action potentials and the wider range of conduction velocities in sensory axons. The difficulties of detection of sensory conduction block using standard nerve conduction studies may explain the normal electrodiagnostic findings in some entrapment neuropathies, such as subacute ulnar nerve lesions that manifest with purely sensory symptoms. The identification of conduction block in motor nerve fibres is, nonetheless, fraught with technical issues. In particular, temporal dispersion and phase cancellation in the summated response of a CMAP will result in an apparent reduction in amplitude which could spuriously mimic conduction block. However, dispersion is more likely to occur in longer segments of nerve than are typically affected in common entrapment neuropathies. Measurement of the area underlying the CMAP overcomes some of the technical problems of temporal dispersion and phase cancellation.

Seddon's classification of nerve injury: electrodiagnostic correlates

Seddon (1943) classified nerve injury as being of three types: neurapraxia, axonotmesis and neurotmesis. In their pure form, these three types of lesion show distinct electrophysiological features (Table 19.2). However, the distinction between neurapraxia and axonal degeneration of partial or complete degree is difficult in the acute stages of nerve injury, prior to evidence of denervation in the form of fibrillation potentials on EMG. Therefore, electrodiagnostic tests cannot reliably differentiate a neurapraxic lesion from one with Wallerian degeneration in the first few days after nerve injury.

LOCALISATION OF LESIONS

The combination of SAP recording and EMG sampling allows delineation of the anatomical site of nerve lesions. Thus, in a patient who presents with unilateral foot drop, an absent superficial peroneal sensory nerve potential and denervation in the tibialis anterior, peroneus longus and tertius indicate a lesion of the common peroneal nerve at the level of the knee. The presence of denervation in the short head of the biceps femoris would signify a more proximal lesion, i.e. one involving the peroneal component of the sciatic nerve. A normal superficial peroneal SAP and denervation in tibialis anterior and tibialis posterior indicates L5 root pathology, as radicular lesions most commonly affect the portion of the root that is proximal to the dorsal root ganglion, and thus the cell bodies and distal axons of sensory nerves are preserved. Sensory nerve recording is therefore of great value in distinguishing between a root lesion and pathology at a more distal site, and this is of particular importance when there is suspicion of root avulsion. The electrodiagnostic triad of root avulsion is:

- a normal SAP (Bonney & Gilliatt 1958) and preserved histamine response
- denervation in paraspinal muscles
- absence of somatosensory evoked potentials, together with fibrillations and absence of voluntary MUPs in peripheral muscles supplied by the root.

The anatomical derivations for sensory nerves and muscles commonly studied in a neurophysiology laboratory are given in Tables 19.3 and 19.4.

Table 19.2 Electrodiagnostic features of nerve injury

Nerve injury type	SAP	CMAP	Conduction velocity	EMG
Neurapraxia	Reduced amplitude proximal to block. Normal amplitude distal to block		Usually preserved	No/sparse fibrillations. Characteristic IP of normal MUPs firing at rapid rates, with reduced interference pattern
Axonotmesis	↓	↓	Normal/reduced to a degree dependent on severity of axonal degeneration and fibre type involved	Fibrillations. Reduced IP, ↑ firing rate of MUPs. Evidence of reinnervation dependent on age of lesion (see Table 19.1)
Neurotmesis	A	A	Unmeasurable	Profuse fibrillations. No voluntary MUPs

↑, increased; ↓, decreased; A, absent; CMAP, compound muscle action potential; IP, interference pattern; MUP, motor unit potential; SAP, sensory action potential.

Table 19.3 Derivation of sensory nerves used in electrodiagnosis

SAP	Root	Brachial plexus		
		Trunk	*Cord*	*Nerve*
Upper limb (peripheral)				
Median digit 1	C6	Upper	Lateral	
Median digit 2	C6/7	Middle	Lateral	Median
Median digit 3	C7	Middle	Lateral	
Ulnar digit 5	C8	Lower	Medial	Ulnar
Superficial radial	C7	Middle > upper	Posterior	Radial
Lateral antebrachial cutaneous	C6	Upper	Lateral	Musculocutaneous
Medial antebrachial cutaneous	C7/8	Lower	Medial	
Lower limb		*Peripheral nerve*		
Saphenous	L2–L4		Femoral	
Superficial peroneal	L5		Sciatic	Common peroneal
Medial plantar	L5		Sciatic	Tibial
Lateral plantar	L5		Sciatic	Tibial
Sural	S1		Sciatic	Tibial

Table 19.4 Nerve and main root supply of muscles commonly used in EMG

Muscle	Nerve	Root
Upper limb		
Trapezius	Spinal accessory	C3,4
Rhomboids	Dorsal scapular	C5
Serratus anterior	Long thoracic	C5,6,7
Supraspinatus	Suprascapular	C5,6
Infraspinatus	Suprascapular	C5,6
Latissimus dorsi	Thoracodorsal	C7
Deltoid	Axillary	C5,6
Biceps	Musculocutaneous	C5,6
Triceps	Radial	C6,7
Brachioradialis	Radial	C6
Extensor carpi radialis	Radial	C6,7
Extensor carpi ulnaris	Posterior interosseous	C7
Extensor digitorum communis	Posterior interosseous	C7
Extensor pollicis brevis	Posterior interosseous	C7
Extensor indicis proprius	Posterior interosseous	C7
Pronator teres	Median	C6,7
Flexor digitorum superficialis	Median	C7,8
Abductor pollicis brevis	Median	C8, T1
Opponens pollicis	Median	C8, T1
Flexor pollicis brevis	Median	C8, T1
Flexor digitorum profundus (1 + 2)	Anterior interosseous	C8
Flexor pollicis longus	Anterior interosseous	C8
Pronator quadratus	Anterior interosseous	C8
Flexor carpi ulnaris	Ulnar	C8
Flexor digitorum profundus (3 + 4)	Ulnar	C8
Abductor digiti minimi	Ulnar	C8, T1
Dorsal interossei	Ulnar	C8, T1
Lumbricals (3 + 4)	Ulnar	C8, T1

Table 19.4 *(cont'd)*

Muscle	Nerve	Root
Lower limb		
Iliopsoas	Femoral	L1,2
Vastus lateralis, medialis	Femoral	L3,4
Adductor longus, magnus	Obturator	L2,3
Gluteus medius, minimus	Superior gluteal	L4,5
Gluteus maximus	Inferior gluteal	L5, S1
Biceps femoris (long head)	Sciatic (tibial division)	S1
Gastrocnemius	Sciatic/tibial	S1
Soleus	Sciatic/tibial	S1
Tibialis posterior	Sciatic/tibial	L5
Abductor hallucis	Sciatic/tibial	S1
Biceps femoris (short head)	Sciatic (peroneal division)	L5, S1
Tibialis anterior	Sciatic/deep peroneal	L4, 5
Extensor digitorum brevis	Sciatic/deep peroneal	L5, S1
Peroneus tertius	Sciatic/deep peroneal	L5, S1
Peroneus longus	Sciatic/superficial peroneal	L5, S1
Peroneus brevis	Sciatic/superficial peroneal	L5, S1

NORMAL VARIANTS OF INNERVATION

Innervation anomalies in the upper and lower limbs have implications for clinical practice and interpretation of neurophysiological findings (Sonck et al 1991). Some of these anomalies are relatively common. The Martin–Gruber anastomosis between the median and ulnar nerves in the forearm is estimated to occur in 20% of the population. In this anastomosis, median nerve fibres leave the main nerve trunk or the anterior interosseous branch in the forearm, cross over to the ulnar nerve, and terminate in intrinsic hand muscles normally supplied by the ulnar nerve. This will manifest as a reversal of the usual pattern of CMAP amplitude evoked by median nerve stimulation at the wrist and elbow. In subjects without anomalous innervation, the CMAP produced at the wrist is slightly larger than that at the elbow. When a significant anastomosis is present, the CMAP will be larger at the elbow. The morphology of the CMAP is often anomalous, showing an initial positive deflection. The Martin–Gruber anastomosis can present diagnostic difficulties when a carpal tunnel syndrome is present, because some median fibres will be spared from compression at the wrist. Stimulation of the median nerve at the elbow may produce a response which has a similar or shorter latency compared with the distal latency at the wrist, and the conduction velocity in the forearm segment of the median nerve will be spuriously fast. A Martin–Gruber anastomosis may also affect electrodiagnosis of ulnar neuropathies at the elbow. A complete or severe lesion at this site may appear to be partial because of the minimal involvement of intrinsic hand muscles which are anomalously innervated by the crossed median fibres.

Other anomalous innervations include the "all median" and "all ulnar" hands, variations in sensory innervation on the dorsal side of the hand, and the accessory deep peroneal nerve. This is a branch of the deep peroneal nerve which runs around the lateral malleolus to innervate part or all of the extensor digitorum brevis (EDB) muscle in the foot. The CMAP from EDB evoked by stimulation of the peroneal nerve at the ankle will be smaller than that evoked by stimulation at the knee in the presence of an accessory branch.

ELECTRODIAGNOSIS OF ENTRAPMENT NEUROPATHIES

Nerve conduction studies are an essential component of the preoperative evaluation of entrapment neuropathies in confirming the site, nature and severity of nerve compression. These conditions form one of the commonest reasons for referral for electrodiagnostic tests.

Median neuropathies

Carpal tunnel syndrome

Median nerve compression within the carpal tunnel at the wrist is the most well defined of entrapment neuropathies, but the clinical symptoms and signs of carpal tunnel syndrome (CTS) can be atypical, and nerve conduction studies (NCS) should be performed in all cases to confirm the diagnosis and exclude other conditions, such as a radiculopathy or proximal median nerve lesion (Clarke Stevens 1987). The pathophysiological basis of CTS is focal compression and demyelination of the median nerve in the region of the carpal ligament, and thus electrodiagnosis depends on the demonstration of a delay in sensory and/or motor latency in the segment of the nerve which traverses the carpal tunnel. Sensory latency testing is more sensitive than motor studies (Jablecki et al 1993), although 2–3% of cases manifest with abnormal conduction confined to the motor fibres of the median nerve (Johnson & Shrewsbury 1970). The extent of NCS abnormality depends on the degree of nerve compression and NCS can therefore be used to give an indication of the severity of median nerve entrapment. In *mild* or *moderate* cases, the SAP from median digits is of reduced size and sensory latency is prolonged. Stimulation of the thumb or third finger may be more sensitive than that of the second digit (Macdonell et al 1990). There is no significant difference between orthodromic and antidromic sensory nerve conduction (Tackmann et al 1981), and the orthodromic method of median sensory testing is preferred, being technically easier. In the motor study, some slowing of motor conduction may occur across the wrist, although the distal latency to the abductor pollicis brevis (APB) does not usually exceed 5 ms in mild or moderate cases. Motor conduction in the segment of the nerve above the carpal tunnel should be normal and denervation of APB is not present, but there may be some reduction in size of the CMAP and motor unit recruitment as a consequence of conduction block, if present. Rarely, low-frequency repetitive firing of motor nerve fibres is seen on EMG (Fig. 19.6). This phenomenon was first observed by Simpson (1956), and is probably directly related to demyelination or hyperexcitable regenerating fibres.

In *severe* cases of CTS, the sensory potentials are very small or absent, and motor studies are then essential to demonstrate delayed conduction; usually, the distal latency will be considerably above 5 ms. There may also be slight slowing of conduction in the forearm segment of the median nerve (45–55 m/s). The evoked response from APB will usually be below 4 mv (Kimura & Ayyar 1985). Fibrillations and other evidence of denervation may be present on needle examination of APB, signifying a component of axonal degeneration.

Routine nerve conduction studies will identify abnormalities in 60–70% of patients with CTS. Those in whom routine tests show no definite abnormality usually have mild symptoms, and these cases present a particular electrodiagnostic challenge, especially as the trend is towards earlier diagnosis and treatment. Much recent work has gone into the development of neurophysiological tests that have greater sensitivity and specificity to improve diagnosis in clinically mild CTS. Palmar stimulation (Mills 1985) assesses conduction velocity in median palm–wrist fibres, the segment in which the major slowing of conduction is known to occur. Up to 15–20% more patients show abnormalities on palm–wrist studies compared with standard digital nerve sensory studies. Comparison of sensory conduction in the palmar cutaneous branch and first digital branch of the median nerve has also been shown to increase diagnostic yield (Chang & Lien 1991). Other techniques include inching (Kimura 1979), whereby serial stimulation at 0.5–1 cm intervals along the median nerve from lower forearm to palm localises sensory slowing to the distal edge of the carpal ligament in about half of cases, the remainder showing more diffuse slowing. More sensitive measures of motor conduction include the comparison of latency to the second lumbrical and first dorsal interosseous muscles (Preston & Logigan 1992, Sheean et al 1995) which is of value when sensory tests are equivocal, in severe cases when standard responses are unobtainable or in coexistent neuropathies where localisation of conduction abnormality at the wrist is otherwise difficult. The majority of these additional methods utilise measurement of conduction in relatively short segments of nerve, given that location of conduction delay or block resulting from a small demyelinating lesion can be difficult to identify when the distance between the stimulating and recording electrode is relatively long. Gilliatt and Meer (1990) used a different approach in measuring the refractory period of transmission in the median nerve, defined as the maximum interval between two impulses at which there is failure of a nerve fibre to conduct the second impulse. An increase in the refractory period of transmission could be a more sensitive indicator of a small or localised area of nerve demyelination. Patients with CTS frequently showed loss of impulse transmission at the wrist, whereas median nerve fibres at the elbow retained the ability to conduct a second impulse. This technique has not yet achieved widespread clinical application.

Although these more sensitive techniques appear to improve the yield of diagnosis in CTS, there may be loss of specificity, with a high rate of false positive results

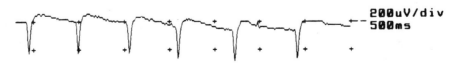

200uV/div
500ms

Fig. 19.6 Low-frequency repetitive discharges in a patient with severe chronic median nerve compression at the wrist.

(Redmond & Rivner 1988). Thus, abnormalities may be seen in otherwise normal subjects, in the contralateral and asymptomatic hand in patients with CTS, or in patients without a history indicative of CTS. Caution must therefore be applied when electrodiagnostic findings appear to indicate CTS in patients without symptoms or in whom the history is very atypical, particularly if more sensitive tests are employed.

Routine testing for CTS should include measurement of the sensory latency and amplitude of at least one other nerve, such as the ulnar or radial, for comparison with the median nerve, and also to identify a more extensive or diffuse neuropathy. Measurement of lower limb or sural potentials has not been found to be useful on a routine basis, and is only necessary when there is suspicion of a generalised neuropathy, such as in a diabetic patient.

The decision to operate is essentially a clinical one, but certain electrodiagnostic abnormalities are strong indicators for surgery. These are absence of the median digital SAP, a prolonged distal motor latency (particularly > 5 ms) or evidence of denervation in APB. The degree of preoperative abnormality is a reasonable guide to the rate and amount of postoperative recovery. When the preoperative findings indicate conduction block only, full and rapid response to median nerve decompression is to be expected. If axonal injury has supervened, improvement will be slower and probably less complete. Goodman and Gilliatt (1961) studied the effect of treatment in patients with CTS and found that where median nerve compression was severe prior to surgery (distal motor latency of > 10 ms), motor latency took up to 18 months to show recovery and residual abnormalities were common (Fig. 19.7). In moderate cases (distal motor latency 7–10 ms), a more rapid and complete recovery occurred over 8–12 months after surgery. Mild cases (distal motor latency 5–7 ms) showed normal motor conduction within 6 months.

The sensory studies showed variable response to surgery, with mild cases usually returning to normal within a few months of operation and severe cases showing persistent abnormality. Electrodiagnostic evaluation of patients with residual symptoms after carpal tunnel decompression can be difficult, and studies are virtually uninterpretable if preoperative data are not available for comparison. Goodman and Gilliatt also looked at the effect of splinting on median nerve conduction and, interestingly, found that most cases showed no change or even a slight deterioration in sensory and motor conduction, despite symptomatic relief.

Proximal median neuropathies

Proximal median neuropathies are uncommon compared with median nerve compression at the wrist. High lesions of the median nerve involve its main trunk at or just proximal to the pronator teres muscle, or the anterior interosseous branch. In general, electromyography is much more useful

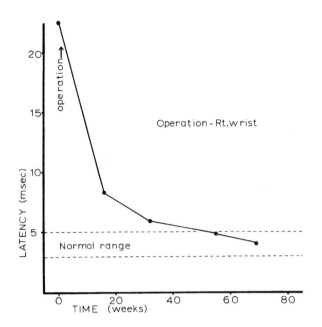

Fig. 19.7 Severe carpal tunnel syndrome: recovery of motor conduction following nerve decompression. Distal motor latency to APB prior to surgery was > 20 ms. Following operation, there was a rapid fall in latency to 7 ms over a period of about 10 weeks. Subsequent improvement in conduction occurred more gradually, with normal latency at 1 year after surgery.

than nerve conduction studies in establishing the level of proximal median neuropathies (Buchthal et al 1974). In one study (Gross & Royden Jones 1992), only 5 of 14 patients with main trunk lesions had abnormalities of nerve conduction, including small median sensory amplitudes, a reduced CMAP from APB or abnormal motor velocity in the forearm segment. Conduction block localised to the antecubital fossa was seen in only one patient. However, all cases had acute or chronic denervation in median innervated forearm muscles, including the pronator teres. EMG was not helpful in distinguishing between median nerve entrapment at the level of pronator teres from more proximal lesions. In the same study, no patients with an anterior interosseous syndrome had abnormal nerve conduction studies, but EMG identified denervation confined to muscles supplied by this branch – namely, the flexor pollicis longus, the pronator quadratus and the median part of flexor digitorum profundus. In any suspected case of the anterior interosseous nerve, extensive EMG should be performed, as the lesion may be a presentation of neuralgic amyotrophy (England & Summer 1987). Thus, proximal muscles, including the spinati, rhomboids and serratus anterior, should be examined in addition to forearm muscles innervated by the median nerve. In patients with anterior interosseous entrapment in the presence of a Martin–Gruber anastomosis between the median and ulnar trunks in the forearm, denervation in intrinsic hand muscles (first dorsal interosseous, adductor pollicis, abductor digiti minimi) may be seen (Wertsch 1992).

Ulnar neuropathies

Lesions at the elbow

Ulnar neuropathies in the region of the elbow are the second commonest type of entrapment neuropathy, although the pathophysiology is more complex than in carpal tunnel syndrome. Electrodiagnosis in mild lesions of the ulnar nerve, manifesting with sensory symptoms alone, can be particularly difficult, and routine nerve conduction studies are often normal or equivocal in these cases. However, most ulnar neuropathies show motor involvement in addition to sensory symptoms, and electrodiagnosis depends on the demonstration of slowing of motor velocity or conduction block to localise lesions at specific sites. Ulnar neuropathies at the elbow can be divided into two main types: lesions in the medial epicondylar groove, which are often chronic and include the tardy ulnar palsy; and entrapment of the nerve by the aponeurosis of the flexor carpi ulnaris muscle in the region of the cubital tunnel. Involvement of the nerve in the medial epicondylar groove results in a small or absent ulnar SAP and mixed nerve action potential (NAP); more subtle abnormalities may be manifest by a reduction in amplitude of the SAPs and NAPs of the order of greater than 50% of the response at the elbow compared with that at the wrist. When the NAP is absent at the elbow, it may be helpful to show that the NAP above the elbow is normal by stimulating the nerve above the sulcal groove and recording from the trunk of the ulnar nerve in the region of the axilla. Localisation to the medial epicondylar groove is dependent on the demonstration of slow motor and/or sensory conduction in the sulcal segment of the ulnar nerve (Payan 1969). It is uncommon to find conduction block in medial epicondylar lesions, in part because they are usually chronic and axonal in type. Denervation will be present in hypothenar muscles and the first dorsal interosseous (FDIO); the flexor carpi ulnaris (FCU) is often spared, either because its branch leaves the main trunk above the level of the medial epicondyle or as a consequence of the fascicular arrangement of the ulnar nerve. Fascicles which innervate more distal muscles lie medially in the ulnar nerve trunk and are therefore more susceptible to compression by adjacent bony structures.

Given that identification of medial epicondylar lesions is dependent on identification of slow conduction in a short segment of the ulnar nerve, the technical difficulties of accurate measurement of nerve length are of particular concern in electrodiagnosis of ulnar neuropathies at the elbow. Small errors in measurement of short lengths of a nerve produce relatively large errors in calculation of nerve conduction. The surface measurement of the ulnar nerve

at the elbow underestimates its length and results in an erroneously low velocity; furthermore, the length of the nerve is affected by elbow position. Rigorous accuracy in measurement and study of the nerve in a standard flexed elbow position (Checkles et al 1971) helps to minimise these errors.

In the cubital tunnel syndrome, compression of the ulnar nerve is identified by the demonstration of conduction block localised to the region of the cubital tunnel. This will be manifest as a reduction of more than 25% in the amplitude of the CMAP from the abductor digiti minimi (ADM) or FD10 (Fig. 19.8), or, occasionally, dispersion of the response (Miller 1979). Stewart (1987) has shown that abnormalities are more likely to be found if recordings are made from FDIO, although in some cases there may be selective involvement of one or other of these muscles, and both should be examined for evidence of conduction block. The preferential involvement of FDIO is thought again to be a consequence of the fascicular arrangement of ulnar nerve fibres at the elbow. Patients with cubital tunnel syndrome will also show abnormalities of the ulnar SAP (small or absent), and on EMG of muscles innervated by the ulnar nerve below the branch to the FCU. These may be confined to evidence of conduction block (i.e. a reduction of motor unit recruitment and increase in firing rates, but normal motor unit morphology and absence of fibrillations), or denervation if axonal degeneration has occurred. Precise localisation of conduction block in cubital tunnel syndrome has been advocated using the technique of inching, whereby the ulnar nerve is stimulated serially at intervals of 1 or 2 cm (Smaje 1983, Campbell et al 1992). However, the exact point of stimulation of the nerve may be uncertain, as a result of local spread of current. The electrophysiologist must also be aware of the variation in anatomy of the cubital tunnel: cadaveric studies have shown that the intramuscular

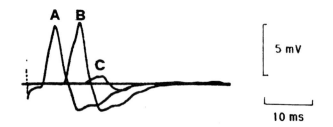

Fig. 19.8 Conduction block in an ulnar neuropathy. CMAPs from the ADM evoked by stimulation at the wrist (A), 5 cm below the elbow (B) and 5 cm above the elbow (C). A marked drop in amplitude of the CMAP is seen with stimulation above the elbow in this patient with tardive dyskinesia induced by neuroleptic treatment. The ulnar neuropathy was thought to be due to repetitive flexion and extension movements of the elbow of a dystonic nature. Management was conservative, with advice to avoid prolonged elbow flexion. The conduction block recovered after 4 months with a normal ulnar nerve study, other than a slightly small ulnar SAP from the little finger of 5 μV.

course of the ulnar nerve through the FCU ranges from 18 to 70 mm, and the nerve exits the FCU at a distance of 28–69 mm from the medial epicondyle (Campbell et al 1991). If a cubital tunnel syndrome is identified, the opposite limb should be examined, as some cases are bilateral (Miller 1991).

The results of surgery for ulnar nerve lesions at the elbow are generally less satisfactory than in carpal tunnel syndrome. If a neurapraxic lesion is identified, with evidence of conduction block on electrophysiological studies, there may be spontaneous recovery, as in ulnar nerve lesions developing after surgical procedures (Watson et al 1992), with return of conduction to normal within a few weeks. In more persistent neurapraxic lesions in the cubital tunnel, decompression may be necessary. Surgical treatment of the chronic axonal ulnar neuropathy in the medial epicondylar groove is relatively disappointing and residual abnormalities of nerve conduction are found after transposition (Payan 1970).

As with other apparent mononeuropathies, an underlying predisposing neuropathy may be present in patients with ulnar nerve lesions, and electrodiagnostic assessment should include examination of at least one other upper limb nerve. The differential diagnosis of an ulnar neuropathy at the elbow includes a lower trunk plexopathy, in which there will be denervation in other C8/T1 muscles including APB; and C8 radiculopathy, with denervation in the C8 myotome and a normal ulnar SAP and NAP. Lesions of the ulnar nerve in the upper arm above the elbow cannot reliably be distinguished from more distal lesions on EMG grounds. Distinction of a high ulnar neuropathy from a more proximal lesion in the brachial plexus should be possible by measuring the medial antebrachial cutaneous SAP, which derives from the C8 root, and by examination of non-ulnar-innervated C8 muscles.

Distal ulnar nerve lesions

Entrapment at the wrist is an important, albeit relatively rare, site of ulnar nerve lesions. The most commonly reported types of distal ulnar neuropathies are compression of the deep branch to the FDIO (Hunt 1911) and lesions of the nerve within Guyon's canal. Other motor branches may be affected in the palm, such as that to the ADM, or there may be a pure sensory lesion.

The characteristic finding in a lesion affecting the deep branch of the ulnar nerve is a relatively prolonged distal motor latency to FDIO, typically by 1 ms or more than the latency to ADM (Ebeling et al 1960). Denervation is present in FDIO, but not in hypothenar muscles. Occasionally, there may be some slowing of conduction in the ulnar nerve in the forearm, if FDIO is used to evaluate this. The ulnar sensory study (SAP from digit 5) is normal in lesions of the deep palmar branch. EMG examination outside the hand may be necessary to exclude a diffuse neurogenic disorder such as anterior horn cell disease, or a C8 radiculopathy.

Entrapment within Guyon's canal involves both distal motor and sensory branches, resulting in loss or reduction of the ulnar digital SAP and denervation of all intrinsic hand muscles innervated by the ulnar nerve. Measurement of the dorsal cutaneous ulnar SAP is a useful technique when distinguishing a distal ulnar lesion from one at the elbow. This sensory branch exits the ulnar nerve approximately 8 cm above Guyon's canal and a normal response will be found in distal ulnar neuropathies, whereas the SAP will be lost or reduced in lesions affecting the nerve at the elbow.

Radial nerve lesions

These are the least common of the upper limb entrapment neuropathies. The radial nerve can be compressed in the upper arm, or around the elbow; occasionally, a lesion may affect the superficial sensory branch in the forearm or at the wrist. The most frequently encountered radial neuropathy is "Saturday night palsy", when the nerve is compressed within the spiral groove of the humerus bone. Although the lesion is primarily of neurapraxic type (Watson & Brown 1992), additional mild denervation in the form of fibrillations and positive sharp waves is often seen in combination with reduced recruitment and increased firing rates of motor units in the extensor digitorum communis, extensor pollicis longus (EPL), supinator and extensor carpi radialis. Occasionally, there may be involvement of the lateral head of the triceps muscle, depending on the exact point of compression of the nerve. The radial SAP will be reduced in size, although often by less than half that of the unaffected limb. It is sometimes possible to locate the site of conduction block in the spiral groove by measuring CMAPs from the EPL or extensor indicis proprius, stimulating above, below and at the level of the spiral groove. If the amplitudes of the CMAP and radial SAP are reduced by more than 50% distal to the site of compression, recovery may be protracted beyond several months and eventually incomplete (Brown & Watson 1993). These measurements are therefore of some value in determining prognosis.

The differential diagnosis of a high radial nerve lesion includes a C7 radiculopathy, in which abnormalities will be found on EMG in other C7 muscles, such as the serratus anterior, latissimus dorsi and cervical paraspinal muscles. Radial sensory and motor conduction studies will be normal in a C7 root lesion. More extensive denervation is also seen in brachial plexopathies involving the middle trunk or posterior cord.

The posterior interosseous nerve is a motor branch of the radial nerve which leaves the main trunk just below the elbow, to enter the supinator muscle under the arcade of Frohse. Compression of this nerve results in wrist and finger drop, but weakness of wrist extension is only partial, because the extensors carpi radiales (ECR L & B) are usually spared. Electromyographic abnormalities are seen in all muscles innervated by the branch; normal EMG of the supinator, ECR L & B and other proximal muscles distinguishes a posterior interosseous neuropathy from a high radial nerve lesion. The superficial radial sensory response is unaffected or minimally reduced in amplitude in posterior interosseous compression. Demonstration of conduction block or focal slowing in neurapraxic posterior interosseous lesions is technically difficult, but it is sometimes possible to show this across the arcade of Frohse.

Pure lesions of the superficial radial nerve are rare, and are usually due to direct compression such as from handcuffs. However, symptoms may be misleading, and some cases are misdiagnosed as De Quervain's tenosynovitis. Diagnosis is established by showing an abnormality of the superficial radial sensory potential, either by comparison with the radial SAP in the unaffected arm, or by comparing conduction with the lateral antebrachial cutaneous nerve on the same side (Spindler & Dellon 1990). Typically, there will be reduction in amplitude of the superficial radial SAP, and perhaps slowing of sensory conduction.

A radial neuropathy is sometimes considered in patients with resistant "tennis elbow" or pain on repeated supination and pronation of the elbow. Variable electrophysiological abnormalities have been reported in these cases. In a series of 28 patients, Rosen & Werner (1980) found that routine radial motor conduction studies were of no value, but an increase in motor latency of > 0.5 ms was seen when conduction studies were repeated during forced supination of the arm. Inconclusive abnormalities were found on EMG of muscles innervated by the posterior interosseous nerve. Whether these cases represent a true compression neuropathy syndrome is uncertain.

Lower limb entrapment neuropathies

Peroneal nerve lesions

Lesions of the peroneal nerve may involve the main trunk, or common peroneal nerve, and its deep or superficial branches. The common peroneal nerve is most vulnerable to compression around the neck of the fibular head, just above the division of the main trunk into its two branches. Lesions of the common peroneal nerve manifest electrophysiologically with reduction in size or loss of the superficial peroneal SAP, a small or absent common peroneal NAP (Fig. 19.9), and abnormalities of motor conduction. Recording of the CMAP from extensor digitorum brevis permits localisation of conduction block in neurapraxic lesions, with a drop in amplitude of the response at the fibular head. Motor conduction may be slowed in the segment of the nerve around the fibular head, or more diffusely. Measurement of sensory conduction using the

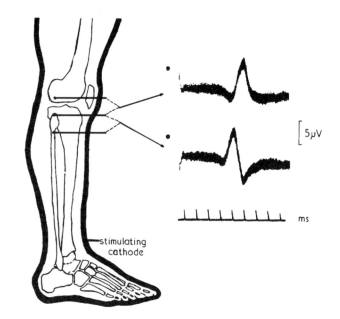

Fig. 19.9 Common peroneal nerve action potential. The NAP is recorded at and above the fibula head, with stimulation distally at the ankle. There is normal conduction around the fibula head.

superficial peroneal nerve or the common peroneal NAP is said to be a more sensitive and reliable method of demonstrating focal slowing (Gilliatt et al 1961). Up to two-thirds of patients with peroneal palsy will show slowing of conduction or focal conduction block if both sensory and motor conduction studies are used (Singh et al 1974).

Denervation is found in the tibialis anterior, peroneal, and extensor digitorum brevis (EDB) muscles, depending on the degree of axonal degeneration. Muscles innervated by the deep peroneal branch are more likely to show denervation in common peroneal palsies, probably as a consequence of fascicular arrangement within the main nerve trunk. Evidence of axonal involvement should not be based on abnormalities confined to EDB, as this and other intrinsic foot muscles may show fibrillations and other evidence of denervation in otherwise normal subjects in middle and old age. Sequential electrodiagnostic studies are valuable in peroneal nerve lesions, as signs of reinnervation are detectable on EMG prior to evidence of clinical recovery.

An important clinical problem is the distinction between a lesion of the common peroneal nerve and the peroneal division of the sciatic nerve. This may arise in patients undergoing hip replacement who develop foot drop following surgery. Electrodiagnosis is unhelpful in the first few days after operation, prior to the appearance of denervation in affected muscles, unless clear evidence of conduction block or slowing is present at the fibular head signifying a focal common peroneal nerve lesion. Once degeneration has taken place (approximately 10–14 days after surgery), EMG examination of the short head of biceps femoris is the most useful test in differentiating between a common peroneal and sciatic neuropathy (Katirji & Wilbourn 1994). If the short head is affected, the lesion must involve the peroneal division of the sciatic nerve; if it is spared, the lesion is confined to the common peroneal nerve. EMG examination of muscles innervated by the tibial division of the sciatic nerve is also helpful, as these are often abnormal in a sciatic neuropathy, even when there is preferential involvement of the peroneal division. Measurement of the sural nerve SAP can be useful, as the response may be unilaterally reduced or absent in sciatic lesions. However, the value of sural recording is limited by age-related changes in sural potentials, and the significant number of patients with sciatic neuropathies in whom the sural SAP shows no abnormality (see p. 469).

EMG studies will also differentiate between foot drop caused by L5 radiculopathy and a common peroneal nerve lesion. In the former, denervation is seen in the tibialis posterior in addition to the tibialis anterior, but the superficial peroneal SAP is unaffected and there will be no focal slowing at the fibular head.

Selective damage to the deep peroneal nerve may occur in anterior compartment syndrome. In such cases, denervation will be confined to muscles innervated by this branch, and the superficial peroneal SAP is preserved.

Sciatic nerve lesions

Sciatic neuropathies are relatively uncommon, although the causes are diverse. Prior to the report of 100 consecutive sciatic nerve lesions by Yuen et al (1995), there had been no large series looking at the value of different electrophysiological measures in determining diagnosis and prognosis. The aetiology in these 100 patients was heterogeneous; the major causes were: hip replacement in 22, acute external compression (from prolonged surgery, bed rest or drug-induced coma) in 18, trauma due to gunshot wounds in 11 and nerve infarction in 10. The most notable electrophysiological finding was the overwhelming proportion of patients who showed evidence of significant axonal loss, based on low-amplitude SAPs and CMAPs, and denervation on EMG. A demyelinating lesion was seen in only seven patients, most of whom had external compressive injury. Demyelination was not found in any of the cases with a presumed stretch lesion of the nerve following hip replacement or dislocation. However, as already stated, identification of a small or localised area of demyelination or conduction block is technically difficult in proximal nerve lesions, even when near-nerve needle stimulation and recording, or high-voltage stimulators are used to achieve supramaximal stimulation of deeply sited nerves. Recording of F responses or H reflexes probably adds little to the evaluation of a possible sciatic neuropathy, as neither of these techniques can distinguish lesions at different sites within the sciatic nerve or at the level of the root.

Preferential involvement of the peroneal division is a long recognised feature of sciatic nerve lesions, and was seen in 64% of the cases described by Yuen et al (1995). Only 8 of the 100 patients had predominant involvement of the tibial division; most of these were cases in which direct thigh trauma had occurred. A normal sural potential does not exclude tibial division involvement, as nearly a third of Yuen's cases had normal sural SAP amplitudes. The preferential susceptibility of the peroneal part of the sciatic nerve to damage probably depends on a number of factors: the common peroneal nerve is relatively fixed at the level of the knee, and the peroneal fibres are therefore more vulnerable to stretch injury; and there may be less supportive connective tissue within the peroneal division, and its position is superficial to the tibial division in the proximal part of the sciatic nerve.

Certain measures may be of prognostic value in sciatic neuropathies. In an earlier study, Yuen et al (1994) identified the presence of a recordable CMAP from extensor digitorum brevis as being the best predictor of prognosis. Those with CMAPs had faster and more complete recovery. The timing of reinnervation was approximately 5 months in biceps femoris (short head), 11 months in tibialis anterior, and 15 months in calf muscles (Yuen et al 1995).

Compression of the sciatic nerve occurs in the piriformis syndrome, in which there is an anatomical variation in the course of the nerve as it crosses the piriformis muscle. The anomaly, which usually involves the peroneal division, has been identified in 5% of cadavers (Pecina 1979), suggesting that piriformis syndrome may be an under-recognised condition. It has no specific electrodiagnostic features.

Femoral neuropathies

As with sciatic mononeuropathies, femoral nerve lesions have many causes, although there are no reported cases of pure entrapment within or by a specific anatomical structure. Most cases are due to vascular lesions, diabetes or stretch injury from excessive hip abduction in the lithotomy position. The nature of the nerve lesion will depend on the cause. Most result in axonal damage, but excess stretch can produce focal demyelination, which accounts for the relatively good prognosis of femoral neuropathy from a prolonged lithotomy position during childbirth (Hakim & Katirji 1993). Electrodiagnostic tests which are useful in femoral nerve lesions include: measurement of the saphenous SAP; CMAP recording from a quadriceps muscle, such as vastus medialis; and EMG examination, which is essential to identify whether denervation is confined to, or extends beyond, the territory of the femoral nerve. It is sometimes possible to localise conduction abnormalities to the inguinal ligament, although slow conduction does not reliably distinguish demyelinating lesions from those which are primarily axonal or degenerative (Gassel 1963). The main differential diagnosis of a femoral neuropathy is a lesion in the lumbar plexus or a radiculopathy. In a radicular lesion, the saphenous SAP is normal, and denervation may be seen in lumbar paraspinal muscles. Abnormal EMG of muscles outside the territory of the femoral nerve will be seen in a plexopathy. Most patients with diabetic amyotrophy, which is often erroneously considered to be a femoral mononeuropathy, have extensive denervation involving several muscles in different myotomes. Although the precise level of the pathology in diabetic amyotrophy is unknown (Chokroverty 1987), it is likely to be a polyradiculopathy or radiculoplexopathy, and in many cases there will also be evidence of a peripheral sensorimotor neuropathy on nerve conduction studies.

Uncommon entrapment neuropathies

There are a number of rare entrapment syndromes affecting single nerves in the upper and lower limbs, in which electrodiagnostic characteristics have been described. Evaluation of conduction in some of these nerves is technically challenging, and apparent abnormalities can be difficult to interpret. Comparison with the uninvolved nerve in the contralateral limb is essential, although less valuable when symptoms are bilateral.

In *tarsal tunnel syndrome*, the tibial nerve is entrapped within the tunnel, usually at the level of the medial malleolus. Electrodiagnostically, the syndrome presents with abnormal sensory conduction in the medial (Guiloff & Sherratt 1977) and lateral plantar nerves, and a small CMAP and prolongation of distal motor latency in the abductor hallucis (a difference of more than 1 ms compared with the unaffected foot being considered as significant). There is usually denervation in intrinsic foot muscles innervated by the tibial nerve. Following decompressive surgery, motor conduction returns to normal values, but minor abnormalities of sensory conduction may persist indefinitely, despite symptomatic improvement (Oh et al 1991).

Meralgia paraesthetica is most often due to entrapment of the lateral femoral cutaneous nerve as it passes underneath the inguinal ligament near to the anterior superior iliac spine. A number of electrophysiological tests have been described as being useful in diagnosis: comparison of SAP amplitude in the affected and unaffected leg, measurement of sensory conduction velocity, and recording of somatosensory responses (SEPs) evoked by stimulation of the lateral femoral cutaneous nerve. The latter is probably the most technically robust, as SAP recording using skin electrodes can be difficult in the well-built thighs of many patients with meralgia paraesthetica. However, a recent study suggested that SAP amplitude comparison was most sensitive (Lagueny et al 1991) although no test appeared to be helpful in predicting outcome and recovery.

Suprascapular nerve entrapment should be considered in patients with unexplained shoulder pain. The nerve is most commonly trapped within the suprascapular notch, resulting in denervation of both the infraspinatus and supraspinatus muscles. Very rarely, the entrapment is more distal at the spinoglenoid notch, and the infraspinatus alone is affected (Kiss & Komar 1990). Chronic partial denervation will be seen on EMG; fibrillations and other evidence of acute denervation are not usually found, as a diagnosis of suprascapular entrapment is often a late consideration. Conduction studies may be helpful in cases where distinction from a brachial plexopathy or C5 radiculopathy is not clear on EMG.

Isolated lesions of the *musculocutaneous nerve* are uncommon, but result in well-defined electrodiagnostic abnormalities: evidence of denervation on EMG of biceps, brachialis and coracobrachialis; and a reduction in size or absence of the lateral antebrachial cutaneous SAP, which is the sensory termination of the musculocutaneous nerve. Measurement of sensory and motor conduction has been reported as being useful in differentiating lesions of the musculocutaneous nerve from brachial plexopathies or root avulsion (Trojaborg 1976).

Most cases of *axillary nerve* lesions have a traumatic basis. A retrospective study of 94 patients with a traumatic aetiology revealed partial axonotmesis in nearly 70%; one-fifth had complete lesions and the remainder had neurapraxic lesions (Degrande et al 1995). Full recovery was seen in some 80% of those with a neurapraxic injury; nearly half of those with partial axonal damage had incomplete recovery. Unsurprisingly, given the anatomical location of the nerve and the nature of the trauma resulting in axillary nerve injury, associated nerve lesions were seen in one-third of patients, these most commonly involving the suprascapular nerve. EMG in axillary nerve lesions will reveal denervation in the deltoid and teres minor; more extensive examination of other muscles is necessary to exclude lesions of the brachial plexus or other nerves.

Iatrogenic injury during minor surgical procedures, such as lymph node biopsy in the neck, is the commonest cause of a lesion of the *spinal accessory nerve* in its extracranial course. In many cases, weakness and denervation is confined to the trapezius; involvement of the sternocleinomastoid muscle is uncommon. Intraoperative electrophysiological studies can be helpful in revealing evidence of lesions in continuity, with NAPs being recorded beyond the lesion or trapezius contraction on direct stimulation of the nerve (Donner & Kline 1993).

PLEXOPATHIES

Lesions of the brachial plexus

Diverse pathologies affect the brachial plexus, including trauma, neoplastic infiltration, radiation damage, neuralgic amyotrophy, hereditary pressure palsies, compression due to cervical ribs or bands and, in neonates, injury to the plexus at birth. The principal role of electrodiagnosis is to identify the level of nerve pathology and to give some indication of the type of nerve injury, and thus of the prognosis. The level of the lesion is established using a combination of nerve conduction studies and EMG (Wilbourn 1985). Ferrante and Wilbourn (1995) have investigated the utility of several sensory nerve studies in assessing brachial plexopathies. Cases with an upper trunk lesion had absent or small lateral antebrachial cutaneous and first digital median SAPs; the ulnar SAP was normal. Lower trunk lesions showed abnormal ulnar, dorsal cutaneous and medial antebrachial cutaneous SAPs. In the single case of a medial trunk lesion, the third digit median SAP was the only abnormal sensory response.

Muscles innervated by the upper trunk include the spinatii, biceps, deltoid, triceps, pronator teres and ECR. Abnormalities on EMG in the ECR, extensor carpi ulnaris, extensor digiti communis and extensor indicis proprius indicate a lesion of the middle trunk; EMG abnormalities of the flexor carpi ulnaris and intrinsic hand muscles indicate a lesion of the lower trunk. Identification of lesions proximal to the upper trunk is aided by EMG examination of the rhomboid muscles, innervated by the dorsal scapular nerve which branches directly from C5. Similarly, examination of serratus anterior is useful in localisation of lesions of the C7 root, as the long thoracic nerve leaves the plexus proximal to the upper and medial trunks. The pattern of neurophysiological abnormality in brachial plexopathy may sometimes suggest a mononeuropathy or mononeuritis multiplex, particularly in cases of neuralgic amyotrophy. The posterior interosseous, anterior interosseous and long thoracic nerves are most often affected in this way (England & Sumner 1987).

Nerve conduction studies and EMG can be helpful in brachial plexus lesions where the differential diagnosis lies between recurrent carcinoma and radiation plexopathy. Patients with radiation damage are more likely to have abnormalities of sensory and motor conduction, and characteristically show myokymic discharges on EMG (Lederman & Wilbourn 1984).

Traumatic brachial plexus lesions in adults

With an increasing trend towards early operative intervention, particularly in cases where there is associated vascular or bony injury, electrodiagnosis has a limited role in preoperative assessment in adults with brachial plexus lesion of traumatic origin, as abnormalities will not be manifest within the first 24–48 hours after injury (Smith 1996). However, electrodiagnosis is still valuable for the distinction between a postganglionic lesion of the plexus and preganglionic injury or root avulsion. The neurophysiological triad indicative of root avulsion has been described above (normal SAP and preserved histamine response; absence of somatosensory evoked potentials; and denervation of cervical paraspinal muscles and distal muscles innervated by the root). Intraoperative studies using direct nerve stimulation and SEP recording provide further evidence of whether a root is in continuity (Hetreed et al 1994).

If the role of preoperative electrodiagnosis in traumatic brachial plexopathy in adults is now limited, sequential neurophysiological studies remain useful in establishing the rate of postoperative recovery, particularly for identification of early reinnervation. This will be seen on EMG prior to signs of clinical recovery. The most reliable method of quantifying reinnervation is to measure evoked CMAPs, although analysis of motor unit territory and fibre density using macro-EMG may also be helpful.

Obstetric brachial plexopathy

Obstetric brachial plexopathy (OBP) remains an important clinical problem, despite advances in obstetric care which have occurred in recent decades (see Ch. 10). Most reports or descriptions of this condition have characterised the lesion in terms of its anatomical distribution, with three main patterns of involvement: damage to the C5 and C6 roots or upper trunk (Erb's palsy); entire plexus involvement; and injury confined to the lower trunk (Klumpke's paralysis). The nature or type of nerve injury has received less consideration, even though this has important implications for prognosis and need for surgical intervention. The nature of the lesion has usually been inferred from features at presentation, and the degree, if any, of clinical improvement within the first few months after birth. For example, it has been recognised for many years that the primary lesion in a proportion of cases of OBP is neurapraxia, and in these cases, the natural history and long-term outlook is favourable, with full recovery expected. In the few cases of presumed neurapraxia in which EMG has been performed, the findings have usually been reported as "normal" (Eng et al 1978); but there have been no reports documenting clear evidence of the pathophysiological process underlying neurapraxia, i.e. conduction block. Indeed the role of electrodiagnosis in preoperative assessment of OBP is viewed by some as being very limited, adding little to careful clinical evaluation (Slooff 1993). In determining the severity of the lesion, and thus the need for surgery to optimise outcome, the clinical picture is considered to be most reliable – in particular, whether there is recovery of function in biceps by the age of 3 months (Gilbert & Tassin 1984). Thus, less severe lesions, which may include cases of neurapraxia or conduction block, would be expected to recover within a few months of birth, through resolution of the conduction block or as a consequence of reinnervation in partial axonal injury. More severe lesions in which there is avulsion or little potential for reinnervation will not show early recovery. However, this is an oversimplification of the complex types of damage that may occur in OBP (as in adult traumatic brachial plexopathy), and does not take into account the different degrees of involvement of individual roots and trunks at the pre- and postganglionic level. Evaluation of a consecutive series of 50 cases of OBP by two of the authors (S.J.M.S. and R.B.) suggests that detailed electrodiagnosis adds significantly to clinical assessment in determining the nature and level of the lesion, and, furthermore, can predict prognosis and need for surgery in individual cases.

The infants were assessed using a combination of mixed nerve action potential (NAP) recording in the median and ulnar nerves in the forearm, together with EMG examination of several muscles (biceps, deltoid, infraspinatus, triceps, extensor and flexor muscles in the forearm; and, in some cases, small hand muscles). On the basis of the predominant findings on EMG, lesions were characterised into three groups. Type A (six infants, with a mean age at time of neurophysiological study of 5 months) had features on EMG in the biceps, deltoid and infraspinatus that suggested conduction block – absence of spontaneous activity and a reduced number of motor units of normal morphology, but increased firing rates. The median and ulnar NAPs were of normal amplitude, as expected in nonaxonal injury. Thus, these infants had documented evidence for a neurapraxic lesion, and notably this was seen at 6 and 10 months of age in two cases. Management in all six cases was conservative, and all went on to have full recovery of arm function. These infants were clinically indistinguishable from those with severe axonal damage described below; furthermore, in having no or minimal recovery of biceps function by the age of 3 months, they would have fulfilled Gilbert's criteria for early surgical intervention.

The neurophysiological findings in the remaining infants indicated that axonal damage or degeneration had occurred. The pattern of EMG and NAP abnormality could be used to predict the severity of axonal damage, and thus the likely prognosis. Two further groups of lesions were identified. The type B lesion was characterised by an EMG pattern of relatively good motor unit recruitment, with a mixture of normal units and potentials showing evidence of collateral reinnervation in affected muscles (Fig. 19.10). The lesion was further characterised by the NAP features. If this was of normal or slightly reduced amplitude compared with the unaffected limb, the findings suggested a favourable lesion with little axonal damage. Infants with lesions of this type were managed conservatively and went on to have excellent recovery of arm function, including cases in whom the clinical impression had been of a more severe lesion. Significant reduction in size (i.e. amplitude less than 50% of the opposite arm) or absence of NAP was considered to indicate a less

favourable nerve injury or lesion, and thus a need for surgical exploration. The neurophysiological findings predicted a lesion in continuity, which was confirmed at operation. Typically, there was a soft fusiform neuroma, across which evoked responses could be obtained, using SEP recording and direct nerve stimulation. The surgical procedure in these cases is limited to neurolysis. Functional outcome in these infants was very good, with recovery of muscle strength to at least Medical Research Council (MRC) grade 4. In lesions of type B, the amplitude of the NAP appears to be the most useful predictor of severity of axonal injury and need for surgical intervention.

In type C lesions, EMG usually revealed poor motor recruitment and no evidence for collateral reinnervation. The NAP was either absent or substantially reduced in size, suggesting relatively severe axonal injury (Fig. 19.11). This was confirmed at operation, with the finding of considerable scarring in the posterior triangle and hard neuromata of three or more times the size of the normal trunk. However, preservation of some SEP responses or distal muscle contraction showed that the lesions were usually not complete. Grafting was undertaken in these cases. In some infants, there was evidence of root avulsion – spontaneous activity and absence of voluntary motor unit potentials, together with preservation of the NAP response, indicating preganglionic injury. Root avulsion could be seen in combination with lesser degrees of injury at other levels, as illustrated in the following case.

Case report. A male infant was seen at the age of 3 months. At birth, there had been a complete lesion of the left brachial plexus, and at the time of examination, the only recovery was that of shoulder abduction. Neurophysiological findings were as follows:

	Right arm	Left arm
Median NAP (μV)	40	20
Ulnar NAP (μV)	34	25

EMG in the left deltoid and infraspinatus showed no fibrillations and a very good degree of motor unit recruitment, with no abnormality of morphology. In the biceps, the recruitment pattern was very reduced, with no definite reinnervation. Only nascent units were seen in the triceps. The extensor and flexor muscle groups in the forearm, and the FDIO in the hand, showed profuse fibrillations and complete absence of voluntary potentials.

These findings indicate: minimal involvement of the C5 root (near-normal EMG in the deltoid and infraspinatus); severe axonal injury of C6 (nascent units in the triceps and poor recruitment in the biceps, together with a relative reduction in the median NAP); and avulsion of the C8 and T1 roots (characteristic EMG and preservation of the ulnar NAP).

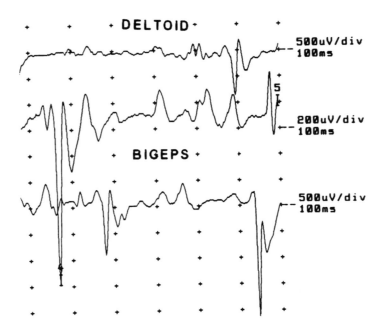

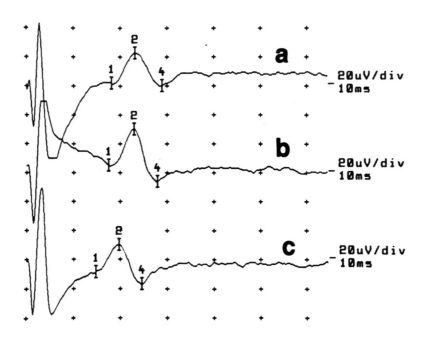

Fig. 19.10 Type B lesion in obstetric brachial plexopathy. (Top) Good EMG recruitment (> 50% of normal) in the biceps and deltoid muscle, with a mixture of normal units and evidence of collateral reinnervation. (Bottom) The median (a) and ulnar (b) NAPs were normal in this case, indicating a favourable lesion. Median NAP in unaffected arm shown in trace (c).

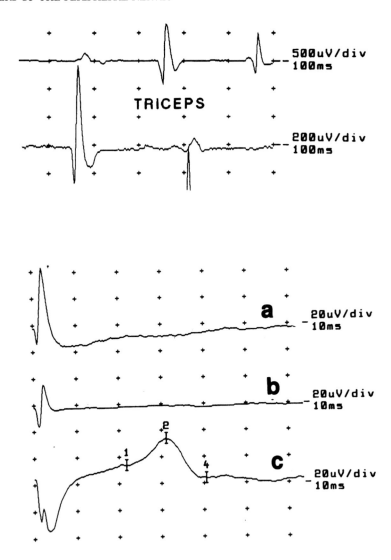

Fig. 19.11 Type C lesion in obstetric brachial plexopathy. An infant aged 4 months, with Gilbert group 3 (C5–8 involvement). EMG in triceps shows very limited activity (top), with motor units firing in isolation and little evidence of reinnervation. The NAPs (bottom) were absent. Median NAP in unaffected arm shown in trace (c).

The preoperative findings in the above 50 cases suggest an important role for electrodiagnosis in OBP: firstly to determine the extent and level of involvement of individual components of the plexus; secondly to identify root avulsion; and thirdly, to define the nature of the lesion in terms of neurapraxic, axonotmetic and neurotmetic injury, and thus to assist in making a prognosis.

Thoracic outlet syndrome

True neurogenic thoracic outlet syndrome (TOS) is rare, with an estimated incidence of 1 per million of the population (Wilbourn 1982). It has a well-defined clinical picture, with characteristic electrodiagnostic features (Gilliatt et al

1970). These reflect a predominantly axonal lesion of the lower trunk of the brachial plexus, and thus comprise:

- a small or absent ulnar SAP, i.e. a postganglionic lesion of C8 sensory fibres
- a low-amplitude CMAP from abductor pollicis brevis
- denervation, typically of chronic neurogenic type, in muscles innervated by the lower trunk.

The CMAP from ADM is usually of normal size, and motor conduction velocities in the forearm segments of the median and ulnar nerve should fall within the normal range, although some slowing may be seen if atrophy is marked. The degree of reduction in amplitude of both sensory and motor responses may depend on the severity and duration of neurogenic TOS. In the seminal study of nine patients by Gilliatt and colleagues, four had absent ulnar SAPs, in one case the amplitude was reduced, but in three the response was of normal size.

There have been several descriptions of additional techniques for diagnosis of neurogenic TOS, directed towards better localisation through measurement of nerve conduction across the site of the lesion. Wulff and Gilliatt (1979) used F wave recording from hypothenar muscles evoked by stimulation of the ulnar nerve at the wrist, and found prolongation of latency in the affected hand compared with the opposite limb. In the majority of cases, the latency remained abnormally long after surgery, suggesting degeneration of faster conducting fibres. However, in one case, the amplitude of the F responses increased, and the latency decreased after removal of the cervical band, implying recovery of localised proximal conduction block. The technique described by Urschel and Razzuk (1972), whereby conduction studies at progressively more proximal points along the length of the ulnar nerve appeared to identify localised slowing across the thoracic outlet, has now been largely discredited (Wilbourn & Lederman 1984). Somatosensory evoked potentials (SEPs) have been used to demonstrate abnormalities of proximal sensory conduction in the region of the brachial plexus. The plexus or N9 response evoked by stimulation of the median nerve is normal, whereas the amplitude of the ulnar nerve N9 is reduced and its latency prolonged (Jerret et al 1984). In combination with F responses, as a measure of proximal motor conduction, SEPs appear to be a reliable and sensitive diagnostic tool, although they may not be helpful in early cases (Newmark et al 1985).

Because of the variable presentation and symptoms encountered in patients with neurogenic TOS, other diagnostic possibilities must be considered, and neurophysiological studies should include examination for carpal tunnel syndrome and other common upper limb entrapment neuropathies, and exclusion of anterior horn cell disease or radiculopathy, particularly in cases where the ulnar SAP is relatively unaffected.

Lumbosacral plexopathy

The principles of electrophysiological investigation in lumbosacral plexopathies are similar to those in the evaluation of brachial plexus lesions: diagnosis depends on demonstration of EMG abnormalities in muscles innervated by the lumbar and sacral trunks, and reduction of sensory potentials in the sural and superficial peroneal nerves. The saphenous SAP may be affected, depending on the level of the lesion. Paraspinal muscles are spared, in contrast to the case in lumbar or sacral radiculopathies. The superior and/or inferior gluteal nerves can be involved in plexus lesions at the level of the pelvic rim, resulting in denervation of the glutei in addition to other muscles.

This has been described in plexus injuries occurring during labour and delivery, in which the descending fetal head is thought to cause direct compression of the plexus (Feasby & Hahn 1992).

However, electrophysiological distinction of lumbosacral plexopathies from distal lesions of the peripheral nerves, or proximal lesions of the roots, is often difficult in practice. Sensory fibres can be affected to a variable degree in lumbosacral plexopathies, and motor involvement is often the predominant feature. Furthermore, some cases of plexopathy are properly considered as radiculoplexopathies, since the underlying pathological process, notably in cases of neoplastic infiltration and radiation damage, affects the extraspinal and sometimes the intradural extramedullary roots, in addition to the plexus.

As in brachial plexopathy, the finding of myokymia on EMG is specifically helpful in the differential diagnosis of tumour and radiation-induced lumbosacral plexopathy. Thomas et al (1985) found myokymic discharges in 57% of patients with radiation damage, but in none of their cases with neoplastic infiltration of the lumbosacral plexus. Myokymia was most likely to be seen in proximal muscles, including the paraspinals, gluteal muscles and the knee extensor and flexor groups in the thigh.

RADICULOPATHIES

Although the investigation of radicular disease has been considerably enhanced by the advent of anatomical imaging techniques such as computed tomography (CT) scanning and magnetic resonance imaging (MRI), electrophysiological evaluation continues to have a role in diagnosis, given that root entrapment or disc protrusion is a common radiological finding and its clinical or functional significance may be uncertain. The electrophysiological features which permit a diagnosis of a radiculopathy or preganglionic lesion are:

- normal sensory nerve responses
- denervation in a myotomal distribution (at least two muscles from a single myotome should be examined, preferably those with the same root but different peripheral nerve supply)
- denervation in paraspinal muscles.

In up to one-third of cases, EMG abnormalities may be confined to the paraspinal muscles. Measurement of limb CMAPs may be helpful in anatomical localisation of polyradiculopathy. McGonagle et al (1990) found that patients with intradural–extra-axial lesions are more likely to show a reduction in CMAP amplitude than are those with extradural or intra-axial disease.

Nerve conduction studies have a relatively minor role in the diagnosis of radiculopathies, beyond exclusion of a peripheral or distal lesion. Some patients may have dual lesions, such as median nerve compression in the carpal tunnel and a C6 radiculopathy. This has been called the "double crush syndrome" – a lesion at one level is thought to predispose to a second at another level. However, opinion has varied over the years as to the clinical significance of this concept (Roger Gilliatt, personal communication). Techniques for measuring proximal conduction, such as the H reflex and F response, have been used in root lesions, but EMG is probably more sensitive, and the utility of these techniques is limited by the difficulty of detection of small regions of demyelination in a long length of nerve, and the probable pathophysiological changes in most radicular lesions due to chronic disc disease, i.e. axonal degeneration or a combination of axonopathy and focal demyelination.

There are several limitations to electrodiagnosis in radicular disease. Symptoms arising from a root lesion are usually painful or predominantly sensory in type, whereas EMG assesses motor fibres only. Abnormalities on EMG may not be manifest until a certain number of motor axons have been lost, and thus EMG is less sensitive or valuable in early cases. The amount of denervation in individual muscles within a myotome can vary, with profuse fibrillations in one muscle and relatively little abnormality in another. Furthermore, anatomical and other studies in man suggest a greater variability in the segmental innervation of cervical and lumbosacral myotomes than is usually indicated in standard textbooks. Levin et al (1996) compared surgical and electromyographic localisation of single cervical root lesions, and found that the pattern of muscle involvement was fairly stereotyped in C5, C7 and C8 root lesions, whereas it varied in C6 radiculopathies. In half these cases, the muscles affected were similar to those in C5 root lesions, but with the additional involvement of pronator teres; in the remainder, the pattern resembled that of a C7 radiculopathy. Stimulation studies in children (Phillips & Park 1991) have revealed that asymmetries in the segmental innervation of lower limb muscles are common, suggesting that attribution of a particular pattern of EMG abnormality to a specific spinal root may be misleading. Localisation using paraspinal muscles is also difficult, given that there are often uncertainties as to the precise segmental level in both the cervical and lumbosacral regions. Finally, persistence of EMG changes due to surgery (spontaneous activity and abnormalities of motor units) limits electrodiagnostic interpretation in patients following a laminectomy (Johnson et al 1972).

The role of SEPs in the diagnosis of radicular disease is controversial. Although SEPs assess the proximal sensory pathways, including the preganglionic portion of the root, relatively short segments of demyelination may not manifest as a significant increase in latency of the SEP. The amplitude of individual components of the SEP is variable and insufficiently robust to permit reliable identification of focal conduction block in sensory roots. Furthermore,

many peripheral nerves are multisegmental – the median nerve, for example, contains fibres from C6, C7, C8 and T1. This limits the utility of SEPs evoked by peripheral nerve trunk stimulation for identification of a root lesion at a single level. SEPs can be recorded using dermatomal stimulation, but reports have varied as to the sensitivity of this technique. Aminoff et al (1985) found that only 25% of cases had abnormal dermatomal SEPs, whereas 75% showed abnormal EMG. Others have found a much higher sensitivity, with 95% of patients showing abnormal dermatomal responses (Kilifi & Sedgwick 1987). The difference in sensitivity is almost certainly a reflection of the wider criteria for abnormality used by Kilifi and Sedgwick. Use of magnetic stimulation of roots to measure latency of motor evoked responses (Chokroverty et al 1989) is limited by uncertainty as to the exact site of stimulation, and the method is probably no less discomforting to the patient than high voltage electrical stimulation over the spine.

Relatively little work has been done on the sensitivity and specificity of functional and anatomical techniques for detection of radicular lesions. There is no "gold standard" against which to compare the diagnostic methods, other than the operative appearance of the roots and surrounding structures, and these may be unreliable. Series in which EMG has been compared with myelography and/or CT scanning (Knutsson 1961, Khatri et al 1984, Katiriji et al 1988) generally indicate a sensitivity of about 65% for EMG, providing a detailed examination is undertaken; furthermore, the false-positive rate for EMG is less than that for CT scanning. The findings at EMG may also be more reliable with regard to prognosis. Katirji et al (1988) identified five patients with disc protrusion on CT who had normal EMG; all of these recovered with conservative management. Nine cases with abnormal EMG but no evidence for disc disease on CT had a more mixed outcome: four of six managed conservatively showed no change in symptoms or signs at follow-up, whereas the three patients who had undergone intervention were clinically improved.

There are no specific electrophysiological features of lumbar canal stenosis, although the presence of bilateral abnormalties may be a helpful pointer to this diagnosis. Conditions that mimic root lesions or polyradiculopathy include: plexopathies, in which SAP abnormalities should be found; and multifocal motor neuropathy, which is identified by the finding of multiple sites of conduction block in peripheral nerves, including sites where entrapment does not usually occur, such as the mid-forearm; and anterior horn cell disease. The latter can be extremely difficult to differentiate electrophysiologically from polyradiculopathy, but the clinical presentation and presence of upper motor neuron features usually clarifies the differential diagnosis.

DIFFUSE PROBLEMS

The electrophysiologist must always consider the possibility of a widespread disorder, such as an underlying polyneuropathy in patients who present with what appears to be a single compressive nerve lesion, or anterior horn cell disease in cases of muscle atrophy in the hands or one leg. The extent of the electrodiagnostic examination in the individual case will be determined by a careful clinical history and examination. Detailed electrophysiological evaluation may reveal a condition unsuspected by the referring doctor.

Case report. A 64-year-old woman presented with paraesthesia in a median nerve distribution in her right hand. She underwent decompression of the carpal tunnel, but symptoms persisted after operation. The finding of a positive Tinel sign over the median nerve at the elbow led to operation at this site, again without improvement in the sensory disturbance. Prior to further operation on the median nerve in the region of the axilla, the surgeon requested nerve conduction studies for the first time. These revealed absent median and ulnar SAPs in both hands, a small superfical radial SAP of 9 μV, and an absent sural SAP. Distal motor latencies and motor conduction velocities were slow in several upper and lower limb nerves, with patchy involvement of different nerve segments, and conduction block was seen in the ulnar nerves at the elbow and in the lateral popliteal nerve at the knee.

	Median nerve	Ulnar nerve	
	Right	Right	Left
Distal motor latency (ms)	6.6	7.6	8.0
CMAP wrist (mV)	0.7	4.0	1.4
CMAP elbow	0.4	1.1	0.8
CMAP axilla	–	0.8	Absent
CV wrist–elbow (m/s)	18	35	27
CV elbow–axilla		21	–
F response (ms)	Absent	Absent	38

Mild chronic partial denervation was seen in distal limb muscles.

The nerve conduction studies showed a generalised demyelinating neuropathy, and the patchy nerve involvement suggested an inflammatory cause, i.e. chronic inflammatory polyneuropathy. The cerebrospinal fluid protein was elevated (1.2 g) and inflammation was confirmed on nerve biopsy.

Nerve conduction studies in peripheral neuropathies are directed towards assessing involvement of sensory and motor nerve fibres, and determination of whether the neuropathy is of axonal or demyelinating type. The distribution of nerve abnormality reveals whether the neuropathy is symmetrical or multifocal (mononeuritis multiplex). Preferential involvement of the longest or lower limb nerves is seen in distal dying back neuropathies, which typically have a metabolic or toxic cause. Characterisation of the type and pattern of a neuropathy is of importance in suggesting likely aetiologies, and thus allowing a more focused approach to further investigation.

Anterior horn cell disorders (poliomyelitis, motor neuron disease, spinal muscular atrophy) produce acute and chronic partial denervation on EMG – fibrillations, positive sharp waves, fasciculations, and motor units which show denervation and reinnervation characteristics. Striking abnormalities can be seen in clinically asymptomatic muscles. A diagnosis of anterior horn cell disease should not be made unless there is clear evidence of denervation in at least three limbs. In cases with a presentation that is predominantly bulbar, fibrillations and abnormal motor units are seen in tongue muscles. Although there is pathological evidence for involvement of sensory pathways in anterior horn neuronopathies, SAPs and SEPs are normal in the majority of cases, except in the X-linked form of bulbospinal muscular atrophy, which is associated with reduced or absent SAPs (Wilde et al 1987).

Myopathic disorders present with weakness, fatiguability and muscle atrophy. Although there is a characteristic appearance of myopathic motor units on EMG, the abnormality is not specific to primary muscle disease, and similar changes may be seen in disorders of the neuromuscular junction and, occasionally, in neurogenic lesions. The distribution of muscle involvement is usually the clue to the type of disorder in muscular dystrophies. Thus the facial, sternomastoid, spinati and upper arm muscles are affected in facioscapulohumeral dystrophy, whereas EMG abnormalities are seen in proximal girdle muscles in limb girdle dystrophies. Myotonic discharges are the diagnostic EMG finding in myotonic dystrophies, such as dystrophia myotonica and Thomsen's disease. The discharges occur spontaneously, and can also be provoked by movement of the EMG needle or by muscle contraction. Some patients with dystrophia myotonica have evidence of a sensorimotor neuropathy on nerve conduction studies, with slow conduction velocity (Olson et al 1978). Inflammatory muscle disorders (polymyositis, dermatomyositis) characteristically show fibrillations on EMG, although the amount of spontaneous activity is poorly correlated with disease activity. Muscle involvement can be quite patchy in these inflammatory disorders, and EMG can be helpful in guiding muscle biopsy. Myopathic motor unit abnormalities in inflammatory muscle disease may be most evident in proximal muscles, such as the iliopsoas and paraspinal groups. There are no EMG features that allow distinction between relapse of myositis and drug-induced myopathy in patients who have been treated with steroids.

Detailed investigation using repetitive nerve stimulation and single-fibre EMG is required for diagnosis of disorders of the neuromuscular junction, such as myasthenia gravis and the myasthenic syndrome. Single-fibre EMG is the most sensitive test for identifying abnormalities of the neuromuscular junction, but increased jitter and blocking may be seen in almost any neurogenic or myopathic condition. Although repetitive nerve stimulation is less sensitive, the pattern of CMAP amplitude change with trains of low- and high-frequency stimuli pre- and post-exercise shows specific changes which allow distinction between a presynaptic disorder (i.e. the myasthenic or Lambert–Eaton syndrome) and a postsynaptic disorder (myasthenia gravis). The degree of abnormality on repetitive nerve stimulation shows good correlation with disease severity and is helpful in determining adequacy of treatment.

References

Abdulla S, Bowden R E M 1960 The blood supply of the brachial plexus. Proceedings of the Royal Society of Medicine 53: 203–205

Abernathy C D, Onofrio B, Scheithauer B et al 1986 Surgical management of giant sacral schwannomas. Journal of Neurosurgery 65: 286–295

Abse D W 1987 Hysteria and related mental disorders. Wright, Bristol, p 25

Ad hoc Subcommittee of the American Academy of Neurology Aids Task Force 1991 Research criteria for diagnosis of chronic inflammatory demyelinating polyneuropathy (CIDP). Neurology 41: 617–618

Adams J A 1980 The pyriformis syndrome. Report of four cases and review of the literature. South African Medical Journal 18: 13–18

Adams J C 1980 Standard orthopaedic operations, 2nd edn. Churchill Livingstone, Edinburgh

Adams J E 1976 Naloxone reversal of analgesia produced by brain stimulation in the human. Pain 2: 161–166

Adams J T, De Weise J A, Mahoney E B, Rob C G 1968 Intermittent subclavian vein obstruction without thrombosis. Surgery 63: 147–165

Adamson J E, Srouji S J, Horton C E et al 1971 The acute carpal tunnel syndrome. Plastic and Reconstructive Surgery 47: 332–336

Adar R 1979 Iatrogenic brachial plexus injuries. Mayo Clinic Proceedings 54: 277

Adler J B, Patterson R L 1967 Erb's palsy: long term results of treatment in 88 cases. Journal of Bone and Joint Surgery 49A: 1052–1064

Adrian E D 1916 The electrical reactions of muscles before and after nerve injury. Brain 39: 1–35

Adrian E D 1917 Physiological basis of electrical tests in peripheral nerve injury. Archives of Radiology and Electrotherapy 21: 379–392

Adrian E D 1925 Interpretation of the electromyogram: Oliver–Sharpey lecture. Lancet 13 June

Adson A W 1947 Surgical treatment for symptoms produced by cervical rib and the scalenus anticus muscle. Surgery, Gynecology and Obstetrics 85: 687–700

Adson A W 1951 Symptoms, differential diagnosis for section of the insertion of the scalenus anticus muscle. Journal of International College of Surgeons 16: 546–559

Adson A W, Brown G E 1929 The treatment of Raynaud's disease by resection of the upper thoracic and lumbar sympathetic ganglia and trunks. Surgery, Gynecology and Obstetrics 48: 577–603

Adson A W, Coffey J R 1927 Cervical rib. A method of anterior approach for relief of symptoms by division of the scalenus anticus. Annals of Surgery 85: 839–857

Agee J, Tortosa R, Berry D et al 1990 Endoscopic release of the carpal tunnel; a randomised prospective multicenter study. Presented at the 45th Annual Meeting of the American Society for the Study of the Hand, Toronto, September 1990

Aho K, Sainio K, Kianta M et al 1983 Pneumatic tourniquet paralysis. Journal of Bone and Joint Surgery 65B: 441–443

Aitken J 1952 Deformity of the elbow joint as a sequel to Erb's obstetrical paralysis. Journal of Bone and Joint Surgery 34B: 352–365

Akasaha Y, Hara T 1996 111 cases of free muscle transfer for elbow flexion and wrist extension in brachial plexus injury. Personal communication

Akasaha Y, Hara T, Takahishi M 1991 Free muscle transplantation combined with intercostal nerve crossing for reconstruction of elbow flexion and wrist extension in brachial plexus injuries. Microsurgery 12: 346–351

Akoev G N 1981 Catecholamines, acetylcholine and excitability of mechanoreceptors. Progress in Neurobiology 15: 269–294

Albe-Fessard D, Lombard M C 1983 Use of an animal model to evaluate the origin of and protection against deafferentation pain. In: Bonica J J, Lindblom U, Iggo A (eds) Advances in pain research and therapy. Raven Press, New York, vol 5, p 691–700

Albert H H von, Mackert B 1970 Eine neue Behandlungsmöglichkeit strahlenbedingter Armplexusparesen nach Mammakarzinomoperation. Deutsche Medinizinische Wochenschrift 95: 2119–2122

Alberty R E, Goodfried G, Boyden A M 1981 Popliteal artery injury with fracture dislocation of the knee. American Journal of Surgery 142: 36–40

Albrektsson B, Rydholm A, Rydholm V 1982 The tarsal tunnel syndrome in children. Journal of Bone and Joint Surgery 64B: 215–217

al Hakim M and Katirji M B 1993 Femoral mononeuropathy induced by the lithotomy position: a report of 5 cases with a review of the literature. Muscle and Nerve 16: 891–895

Allan S G, Towla H M A, Smith C C et al 1982 Painful brachial plexopathy: an unusual presentation of polyarteritis nodosa. Postgraduate Medical Journal 58: 311–313

Allieu Y 1975 Exploration et traitement direct des lésions nerveuses dans les paralysies traumatiques par élongation du plexus brachial chez l'adulte. Revue de Chirurgie Orthopedique 63: 107

Allieu Y 1989 Les neurotisations par le nerf spinal dans les avulsions du plexus brachial de l'adulte. In: Alnot J Y, Narakas A (eds) Les paralysies du plexus brachiale. Monographies du Groupe de l'étude de la Main. Expansion Scientifique, Paris, p 173–179

Allieu Y, Connes H, Ruscayret Ch et al 1977 Les accidents neurologiques périphériques des traitements anticoagulants. Annales Orthopédiques de l'Ouest. 9: 67–72

Allieu Y, Asencio G, Mailhe D et al 1983 Syndrome du canal carpien chez l'hémodialyse chronique. Approche étio-pathogénique. Revue de Chirurgie Orthopédique 69: 233–238

Allieu Y, Gomis R, Asencio G et al 1986 Sciatic paralysis following hip surgery. Peripheral Nerve Repair and Regeneration 4: 27–31. Liviano Press Padua.

Alnot J Y 1988. Traumatic brachial plexus palsy in the adult. Clinical Orthopaedics and Related Research 237: 9–16

Alnot J Y, Abols Y 1984 Réanimation de la Flexion du Coude par Transferts Tendineux dans les Paralysies Traumatiques du Plexus Brachial de l'Adulte. Revue de Chirurgie Orthopédique 70: 313–323

Alnot J Y, Jolly A, Frot B 1981 Traitement direct de lésions nerveuses dans les paralysies traumatique du plexus brachial chez l'adulte. Orthopädie (Berlin) 5: 151–168

Alnot J Y, Narakas A (eds) 1989 Les Paralysies du Plexus Brachial. Expansion Scientifique Française, Paris

Alnot J Y, Narakas A (eds) 1996 Traumatic Brachial Plexus Injuries. Expansion Scientifique Française, Paris

Alnot J Y, Oberlin C 1993 Tendon transfers in palsies of flexion and extension of elbow. In: Tubiana R (ed) The hand. W B Saunders, Philadelphia, vol IV, p 134–146

Alnot J Y, Oberlin Ch 1995 Les nerfs utilisables pour une neurotisation. In: Alnot J-Y, Narakas A (eds) Les paralysies du plexus brachial, 2nd edn. Monographie de la Société Française de Chirurgie de la Main, p 33–38

Alnot J Y, Rostoucher P, Houvet P 1995 Paralysie de la flexion du coude. 239–242. In: Alnot J Y, Narakas A (eds) Les paralysies du plexus brachial, 2nd edn. Expansion Scientifique Française, Paris

Alter M 1975 Statistical aspects of spinal cord tumours. In: Vinken P J, Bruyn G W (eds) Handbook of clinical neurology, vol 19, Tumours of the spine and spinal cord, Part I. North Holland, Amsterdam

Amadio P C 1985 Pyridoxine as an adjuvant in the treatment of carpal tunnel syndrome. Journal of Bone and Joint Surgery 10A: 237–241

Amarenco G, Lanoë Y, Perrigot M et al 1987 Un nouveau syndrome canalaire: la compression du nerf honteux interne dans le canal d'Alcock ou paralysie perinéale du cycliste. La Presse Médicale 16: 399

Amarenco G, Lanoë Y, Ghnassia R T et al 1988 Syndrome du canal d'Alcock et névralgie périnéale. Revue Neurologique 144: 523–526

Aminoff M J, Goodin D S, Parry G J et al 1985 Electrophysiological evaluation of lumbosacral radiculopathies: electromyography, late responses and somatosensory evoked potentials. Neurology 35: 1514–1518

Anand P 1986 Post-sympathectomy pain and sensory neuropeptides. Letter to Lancet Vol 1: 512

Anand P 1992 Lack of chronic pain and autotomy in young children and rats after peripheral nerve injury: the basis of a new plasticity theory of chronic pain. Journal of Neurology 239: 512

Anand P 1995 Nerve growth factor and nociception. British Journal of Anaesthesia. 75: 201–208

Anand P, Rudge P, Mathias C J et al 1991 New autonomic and sensory function with loss of adrenergic sympathetic function and sensory neuropeptides. Lancet 337: 1253–1254

Anand P, Pandya S, Ladiwake U et al 1994a Depletion of nerve growth factor in leprosy. Lancet 344: 129–130

Anand P, Warner G, Parrett A et al 1994b Nerve growth factor related small fibre dysfunction in human diabetic neuropathy. Annals of Neurology 36: 284A

Anand P, Birch R, Parrett A et al 1994d Nerve growth factor and ciliary neurotrophic factor in human peripheral nerves after injury. Annals of Neurology 36: 319A

Anand P, Terenghi G, Warner G, Kopelman P, Williams-Chestnut RE, Sinicropi DV 1996 The role of the endogenous growth factor in human diabetic neuropathy. Nature Medicine 2: 703–707

Anderson N E, Rosenblum M K, Graus F et al 1988 Auto-antibodies in para-neoplastic syndromes associated with small cell lung cancer. Neurology 38 (9): 1391–1398

Anderson S D, Basbaum A I, Fields H I 1977 Response of medullary raphe neurons to peripheral stimulation and to systemic opiates. Brain Research 123: 363–368

Angus P D, Cowell H R 1986 Triple arthrodesis. A critical long term review. Journal of Bone and Joint Surgery 68B: 260–265

Antia N H, Enna C D, Daver B M 1992 The surgical management of deformities in leprosy. Oxford University Press, Oxford

Aoike I, Gejyo F, Arakawa M and Niigata Research Programme for β_2-M Removal Membrane 1995 Learning from Japanese Registry: how will we prevent long-term complications? Nephrology Dialysis Transplantation 10 (suppl 7): 7–15

Aramburo F 1986 Exposure of the lumbo-sacral plexus. Peripheral Nerve Repair and Regeneration 4: 13–15

Archer D R, Griffin J W 1993 "Bystander" proliferation of cells in the sciatic nerve is induced by lumbar ventral radiculotomy. Cited by Griffin J W, Hoffman P N. In: Dyck P J, Thomas P K (eds) Peripheral Neuropathy, 3rd edn. W B Saunders, Philadelphia, p 365

Armstrong J R 1948 Traumatic dislocation of the hip. Journal of Bone and Joint Surgery 30B: 430–445

Asbury A K, Baringer J R, Cox S E 1972 Renaut bodies – an ultrastructural study. Presented at the Annual Meeting of the American Association of Neuropathologists, June 9–11

Ashbell G R, Lipscomb P R 1967 The changing treatment of Volkmann's ischaemic contracture from 1955 to 1965 at the Mayo Clinic. Clinical Orthopedics and Related Research 50: 215–223

Asher R 1951 Munchausen's Syndrome. Lancet i: 339–341

Aspden R M, Porter R W 1994 Nerve traction during correction of knee deformity. Journal of Bone and Joint Surgery 76B: 471–473

Atkins H J B 1949 Peraxillary approach to the stellate and upper thoracic ganglia. Lancet ii: 1152.

Atweh S F, Kuhar M J 1977 Autoradiographic localization of opiate receptors in rat brain. II. The brain stem. Brain Research 129: 1–12

Augustijn P, Vannesti J 1992 The tarsal tunnel syndrome after a proximal lesion. Journal of Neurology, Neurosurgery and Psychiatry 55: 65–67

Baba M, Fowler C J, Jacobs J M et al 1982 Changes in peripheral nerve fibres distal to a constriction. Journal of the Neurological Sciences 54: 197–208

Bach S, Noreng M F, Tjellden N U 1988 Phantom limb pains in amputees during the first twelve months following limb amputation, after peri-operative epidural blockade. Pain 33: 297–301

Badger F G 1959 Fractures near or involving joints of the lower limb. In: Clarke A R, Badger F G, Sevitt S (eds) Modern trends in accident surgery and medicine. Butterworth, London, p 176–195

Bainbridge L C 1996 Brachial plexus neuropathy after radiotherapy can be treated by specialist surgeons. British Medical Journal 312: 780.

Baker A S, Bitounis V C 1989 Abductor function after total hip replacement. Journal of Bone and Joint Surgery 71B: 47–50

Baker A S, Scotland T R 1995 Entrapment neuropathy of the common peroneal nerve by a fabella. Orthopaedics 3: 77–78

Baker R H, Cox W A, Scully T J et al 1973 Causalgia and transthoracic sympathectomy. Plastic and Reconstructive Surgery 52: 322

Ballantyne J P and Campbell M J 1973 Electrophysiological study after surgical repair of sectioned human peripheral nerves. Journal of Neurology, Neurosurgery and Psychiatry 36: 797–805

Bandi S, De Smet L, Fabry G 1994 Endoscopic versus open carpal tunnel release. Journal of Hand Surgery 19B: 14–17

Banerjee T, Hall C D 1976 Sciatic entrapment neuropathy. Journal of Neurosurgery 45: 216–217

Banerjee T, Koons D D 1981 Superficial peroneal nerve entrapment. Journal of Neurosurgery 55: 991–992

Banks R W, Barker D, Stacey M J 1982 The sensory innervation of cat muscle spindles. Philosophical Transactions of the Royal Society of London, Series B 299: 329–364

Banzet P, Brocheriou C 1985 Sarcomes neurogéniques survenant au cours de la maladie de Von Recklinghausen. Archives d'Anatomie et de Cytologie Pathologique 33: 5–16

Baratta J B, Lim V, Mastromonaco E et al 1983 Axillary artery disruption secondary to anterior dislocation of the shoulder. Journal of Trauma 13: 1009–1011

Barbut D, Blah J M, Wall P D 1981 Substance P in spinal cord dorsal horn decreases following peripheral nerve injury. Brain Research 205: 289–298

Baring-Gould W S (ed) 1968 The adventure of the lion's mane (1909). In: The annotated Sherlock Holmes. J Murray, London, p 776–789

Barker D, Scott J J A, Stacey M J 1986 Re-innervation and recovery of cat muscle receptors after long term denervation. Experimental Neurology 94: 184–202

Barker D, Berry R B, Scott J J A 1990 The sensory reinnervation of muscles following immediate and delayed repair in the cat. British Journal of Plastic Surgery 43: 107–111

Barkhaus P E, Means E D, Sawaya R 1987 Ligature injury to the accessory nerve. Journal of Neurology, Neurosurgery and Psychiatry 50: 1382–1383

Barnes M P 1993 Organisation of neurological rehabilitation services. In: Greenwood R, Barnes M P, McMillan T M, Ward C D (eds) Neurological rehabilitation. Churchill Livingstone, London, p 29–40

Barnes R 1949 Traction injuries of the brachial plexus in adults. Journal of Bone and Joint Surgery 31: p 10–16

Barnes R 1953 The role of sympathectomy in the treatment of causalgia. Journal of Bone and Joint Surgery 35B: 2: 172–180

Barnes R 1954a Causalgia: a review of 48 cases. In: Seddon H J (ed) Peripheral nerve injuries. HMSO, London, p 156–185

Barnes R 1954b Peripheral nerve injuries. Medical Research Council Special Report Series No. 282. HMSO, London

Barnes R, Bacsich P, Wyburn G M et al 1946 A study of the fate of nerve grafts in man. British Journal of Surgery 34: 34–41

Barnett H G, Connolly E S 1975 Lumbosacral nerve root avulsion: report of a case and review of the literature. Journal of Trauma 15: 532–535

Baron R, Maier C 1995 Phantom limb pain; are cutaneous nociceptors and spinothalamic neurons involved in the signalling and maintenance of spontaneous and touch-evoked pain? A case report. Pain 60: 223–228

Baron R, Blumberg H, Jänig W 1996 Clinical characteristics of patients with complex regional pain syndrome in Germany with special emphasis on vaso-motor function. Progress in Pain Research and Management 6: 25–48

Barr L C, Kissin M W 1987 Radiation-induced brachial plexus neuropathy following breast conservation and radical radiotherapy. British Journal of Surgery 74: 855–856

Barros D'Sa A A B 1982 A decade of missile-induced vascular trauma. Annals of the Royal College of Surgeons of England 64: 37–44

Barros D'Sa A A B 1989 The rationale for arterial and venous shunting in the management of limb vascular injuries. European Journal of Vascular Surgery 3: 471–474

Barros D'Sa A A B 1992a Radiation injury of arteries. In: Eastcott H H G (ed) Arterial surgery, 3rd edn. Churchill Livingstone, Edinburgh, p 355–414

Barros D'Sa A A B 1992b Arterial spasm. In: Eastcott H H G (ed) Arterial surgery, 3rd edn. Churchill Livingstone, Edinburgh, p 369

Barros D'Sa A A B 1992c Arterial spasm. In: Eastcott H H G (ed) Arterial surgery, 3rd edn. Churchill Livingstone, Edinburgh, p 397

Barros D'Sa A A B 1992d Arterial spasm in children. In: Eastcott H H G (ed) Arterial Surgery, 3rd edn. Churchill Livingstone, Edinburgh, p 380

Barros D'Sa A A B 1992e Intra-arterial injection. In: Eastcott H H G (ed) Arterial surgery, 3rd edn. Churchill Livingstone, Edinburgh, p 379

Barros D'Sa A A B 1992f Arterial injuries. In: Eastcott H H G (ed) Arterial surgery, 3rd edn. Churchill Livingstone, Edinburgh, p 355–413

Barros D'Sa A A B, Moorhead R J 1989 Combined arterial and venous intraluminal shunting in major trauma of the lower limb. European Journal of Vascular Surgery 3: 577–581

Basbaum A I, Clanton L H, Fields H L 1977a Three bulbospinal pathways from the rostral medulla of the cat. Journal of Comparative Neurology 178: 209–224

Basbaum A I, Marley N J, O'Keefe J et al 1977b Reversal of morphine and stimulation-produced analgesia by subtotal spinal cord lesions. Pain 3: 43–56

Bates T, Evans R G B 1995 Brachial neuropathy following radiotherapy for breast cancer. Report of the independent review commissioned by the Royal College of Radiologists

Batten F B 1897 The muscle-spindle under pathological conditions. Brain 20: 138–179

Baudet J, Guimberteau J C, Nacimento E 1976 Successful clinical transfer of two free thoracodorsal axillary flaps. Plastic and Reconstructive Surgery 58: 680–688

Baumel J J 1974 Trigeminal–facial nerve connections. Their function in facial muscle innervation and re-innervation. Archives of Otolaryngology 99: 34–44

Becker C, Gueuning C, Gilbert A et al 1989 Increase of muscle regeneration after repair of divided motor nerve with neurotrophic factor containing glue. Archives Internationales de Physiologie et de Biochimie 97: 521–529

Beecher H K 1946 Pain of men wounded in battle. Annals of Surgery 123: 96–105

Beghi B, Kurland L T, Mulder D W, Nicolosi A 1985 Brachial plexus neuropathy in the population of Rochester, Minnesota 1970–1981. Annals of Neurology 18: 320–323

Behse F, Buchtal F, Carlsen F, Knappeis G B 1972 Hereditary neuropathy with liability to pressure palsies. Brain 95: 777–794

Bell J, Burford W 1982 The force time relationship of clinically used sensory testing instruments. Presented at American Society for Surgery of the Hand 37th Annual Meeting, New Orleans

Bell M A, Weddell A G M 1984 A descriptive study of the blood vessels of the sciatic nerve in the rat, man and other animals. Brain 107: 871–898

Bell R, Di Tunno J, Northrup B 1995 Vertebral artery injury after acute cervical spine trauma: rate of occurrence as detected by MR angiography and assessment of clinical consequence. American Journal of Roentgenology 164: 448–449

Bellini F, Buitoni P 1963 Paralisi ostetrica con sindryome di Duchenne-Erb. Clinica Paediatrica, Bologne 45: 319–338

Belloc H 1940 Henry King. In: Cautionary verses. Duckworth, London, p 13–16

Bence Y, Commandre F, Revelli G et al 1978 Données électromyographiques dans les épicondylalgies. Étude a propos de 122 patients. Rhumatologie 91: 87–98

Bennet C C, Harrold A J 1976 Prognosis and early management of birth injuries to the brachial plexus. British Medical Journal 1: 1520–1521

Bennett M I, Tai Y M A 1994 Cervical dorsal column stimulation relieves pain of brachial plexus avulsion. Journal of the Royal Society of Medicine: 87 5–7

Bergentz S-E, Hansson L O, Norback B 1966 Surgical management of complications of arterial puncture. Annals of Surgery 164: 1021–1026

Beric A, Dimitrijevic M R, Lundblom U 1988 Central dysaesthesia syndrome in spinal cord injury patients. Pain 304: 109–116

Berkeley C, Bonney V 1920 Violet-green antiseptic paint. In: A textbook of gynaecological surgery, 2nd edn. Cassell, London, p 35

Berman J S, Taggart M, Anand P et al 1995 The effect of surgical repair on pain relief after brachial plexus injuries. Proceedings of the British Neurological Association, p 44 (abstract)

Berman J, Anand P, Chen L, Taggart M 1996 Pain relief from preganglionic injury to the brachial plexus by later intercostal transfer. Journal of Bone and Joint Surgery 78B: 759–760

Bernhardt M 1895 Ueber isolirt im Gebiet des N cutaneus femoris externus vorkommende Parästhesien. Neurologisches Centralblatt 14: 242–244

Berthold C H, Carlstedt T, Corneliuson O 1993 Anatomy of the mature transitional zone. In: Dyck P J, Thomas P K, Griffin J W, Low P A, Poduslo J F (eds) Peripheral neuropathy, 3rd edn. W B Saunders, Philadelphia, p 75–80

Besse D, Lombard M C, Zakac J M et al 1990 Pre and post-synaptic distribution of mu, delta and kappa opioid receptors in the superficial layers of the cervical dorsal horn of the rat spinal cord. Brain Research 521: 15–22

Betcher A M, Bean G, Casten D F 1953 Continuous procaine blocks of paravertebral sympathetic ganglions: observations in 100 patients. Journal of the American Medical Association 151: 288–292

Betts L O 1940 Morton's metatarsalgia: neuritis of the fourth digital nerve. Medical Journal of Australia 1: 514–515

Beverly M C, Fearn C B 1984 Anterior interosseous nerve palsy and dislocation of the elbow. Injury 6: 126–128

Bickford R G 1939 The fibre dissociation produced by cooling human nerves. Clinical Science 4: 159–164

Biesalski K, Mayer L 1916 Die Physiologische Sehnenverpflanzung. Springer, Berlin. p 330

Bigenzahn W, Balogh N, Zrunek M et al 1991 Funktionelle und elektromyographische langzeitergebnisse nach primärer mikrochirurgischer Versorgung des N. laryngeus recurrens. Laryngootologie 70: 508–510

Bigliani L U, Perez-Sanz J R, Wolfe I N 1985 Treatment of trapezius paralysis. Journal of Bone and Joint Surgery 67A: 871–877

Bigliani L U, Craig E V, Butters K P 1991 Fractures of the shoulder. In: Rockwood C A, Green D P and Bucholz R W (eds) Fractures in adults, 3rd edn. J B Lippincott, Philadelphia, p 871–1020

Birch R 1984 The primary and secondary repair of divided peripheral nerves. In: Birch R, Brooks D M The Hand, in Rob and Smith's Operative Surgery, 4th edn. Butterworths p 168–177

Birch R 1986 Lesions of peripheral nerves: the present position. Journal of Bone and Joint Surgery 68B: 2–8

Birch R 1987 The place of microsurgery in orthopaedics. In: Catterall A (ed) Recent Advances in Orthopaedics 5: 165–186

Birch R 1989 The repair of peripheral nerves: experimental and clinical observations. Master of Surgery Thesis, University of Cambridge, Cambridge

Birch R 1991a Major neurovascular bundles. In: Colton C L, Hall A J (eds) Atlas of orthopaedics: surgical approaches. Butterworth-Heinemann, Oxford, p 120–133

Birch R 1991b Repair of damaged peripheral nerves. In: Dudley H, Carter D, Russel R C G (eds) Rob and Smith's operative surgery. Orthopaedics, Part 1, 4th edn. Butterworth-Heinemann, Oxford, p 24–38

Birch R 1992 Day surgery. Journal of the Medical Defence Union 8: 71

Birch R 1993a Peripheral nerve tumours. In: Dyck P J, Thomas P K, Griffin J W, Low P A, Poduslo J F (eds) Peripheral neuropathy. W B Saunders, London, p 1627–1628

Birch R 1993b Management of brachial plexus injuries. In: Greenwood R, Barnes M P, McMillan T M, Ward C D (eds) Neurological rehabilitation. Churchill Livingstone, Edinburgh, p 587–606

Birch R 1995a Nerves of the thoracoscapular and gleno-humeral joints. In: Copeland S (ed) Operative shoulder surgery. Churchill Livingstone, New York, p 331–356

Birch R 1995b Obstetrical brachial plexus palsy. Clinical risk 1: 71–73

Birch R 1996 Brachial plexus injuries. Journal of Bone and Joint Surgery 78B: 986–992

Birch R, Chen L 1996 The medial rotation contracture of the shoulder in obstetric brachial plexus palsy. Journal of Bone and Joint Surgery 73B (suppl 1): 68

Birch R, Raji A R M 1991 Repair of median and ulnar nerves. Journal of Bone and Joint Surgery 73B: 154–157

Birch R, St Clair Strange F G 1990 A new type of peripheral nerve lesion. Journal of Bone and Joint Surgery 72B: 312–313

Birch R, Dunkerton M, Bonney G, Jamieson A M 1988 Experience with the free vascularised ulnar nerve graft in repair of supraclavicular lesion of the brachial plexus. Clinical Orthopaedics and Related Research 237: 96–104

Birch R, Bonney G, Marshall R W 1990 A surgical approach to the cervico-dorsal spine. Journal of Bone and Joint Surgery 72B: 904–907.

Birch R, Bonney G, Dowell J et al 1991a Iatrogenic injuries of peripheral nerves. Journal of Bone and Joint Surgery 73B: 280–282

Birch R, Jessop J, Scott G 1991b Brachial plexus palsy after manipulation of the shoulder. Journal of Bone and Joint Surgery 73: 172

Birch R, Jessop J, Scott G 1991c Iatrogenic injuries of peripheral nerves. Journal of Bone and Joint Surgery 73B: 280–282

Birch R, Wilkinson M C P, Vijayan K P et al 1992 Cement burn of the sciatic nerve. Journal of Bone and Joint Surgery 74B: 731–733

Birnstingl M 1982 Vascular injuries. In: Watson-Jones R (ed) Fractures and joint injuries, 6th edn. Churchill Livingstone, Edinburgh, p 211–241

Bjik K D, Bellamy R F 1984 Editorial. A note on combat casualty statistics. Military Medicine 149: 229–230

Bland-Sutton J 1920 Humeral foramina. In: Selected Lectures and Essays. Heinemann, London, p 4–5

Bland-Sutton J 1930 Injuries of the peripheral nerves. In: The story of a surgeon. Methuen, London, p 34–37

Blix M 1884 Experimentelle Beitrage zur Lösung der Frage über die specifische Energie der Hautnerven. Zeitschrift für Biologie 20: 141–156

Blom S, Dahlback L O 1970 Nerve injuries in dislocation of the shoulder joint and fractures of the neck of the humerus. Acta Chirurgica Scandinavica 136: 461–466

Blom S, Hele P, Parkman L 1971 The supinator channel syndrome. Scandinavian Journal of Plastic and Reconstructive Surgery 5: 71–75

Boivie J 1994 Central pain. In: Wall P D, Melzack R M (eds) Textbook of pain. Churchill Livingstone, Edinburgh, p 871–902

Bolam vs Friern Hospital Management Committee 1957 All England Reports 118

Bolton J S, Vauthey J-N, Farr G H et al 1989 Is limb sparing surgery applicable to neurogenic sarcomas of the extremities? Archives of Surgery 124: 118–121

Bonicka J J, Lundblom U 1983 Advances in Pain. Research and Therapy Series. World Congress in Pain (3rd Edinburgh Proceedings) Lipencott-Raven

Bonica J J 1990 Causalgia and other reflex sympathetic dystrophies. In: Bonica J J (ed) The management of pain. Lea & Febiger, Philadelphia, vol 2, p 220–243

Bonnard C, Narakas A 1985 Syndromes douloureux et lésions post-traumatiques du plexus brachial. Helvetica Chirurgica Acta 52: 621–632

Bonnel F 1989 Anatomie du plexus brachial chez le nouveau-né et l'adulte. In: Alnot J Y, Narakas A. (eds) Les paralysies du plexus brachial. Monographies du Groupe d'Étude de la Main. Expansion Scientifique, Paris, p 3–13

Bonnel F, Allieu Y, Sugata Y et al 1979 Bases anatomo-chirurgicales des neurotisations pour avulsion radiculaires du plexus brachial. Anat Clin. 1: 291–196

Bonellie S R, Raab G M 1997 Why are babies getting heavier? Comparison of Scottish births from 1980 to 1992. British Medical Journal 315: 1205

Bonney G 1954 The value of axon responses in determining the site of lesion in traction lesions of the brachial plexus. Brain 77: 588–609

Bonney G 1959 Prognosis in traction lesions of the brachial plexus. Journal of Bone and Joint Surgery 41B: 4–35

Bonney G 1963 Thrombosis of the femoral artery complicating fracture of the femur. Journal of Bone and Joint Surgery 47B: 28–272

Bonney G 1965 The scalenus medius band: a contribution to the study of the thoracic outlet syndrome. Journal of Bone and Joint Surgery 47B: 268–272

Bonney G 1973 Causalgia. British Journal of Hospital Medicine 9: 593–596

Bonney G 1977 Some lesions of the brachial plexus. Annals of the Royal College of Surgeons, England 59: 298–306

Bonney G 1983 Peripheral nerve lesions. In: Harris N H (ed) Clinical orthopaedics. Wright, Bristol, p 726

Bonney G 1986 Iatrogenic injuries of nerves. Journal of Bone and Joint Surgery 68B: 9–13

Bonney G 1990 The function of the defence societies. In: Powers M J, Harris N H (eds) Medical negligence. Butterworths, Oxford, p 44–45

Bonney G 1991 Nerve root, plexus and peripheral nerve trauma. In: Swash M, Oxbury J (eds) Clinical neurology. Churchill Livingstone, Edinburgh, p 760

Bonney G 1992 Pitfalls in "day-case" operating. Journal of the Medical Defence Union 8: 4–5

Bonney G, Gilliatt R W 1958 Sensory nerve conduction after traction lesion of the brachial plexus. Proceedings of the Royal Society of Medicine 51: 365–367

Bonney G, Jamieson A 1979 Reimplantation of C7 and C8. Communication au symposium sur le plexus brachial. International Microsurgery 1: 103–106

Bonney G, Birch R, Jamieson A M et al 1984 Experience with vascularised nerve grafts. Clinics in Plastic Surgery 11: 137–142

Bonney V 1947 A textbook of gynaecological surgery, 5th edn. Cassell, London, p 55

Bonnin J G 1945 Sacral injuries and injuries of the cauda equina. Journal of Bone and Joint Surgery 27: 112–127

Boo N Y, Lye M S, Kanchanala M et al 1991 Brachial plexus lesions in Malaysian neonates: incidence and associated risk factors. Journal of Tropical Paediatrics 37: 327–330

Bostock H 1993 Impulse propagation in experimental neuropathy. In: Dyck P J, Thomas P K, Griffin J W, Low P A, Poduslo J F (eds) Peripheral neuropathy, 3rd edn. W B Saunders, London, p 109–120

Bostwick J, Nahai F, Wallace J G, Vasconez L O 1979 Sixty latissismus dorsi flaps. Plastic and Reconstructive Surgery 63: 31–41

Bottoms S F, Rosen M G, Sokol R J 1980 The increase in Cesarean birth rate. New England Medical Journal 302: 559–563

Bowden R E M, Gutmann E 1944 Denervation and re-innervation of human voluntary muscle. Brain 67: 273–313

Bowden R E M, Napier C 1961 Assessment of hand function. Journal of Bone and Joint Surgery 43B: 481–492

Bowen J, Gregory R, Squier M et al 1996 The post-irradiation lower motor neuron syndrome. Neuronopathy or radiculopathy? Brain 119: 1429–1439

Bowen T L, Stone K H 1966 Posterior interosseous nerve paralysis caused by a ganglion at the elbow. Journal of Bone and Joint Surgery 48B: 774–776

Bowsher D 1976 Role of the reticular formation in response to noxious stimulation. Pain 2: 361–378

Bowsher D 1996 Central pain: clinical and physiological characteristics. Journal of Neurology, Neurosurgery and Psychiatry 61: 62–69

Boyd I A 1962 The structure and function of the nuclear bag muscle fibre system and the nuclear chain muscle fibre system in mammalian muscle spindle. Philosophical Transactions of the Royal Society of London, Series B 245: 81–136

Boyd I A 1966 The behaviour of isolated mammalian muscle spindles with intact innervation. Journal of Physiology, London 186: 109P–110P.

Boyd I A 1976 The response of fast and slow nuclear bag fibres and nuclear chain fibres in isolated cat muscle spindles to fusiform stimulation, and the effect of intrafusal contraction on the sensory endings. Quarterly Journal of Experimental Physiology 61: 203–254

Boyd I A 1983 Muscle spindles and stretch reflexes. In: Swash M, Kennard C (eds) The scientific basis of clinical neurology. Churchill Livingstone, London, p 74–77

Boyd I A, Smith R S 1984 The muscle spindle. In: Dyck P J, Thomas P K, Lambert E H, Burge R (eds) Peripheral neuropathy, 2nd edn. W B Saunders, London, p 171–202

Boyer G F 1911 The complete histopathological examination of the nervous system of an unusual case of obstetrical paralysis 41 years after birth and a review of the pathology. Proceedings of the Royal Society of Medicine (5): 31–58

Boyes J H 1960 Tendon transfers for radial palsy. Bulletin of the Hospital for Joint Diseases 21: 97–105

Brady S T, Lasek R J, Allen R D 1982 Fast axonal transport in extruded axoplasm from squid giant axon. Science 218: 1129–1131

Brain W R, Wright A D, Wilkinson M 1947 Spontaneous compression of both median nerves in the carpal tunnel. Lancet i: 277–282

Braithwaite B, Quinones-Baldrich W, Earnshaw J 1995 Skeletal muscle reperfusion syndrome. Hospital Update 21: 27–33

Braithwaite I, Klenerman L 1996 Burns under tourniquets – Bruner's ten rules revisited. Journal of the Medical Defence Union 12: 14–15

Bramwell E, Struthers J W 1903 Paralysis of the serratus magnus and lower part of the trapezius muscles. Review of Neurology and Psychiatry 1: 717–730

Brand P W 1958 Paralytic claw hand. Journal of Bone and Joint Surgery 40B: 618–632

Brand P W 1985 Clinical mechanics of the hand. C V Mosby, St Louis, 61–191

Brand P W 1987 Biomechanics of tendon transfer. In: Lamb D W (ed) The paralysed hand. Churchill Livingstone, Edinburgh, p 190–214

Brannon E W 1963 Cervical rib syndrome. Journal of Bone and Joint Surgery 45A: 977–988

Breidenbach W C 1988 Vascularised nerve grafts. Orthopaedic Clinics of North America 19: 81–89

Bremer F, Titica J 1946 Étude oscillographique de la paralysie thermique du nerf. Archives Internationales de Physiologie 54: 237–272

Brewer P L, Schramel R J, Menendez C V et al 1969. Injuries of the popliteal artery. American Journal of Surgery 118: 36–42

Bristol D C, Fraher J P 1989 Experimental traction injuries of ventral spinal nerve roots. A scanning electron microscopic study. Neuropathology and Applied Neurobiology 15: 549–561

British National Formulary 1997 No 33 British Medical Association and Royal Pharmaceutical Society of Great Britain, London, pp 531, 563, 571

Britz G W, Haynor D R et al 1996 Ulnar nerve entrapment at the elbow: correlation of magnetic resonance imaging, clinical, electrodiagnostic and intraoperative findings. Journal of Neurosurgery 38: 458–465

Britz G W, Haynor D R, Kuntz C et al 1995 Carpal tunnel syndrome: correlation of magnetic resonance imaging, clinical, electrodiagnostic and intraoperative findings. Journal of Neurosurgery 37: 1097–1103

Brodal A 1981a The spinal accessory nerve. In: Neurological anatomy. Oxford University Press, New York, p 458

Brodal A 1981b Neuron theory. Ibid, p 9

Brodal A 1981c Extrapyramidal tracts. Ibid, p 194–211

Brodal A 1981d The fibers in the dorsal funiculi and the medial lemniscus. Ibid, p 74–84

Brodal A 1981e The segmental sensory innervation. In: Neurological anatomy. Oxford University Press, New York, p 69–74

Brodeur G M, Green A A, Hayes F A 1980 Cytogenetic studies of primary human neuroblastoma. In: Evans A E (ed) Advances in Neuroblastoma Research. Raven, New York

Bromwich P 1986 Big babies. British Medical Journal 293: 1387–1388

Brooke H, Barton A 1994 Consent to treatment. In: Powers M J, Harris N H (eds) Medical negligence, 2nd edn. Butterworths, London, p 304–326

Brooks B 1922 Pathologic changes of muscle as a result of disturbance of circulation. Archives of Surgery 5: 188

Brooks D M 1952 Nerve compression by simple ganglia. Journal of Bone and Joint Surgery 34B: 391–400

Brooks D M 1954 Open wounds of the brachial plexus. In: Seddon H J (ed) Peripheral nerve injuries. Medical Research Council special report. HMSO, London, p 418–429

Brooks D M 1984a Tendon transfer for paralysis. In: Birch R, Brooks D M (eds) Rob and Smith's operative surgery. The Hand, 4th edn. Butterworths, London, p 310–317

Brooks D M 1984b Volkmann's contracture. In: Birch R, Brooks D M (eds) Rob and Smith's operative surgery. The Hand, 4th edn. Butterworths, London, p 235–241

Brooks D M 1984c Clinical presentation and treatment of peripheral nerve tumours. In: Dyck P J, Thomas P K, Lambert E H, Bunge R (eds) Peripheral neuropathy, 2nd edn. W B Saunders, Philadelphia, p 2236–2252

Brooks D M, Seddon H J 1959 Pectoral transplantation for paralysis of the flexors of the elbow. A new technique. Journal of Bone and Joint Surgery 41B: 36–43

Brooks J S J, Freeman M, Enterline H T 1985 Malignant "triton" tumours. Cancer 55: 2543–2549

Brown H, Burns S, Kaiser C W 1988 The spinal accessory nerve plexus, the trapezius muscle, and shoulder stabilization after radical neck cancer. Annals of Surgery 208: 654–661

Brown H A 1969 Internal neurolysis in the treatment of peripheral nerve injuries. Clinical Neurosurgery 17: 99–110

Brown M J, Martin J R, Asbury A K 1976 Painful diabetic neuropathy: a morphometeric study. Archives of Neurology 33: 164

Brown P W 1970 The time factor in surgery of upper extremity peripheral nerve injury. Clinical Orthopaedics and Related Research 68: 14–21

Brown W F and Bolton C F 1993 Clinical electromyography, 2nd edn. Butterworth-Heinemann, Oxford

Brown W F and Watson B V 1993 Acute retrohumeral radial neuropathies. Muscle and Nerve 16: 706–711

Brown W F, Ferguson S G, Jones M W et al 1976 The location of conduction abnormalities in human entrapment neuropathies. Canadian Journal of Neurological Science 3: 111–122

Brunelli G 1964 Lipoma interfibrillare del nervo mediano con sindrome da compressione nel canale del carpo. Minerva Ortopedica 15: 211–217

Brunelli G 1980a Nerve suture. International Surgery 65: 499–501

Brunelli G 1980b Neurotization of avulsed roots of the brachial plexus by means of anterior nerves of the cervical plexus. International Journal of Microsurgery 2: 55–58

Brunelli G A, Brunelli G R 1991 A fourth type of brachial plexus lesion: the intermediate (C7) palsy. Journal of Hand Surgery 16: 492–494

Brunelli G, Brunelli F 1995 Anatomie de la troisième anse du plexus cervical et son intérêt chirurgical. In: Alnot J-Y, Narakas A (eds) Les Paralysies du plexus brachial, 2nd edn. Monographie De La Société Française De Chirurgie De La Main. p 39–42

Brunelli G, Monini L 1985 Direct muscular neurotisation. Journal of Hand Surgery 10A: 993–994

Brunelli G, Vigasio A 1986 Lumbar plexus surgery. Peripheral Nerve Repair and Regeneration. Liviana Press, Padua, p 21–25

Brunelli G, Fontana G, Jager C et al 1987 Chemotacic arrangement of axons inside and distal to a vein graft. Journal of Reconstructive Microsurgery 3: 87–89

Bruner J M 1951 Safety factors in the use of pneumatic tourniquet in surgery of the hand. Journal of Bone and Joint Surgery 33A: 221–224

Brushart T M E, Mather V, Sood R et al 1995 Dispersion of regenerating axons across enclosed neural gaps. Journal of Hand Surgery 20A: 557–564

Brushart T M E 1988 Preferential reinnervation of motor nerves. Journal of Neurosciences 8: 1026–1031

Brushart T M E, Seiler W A 1987 Selective innervation of distal motor stumps by peripheral motor axons. Experimental Neurology 97: 289–300

Buchthal F, Rosenfalck A 1971 Sensory conduction from digit to palm and from palm to wrist in the carpal tunnel syndrome. Journal of Neurology, Neurosurgery and Psychiatry 34: 243–252

Buchthal F, Guld C and Rosenfalck A 1957 Multielectrode study of the territory of a motor unit. Acta Physiologica Scandinavica 39: 83–104

Buchthal F, Rosenfalck A and Trojaborg W 1974 Electrophysiological findings in entrapment of the median nerve at wrist and elbow. Journal of Neurology, Neurosurgery and Psychiatry 37: 340–360

Buchthal F, Rosenfalck A and Behse F 1984 Sensory potentials in normal and diseased nerves. In: Dyck P J, Thomas P K, Lambert E H, Bunge R (eds) Peripheral neuropathy, 2nd edn. W B Saunders, Philadelphia, p 981–1015

Buck-Gramcko D, Lugahn J D 1993 The Hoffman–Tinel sign. Journal of Hand Surgery 18B: 800–805

Budny P H G, Regan P J, Roberts A H N 1992 Localised nodular synovitis: a rare cause of ulnar nerve compression in Guyon's canal. Journal of Hand Surgery 17A: 663–664

Bufalini C, Pescatori G 1969 Posterior cervical electromyography in the diagnosis and prognosis of brachial plexus injuries. Journal of Bone and Joint Surgery 51B: 627–631

Buncke H J, Buncke G M, Valauri F A 1991. In: Meyer V E, Black M J M (eds) Microsurgical procedures. Hand and upper limb series, vol 7. Churchill Livingstone, Edinburgh, p 1–8

Bunge, M B, Wood P M, Tynan L B et al 1989 Perineurium originates from fibroblasts: demonstration in vitro with a retroviral marker. Science 243: 229–231

Bunnell S 1928 Repair of nerves and tendons of the hand. Journal of Bone and Joint Surgery 10: 1–26

Bunnell S 1938 Opposition of the thumb. Journal of Bone and Joint Surgery 20: 269–284

Bunnell S 1953 Restoring flexion to the paralysed elbow. Journal of Bone and Joint Surgery 33A: 566–571

Burn S 1996 Access to civil justice: Lord Woolf's visionary new landscape. British Medical Journal 313: 242–243

Burns R J 1978 Delayed radiation-induced damage to the brachial plexus. Clinical and Experimental Neurology 15: 221–227

Burnstock G, Evans B, Gannon B J et al 1971 New method of destroying adrenergic nerves in adult animals using guanethidine. British Journal of Pharmacology 43: 259–301

Burton A C 1951 On the physical equilibrium of small blood vessels. American Journal of Physiology 164: 319–329

Busa A, Adani R, Marcuzzi A et al 1995 Acute posterior interosseous nerve palsy caused by a synovial haemangioma of the elbow joint. Journal of Hand Surgery 20B: 652–654

Butler M J, Lane R H S, Webster J H H 1980 Irradiation injury to large arteries. British Journal of Surgery 67: 341–343

Cabaud H E, Rodky G, Nemeth T J 1982 Progressive ultrastructural changes after peripheral nerve transection and repair. Journal of Hand Surgery 7: 353–365

Cahill B R, Palmer R E 1983 Quadrilateral space syndrome. Journal of Hand Surgery 8: 65–69

Calandruccio R A 1980 Nerve injuries in hip arthroplasty. In: Edmondson A S, Crenshaw A H (eds) Campbell's operative orthopaedics, 6th edn. C V Mosby, St Louis, p 2329

Calder J S, Green C J 1996 Nerve–muscle sandwich grafts: the importance of Schwann cells in peripheral nerve regeneration through muscle basal lamina conduits. Journal of Hand Surgery 20B: 423–428

Calder J S, Norris R W 1993 Repair of peripheral nerves using muscle autografts: a preliminary communication. British Journal of Plastic Surgery 46: 557–564

Calvert P T, Edgar M A, Webb P J 1985 Neurofibromatosis and scoliosis. Journal of Bone and Joint Surgery 67B: 500

Calvet J, Leroy M, Lacroix L 1942 Luxations de l'épaule et lesions vasculaires. Journal de Chirurgie 58: 337–346

Calvin W H, Devor M, Howe J F 1982 Can neuralgias arise from minor demyelination? Spontaneous firing mechanosensitivity and after discharge from conductory axons. Experimental Neurology 75: 755–763

Campbell J A, Lipton S 1983 Somatosensory evoked potentials recorded from within the antero-lateral quadrant of the human spinal cord. In: Bonica J J, Lundblom (eds) Advances in Pain Research and Therapy. vol 5. Proceedings of the Third World Congress on Pain

Campbell J A, Miles J 1984 Evoked potentials as an aid to lesion making in the dorsal root entry zone. Neurosurgery 15: 951–952

Campbell J N, LaMotte R H 1983 Latency to detection of first pain. Brain Research 266: 203–208

Campbell J N, Raja S N, Meyer R A et al 1988 Myelinated afferents signal the hyperalgesia associated with nerve injury. Pain 32: 89–94

Campbell M J, Patey D W 1974 Carcinomatous neuropathy. 1. Electrophysiological studies. Journal of Neurology, Neurosurgery and Psychiatry 37: 131–141

Campbell W W, Sahni S K, Pridgeon R M et al 1988 Intraoperative electroneurography: management of ulnar neuropathy at the elbow. Muscle and Nerve 11: 75–81

Campbell W W, Pridgeon R M, Riaz G et al 1991 Variations in anatomy of the ulnar nerve at the cubital tunnel: pitfalls in the diagnosis of ulnar neuropathy at the elbow. Muscle and Nerve 14: 733–738

Campbell W W, Pridgeon R M, Sahni S K 1992 Short segment incremental studies in the evaluation of ulnar neuropathy at the elbow. Muscle and Nerve 15: 1050–1054

Campbell-Reid D A 1984 Capsulectomy of the metacarpophalangeal joint and proximal interphalangeal joints. In: Brooks D M, Birch R (eds) Rob and Smiths operative surgery. The Hand, 4th edn. Butterworths, London, p 226–234

Camus M, Lefebvre G, Veron P et al 1995 Traumatisme obstétrique du nouveau né. Journal de Gynecologie, Obstetrique et Biologie de la Reproduction 14: 1033–1044

Canale S T 1991 Fractures of the pelvis. In: Rockwood C A, Wilkins K E, King R E (eds) Fractures in Children, 3rd edn. J B Lippincott, Philadelphia, p 992–1046

Cannon B W, Love J G 1946 Tardy median nerve palsy: median neuritis: median thenar neuritis amenable to surgery. Surgery 20: 210–216

Capener N 1966 The vulnerability of the posterior interosseous nerve in the forearm. Journal of Bone and Joint Surgery 48B: 770–773

Carlioz H, Brahimi L 1986 La place de la désinsertion interne du sous-scapulaire dans le traitement de la paralysie obstétricale du membre supérieur chez l'enfant. Chirurgie Pédiatrique 12: 159–167

Carlstedt T 1991 Experimental studies on surgical treatment of avulsed spinal nerve roots in brachial plexus injury. Journal of Hand Surgery 16B: 477–482

Carlstedt T, Lindå H, Cullheim S et al 1986 Reinnervation of hind limb muscles after ventral root avulsion and implantation in the lumbar spinal cord of the adult rat. Acta Physiologica Scandinavica 128: 645–646

Carlstedt T, Risling M, Lindå H et al 1990 Regeneration after spinal nerve root injury. Restorative Neurology and Neuroscience 1: 289–295

Carlstedt T, Hallin R G, Hedström K G et al 1993 Functional recovery in primates with brachial plexus injury after spianl cord implantation of avulsed ventral roots. Journal of Neurology, Neurosurgery and Psychiatry 56: 649–654

Carlstedt T, Grane P, Hallin R G et al 1995 Return of function after spinal cord implantation of avulsed spinal nerve roots. Lancet 346: 1323–1325

Carr D B, Todd D P 1991 Therapeutic blocks and continuous infusion in the treatment of chronic pain. In: Gelberman R H (ed) Operative nerve repair and reconstruction. J B Lippincott, Philadelphia, p 1563–1569

Carrel A 1902 La technique opérative des anastomoses vasculaires et la transplantation des viscères. Lyon Médicale 98: 859–864

Carroll R E, Green D P 1972 The significance of the palmar cutaneous nerve at the wrist. Clinical Orthopaedics and Related Research 83: 24–28

Carroll R E, Hill N A 1970 Triceps transfer to restore elbow flexion. Journal of Bone and Joint Surgery 52A: 239–244

Carstens H, Schrodt G 1969 Malignant transformation of a benign encapsulated neurilemmoma. American Journal of Clinical Pathology 51: 144–149

Casagrande P A, Dahany P R 1971 Delayed sciatic nerve entrapment following the use of self curing acrylic. Journal of Bone and Joint Surgery 53A: 167–169

Cassinari V, Pagni C A 1969 Central pain. A neurosurgical survey. Harvard University Press, Cambridge, MA

Castagno A A, Shuman W P 1987 M R imaging in clinically suspected brachial plexus tumor. American Journal of Roentgenology 148: 1219–1222

Castaigne P, Cathala H-P, Dry J, Mastropaola C 1966. Les responses des nerfs et des muscles à des stimulations électriques au course d'une épreuve de garrot ischémique chez l'homme normal et chez diabétique. Revue Neurologique 115: 61–66

Castaigne P, Laplane D, Augustin P et al 1969 A propos des paralysies du plexus brachial après cancer du sein. Presse Médicale 77: 1801–1804

Causey G 1948 The effect of pressure on nerve fibres. Journal of Anatomy 82: 262–270

Causey G, Palmer F 1952 Early changes in degenerating mammalian nerves. Proceedings of the Royal Society, London, Series B 139: 597–609

Cavanagh J B 1968a Prior irradiation and the cellular response to nerve crush: duration and effect. Experimental Neurology 22: 253–258

Cavanagh J B 1968b Effects of irradiation on the proliferation of cells in peripheral nerve during Wallerian degeneration. British Journal of Radiology 41: 275–281

Cavanagh S P, Bonney G, Birch R 1987 The infraclavicular brachial plexus: the case for primary repair. Journal of Bone and Joint Surgery 69B: 489

Celli L, Rovesta C 1987 Electrophysical intraoperative evaluations of the damaged root in traction of the brachial plexus. In: Terzis J K (ed) Microreconstruction of nerve injuries. W B Saunders, Philadelphia, 473–482

Chakravorty B G 1969 Arterial supply of the spinal cord and its relation to the cervical myelopathy in spondylosis. Annals of the Royal College of Surgeons of England 45: 232–251

Chalk C H, Dyck P J 1993 Ischemic neuropathy. In: Dyck P J, Thomas P K, Griffin J W, Low P A, Poduslo J F (eds) Peripheral neuropathy, 3rd edn. p 980–989

Chammas M, Allieu Y, Meyer Z U et al 1995 L'arthrodèse de l'épaule. In: Alnot J Y, Narakas A (eds) Les Paralysies du Plexus Brachial, 2nd edn. Monographie de la Société Française de Chirurgie de la Main, Paris, p 190–214

Chang C-W, Lien I-N 1991 Comparison of sensory nerve conduction in the palmar cutaneous branch and first digital branch of the median nerve: a new diagnostic method for carpal tunnel syndrome. Muscle and Nerve 14: 1173–1176

Chang T S, Wang W 1984 Application of microsurgery in plastic and reconstructive surgery. Journal of Reconstructive Microsurgery 1: 55–63

Chapon F, Lechevalier B, Da Silva D C et al 1985 Neuropathies à la thalidomide. Revue Neurologique 141: 719–728

Chaudhry V, Cornblath D R 1992 Wallerian degeneration in human nerves: serial electrophysiological studies. Muscle and Nerve 15: 687–693

Chaudhry V, Cornblath D R, Mellits E D et al 1991 Inter- and intra-examiner reliability of nerve conduction measurements in normal subjects. Annals of Neurology 30: 841–843

Chaudry V, Corse A M, Freimer M L et al 1994 Inter- and intra-examiner reliability of nerve conduction measurements in patients with diabetic neuropathy. Neurology 44: 1459–1462

Checkles N S, Russakov A D, Peiro D L 1971 Ulnar nerve conduction velocity effect of elbow position on measurement. Archives of Physical and Medical Rehabilitation 52: 362–365

Chen C W, Ch'en Y C, Pao Y S 1963 Salvage of the forearm following complete traumatic amputation: case report. Chinese Medical Journal 82: 632

Chen C W, Ch'en Y C, Pao Y S et al 1965 Further experience in the restoration of amputated limbs. Chinese Medical Journal 3: 225

Chen L 1996 C7 versus phrenic nerve, and vascularised versus non vascularised nerve grafts in reinnervation of rat biceps muscle. Shanghai International Brachial Plexus Symposium

Chen L, Gu Y D 1994 An experimental study of contralateral C7 root transfer with vascularised nerve grafting to treat brachial plexus root avulsion. Journal of Hand Surgery 19B: 60–66

Chen Z W, Meyer V E, Kleinert H E, Beasley R W 1981 Present indications and contraindications for replantation as reflected by long-term functional results. Orthopedic Clinics of North America 12: 849–870

Cherington M, Happer I, Machanic B et al 1986 Surgery for thoracic outlet syndrome may be hazardous to your health. Muscle and Nerve 9: 632–634

Chestnut R E 1994 Depletion of nerve growth factor in leprosy. Lancet 344: 129–130

Chiasserini A 1934 Tentantivi di cura in casi di paraplegia da lesione de midollo lombare consecutiva a frattura vertebrale (anastòmosi radiculo-intercostale). Il Policlinico 12: 603–607

Childress H M 1975 Recurrent ulnar–nerve dislocation at the elbow. Clinical Orthopaedics and Related Research 108: 168–173

Chokroverty S 1987 Diabetic amyotrophy. Muscle and Nerve 10: 679–684

Chokroverty S, Sachdeo R, Dilullo J et al 1989 Magnetic stimulation in the diagnosis of lumbosacral radiculopathy. Journal of Neurology, Neurosurgery and Psychiatry 52: 767–772

Chow J 1989 Endoscopic release of the carpal ligament. A new technique for carpal tunnel syndrome. Arthroscopy 5: 19–24

Citron N, Taylor J 1987 Tendon transfer in partially anaesthetic hands. Journal of Hand Surgery 12B: 14–18

Clagett O T 1962 Research and prosearch. Journal of Thoracic and Cardiovascular Surgery. 43B: 152–156

Clark J M P 1956 Muscle and tendon transposition in poliomyelitis. In: Platt H (ed) Modern trends in orthopaedics, 2nd ser. Butterworths, London, p 116–143

Clark K 1961 Ganglion of the lateral popliteal nerve. Journal of Bone and Joint Surgery 43B: 778–783

Clark K, Williams P, Willis W et al 1969 Injection injury of the sciatic nerve. Clinical Neurosurgery 17: 111–125

Clark L P, Taylor A S, Prout T P 1905 A study in brachial birth palsy. American Journal of Medical Science 130: 670–707

Clark W L, Trumble T E, Swiontowski M F et al 1992 Nerve tension and blood flow in a model of immediate and delayed repairs. Journal of Hand Surgery 17A: 677–687

Clark R A 1959 Principles and technique of wound surgery. In: Clark R A, Badger F C, Sevitt S (eds) Modern trends in accident surgery and medicine. Butterworth, London, p 107–122

Clarke E, Bearn J S 1972 The spiral nerve bands of Fontana. Brain 95: 1–20

Clarke Stevens J 1987 The electrodiagnosis of carpal tunnel syndrome. Muscle and Nerve 10: 99–113

Clausen E G 1942 Postoperative "anaesthetic" paralysis of the brachial plexus. Surgery 12: 933–942

Claustre J, Simon L 1978 La maladie de Thomas Morton. Syndrome canalaire. Rhumatologie 91: 283–287

Clawson D K, Seddon H J 1960a The results of repair of the sciatic nerve. Journal of Bone and Joint Surgery 42B: 205–212

Clawson D K, Seddon H J 1960b The late consequences of sciatic nerve injury. Journal of Bone and Joint Surgery 42B: 213–225

Clifton G L, Coggeshall R E, Vance W H et al 1976 Receptive fields of unmyelinated ventral root afferent fibres in the cat. Journal of Physiology, London 256: 573–600

Cloward R B 1964 Cervical cordotomy by the anterior approach. Journal of Neurosurgery 21: 19–25

Cobb C A, Moiel R H 1974 Ganglion of the peroneal nerve. Journal of Neurosurgery 41: 255–259

Cobbett J R 1969 Free digital transfer. Journal of Bone and Joint Surgery 51B: 677–679

Cockett S A, Kiernan J A 1973 Acceleration of peripheral nervous regeneration in the rat by exogenous tri-iodothyronine. Experimental Neurology 39: 389–394

Codavilla A 1899 Tendon transplants in orthopaedic practice [Ferrara J D, trans]. Clinical Orthopaedics and Related Research 1976, 118: 2

Coene L N J E M, Narakas A O 1992 Operative management of lesions of the axillary nerve isolated or combined with other lesions. Clinical Neurology and Neurosurgery 94 (suppl): S64–66

Coggeshall R B, Coulter J D, Willis W D 1974 Unmyelinated axons in the ventral roots of the cat lumbosacral enlargement. Journal of Comparative Anatomy 153: 39–58

Cohen S, Levi-Montalcini R, Hamburger V 1954 A nerve growth stimulating factor isolated from sarcomas 37 and 180.

Proceedings of the National Academy of Sciences of the USA 40: 1014–1018

Cohen S, Levi-Montalcini R 1956 A nerve growth-stimulating factor isolated from snake venom. Proceedings of the National Academy of Sciences of the USA 42: 571–574

Cohen S M 1948 Accidental intra-arterial injection of drugs. Lancet 11: 409–416

Collins H A, Jacobs J K 1961 Acute arterial injuries due to blunt trauma. Journal of Bone and Joint Surgery 43A: 193–197

Comtet J J 1993 Nerve compression syndromes. In: Tubiana R (ed) The Hand. W B Saunders, Philadelphia, vol IV, p 319–327

Comtet J J Herzberg G, Alnaasan I 1993a Biomechanics of the shoulder and the scapulothoracic girdle. In: Tubiana R (ed) The hand. W B Saunders, Philadelphia, vol IV, p 995

Confino-Cohen R, Lishner R M, Savin H et al 1991 Response of carpal tunnel syndrome to hormone replacement therapy. British Medical Journal 303: 1514

Conley J, Janecka S 1973 Neurilemmomas of the facial nerve. Plastic and Reconstructive Surgery 52: 55–60

Connell J L 1962 Vascular trauma. Australian and New Zealand Journal of Surgery 32: 42–50

Constant C R 1997 Assessment of shoulder function. In: Copeland S (ed) Shoulder Surgery. W B Saunders Co. Ltd, London, Philadelphia, Toronto, Sydney, Tokyo

Constant C R, Murley A H G 1987 A clinical assessment of the shoulder. Clinical Orthopaedics and Related Research 214: 160–164

Cooke E D, Ward C 1990 Vicious circles in reflex sympathetic dystrophy – a hypothesis: discussion paper. Journal of the Royal Society of Medicine 83: 96–99

Cooke E D, Steinberg M D, Pearson R M et al 1993 Reflex sympathetic dystrophy and repetitive strain injury: temperature and microcirculatory changes following mild cold stress. Journal of the Royal Society of Medicine 86: 690–693

Cooke J, Powell S, Parsons C 1988 The diagnosis by computed tomography of brachial plexus lesions following radiotherapy for carcinoma of the breast. Clinical Radiology 39: 602–606

Cooper A 1821 On exostosis. In: Cooper A, Travers B (eds) Surgical essays, 2nd American edn. James Webster, Philadelphia

Cooper A, Travers B 1817 On Exostosis. In: Cooper A, Travers B (eds) Surgical essays. 2nd edn. London: Cox and Son, Longman, Hunt, Rees, Orme Brown, Edinburgh: A. Constable, Glasgow: Smith and Son, Dublin: Hodges and McArthur

Cooper D E 1991 Injuries of the brachial plexus during cardiac surgery. In: Gelberman R H (ed) Operative nerve repair and reconstruction. J B Lippincott, Philadelphia, p 1231–1242

Cooper D E, Jenkins R S, Bready L et al 1988 The prevention of injuries of the brachial plexus secondary to malposition of the patient during surgery. Clinical Orthopaedics and Related Research 228: 33–41

Cooper G J, Ryan J M 1990 Interaction of penetrating missiles with tissues: some common misapprehensions and implications for wound management. British Journal of Surgery 77: 606–610

Cooper S 1953 Muscle spindles in the intrinsic muscles of the human tongue. Journal of Physiology 67: 1–13

Cooper S, Daniel P M 1963 Muscle spindles in man: their morphology in the lumbricals and the deep muscles of the neck. Brain 86: 563–586

Coote H 1861 Exostosis of the left transverse process of the seventh cervical vertebra, surrounded by blood vessels and nerves, successful removal. Lancet i: 360–361

Copeland S A 1995a Surgical approaches to the shoulder. In: Copeland S A (ed) Operative shoulder surgery. Churchill Livingstone, New York, p 2–3

Copeland S A 1995b Decompression of the suprascapular nerve. In: Copeland S A (ed) Operative shoulder surgery. Churchill Livingstone, New York, p 325–350

Copeland S A 1995c Thoracoscapular fusion. In: Copeland S A (ed) Operative shoulder surgery. Churchill Livingstone, New York, p 297–308

Copeland S A 1995d Glenohumeral arthrodesis. In: Copeland S A (ed) Operative shoulder surgery. Churchill Livingstone, New York, p 267–278

Copeland S A, Howard R C 1978 Thoracoscapular fusion for facio-scapulo-humeral dystrophy. Journal of Bone and Joint Surgery 60B: 547–551

Corbin K B, Gardner E D 1937 Decrease in number of myelinated nerve fibres in human spinal roots with age. Anatomical Record 68: 63–74

Cormier P J, Matalon T A S, Wolin P M 1988 Quadrilateral space syndrome: a rare cause of shoulder pain. Radiology 167: 797–798

Cornblath D R 1990 Electrophysiology in Guillain–Barré syndrome. Annals of Neurology 27 (suppl): S17–S20

Cosman E R, Nashold B S Jr, Ovelmen-Levitt J 1984 Theoretical aspects of radio frequency lesions in the dorsal root entry zone. Neurosurgery 15: 945–950

Cottrell L 1940 Histologic variations with age in apparently normal nerve trunks. Archives of Neurology and Psychiatry (Chicago) 43: 1138–1150

Coupland R M 1993 War wounds of limbs. Butterworth-Heinemann, Oxford

Cox C L, Cocks G R 1973 Headaches treated by anterior scalenotomy. Journal of the Medical Association of the State of Alabama 43: 385–387

Cox R A F 1996 Avoiding discrimination against disabled people. British Medical Journal 313: 1346–1347

Cragg B, Thomas P K 1961 Changes in conduction velocity and fibre size proximal to peroneal nerve lesions. Journal of Physiology 157: 315–327

Cravens G, Kline D G 1990 Posterior interosseous nerve palsies. Neurosurgery 27: 397–402

Crockard H A, Bradford R 1985 Transoral transclival removal of a schwannoma anterior to the cranio-vertebral junction. Journal of Neurosurgery 62: 293–295

Croft P B, Wilkinson M 1969 The course and prognosis in some types of carcinomatous neuromyopathy. Brain 92 (1): 2–8

Croft P D, Henson R A, Urich H, Wilkinson P C 1965 Sensory neuropathy with bronchial carcinoma: a study of four cases showing neurological abnormalities. Brain 88: 501–514

Cros D, Shahani B 1991 Compression and entrapment neuropathies. In: Swash M, Oxbury J (eds) Clinical neurology. Churchill Livingstone, Edinburgh, p 1204–1213

Cullheim S, Carlstedt T, Lindå H et al 1989 Motoneurons reinnervate skeletal muscle after ventral root implantation into the spinal cord of the cat. Neuroscience 29: 725–733

Curtis B N, Fisher R L, Butterfield W L et al 1969 Neurofibromatosis with Paraplegia. Journal of Bone and Joint Surgery 51A: 843–861

Cushing H, Wolback S B 1927 Sympathoblastoma into benign gangiioneuroma. American Journal of Pathology 3: 203–216

D'Agostino A N, Soule E H, Miller R H 1963 Primary malignant neoplasms of nerves (malignant neurilemmomas) in patients without manifestations of multiple neurofibromatosis (von Recklinghausen's disease). Cancer 16: 1003–1014

Dahlin L B, Rydevik B, McLean W G et al 1984 Changes in fast axonal transport during experimental nerve compression at low pressures. Experimental Neurology 84: 29–36

Dahlin L B, Meiri K F, McLean W G et al 1986a Effects of nerve compression on fast axonal transport in streptozotocin – induced diabetes mellitus. Diabetologica 29: 181–185

Dahlin L B, Rydevik B, Lundborg G 1986b Pathophysiology of nerve entrapments and nerve compression injuries. In: Hargens A R (ed) Tissue nutrition and viability. Springer, Berlin, p 135–160

Dahlström A, Fuxe K 1964a A method for the demonstration of monoamine-containing nerve fibres in the central nervous system. Acta Physiologica Scandinavica 60: 293–294

Dahlstrom A, Fuxe K 1964b Evidence for the existence of monoamine neurons in the central nervous system. II. Experimental demonstration of monoamines in the cell bodies of brainstem neurons. Acta Physiologica Scandinavica 62B: suppl 232: 1–55

Dahners L E, Wood F M, Hill C 1984 Anconeus epitrochlearis, a rare cause of cubital tunnel syndrome: a case report. Journal of Hand Surgery 9A: 579–580

Dailey A T, Tsuruda J S, Goodkin R et al 1996 Magnetic resonance neurography for cervical radiculopathy: a preliminary report. Journal of Neurosurgery 38: 488–492

Danielsen N, Dahlin L B, Ericson L E et al 1986 Experimental hyperthyroidism stimulates axonal growth in mesothelial chamber. Experimental Neurology 94: 54–65

Danyou M 1851 Paralysie du membre supérieur chez le nouveau – né. Bulletin de la Societe de Chirurgie 2: 148–151

Das Gupta T K, Brasfield R D, Strong E W et al 1969 Benign solitary schwannomas (neurilemmomas). Cancer 24: 355–366

Das Gupta T K, Brasfield R D 1970 Solitary malignant schwannoma. Annals of Surgery 171: 419–428

Daube J R 1991 Needle examination in clinical electromyography. Muscle and Nerve 14: 685–700

Dautry F, Apoil A, Moinet F et al 1977 Paralysie radiculaire supérieure du plexus brachial, traitement par transpositions musculaires associées. Revue de Chirurgie Orthopedique 63: 399–407

Dav R, Ariely D, Frenk M 1995 Effect of past injury on pain threshold and tolerance. Pain 60: 189–193

Davar G, Maciewicz R 1991 Pain pathways and responses to pain. In: Gelberman R H (ed) Operative nerve repair and reconstruction Vol 11. J B Lippincott, Philadelphia, vol 11, p 1479–1488

Davidoff G, Roth E J 1991 Clinical characteristics of central dysnesinctic pain in spinal cord injury patients. In: Casey K L (ed) Pain and central nervous system disease: the central pain syndromes. Raven Press, New York, p 77–83

Davies D M 1954 Recurrent peripheral nerve palsies in a family. Lancet ii: 266–268

Davis E R, Sutton D, Bligh A S 1966 Myelography in brachial plexus injury. British Journal of Radiology 39: 362–371

Davison C, Schick W 1935 Spontaneous pain and other sensory disturbances. Archives of Neurology and Psychiatry 34: 1204–1237

Davlin L B, Aulicino P L, Bergfield T G 1991 Sensory neural loop of the median nerve at the carpal tunnel. Journal of Hand Surgery 16a: 863–865

Dawson D M, Hallett M, Millender L H 1990a Thoracic outlet syndrome. In: Entrapment neuropathies, 2nd edn. Little Brown, Chicago, p 237

Dawson D M, Hallett M, Millender L H 1990b Quadrilateral space syndrome. In: Entrapment neuropathies, 2nd edn. Little Brown, Chicago, p 312

Dawson D M, Hallett M, Millender L H 1990c Sciatic nerve entrapment. In: Entrapment neuropathies, 2nd edn. Little Brown, Chicago, p 270

Dawson D M, Hallett M, Millender L H 1990d Lateral femoral cutaneous nerve. Ibid, p 301

Dawson G D, Scott J W 1949 The recognition of nerve action potentials through the skin in man. Journal of Neurology, Neurosurgery and Psychiatry 12: 259–267

DeBakey M E, Simeone F A 1946 Battle injuries of the arteries in World War II. Annals of Surgery 123: 534–579

DeBakey M E, Simeone F A 1955 Acute battle incurred arterial injury. In: Surgery and World War Two, vascular surgery. Medical Department US Army, US Government Printing Office, Washington, DC, p 60–148

Dederich R 1963 Plastic treatment of the muscles and bone in amputation surgery. Journal of Bone and Joint Surgery 45B(1): 60–66

Degrande J, Lissens M A, Vanderstraeten G G 1995 Traumatic axillary nerve lesions: retrospective study of 94 patients. Electroencephalography and Clinical Neurophysiology 97: S136

Déjerine P J 1901 Sémiologie du systéme nerveux. In: Traité pathologie générale. Masson, Paris, p 559

Déjerine P J, Roussy G 1906 Le syndrome thalamique. Revue Neurologique (Paris) 14: 521–532

Dekel S, Rushworth G 1993 The etiology of idiopathic carpal tunnel syndrome. In: Tubiana R (ed) The hand. W B Saunders, Philadelphia, vol IV, p 450–462

De Laat E A T, Visser C P J, Coene L N J E M et al 1994 Nerve lesions in primary shoulder dislocations and humeral neck fractures. A prospective clinical and EMG study. Journal of Bone and Joint Surgery 76B: 381–383

De Lee J 1991 Fractures and dislocations of the hip. In: Rockwood A C, Green D P, Bucholz R W (eds) Fractures, 3rd edn. J P Lippincott, Philadelphia, vol 1, p 1609–1610

Dellon A L, Curtis R M, Edgerton M T 1974 Reeducation of sensation in the hand after nerve injury and repair. Plastic and Reconstructive Surgery 53: 297–305

DeLisa J A, Mackinnon K, Baran E M 1987 Manual of nerve conduction velocity and somatosensory evoked potentials, 2nd edn. Raven Press, New York

DeLisa J A, Lee H J, Bran E M et al 1994 Macroelectromyography. In: Manual of Nerve Conduction Velocity and Clinical Neurophysiology, 3rd edn. Raven Press, New York, p 465

Dellemijn P L I, Fields H L, Allen R R et al 1994 The interpretation of pain relief and sensory changes following sympathetic blockade. Brain 117: 1475–1487

Dellon A L 1976 Reinnervation of denervated Meissner's corpuscles. A sequential histologic study in the monkey following fascicular repair. Journal of Hand Surgery 1: 98–109

Dellon A L 1978 The moving two-point discrimination test: clinical evaluation of the quickly-adapting fiber receptor system. Journal of Hand Surgery 3: 474–481

Dellon A L 1980 Clinical use of vibratory stimuli to evaluate peripheral nerve injury and compression neuropathy. Plastic and Reconstructive Surgery 65: 466–476

Dellon A L 1981 Results of nerve repair in the hand. In: Dellon A L (ed) Evaluation of sensibility and re-education of sensation in the hand. Williams & Wilkins, Baltimore, p 193–202

Dellon A L 1991 Sensory receptors and their fibres. In: Gelberman R H (ed) Operative nerve repair and reconstruction. J B Lippincott, Philadelphia, p 135–138

Dellon A L, Mackinnon S E 1986 Treatment of painful neuroma by neuroma resection and muscle implantation. Plastic and Reconstructive Surgery 77: 427–436

Dellon A L, Mackinnon S E 1988 Human ulnar neuropathy at the elbow: clinical, electrical and morphological correlations. Journal of Reconstructive Microsurgery 4: 179–184

Dellon A L, Munger B L 1983 Correlation of histology and sensibility after nerve repair. Journal of Hand Surgery 8: 871–875

Dellon A L, Mackinnon S E, Pestronk A 1984 Implantation of sensory nerve into muscle: preliminary clinical and experimental observations on neuroma formation. Annals of Plastic Surgery 12: 30–40

Delorme E 1915 The treatment of gunshot wounds of nerves. British Medical Journal 1: 853–855

De Mello W, Khan F 1990 Extensive femoral vessel damage after blunt injury. Injury 21: 412–413

Demos N J, Rubenstein H, Restivo C 1980 Role of scalenotomy for relief of positional vertebro-basilar ischaemia. Journal of the Medical Society of New Jersey 6: 419–422

Denman E E 1978 The anatomy of the space of Guyon. The Hand 10: 69–76

Denny-Brown D 1948 Primary sensory neuropathy with muscular changes associated with carcinoma. Journal of Neurology, Neurosurgery and Psychiatry 11: 73–87

Denny-Brown D, Brenner C 1944 The effect of percussion on nerve. Journal of Neurology, Neurosurgery and Psychiatry 7: 76–95

Denny-Brown D E, Adams R D, Brenner G et al 1945 The pathology of injury to nerve induced by cold. Journal of Neuropathology and Experimental Neurology 4: 305–323

Denys E H 1991 The influence of temperature in clinical neurophysiology. Muscle and Nerve 14: 795–811

De Reuck J 1974 The pathology of human muscle spindles. Acta Neuropathologica 30: 43–50

De Smet L, Fabry G 1995 Transection of the motor branch of the ulnar nerve as a complication of two-portal endoscopic carpal tunnel release. Journal of Hand Surgery 20A: 18–19

Devor M 1991 Neuropathic pain and injured nerve: peripheral mechanisms. British Medical Bulletin 47: 619–630

Devor M, Janig W 1981 Activation of myelinated afferents ending in a neuroma by stimulation of the sympathetic supply in the rat. Neuroscience Letters 24: 43–47

Di Vincenti F C, Moncrieff J A, Pruitt B A 1969 Electrical injuries: a review of 65 cases. Journal of Trauma 9: 497–507

Dickensen A H 1995 Spinal cord pharmacology of pain. British Journal of Anaesthesia 75: 193–200

Dickensen A H, Sullivan A F 1986 Electrophysiological studies in the effects of intrathecal morphine on nociceptive neurones in the rat dorsal horn. Pain 24: 211–222

Di Stefano V, Sack J T, Whittaker R et al 1972 Tarsal tunnel syndrome. Clinical Orthopaedics and Related Research 88: 76–79

Dodge H W, Craig W McK 1957 Benign tumours of peripheral nerves and their masquerade. Minnesota Medicine 40(5): 294–301

Dodt E 1953 Differential sensitivity of mammalian nerve fibres. Acta Physiologica Scandinavica 29: 91–108

Doi K, Kuwata N, Sakai K et al 1987 A reliable technique of free vascularized sural nerve grafting and preliminary results of clinical applications. Journal of Hand Surgery 12A: 677–684

Doi K, Tamaru K, Sakai K et al 1992 A comparison of vascularized and conventional sural nerve grafts. Journal of Hand Surgery 17A: 670–676

Dolenc V V 1987 Intercostal neurotisation of the peripheral nerves in avulsion plexus injuries. In: Terzis J K (ed) Microreconstruction of nerve injuries. W B Saunders, Philadelphia, p 425–434

Donaghy M J 1996 Vincristine and neuropathies. Prescribers' Journal 36: 116–119

Donn S M, Faix R G 1983 Long term prognosis for the infant with severe birth trauma. Clinics in Perinatology 10: 507–520

Donner T R, Kline D G 1993 Extracranial spinal accessory nerve injury. Neurosurgery 32: 907–911

Donoso R S, Ballantyne J P, Hansen S 1978 Regeneration of human peripheral nerves: an electrophysiological study. Journal of Neurology, Neurosurgery and Psychiatry 42: 97–106

Donovan D L, Sharp W V 1984 Blunt trauma to the axillary artery. Journal of Vascular Surgery 1: 681–683

Doriguzzi C, Palmucci, Troni W 1982 Isolated accessory nerve injury. Case Report. Italian Journal of Neurological Science 2: 135–138

Douglas W W, Malcolm J L 1955 The effect of localized cooling on conduction in cat nerves. Journal of Physiology 130: 63–71

Doupe J, Cullen C H, Chance G Q 1944 Post-traumatic pain and the causalgic syndrome. Journal of Neurology, Neurosurgery and Psychiatry 7: 33–48

Downey D B, Breatnach E S, Foley-Nolan D R et al 1989 Large schwannoma of the psoas: a rare but treatable cause of back pain. Journal of the Royal Society of Medicine 82: 504

Drago J, Kilpatrick T J, Koblar S A et al 1994 Growth factors: potential therapeutic applications in neurology. Journal of Neurology, Neurosurgery and Psychiatry 57: 1445–1450

Dray A 1995 Inflammatory mediation of pain. British Journal of Anaesthesia 75: 125–131

Dreyfuss U, Kessler I 1978 Snapping elbow due to dislocation of the medial head of triceps. Journal of Bone and Joint Surgery 60B: 56–57

Drury K, Scullion J E 1980 Vascular complications of anterior dislocation of the shoulder. British Journal of Surgery 67: 579–581

Dubuisson A S, Kline D G, Weinshel S S 1993 Posterior subscapular approach to the brachial plexus. Journal of Neurosurgery 79: 319–330

Ducatman B S, Scheithaeur B W 1983 Post irradiation neurofibrosarcoma. Cancer 51: 1028–1033

Ducatman B S, Scheithauer B W, Piepgras D G et al 1986 Malignant peripheral nerve sheath tumour: a clinicopathological study of 120 cases. Cancer 57: 2006–2021

Duchenne G B A 1872 De l'élèctrisation localisée et de son application à la pathologie et à la thérapeutique, 2nd edn. J B Ballière, Paris, p 357–362

Dudley H A F, Knight R J, McNeur J C et al 1968 Civilian battle casualties in South Vietnam. British Journal of Surgery 55: 337–341

Dumontier C, Sokolow C, Leclerq C et al 1995 Early results of conventional versus two-portal endoscopic carpal tunnel release. Journal of Hand Surgery 20B: 658–662

Dunkerton M C D, Boome R 1988 Stab wounds involving the brachial plexus. Journal of Bone and Joint Surgery 70B: 566–570

Dunn D W, Engle W A 1985 Brachial plexus palsy: intrauterine onset. Paediatric Neurology 1: 367–369

Dunnett W, Birch R 1994 A ten year experience of the thoracic outlet syndrome. Journal of Bone and Joint Surgery 76B (suppl II/III): 156

Dunnet W, Housden P, Birch R 1995 Results of flexor to extensor tendon transfer. Journal of Hand Surgery 20B (1): 26–28

Dupont C, Cloutier G E, Prevost Y, Dion M A 1965 Ulnar-tunnel syndrome at the wrist. Journal of Bone and Joint Surgery 47A: 757–761

Duthie H L 1957 Radial nerve in osseous tunnel at humeral fracture site diagnosed radiographically. Journal of Bone and Joint Surgery 39B: 746–747

Dutkowsky J P, Kasser J R 1991 Nerve injury associated with fractures in children. In: Gelberman R H (ed) Operative nerve repair and reconstruction. J B Lippincott, Philadelphia, vol 1, p 635–653

Duval P, Guillain G 1898 Pathogénie des accidents nerveux consécutifs aux luxations et traumatisme de l'épaule. Paralysies radiculaires traumatiques du plexus brachial. Archives Générales de Médecine 2: 143–191

Duval P, Guillain G 1901 Les paralysies radiculaire du plexus brachial. G Steinheil, Paris

Dyck P J, Nukada H, Lais C A et al 1984 Permanent axotomy: a model of chronic neuronal degeneration produced by axonal atrophy, myelin remodelling and regeneration. In: Dyck P J, Thomas P K, Lambert E H, Bunge R (eds) Peripheral neuropathy, 2nd edn. W B Saunders, Philadelphia, p 660–690

Dyck P J 1966 Non invasive neurological changes in systemic malignancy. Minnesota Medicine 49: 1629–1636

Dyck P J, Conn D L, Okazaki H 1972 Necrotizing angiopathic neuropathy. Mayo Clinic Proceedings 47: 461–475

Dyck P J, Benstead T J, Conn D L et al 1987 Nonsystemic vasculitic neuropathy. Brain 110: 843–854

Dyck P J, Thomas P K et al (eds) 1993 Peripheral neuropathy, 3rd edn. W B Saunders, Philadelphia

Dyer C 1996 Overhaul of medical negligence litigation announced. British Medical Journal 313: 247

Eames R, Gamble H J 1964 Electron microscopy in human dorsal nerve roots. Journal of Anatomy 98: 478–479

Eames R, Gamble G 1970 Schwann cell relationships in normal human cutaneous nerves. Journal of Anatomy 106: 417–435

Eames R, Lange L S 1967 Clinical and pathological study of ischaemic neuropathy. Journal of Neurology, Neurosurgery and Psychiatry 30: 215–236

Earl C J, Fullerton P M, Wakefield G S et al 1964 Hereditary neuropathy with liability to pressure palsies. Quarterly Journal of Medicine 33: 481–498

Earnshaw J J 1995 Research flows at vascular meeting. Hospital Update 21: 422–423

Eastcott H H G 1962 Reconstruction of the subclavian artery for complications of cervical rib and thoracic-outlet syndrome. Lancet ii: 1243–1246

Eastcott H H G 1965 The management of arterial injuries. Journal of Bone and Joint Surgery 47B: 394–398

Eastcott H H G 1973a Cervical rib and thoracic outlet compression. In: Eastcott H H G (ed) Arterial surgery, 2nd edn. Pitman Medical, London, p 217–235

Eastcott H H G 1973b Arterial injuries. In: Eastcott H H G (ed) Arterial surgery, 2nd edn. Pitman Medical, London, p 236–257

Eastcott H H G (ed) 1992 Arterial surgery, 3rd edn. Churchill Livingstone, Edinburgh

Eastcott H H G, Blaisdell F W, Silver D 1992a. In: Eastcott H H G (ed) Arterial surgery, 3rd edn. Churchill Livingstone, Edinburgh, p 31–54

Eastcott H H G, Veith F J, Bergan J J 1992b Chronic ischaemia. In: Eastcott H H G (ed) Arterial surgery, 3rd edn. Churchill Livingstone, Edinburgh, p 55–151

Eaton R G, Green W T 1972 Epimysiotomy and Fasciotomy in the treatment of Volkmann's Ischaemic Contracture. Orthopaedic Clinics of North America 3: 175–186

Ebeling P, Gilliatt R W, Thomas P K 1960 The clinical and electrical study of ulnar nerve lesion in the hand. Journal of Neurology, Neurosurgery and Psychiatry 23: 1–9

Ebner F, Kressel H Y, Mintz M C et al 1988 Tumour recurrence versus fibrosis in the female pelvis: differentiation with MR imaging at 1.5 T. Radiology 166: 333–340

Edelson J G, Nathan H 1977 Meralgia paraesthetica. An anatomical investigation. Clinical Orthopaedics and Related Research 122: 256–262

Eden K C 1939 The vascular complications of cervical ribs and first thoracic rib abnormalities. British Journal of Surgery 27: 111–139

Eden R 1924 Zur behandlung der Trapezius Lähmung mittels muskelplastik. Deutsche Zeitschrift für Chirurgie 184: 387–397

Edmondson R A, Banarjee A K, Rennie J A 1992 Endoscopic transthoracic sympathectomy in the treatment of hyperhidrosis. Annals of Surgery 215: 289–293

Edshage S 1964 Peripheral nerve suture. A technique for improved intraneural topography. Acta Chirurgica Scandinavica 331 (suppl): 1–104

Eide P K, Jonim E, Stubhang A et al 1994 Relief of post herpetic neuralgia with the N-methyl-D-asparate receptor antagonist ketamine. Pain 58: 347–354

Eide P K, Jørum E, Stenehjem A E 1996 Somatosensory findings in patients with spinal cord injury and central dysaesthesia pain. Journal of Neurology, Neurosurgery and Psychiatry 60: 411–415

Eisenberg K S, Scheft D J, Murray W R 1972 Posterior dislocation of the hip producing lumbosacral nerve root avulsion. Journal of Bone and Joint Surgery 54A: 1083–1086

Elliott J, Templeton J, Barros D'Sa A A B 1984 Combined bony and vascular limb trauma: a new approach in treatment. Journal of Bone and Joint Surgery 66B: 281

Ellis C J, Wallis W E, Caruana M 1994 Peripheral neuropathy with bezafibrate. British Medical Journal 309: 929

Ellis H 1958 Disability after tibial shaft fractures. Journal of Bone and Joint Surgery 40B: 190–197

Ellis J M, Folkers K, Levy M et al 1982 Response of vitamin B_6 deficiency and the carpal tunnel syndrome to pyridoxine. Proceedings of the National Academy of Science USA 79: 7494–7498

Ellis V H 1936 Two cases of ganglion in the sheath of the peroneal nerve. British Journal of Surgery 24: 141–142

Eng G 1971 Brachial plexus palsy in new born infants. Paediatrics 48: 18–28

Eng G D, Koch B, Smokvina M D 1978 Brachial plexus palsy in neonates and children. Archives of Physical Medicine and Rehabilitation 59: 458–464

England J D, Sumner A J 1987 Neuralgic amyotrophy: an increasingly diverse entity. Muscle and Nerve 10: 60–68

Enneking W F 1983 Musculo-skeletal tumor surgery. Churchill Livingstone, New York, vol 2

Enzinger F M, Weiss S W 1988 Soft tissue tumours, 2nd edn. C V Mosby, St Louis

Epstein H C 1980 Traumatic dislocation of the hip. Williams & Wilkins, Baltimore

Erb W 1875 Ueber eine eigenthümliche Lokalization von Lähmungen im Plexus brachialis. Verhandlungen des Naturhistorisch-medizinischen Vereins zu Heidelberg, p 130–136

Erb W H 1876 Diseases of the peripheral cerebro-spinal nerves. In: von Ziemson H (ed) Cyclopedia of the practice of medicine. Samson Low, Marston, Searle and Rivington, London, vol II

Eriksond L, Long D M 1983 Ten year follow up of dorsal column stimulation. In: Bonica J J, Lundblom V, Iggo F (eds) Advances in pain research and therapy. Proceedings of the Third World Congress on Pain. Raven Press, New York, vol 5, p 583–590

Erlandson R A, Woodruff J M 1982 Peripheral nerve sheath tumours. An electron microscopic study of 43 cases. Cancer 49: 273–287

Ewing M R 1950 Postoperative paralysis in the upper extremity. Lancet i: 99–103

Fabre T, Bernez J, De Coucy F et al 1996 Complete femoral nerve division at total hip arthroplasty. Journal of Bone and Joint Surgery 78B: 148–149

Fachinelli A, Masquelet A, Restropo J et al 1981 The vascularized sural nerve. Anatomy and surgical approach. International Journal of Microsurgery 3: 57–62

Fahr L M, Sauser D D 1988 Imaging of peripheral nerve lesions. Orthopaedic Clinics of North America 19: 27–41

Fahrni W H 1950. Neonatal sciatic palsy. Journal of Bone and Joint Surgery 32B: 42–47

Fairbank H A T 1913 Subluxation of shoulder joint in infants and young children. Lancet i: 1217–1223

Falconer M A, Li F W P 1962 Resection of first rib in costo-clavicular compression of the brachial plexus. Lancet ii: 59–63

Falconer M A, Weddell G 1943 Costo-clavicular compression of the subclavian artery and vein. Relation to scalenus syndrome. Lancet ii: 539–543

Falk S J 1994 Radiotherapy and the management of the axilla in early breast cancer. British Journal of Surgery 81: 1277–1281

Fallet G H, Moody J F, Roth G et al 1967 Lésions du plexus brachial survénant après radiothérapie pour cancer du sein. Rhumatologie 19: 199–204

Fantis A, Slezak Z 1965 On the possibility of re-innervation in total lesions of the brachial plexus by intercosto-plexual anastomosis. Céskoslovenska Neurologie 28: 412–418 (summary in English)

Favero K J, Hawkins R M, Jones M W 1987 Neuralgic amyotrophy. Journal of Bone and Joint Surgery 69B: 195–198

Fawcett E 1896 What is Sibson's muscle (scalenus pleuralis)? Journal of Anatomy and Physiology 30: 433–436

Fawcett K J, Dahlin D C 1967 Neurilemmoma of bone. American Journal of Clinical Pathology 47: 759–766

Fearn C B D'A, Goodfellow J W 1965 Anterior interosseous nerve palsy. Journal of Bone and Joint Surgery 47B: 91–93

Feasby T E, Hahn A F 1992 Obstetrical lumbosacral plexus injury. Muscle and Nerve 15937–940

Feasby T E, Bostock, H Sears T A 1981 Conduction in regenerating dorsal root fibres. Journal of Neurological Sciences 49: 439–454

Feasby T E, Brown W F, Gilbert J J et al 1985 The pathological basis of conduction block in human neuropathies. Journal of Neurology, Neurosurgery and Psychiatry 48: 239–244

Fender F A 1939 Foerster's scheme of the dermatomes. Archives of Neurology and Psychiatry 41: 688–693

Fernandez L L 1955 Compresion del tronco inferior del plexo braquial por el escaleno medio. Sociedad Argentina de Cirurgía Ortopédica y Traumatología, Sesion del 25 de Octubre de 1985, p 156–164

Ferrante M A, Wilbourn A J 1995 The utility of various sensory nerve conduction responses in assessing brachial plexopathies. Muscle and Nerve 18: 879–889

Féry A, Sommelet J 1987 La paralysie du grande dentélé. Résultat de traitement de 12 cas dont 9 opérés et revue genérale de la litterature. Revue de Chirurgie Orthopédique 73: 277–288

Fiddian M A, King R J 1984 The winged scapula. Clinical Orthopaedics and Related Research 185: 228–236

Fields R D, Le Beau J M, Longo F M et al 1989 Nerve regeneration through artificial tubular implants. Progress in Neurobiology 33: 87–134

Filler A G, Howe F A, Hayes C E et al 1993 Magnetic resonance neurography. Lancet 341: 659–661

Filler A G, Kliot M, Howe F A et al 1996 Application of magnetic resonance neurography in the evaluation of patients with peripheral nerve pathology. Journal of Neurosurgery 85: 299–309

Finch J, Cowley R 1994 The Law. In: Powers M J, Harris N H (eds) Medical negligence, 2nd edn. Butterworths, London, p 1–21

Fincham R W, Cape C A 1968 Neuropathy in hypothyroidism. Archives of Neurology 19: 464–467

Finney L A, Wulfman W A 1960 Traumatic induced lumbar nerve root avulsion with associated traction injury to the common peroneal nerve. American Journal of Roentgenology, Radium Therapy and Nuclear Medicine 84: 952–957

Finochietto R 1920 Retracción de Volkmann de lomúsculos. Intrinsecos de las manos. Boletines y trabajos, sociedad argentina de circujenos Buenos Aires 4: 31

Fiolle J, Delmas J 1921 In: Cumston C G (trans, ed) The Surgical exposure of the deep seated blood vessels. Heinemann, London, p 61–67

Fisher M A 1992 H reflexes and F waves: physiology and clinical indications. Muscle and Nerve 15: 1223–1233

Fitzgerald B 1978 St Anthony's fire or carpal tunnel syndrome? The Hand 10: 82–86

Flaubert A C 1827 Mémoire sur plusieurs cas de luxation dans les efforts pour la réduction ont été suivis d'accidents graves. Répertoire Générale d'Anatomie et de Physiologie Pathologique 3: 55–79

Fletcher I 1981 Amputations of the upper limb. In: Wynn Parry C B (ed) Rehabilitation of the hand, 4th edn. Butterworths, London, p 331–354

Flor H, Ebert T, Knecht S et al 1995 Phantom limb pain in a perceptual correlate of cortical reorganization following arm amputation. Nature 375: 482–484 (letter)

Flynn J M, Bischoff R, Gelberman R H 1995 Median nerve compression at the wrist due to intracarpal canal sepsis. Journal of Hand Surgery 20A: 864–867

Foerster O 1927 Die Leitungsbahnen des Schmerzgefuehls und die chirurgische Behandlung der Schmerz-zustände. Urban Schwarzenberg, Berlin/Vienna

Foerster O 1933 The dermatomes in Man. Brain 56: 1–39

Fordyce W E, McMahon G, Rainwater S et al 1981 Pain complaint – exercise performance relationship in chronic pain. Pain 10: 311–321

Foster J B 1960 Hydrocortisone and the carpal tunnel syndrome. Lancet i: 454–455

Fowler G J, Sitzoglou K, Ali Z et al 1988 The conduction velocities of peripheral nerve fibres conveying sensations of warming and cooling. Journal of Neurology, Neurosurgery and Psychiatry 51: 1164–1170

Fowler T J, Dunta G, Gilliatt R W 1972 Recovery of nerve conduction after a pneumatic tourniquet: observations in the hind limb of a baboon. Journal of Neurology, Neurosurgery and Psychiatry 35: 638–647

Fragiadakis E G, Lamb D W 1970 An unusual cause of ulnar nerve compression. The Hand 2: 14–16

Francel P C, Koby M, Park T S et al 1995 Fast spin-echo magnetic resonance imaging for radiological assessment of neonatal brachial plexus injury. Journal of Neurosurgery 83: 461–466

Franz D N, Iggo A 1968 Conduction failure in myelinated and non-myelinated axons at low temperatures. Journal of Physiology 199: 319–345

Frazer J E 1920 The anatomy of the human skeleton, 2nd ed. J & A Churchill, London

Frazier C H, Skillern P G 1911 Supraclavicular subcutaneous lesions of the brachial plexus not associated with skeletal injuries. The Journal of the American Medical Association Vol 57 No 25 December 1911 1957–1963

Freeman L W 1952 Observations on spinal nerve root transplantation in the male Guinea baboon. Annals of Surgery 136: 206–210

Freud S 1895 Über die Bernhardt'sche Sensibilitätsstörung am Oberschenkel. Neurologisches Centralblatt 14: 491–492

Frey M, Gruber H 1991 The vascularised nerve graft. In: Meyer V E, Black M J M (eds) Microsurgical procedures (Hand and Upper Limb Series, vol 7). Churchill Livingstone, Edinburgh, p 185–201

Friedman A H, Nashold B S Jr 1986 DREZ lesions for relief of pain related to spinal cord injury. Journal of Neurosurgery 65: 465–475

Friedman D, Flanders A, Thomas C et al 1995 Vertebral artery injury after acute cervical spinal trauma: rate of occurrence as detected by magnetic resonance angiography and assessment of clinical consequences. American Journal of Radiology 164: 443–447

Frohse F, Fränkel M 1908 Die Muskeln des Menschlichen Armes. Fischer, Jena

Frykholm A, Hyde J, Norlen G, Skogland G R 1951 On pain sensations produced by stimulation of the ventral roots in man.

Frykman G K, Cally D 1988 Interfascicular nerve grafting. Orthopedic Clinics of North America 19: 57–69

Frykman G K, Adams J, Bowen W W 1981 Neurolysis. Orthopedic Clinics of North America 12: 325–342

Fullerton P M 1963 The effect of ischaemia on nerve conduction in the carpal tunnel. Journal of Neurology, Neurosurgery and Psychiatry 26: 385–397

Furness J B, Costa M 1980 Types of nerves in the enteric nervous system. Neuroscience 5: 1–20

Futami T 1995 Surgery for bilateral carpal tunnel syndrome. Endoscopic and open release compared in 10 patients. Acta Orthopaedica Scandinavica 66: 153–155

Galardi G, Comi G, Lozza L et al 1990 Peripheral nerve damage during limb lengthening. Journal of Bone and Joint Surgery 72B: 121–124

Gamble H J 1964 Comparative electron-microscopic observations on the connective tissue of a peripheral nerve and a spinal nerve root in the rat. Journal of Anatomy 98: 17–24

Gamble H J, Eames R A 1964 An electron microscope study of the connective tissues of human peripheral nerve. Journal of Anatomy 98: 655–662

Ganzhorn R W, Hocker J T, Horowitz M et al 1981 Suprascapular nerve entrapment. Journal of Bone and Joint Surgery 63A: 492–494

Garcin R 1937 La douleur dans les affections organiques du systéme nerveux central. Revue Neurologique 68: 105–153

Gardner E, Bunge R P 1993 Gross anatomy of the peripheral nervous system. In: Dyck P J, Thomas P K, Griffin J W, Low P A, Poduslo J F (eds) Peripheral neuropathy, 3rd edn. W B Saunders, Philadelphia, p 8–27

Gardner-Medwin J, Powell R J 1994 Clinical experience with thalidomide in the management of severe oral and genital ulceration in conditions such as Behçet's disease; the use of neurophysiological studies to detect thalidomide neuropathy. Annals of the Rheumatic Diseases 53: 828–832

Garrett W E J R 1991 The motor end plate. In: Gelberman R H (ed) Operative nerve repair and reconstruction. J B Lippincott, Philadelphia, p 73–83

Gassel M M 1963 A study of femoral conduction time. Archives of Neurology 9: 607–614

Gasser H F 1955 Properties of dorsal root unmedullated fibres on the two sides of the ganglion. Journal of General Physiology 38: 709–728

Gattuso J M, Davies A H, Glasby M A et al 1988 Peripheral nerve repair using muscle autografts. Journal of Bone and Joint Surgery 70B: 524–529

Gauthier G, Dutertre P 1975 La Maladie de Morton: syndrome canalaire: 74 cas opérés sans résection du nevrome. Lyon Médical 223: 917–921

Gautier Smith P C 1967 Clinical aspects of spinal neurofibromas. Brain 90: 359–393

Gay J R, Love J G 1947 Diagnosis and treatment of tardy paralysis of the ulnar nerve. Journal of Bone and Joint Surgery 29: 1087–1097

Gelberman R H, Rydevik B L, Pess G M et al 1988 Carpal tunnel syndrome. Orthopaedic Clinics of North America 19: 115–124

Gelberman R H, Hergenroeder P T, Hargens A R et al 1981 The carpal tunnel syndrome. A study of carpal canal pressures. Journal of Bone and Joint Surgery 63A: 380–383

Gelberman R H, Eaton R, Urbaniak J R et al 1993 Peripheral nerve compression. Journal of Bone and Joint Surgery 75A: 1854–1878

Gentili F, Hudson A, Kline D G et al 1979 Peripheral nerve injection injury: an experimental study. Neurosurgery 4: 244–253

Gerard J M, Franck N, Moussa Z et al 1989 Acute ischaemic brachial plexus neuropathy following radiation therapy. Neurology 39: 450–451

Geschickter C F 1935 Tumour of the Peripheral Nerves. American Journal of Cancer 25: 377–410

Ghent W R 1959 Meralgia paraesthetica. Canadian Medical Association Journal 81: 633–635

Ghosh B C, Ghosh L, Huvos A G et al 1973 Malignant schwannoma – a clinical study. Cancer 31: 184

Giannini C, Dyck P J 1990 Fragmentation of Schwann cell basal lamina. Quoted by Griffin J W, Hoffman P N. In: Dyck P J, Thomas P K, Griffin J W, Low P A, Poduslo J F (eds) Peripheral neuropathy, 3rd edn. W B Saunders, Philadelphia, 1993, p 367

Gibson W S, Hora J F 1970 Intraparotid facial neuroma. Annals of Otology, Rhinology and Laryngology 79: 412–417

Giddins G E B, Birch R, Singh D, Taggart M 1994 Risk factors for obstetric brachial plexus palsies. Journal of Bone and Joint Surgery 76B (suppl II/III):156

Gilbert A 1993 Personal communication. Evaluation of results in obstetrical brachial plexus palsy. Systems for shoulder Presented to The International Meeting on Obstetric Brachial Plexus Palsy, Heerlen, 1993.

Gilbert A 1987 Vascularised sural nerve graft. In: Terzis J K (ed) Microreconstruction of nerve injuries. W B Saunders, Philadelphia, p 117–126

Gilbert A 1993 Obstetrical brachial plexus palsy. In: Vol. 4. Tubiana R (ed) The Hand. W B Saunders, Philadelphia, vol 4, ch 38, p 576–601 (English translation)

Gilbert A 1995 Paralysie obstétricale du plexus brachial. In: Alnot J-Y, Narakas A (eds) Les paralysies du plexus brachial, 2nd edn. Monographie de la Société Française de Chirurgie de la Main. Expansion Scientifique Française, Paris, p 270–281

Gilbert A, Tassin J L 1984 Réparation chirurgicale du plexus brachial dans la paralysie obstétricale. Chirurgie (Paris) 110: 70–75

Gilbert A, Khouri N, Carlioz M 1980 Exploration chirurgicale du plexus brachial dans la paralysie obstétricale. Revue du Chirurgie Orthopédique 66: 33–42

Gilbert A, Razaboni R, Amar-Khodja S 1988 Indications and results of brachial plexus surgery in obstetrical palsy. Orthopedic Clinics of North America 19 (1): 91–105

Gilbert A, Masquelet A C, Hentz V R 1990 Les Lambeaux artériles pédiculés du membre supérieur. Expansion Scientifique Française, Paris

Gilbert A, Raimondi P 1996 Evaluation of results in obstetric brachial plexus palsy. The elbow. Paper read to the International Meeting on Obstetric Brachial Plexus Palsy Heerlen 1996

Gilliatt R W, Goodman H V, Willison R G 1961 The recording of lateral popliteal nerve action potentials in man. Journal of Neurology, Neurosurgery and Psychiatry 24: 305–318

Gilliatt R W 1961 Nerve conduction: motor and sensory. In: Licht S (ed) Electrodiagnosis and electromyography. Waverley Press

Gilliatt R W 1980 Acute compression block. In: Sumner A J (ed) The physiology of peripheral nerve disease. W B Saunders, Philadelphia, p 287–315

Gilliatt R W 1981 Physical injury to peripheral nerves. Mayo Clinic Proceedings 56: 361–370

Gilliatt R W 1984 Thoracic outlet syndrome. In: Dyck P J, Thomas P K, Lambert E H, Bunge R (eds) Peripheral neuropathy, 2nd edn. W B Saunders, Philadelphia, p 1409–1424

Gilliatt R W, Hjorth R J 1972 Nerve conduction during Wallerian degeneration in the baboon. Journal of Neurology, Neurosurgery and Psychiatry 35: 335–341

Gilliatt R W, Meer J 1990 The refractory period of transmission in patients with carpal tunnel syndrome. Muscle and Nerve 13: 445–450

Gilliatt R W, Sears T A 1958 Sensory nerve action potentials in patients with peripheral nerve lesions. Journal of Neurology, Neurosurgery and Psychiatry 21: 109–118

Gilliatt R W, Taylor J C 1959 Electrical changes following section of the facial nerve. Proceedings of the Royal Society of Medicine 52: 1080–1083

Gilliatt R W, Thomas P K 1960 Changes in nerve conduction with ulnar lesions at the elbow. Journal of Neurology, Neurosurgery and Psychiatry 23: 312–319

Gilliatt R W, Willison R G 1962 Peripheral nerve conduction in diabetic neuropathy. Journal of Neurology, Neurosurgery and Psychiatry 25: 11–18

Gilliatt R W, Wilson T G 1953 A pneumatic-tourniquet test in the carpal tunnel syndrome. Lancet ii: 595–597

Gilliatt R W, LeQuesne P M, Logue V et al 1970 Wasting of the hand associated with the cervical rib or band. Journal of Neurology, Neurosurgery and Psychiatry 33: 615–624

Girgis F L, Wynn Parry C B 1989 Management of causalgia after peripheral nerve injury. International Disability Studies 11: 15–20

Gjörup L 1965 Obstetrical lesion of the brachial plexus. Acta Neurologica Scandinavica 42 (suppl 18): 9–38

Glasby M A 1990 Nerve growth in matrices of orientated muscle basement membrane. Developing a new method of nerve repair. Clinical Anatomy 3: 161–182

Glasby M A, Hems T E J 1993 Basil Kilvington. Unknown pioneer of peripheral nerve repair. Journal of Hand Surgery 18B: 461–464

Glasby M A, Davies A H, Gattuso V M et al 1991 Specificity for homonymous pathways following repair of peripheral nerves with treated skeletal muscle autografts in the primate. British Journal of Plastic Surgery 44: 135–141

Glazer H S, Lee J K T, Levitt R G et al 1985 Radiation fibrosis: differentiation from recurrent tumor by M R imaging. Radiology 156: 721–726

Goddard N 1993 The development of the proximal humerus in the neonate with particular reference to bony lesions about the shoulder. In: Tubiana R (ed) The Hand (English translation). W B Saunders, Philadelphia, vol IV, p 624–631

Godina M 1986 Early microsurgical reconstruction of complex trauma of the extremities. Plastic and Reconstructive Surgery 78: 285–292

Godsall R W, Hansen G A 1971 Traumatic ulnar neuropathy in adolescent baseball players. Journal of Bone and Joint Surgery 53A: 359–361

Goldie B S, Coates C J 1992 Brachial plexus injuries – a survey of incidence and referral pattern. Journal of Hand Surgery 17B: 86–88

Goldie B S, Powell J M 1991 Bony transfixion of the median nerve following Colles fracture. Clinical Orthopaedics and Related Research 273: 275–277

Goldie B S, Coates C J, Birch R 1992 The long term results of digital nerve repair in no-man's land. Journal of Hand Surgery 17B: 75–77

Goldscheider A 1884 Die spezifische Energie der Gefühlsnerven der Haut. Monatshefte für praktische Dermatologie 3: 283–300

Golgi C 1882 Annotazioni intorno all' Istologia normale e patologica dei muscoli volontari. Archivio per le Scienze medichi (Torino) 5: 194–236

Goodman H V, Gilliatt R W 1961 The effect of treatment on median nerve conduction in patients with the carpal tunnel syndrome. Annals of Physical Medicine 6: 137–155

Goodwin G M, McCloskey D I, Matthews P B C 1972 The contribution of muscle afferents to kinaesthesia shown by vibration induced illusions of movement and by the effect of paralysing joint afferents. Brain 95: 705–748

Gordon G, Jukes M G M 1964 Descending influences on the exteroceptive organisations of the cat's gracile nucleus. Journal of Physiology 173: 291–319

Gordon M, Rich H, Deutschberger J, Green M 1973 The immediate and long term outcome of obstetric birth trauma. 1. Brachial plexus paralysis. American Journal of Obstetrics and Gynaecology 117: 51–56

Gorman J F 1968 Combat wounds of the popliteal artery. Annals of Surgery 168: 974–980

Göthberg H, Hyltander A, Claes G 1990 Endoskopisk torakal sympathektomi. Laekartidningen 87: 3318–3319

Gousheh J 1995 The treatment of war injuries in the brachial plexus. Journal of Hand Surgery 20A: 568–576

Gowers W R 1886 A manual of disease of the nervous system. Diseases of the spinal cord and nerves. J A Churchill, London

Gozna E R, Harris R 1979 Traumatic winging of the scapula. Journal of Bone and Joint Surgery 61A: 1230–1233

Gracely R, Lynch S A, Bennett G J 1993 Painful neuropathy: altered central processing maintained dynamically by peripheral input. Pain 52: 251–253

Graham A N J, Lowry K G, McGuigan J A 1993 Anaesthesia for thoracic sympathectomy. British Medical Journal 307: 326

Graham J G, Pye I F, McQueen I N F 1981 Brachial plexus injury after median sternotomy. Journal of Neurology, Neurosurgery and Psychiatry 44: 621–625

Green N E, Allen B L 1977 Vascular injuries associated with dislocation of the knee. Journal of Bone and Joint Surgery 59A: 236–239

Greenfield J G, Carmichael E A 1935 The peripheral nerves in cases of subacute combined degeneration of the cord. Brain 58: 483–491

Greenfield S, Brostoff S, Eylar E H et al 1973 Protein composition of myelin of the peripheral nervous system. Journal of Neurochemistry 20: 1207–1216

Greenwald A G, Schute P C, Shively J L 1984 Brachial plexus palsy: a 10 year report on the incidence and prognosis. Journal of Paediatric Orthopaedics 4: 639–692

Gregg J R, Lubosky D, Harty M et al 1979 Serratus anterior paralysis in the young athlete. Journal of Bone and Joint Surgery 61A: 825–832

Grenet H, Isaac-Georges P, Ladet Mlle 1937 Paralysie radiculaire du plexus brachial et paralysie diaphragmatique. Bulletin de la Societe Pédiatrique, Paris 146: 35–46

Greulich M von 1976 Der zweipunkte-Stern. Hand Chirurgie 8: 97–99

Griffin J W, Hoffman P N 1993 Degeneration and regeneration in the peripheral nervous system. In: Dyck P J, Thomas P K, Lambert E H, Bunge R (eds) Peripheral neuropathy, 3rd edn. W B Saunders, Philadelphia, p 361–376

Griffin J W, Cornblath D R, Alexander E et al 1990 Ataxic sensory neuropathy and dorsal root ganglionitis associated with Sjögrens syndrome. Annals of Neurology 27: 304–315

Griffiths D L 1940 Volkmann's ischaemic contracture. British Journal of Surgery 28: 239–260

Griffiths D L 1964 The "nervous syndrome" of cervical ribs. Journal of Bone and Joint Surgery 46B: 780

Grilli F P 1959 Il trapianto del bicipite brachiale in lunzione pronatoria. Archivio Putti di Chirurzia dejli Organi di Movimento 12: 359–371

Gross P T, Royden-Jones H 1992 Proximal median neuropathies: electromyographic and clinical correlation. Muscle and Nerve 15: 390–395

Gross W S, Yao J S T 1982 Vascular problems. In: Wadsworth T G (ed) The Elbow, 1st edn. Churchill Livingstone, Edinburgh, p 223–241

Gruber B J 1990 Neurologic consequences of electrical burns. Journal of Trauma 30: 254–258

Gruber H, Zenker W 1973 Acetylcholinesterase: histochemical differentiation between motor and sensory nerve fibres. Brain Research 51: 207–214

Gruber H, Freilinger G, Holle J, Mandl H 1976 Identification of motor and sensory funiculi in cut nerves and their selective reunion. British Journal of Plastic Surgery 29: 70–73

Gruber W 1869 Über die Halsrippen des Menschen, mit vergleichend-anatomischen Bemerkungen. Mémoires de l'Académie Impériale de St Pétersbourg, VIIe Serie 13: 1–52

Gruber W 1870 Über die Verbindung des Nervus medianus mit dem Nervus ulnaris am Unterarme der Menschen und der Säugethiere. Archive Anatomie Physiologie Medizin (Leipzig) 37: 501–522

Grunberg E, Divertie M B, Woolner L B 1964 A review of unusual systemic manifestations associated with carcinoma. American Journal of Medicine 36: 106–120

Gschmeissner S E, Pereira J H, Cowley S A 1991 The rapid assessment of nerve stumps. Journal of Bone and Joint Surgery 73B: 688–689

Gu X, Thomas P K, King R H M 1995 Chemotrophins in nerve regeneration studied in tissue culture. Journal of Anatomy 186: 153–163

Gu Y D 1996 Intraoperative electromyographic studies of C7 distribution. In: Shanghai International Brachial Plexus Symposium

Gu Y D, Ma M K 1991 Nerve transfer for treatment of root avulsion of the brachial plexus: experimental studies in a rat model. Journal of Reconstructive Microsurgery 7: 15–22

Gu Y D, Shen L Y 1994 Electrophysiological changes after severance of the C7 nerve root. Journal of Hand Surgery 19B: 69–71

Gu Y D, Wu MM, Zhen Y L et al 1989 Phrenic nerve transfer for brachial plexus motor neurotisation. Microsurgery 10: 287–289

Gu Y D, Zhang G M, Chen D S et al 1992 Seventh cervical nerve root transfer from the contralateral healthy side for treatment of brachial plexus root avulsion. Journal of Hand Surgery 17B: 518–521

Gudden Forel Monakow 1882 Cited by Ramon y Cajal S. In: May R M (trans, ed) Degeneration and regeneration of the nervous system. Oxford University Press, London, vol I, p 5

Guiloff R J, Sherratt R M 1977 Sensory conduction in medial plantar nerve. Journal of Neurology, Neurosurgery and Psychiatry 40: 1168–1181

Gunderson R W, Barrett J N 1979 Neuronal chemotaxis: chick dorsal-root axons turn towards high concentrations of nerve growth factor. Science 206: 1079–1080

Gurdjian E S, Larsen R D, Lindner D W 1965 Intraneural cyst of the peroneal and ulnar nerves. Journal of Neurosurgery 23: 76–78

Guthrie C C 1912 Blood vessel surgery and its applications (reprint 1959). In: Harbison S P, Fisher B (eds). University of Pittsburgh Press, Pittsburgh

Gutmann E, Sanders F K 1943 Recovery of fibre numbers and diameters in the regeneration of peripheral nerves. Journal of Physiology 101: 489–518

Gutmann E, Young J Z 1944 The reinnervation of muscle after various periods of atrophy. Journal of Anatomy 78: 15–43

Guttmann L 1977 Median-ulnar nerve communications and carpal tunnel syndrome. Journal of Neurology, Neurosurgery and Psychiatry 41: 957–959

Guyon F 1861 Note sur une disposition anatomique propre à la face antérieure de la région du poignet et non encore décrite par le docteur. Bulletin de la Société Anatomique de Paris 6: 184–186

Haak R A, Kleinhaus F W, Ochs F 1976 The viscosity of mammalian nerve axoplasm measured by electron spin resonance. Journal of Physiology (London) 263: 115–137

Hadley M N, Sonntag V K H, Pittman H W 1986 Suprascapular nerve entrapment. Journal of Neurosurgery 64: 843–848

Haftek J 1970 Stretch injury of peripheral nerve. Journal of Bone and Joint Surgery 52B: 354–365

Haftek J, Thomas P K 1967 An electron-microscopic study of crush injuries to peripheral nerves. Journal of Anatomy 102: 154–155

Haftek J, Thomas P K 1968 Electron-microscopic observations on the effect of localised crush injuries on the connective tissues of peripheral nerve. Journal of Anatomy 103: 233–243

Hagbarth K E 1983 Microelectrode exploration of human nerves: physiological and clinical implications. Journal of the Royal Society of Medicine 76: 7–15

Hagbarth K E, Torebjörk H E, Wallin B G 1993 Microelectrode exploration of human peripheral nerves. In: Dyck P J, Thomas P K, Griffin J W, Low P A, Poduslo J F (eds) Peripheral neuropathy, 3rd edn. W B Saunders, Philadelphia, p 658–671

Hagen N A, Stevens J C, Michet C J 1990 Trigeminal sensory neuropathy associated with connective tissue diseases. Neurology 40: 891–896

Hall G M, Spector T D, Studd J W W 1992 Carpal tunnel syndrome and hormone replacement therapy. British Medical Journal 304: 382

Hall J B, Denis F, Murray J 1977 Exposure of upper cervical spine for spinal decompression by a mandible and tongue splitting approach. Journal of Bone and Joint Surgery 59A: 121–123

Hall S 1997 Axonal regneration through acellular muscle grafts. Journal of Anatomy 190: 57–71

Hallett J 1981 Entrapment of the median nerve after dislocation of the elbow. Journal of Bone and Joint Surgery 63B: 408–412

Hallin R G, Torebjörk H E 1973 Electrically induced A and C fibre responses in intact human skin nerves. Experimental Brain Research 16: 309–320

Hallin R G, Torebjörk H E 1974 Afferent and efferent sympathetic C units can be differentiated. Acta Physiologica Scandinavica 92: 318–331

Hallin R G, Torebjörk H E, Weisenfeld Z 1981 Nociceptors and warm receptors innervated by C fibres in human skin. Journal of Neurology, Neurosurgery and Psychiatry 45: 313–319

Hallock G G 1992 Fascio-cutaneous flaps. Blackwell Scientific Publications, Oxford

Hallowell 1761 Cited by Lambert 1844. In: Erichson J E (ed) Observations on aneurysm

Hamanaka I, Okutso I, Shimizu K et al 1995 Evaluation of carpal tunnel pressure in carpal tunnel syndrome. Journal of Hand Surgery 20A: 848–854

Handforth A, Nag S, Robertson D M 1984 Polyneuropathy with vagus and phrenic nerve involvement in breast cancer. Archives of Neurology 41: 666–668

Hankinson J, Pearce G W, Rowbotham G F 1960 Stereotactic operations for the relief of pain. Journal of Neurology, Neurosurgery and Psychology 23: 352

Hanlon C R, Ester W L 1954 Fractures in childhood: a statistical analysis. American Journal of Surgery 87: 312–323

Hanlon C R, Paletta F X, Cooper T, Willman V L 1965 Acute arterial occlusion in the lower extremity. Clinical and experimental studies of muscular ischaemia. Journal of Cardiovascular Surgery 6: 11–14

Hannington-Kiff J G 1974 Intravenous regional sympathetic block with guanethidine. Lancet i: 1019–1020

Hannington-Kiff J G 1977 Relief of Sudeck's atrophy by regional intravenous guanethidine. Lancet i: 1132–1133

Hannington-Kiff J G 1979 Relief of causalgia in limbs by regional intravenous guanethidine. British Medical Journal 2: 367–368

Hanson M R, Breuer A C, Furlan A J et al 1983 Mechanism and frequency of brachial plexus injury in open-heart surgery: a prospective analysis. Annals of Thoracic Surgery 36: 675–679

Hardy A E 1981 Birth injuries of the brachial plexus. Journal of Bone and Joint Surgery 63B: 98–101

Hardy E G, Tibbs D J 1960 Acute ischaemia in limb injuries. British Medical Journal 1: 1001–1005

Harii K, Ohmari T, Torii S 1976 Free gracilis muscle transplantation with microneurovascular anastomoses for the treatment of facial paralysis. Journal of Plastic and Reconstructive Surgery 57: 133–143

Harkess J W 1992 Arthroplasty of the hip. In: Crenshaw A H (ed) Campbell's operative orthopaedics. Mosby Year Book, St Louis, p 441–626

Harkin J C, Reed O R 1969 Tumours of the peripheral nervous system. In: Atlas of tumour pathology, 2nd series, fascicle 3. Washington D C Armed Forces Institute of Pathology, Washington, D C

Harper C M, Thomas J E, Cascino T L et al 1989 Distinction between neoplastic and radiation induced brachial neuropathy, with emphasis on the role of EMG. Neurology 39: 502–512

Harrelson J M, Newman N 1975 Hypertrophy of the flexor carpi ulnaris as a cause of compression in the distal part of the forearm. Journal of Bone and Joint Surgery 57A: 554–555

Harriman D G F 1977 Ischaemia of peripheral nerve and muscle. Journal of Clinical Pathology II (suppl 30): 94–99

Harris C M, Tanner E, Goldstein M N et al 1974 The surgical treatment of the carpal-tunnel syndrome correlated with preoperative nerve-conduction studies. Journal of Bone and Joint Surgery 61A: 93–98

Harris N H 1995 Medical negligience in trauma and orthopaedics. In: Powers M J, Harris N H (eds) Medical negligence, 2nd edn. Butterworths, London, p 647–666

Harris W 1904 The true form of the brachial plexus and its motor distribution. Journal of Anatomy and Physiology 38: 399–422

Harris W 1929 Occupational pressure neuritis of the deep palmar branch of the ulnar nerve. British Medical Journal 1: 98

Harris W, Low V W 1903 On the importance of accurate muscular analysis in lesions of the brachial plexus and the treatment of Erb's palsy and infantile paralysis of the upper extremity by cross-union of nerve roots. British Medical Journal 2: 1035–1038

Harrison M J G 1976 Pressure palsy of the ulnar nerve with prolonged conduction block. Journal of Neurology, Neurosurgery and Psychiatry 39: 96–99

Hart F D, Golding J R 1960 Rheumatoid neuropathy. British Medical Journal 1: 1594–1600

Hashizume H, Inque H, Nagashima K et al 1993 Posterior interosseous nerve paralysis related to focal radial nerve constriction secondary to vasculitis. Journal of Hand Surgery 18B: 757–760

Hashizume H, Nishida K, Nanba Y et al 1995a Intraneural ganglion of the posterior interosseous nerve with lateral elbow pain. Journal of Hand Surgery 20B: 649–651

Hashizume H, Nishida K, Yamamoto K et al 1995b Delayed posterior interosseous nerve palsy. Journal of Hand Surgery 20B: 655–657

Hastings H, Misamore G 1987 Compartment syndrome resulting from intravenous regional anaesthesia. Journal of Hand Surgery 12A: 559–562

Haug C E, Sanders R J 1991 Arterial TOS. In: Sanders R J, Haug CE (eds) Thoracic outlet syndrome. J B Lippincott, Philadelphia, p 211–231

Hayashi Y, Kojima T, Kohno T 1984 A case of cubital tunnel syndrome caused by the snapping of the medial head of the triceps brachii muscle. Journal of Hand Surgery 9A: 96–99

Hayden J W 1964 Median neuropathy in the carpal tunnel caused by spontaneous intraneural haemorrhage. Journal of Bone and Joint Surgery 46A: 1242–1244

Head H 1920 Studies in neurology. Oxford University Press, London, vol 2

Head H, Holmes G 1911 Sensory disturbances from central lesions. Brain 34: 102–254

Head H, Sherrin J 1905 The consequences of injury to the peripheral nerves in man. Brain 28: 116–338

Head H, Rivers W H R, Sherrin J 1905 The afferent nervous system from a new aspect. Brain 28: 99–116

Healy C, LeQuesne P M, Lynn B 1996 Collateral sprouting of cutaneous nerves in man. Brain 119: 2063–2072

Heathfield K W G, Williams J R B 1954 Peripheral neuropathy and myopathy associated with bronchogenic carcinoma. Brain 77: 122–137

Hempel G K, Rusher A H, Wheeler C G et al 1981 Supraclavicular resection of the first rib for thoracic outlet syndrome. American Journal of Surgery 141: 213–215

Hems T E J, Glasby M A 1992a Repair of cervical nerve roots proximal to the root ganglia. Journal of Bone and Joint Surgery 74B: 918–922

Hems T E J, Glasby M A 1992b Comparison of different methods of repair of long peripheral nerve defects: an experimental study. British Journal of Plastic Surgery 45: 497–502

Hems T E J, Glasby M A 1993 The limit in graft length in the experimental use of muscle grafts for nerve repair. Journal of Hand Surgery 18B: 165–170

Hems T E J, Clutton R E, Glasby M A 1994 Repair of the avulsed cervical nerve roots. An experimental study in sheep. Journal of Bone and Joint Surgery 76B: 818–823

Henderson W H, Papadimitriou J M, Coleman M 1986 Neural tumours. In: Ultrastructural appearances of tumours, 2nd edn. Churchill Livingstone, Edinburgh, Sec 3

Henegar M M, Kaufman B A 1995 Fast spin-echo magnetic resonance imaging for radiological assessment of neonatal brachial plexus injury. Journal of Neurosurgery 83: 461–466

Hennigan T W, Branfoot A C, Theodorou N A 1992 Ancient neurilemmoma of the pelvis. Journal of the Royal Society of Medicine 85: 416–417

Henry A K 1924 A new method of resecting the left cervicothoracic ganglion of the sympathetic chain in angina pectoris. Irish Journal of Medical Science V: 157–167

Henry A K 1957 Upper limb. In: Extensile exposure, 2nd edn. E S Livingstone, London, p 15–116

Hensel H, Andres K H, von During M 1974 Structure and function of cold receptors. Pflügers Archiv 352: 1–10

Henson G F 1956 Vascular complications of shoulder injuries: a report of two cases. Journal of Bone and Joint Surgery 38B: 528–531

Henson R A, Russell D S, Wilkinson M 1954 Carcinomatous neuropathy and myopathy. Brain 77: 82–121

Hentz V, Narakas A O 1988 The results of microneurosurgical reconstruction of complete brachial plexus palsy. Orthopedic Clinics of North America 19: 107–114

Herndon G H 1961 Tendon transplantation at the knee and foot. In: American Academy of Orthopaedic Surgeons. Instructional Course Lectures 18. C V Mosby, St Louis, p 145–168

Herndon J H, Hess A V 1991 Neuromas. In: Gelberman R H (ed) Operative nerve repair and reconstruction. J B Lippincott, Philadelphia, p 1525–1540

Herndon C H, Strong J M, Heyman C H 1956 Transposition of the tibialis anterior in the treatment of paralytic talipes calcaneus. Journal of Bone and Joint Surgery 38A: 751–760

Herndon J H, Eaton R G, Littler J W 1976 Management of painful neuromas in the hand. Journal of Bone and Joint Surgery 58A: 364–373

Hertz V R, Wikswo J, Abraham G 1986 Magnetic measurement of nerve action currents: a new intra-operation recording technique. Peripheral Nerve Regeneration and Repair 1: 27–36

Hertzer N R, Feldman B J, Beren E C et al 1980 A prospective study of the incidence of injury to the cranial nerves during carotid endarterectomy. Surgery, Gynaecology and Obstetrics 151: 781–784

Herzberg G, Narakas A, Comtet J J 1989 Anatomie et rapports des racines du plexus brachial dans l'espace intertransversaire. In: Alnot J Y, Narakas A (eds) Les Paralysies du plexus brachial. Expansion Scientifique Française pp 19–26

Hess K, Eames R A, Darveniza P et al 1979 Acute ischaemic neuropathy in the rabbit. Journal of the Neurological Sciences 44: 19–43

Hetreed M A, Howard L A, Birch R 1984 Evaluation of peroperative sensory Electroencephalography. Clinical Neurophysiology 58: 220–225

Hetreed M A, Howard L A, Birch R 1992 Evaluation of perioperative sensory evoked potentials recorded from nerve roots to the cervical epidural space during brachial plexus surgery. In: Jones S J, Hetreed M, Boyd S, Smith N J (eds) Handbook of spinal cord monitoring. Kluwer, Dordrecht, p 171–178

Heumann R, Lindholm D, Bandtlow C et al 1987 Differential regulation of MRNA encoding nerve growth factor and its receptor in rat sciatic nerve during development, degeneration and regeneration: role of macrophages. Proceedings of the National Academy of Sciences USA 84: 8735–8739

Hewitt R L, Smith A D, Drapanas T 1973 Acute traumatic arteriovenous fistulas. Journal of Trauma 13: 901–906

Higgs P E, Edwards D, Martin D S et al 1995 Carpal tunnel surgery outcomes in workers: effect of workers' compensation status. Journal of Hand Surgery 20A: 354–360

Highet W B 1954 Quoted by Zachary R B. In: Seddon H J (ed) Peripheral nerve injuries. Medical Research Council Special Report Series No. 282. HMSO, London, p 355

Hill G G 1991 What is risk management? International Journal of Risk and Safety in Medicine 85: 663–668

Hill R M 1939 Vascular abnormalities of the upper limb associated with cervical ribs. British Journal of Surgery 27: 100–107

Hirasawa Y, Oda R, Nakatani K 1977 Sciatic nerve paralysis in posterior dislocation of the hip. Clinical Orthopaedics and Related Research 126: 172–175

Hirschmann J 1943 Der Nervenschussmerz und seine Behandlung. Nervenartz 16: 82–88

Ho K H, Lloyd R E 1987 The lingual nerve entrapment syndrome. British Dental Journal 163: 387

Hoang P, Ford D J, Burke F D 1986 Post mastectomy pain after brachial plexus palsy: metastasis or radiation neuritis? Journal of Hand Surgery 11B: 441–443

Hobby J A E, Laing J E 1988 Electrical injuries of the upper limb. In: Tubiana R (ed) The hand. W B Saunders, Philadelphia, vol III, p 779–787

Hobsley M A 1994 Informed consent for parotidectomy for a lump. Hospital Update 20: 299–300

Hodes R, Larrabee M C, German W 1948 The human electromyogram in response to nerve stimulation and the conduction velocity of motor axons. Archives of Neurology and Psychiatry 60: 240–365

Hodgkinson T 1990a Expert evidence: law and practice. Sweet and Maxwell, p 90

Hodgkinson T 1990b Expert evidence: law and practice. Sweet and Maxwell, p 111

Hoffman P 1915a Über eine Methode, den Erfolg einer Nervennalt zu beurteilen. Medizinische Klinik 11: 359–360

Hoffman P 1915b Weiteres über das Verhalten frisch regenerierter Nerven über die Methode, den Erfolg einer Nervennaht Frühzeitig zu beurteilen. Medizinische Klinik 11: 856–858

Hoffman C F E, Choufoer H, Marani E et al 1993a Ultrastructural study on avulsion effects of the cat cervical motor-axonal pathways in the spinal cord. Clinical Neurology and Neurosurgery 95 (suppl): S39–S47

Hoffman C F E, Thomeer R T W M, Marani E 1993b Reimplantation of ventral rootlets into the cervical spinal cord after their avulsion: an anterior surgical approach. Clinical Neurology and Neurosurgery 95: S112–S118

Holden C E A 1975 Compartment syndrome following trauma. Clinical Orthopaedics and Related Research 113: 95–102

Holden C E A 1979 The pathology and prevention of Volkmann's ischaemic contracture. Journal of Bone and Joint Surgery 618: 296–299

Holle J, Freilinger G, Sulzgruber C 1995 Anatomie chirurgicale des nerfs intercostaux (distribution des fibres motrices et sensitives). In: Alnot J-Y, Narakas A (eds) Les paralysies du plexus brachial, 2nd edn. Monographie de la Société Française de Chirugie De La Main, p 43–45

Hollenbeck P J 1989 The transport and assembly of the axonal cytoskeleton. Journal of Cell Biology 108: 223–227

Hollyday M, Hamburger V 1976 Reduction of the naturally occurring motor neuron loss by enlargement of the periphery. Journal of Comparative Neurology 170: 311–320

Holmes S 1881 A study in scarlet. In: Baring-Gould W S (ed) The annotated Sherlock Holmes. John Murray, London, p 168

Holmes W 1947 Histological observations on the repair of nerves by autografts. British Journal of Surgery 35: 167–173

Holmes W, Highet V B, Seddon H J 1944 Ischaemic nerve lesions occurring in Volkmann's contracture. British Journal of Surgery 35: 259–275

Holt M 1994 Accessory to suprascapular transfer in preganglionic lesions of the brachial plexus. Royal Australasian College of Surgeons. Autumn Scientific Meeting, Brisbane

Holtzmann R N N, Mark M H, Patel M R et al 1984 Ulnar nerve neuropathy in the forearm. Journal of Hand Surgery 9A: 576–578

Hongell A, Mattson H S 1971 Neurographic studies before, after and during operation for median nerve compression in the carpal tunnel. Scandinavian Journal of Plastic and Reconstructive Surgery 5: 103–109

Hoogeveen J F, Wondergem J, Troost D et al 1991 Blood vessel damage followed by wallerian degeneration in the rat sciatic nerve after local hypothermia. Neuropathology and Applied Neurobiology 17: 250–251

Hopkins A, Rudge P 1973 Hyperpathia in the cervical cord syndrome. Journal of Neurology, Neurosurgery and Psychiatry 36: 637–642

Horn J S 1959 Peripheral nerve injuries. In: Clark A R, Badger F G, Sevitt S (eds) Modern trends in accident surgery and medicine. Butterworth, London, p 305–319

Horowitz S H 1985 Brachial plexus injuries with causalgia resulting from trans-axillary rib resection. Archives of Surgery 120: 1189–1191

Horsley V 1897 Short note on sense organs in muscle and on the preservation of muscle spindles in conditions of extreme muscular atrophy. Brain 20: 375–376

Horsley V 1899 On injuries to peripheral nerves. The Practitioner (new series) 10: 131–144

Horwitz M T 1939 The anatomy of (a) the lumbosacral nerve plexus – its relation to variation of vertebral segmentation and (b) the posterior sacral nerve plexus. The Anatomical Record 74: 91–107

Horwitz S 1977 Takayasu's arteritis – a clinical study of 107 cases. American Heart Journal 93: 94–103

Hovelaque A 1927 Anatomie Des Nerfs Carniens Et Rachidiens Et Du Système Grand Sympathetique. Doin, Paris

Hovnanian P 1956 Latissimus dorsi transplantation for loss of elbow flexion or extension at the elbow. Annals of Surgery 143 (4): 493–499

Hromada J 1963 On the nerve supply of the connective tissue of some peripheral nervous system components. Acta Anatomica 55: 343–351

Hruban R H, Shiu M H, Senie R T, Woodruff J M 1990 Malignant nerve sheath tumour in the lower limb — 43 cases. Cancer 66: 1253–1265

Hu Y Y, Lu Y P 1993 Successful extirpation of a huge neurofibroma invading the spinal canal. Orthopaedics International Edition (5): 427–428

Huckstep R L 1971 Neglected traumatic dislocation of the hip. Journal of Bone and Joint Surgery 53B: 355

Huckstep R L 1975 Poliomyelitis. Churchill Livingstone, Edinburgh

Hudson A R 1984 Injection injuries of nerves. In: Dyck P J, Thomas P K, Lambert E H, Burge R (eds) Peripheral neuropathy, 2nd edn. W B Saunders, Philadelphia, p 429–431

Hudson A R 1987 Nerve injection injuries. In: Terzis J K (ed) Microreconstruction of nerve injuries. W B Saunders, Philadelphia, p. 173–180

Hughes C W 1958 Arterial repair during the Korean War. Annals of Surgery 147: 555–561

Hughes C W, Bower W F 1961 Traumatic lesions of peripheral vessel. C C Thomas, Springfield, Il

Hughes J 1975 Isolation of an endogenous compound from the brain with pharmacological properties similar to morphine. Brain Research 88: 295–308

Hughes R A C, Cameron J S, Hall S M et al 1982 Multiple mononeuropathy as the initial presentation of systemic lupus erythematosus. Journal of Neurology 228: 239–247

Huittinen V M 1972 Lumbosacral nerve injury in fracture of the pelvis. A post mortem radiographic and patho-anatomical study. Acta Chirurgica Scandinavica 429 (suppl): 7–43

Huittinen V M, Slätis P 1972 Nerve injury in double vertical pelvic fractures. Acta Chirurgica Scandinavica 138 (6): 571–575

Hunt J R 1911 The thenar and hypothenar types of neuralgic atrophy of the hand. American Journal of Medical Sciences 141: 224–241

Hunter J 1837 In: Palmer J F (ed) Works of John Hunter. Longman, London

Hurst L C, Badalmente M A 1991 Nerve growth factor. In: Gelberman R H (ed) Operative nerve repair and reconstruction. J B Lippincott, London, p. 55–72

Hurst L C, Weissberg D, Carroll R E 1985 The relationship of the double crush to carpal tunnel syndrome. Journal of Hand Surgery 10B: 202–204

Huson S M, Compston D A S, Clark P et al 1989a A genetic study of von Recklinghausen's neurofibromatosis in south east Wales 1.

Prevalence, fitness, mutation rate and effect of parental transmission on severity. Journal of Medical Genetics 26: 704–711

Huson S M, Compston D A S, Harper P C 1989b A genetic study of von Recklinghausen's neurofibromatosis in south east Wales II. Guidelines for genetic counselling. Journal of Medical Genetics 26: 712–721

Hutchinson J 1894 Lectures on injuries to epiphyses and their results. British Medical Journal 1: 669–673

Huxley A F, Stämpfli R 1949 Evidence for saltatory conduction in peripheral myelinated fibres. Journal of Physiology (London) 108: 315–339

Hyllienmark L, Ludvigsson J, Brismar T 1995 Normal values of nerve conduction in children and adolescents. Electroencephalography and Clinical Neurophysiology 97: 208–214

Iggo A 1961 Non-myelinated fibres from mammalian skeletal muscle. Journal of Physiology 155: 52P–53P

Iggo A 1977 Cutaneous and subcutaneous sense organs. British Medical Bulletin 33: 97–102

Iggo A 1985 Cutaneous sensation. In: Swash M, Kennard C (eds) The scientific basis of clinical neurology. Churchill Livingstone, Edinburgh, p 153–162

Iggo A 1986 Cutaneous sensory mechanisms. Journal of Bone and Joint Surgery 68B: 19–21

Ikuta Y, Kubo T, Tsuge K 1976 Free muscle transplantation by microsurgical technique to treat severe Volkmann's contracture. Plastic and Reconstructive Surgery 58: 407–411

Illis L S 1990 Central pain. British Medical Journal 300: 1284–1286

Ilstrup D M 1986 Malignant peripheral nerve sheath tumour: A clinicopathological study of 120 cases. Cancer 57: 2006–2021

Imai H, Tajima T 1985 Analysis of the effect of sensory re-education after median-nerve repair. Japanese Society for the Surgery of the Hand 2: 674–677

Imai H, Tajima T, Natsumi Y 1991 Successful re-education of functional sensibility after median nerve repair at the wrist. Journal of Hand Surgery 16A: 60–66

Inglis A E, Straub L R, Williams C S 1972 Median nerve neuropathy at the wrist. Clinical Orthopaedics and Related Research 83: 48–54

Ishijma B, Yoshimasu N, Fukushima T et al 1975 Nociceptive neurons in the human thalamus. Confinia Neurologica (Basel) 37 (1–3): 99–106

Jàbaley M E 1981 Current concepts of nerve repair. Clinics in Plastic Surgery 8: 33–44

Jàbaley M E 1991 Electrical nerve stimulation in the awake patient. In: Gelberman R H (ed) Operative nerve repair and reconstruction. J B Lippincott, Philadelphia, p. 241–257

Jàbaley M E, Burns J E, Orcutt B S et al 1976 Comparison of histologic and functional recovery after peripheral nerve transection and repair. Journal of Hand Surgery 1: 119–130

Jablecki C K, Andary M T, So Y T et al (AAEM quality assurance committee) 1993 Literature review of the usefulness of nerve conduction studies and electromyography for the evaluation of patients with carpal tunnel syndrome. Muscle and Nerve 16: 1392–1414

Jackson J P, Waugh W 1974 The technique and complications of upper tibial osteotomy. Journal of Bone and Joint Surgery 56B: 236–245

Jackson S T, Hoffer M M, Parish N 1988 Brachial-plexus palsy in the newborn. Journal of Bone and Joint Surgery 70A (8): 1217–1220

Jacobs J M, Love S 1985 Qualitative and quantitative morphology of human sural nerve at different ages. Brain 108: 897–924

Jacobs J S, Dean J 1992 Soft tissue injuries of the face. In: Peterson L J (ed) Principles of oral and maxillofacial surgery. J P Lippincott, Philadelphia, p 346–347

Jacobs L G H, Buxton R A 1989 Course of the superior gluteal nerve in the lateral approach to the hip. Journal of Bone and Joint Surgery 71A: 1239–1243

Jacobs L G H, Buxton R A 1990 Reply to letter from McLelland S J. Journal of Bone and Joint Surgery 72A: 791

Jamal G A, Hansen S, Weir A I, Ballantyne J 1987 The neurophysiological investigation of small fibre neuropathies. Muscle and Nerve 10: 537–545

Jamieson A, Eames R A 1980 Reimplantation of avulsed brachial plexus roots: an experimental study in dogs. International Journal of Microsurgery 2: 75–80

Jamieson A, Hughes 1980 The role of surgery in the management of closed injuries of the brachial plexus. Clinical Orthopaedics and Related Research 147: 210–215

Jancke E J 1958 Late structural and functional results of arterial injuries primarily repaired. Surgery 43: 175–183

Janeiki C J, Dovberg J L 1977 Tarsal-tunnel syndrome caused by neurilemmoma of the medial plantar nerve. Journal of Bone and Joint Surgery 59A: 127–128

Janzen A H, Warren S 1942 Effect of roentgen rays on peripheral nerves of rats. Radiology 38: 333–337

Jaradeh S S, Jacobson R D, Konkol R J et al 1994 Neonatal brachial plexopathy: serial electrophysiological studies in 13 cases. Muscle and Nerve 17: 1079

Jefferson D, Eames R A 1979 Subclinical entrapment of the lateral femoral cutaneous nerve. Muscle and Nerve 2: 145–154

Jefferson D, Neary D, Eames R A 1981 Renaut body distribution at sites of human peripheral nerve entrapment. Journal of the Neurological Sciences 49: 19–29

Jennett R J, Tarby T J, Kreinick C J 1992 Brachial plexus palsy: an old problem revisited. American Journal of Obstetrics and Gynecology 166: 1637–1677

Jenq C B, Jenq L L, Coggeshall R E 1987 Nerve regeneration changes with filters of different pore sizes. Experimental Neurology 97: 662–671

Jepson P N 1926 Ischaemic contracture, an experimental study. Annals of Surgery 84: 785–795

Jepson P N 1930 Obstetrical paralysis. Annals of Surgery 91: 724–730

Jerret S A, Cuzzone L J, Pasternak B M 1984 Thoracic outlet syndrome: electrophysiological reappraisal. Archives of Neurology 41: 960–963

Jessing P 1975 Monteggia lesions and their complicating nerve damage. Acta Orthopedica Scandinavica 46: 601–609

Johnson E W, Burkhart I A, Earl W C 1972 Electromyography in postlaminectomy patients. Archives of Physical Medicine and Rehabilitation 53: 407–409

Johnson J R, Bonfiglio M 1969 Lipofibromatous hamartoma of the median nerve. Journal of Bone and Joint Surgery 5A: 984–990

Johnson M, Spinner M, Shrewsbury M M 1979 Median nerve entrapment in the forearm. Journal of Hand Surgery 4: 48–51

Johnson P C 1977 Haematogenous metastases of carcinoma to dorsal root ganglia. Acta Neuropathologica 38 (2): 171–172

Johnson R K, Shrewsbury M M 1970 Anatomical course of the thenar branch of the median nerve – usually in a separate tunnel through the transverse carpal ligament. Journal of Bone and Joint Surgery 52A: 269–273

Johnston A W 1960 Acroparaesthesiae and acromegaly. British Medical Journal 1: 1616–1620

Jones C A 1989 The assessment of hand function. A clinical view of techniques. Journal of Hand Surgery 14A: 221–228

Jones R 1916 On suture of nerves, and alternative methods of treatment by transplantation of tendons. British Medical Journal 1: 641–643

Jones R 1921 Tendon transplantation in cases of musculospiral injuries not amenable to suture. American Journal of Surgery 35 (11): 333–335

Jones R 1928 Volkmann's ischaemic contracture with special reference to treatment. British Medical Journal 2: 639–642

Jones S J 1987 Diagnostic value of peripheral and spinal somatosensory evoked potentials in traction lesions of the brachial plexus. In: Terzis J K (ed) Microreconstruction of nerve injuries. W B Saunders, Philadelphia, p 463–472

Jordan W R 1936 Neuritic manifestations in diabetes mellitus. Archives of Internal Medicine 57: 307–366

Jordan W R, Randall L O, Bloor W R 1935 Neuropathy in diabetes mellitus. Archives of Internal Medicine 55: 17–41

Joyce J W, Hollier L H 1984 The giant cell arteritides: temporal and Takayusu's arteritis. In: Bergen J J, Yao J S T (eds) Evaluation and treatment of upper and lower extremity circulatory disorders. Grune & Stratton, New York

Józsa L, Renner A, Santha E 1980 The effect of tourniquet ischaemia on intact, tenotomized and motor nerve injured human hand muscles. The Hand 12: 235–240

Kalisman M, Laborde K, Wolff T W 1982 Ulnar nerve compression secondary to ulnar artery false aneurysm at the Guyon's canal. Journal of Hand Surgery 7: 137–139

Kapandji A I 1988 Les plasties d'agrandissement du ligament annulaire du carpe dans le traitement du syndrome du canal carpien. Communication au Congrés Annuel de la Société Française de Chirurgie de la Main, Paris

Kaplan P E 1980 Electrodiagnostic confirmation of long thoracic nerve palsy. Journal of Neurology, Neurosurgery and Psychiatry 43: 50–52

Kaplan P E, Kernahan W T 1981 Tarsal tunnel syndrome. Journal of Bone and Joint Surgery 63A: 96–99

Kasai T, Chiba S 1977 True nature of the muscular arch of the axilla and its nerve supply. Acta Anatomica Nipponica 52: 309–336

Katifi H A, Sedgwick E M 1987 Evaluation of the dermatomal somatosensory evoked potential in the diagnosis of lumbo-sacral root compression. Journal of Neurology, Neurosurgery and Psychiatry 50: 1204–1210

Katirji B, Wilbourn A J 1994 High sciatic lesion mimicking peroneal neuropathy at the fibular head. Journal of Neurological Sciences 121: 172–175

Katirji M B, Agrawal R, Kantra T A 1988 The human cervical myotomes: an anatomical correlation between electromyography and CT/myelography. Muscle and Nerve 11: 1070–1073

Katz J N, Forsel K K, Simmons B D et al 1995 Symptoms and functional status and neuromuscular impairment following carpal tunnel release. Journal of Hand Surgery 20A: 549–555

Keck C 1962 The tarsal tunnel syndrome. Journal of Bone and Joint Surgery 44A: 180–182

Keegan J J, Holyoke E A 1962 Meralgia paraesthetica. An anatomical and surgical study. Journal of Neurosurgery 19: 341–345

Kehoe S, Reid R P, Semple J C 1995 Solitary benign peripheral nerve tumour. Journal of Bone and Joint Surgery 77B: 497–500

Kellgren J H, Ball J, Tutton G K 1952 The articular and other limb changes in acromegaly. Quarterly Journal of Medicine 21: 405–424

Kennedy R 1903 Suture of the brachial plexus in birth paralysis of the upper extremity. British Medical Journal 1: 298–301

Kennedy W F, Byrne T F, Majid H A et al 1991 Sciatic nerve monitoring during total hip arthroplasty. Clinical Orthopaedics and Related Research 264: 223–237

Ker A T 1918 The brachial plexus of nerves in man, the variations in its formation and its branches. American Journal of Anatomy 23: 285–395

Kernohan J, Levack B, Wilson J N 1985 Entrapment of the superfical peroneal nerve. Journal of Bone and Joint Surgery 67B: 60–61

Kessel A L, Rang M 1966 Supracondylar spur of the humerus. Journal of Bone and Joint Surgery 48B: 765–769

Kessler F B 1986 Complications of the management of the carpal tunnel syndrome. Hand Clinics 2: 401–406

Khatri B O, Baruah J, McQuillen M P 1984 Correlation of electromyography with computed tomography in evaluation of lower back pain. Archives of Neurology 41: 594–597

Killer H E, Hess K 1990 Natural history of radiation induced brachial plexopathy compared with surgically treated patients. Journal of Neurology 237: 247–250

Kiloh L G 1950 Brachial plexus lesions after cholecystectomy. Lancet i: 103–105

Kiloh L G, Nevin S 1952 Isolated neuritis of the anterior interosseous nerve. British Medical Journal 1: 850–851

Kilvington B 1907 An investigation on the regeneration of nerves, with regard to surgical treatment of certain paralyses. British Medical Journal 1: 988–990

Kim D H, Kline D G 1995 Surgical outcome for intra- and extrapelvic femoral nerve lesions. Journal of Neurosurgery 63: 783–790

Kim P, Ebersold M J, Onofrio B M et al 1989 Surgery of spinal schwannoma. Risk of neurological deficit after resection of involved root. Journal of Neurosurgery 71: 810–814

Kimura J, Ayyar R 1985 The carpal tunnel syndrome: electrophysiological aspects of 639 symptomatic extremities. Electromyography and Clinical Neurophysiology 25: 151–164

Kimura J 1979 The carpal tunnel syndrome: localization of conduction abnormalities within the distal segment of the median nerve. Brain 102: 619–635

Kimura J 1989 Electrodiagnosis in diseases of nerve and muscle: principles and practice, 2nd edn. F A Davis, Philadelphia

Kimura J 1993 The effects of age. In: Dyck P J, Thomas P K, Griffin J W, Low P A, Poduslo J F(eds) Peripheral neuropathy, 3rd edn. W B Saunders, Philadelphia, p 605

King R J, Dunkerton M 1982 The pronator syndrome. Journal of the Royal College of Surgeons of Edinburgh 27: 142–145

King R J, Morgan F P 1959 Late results of removing the medial humeral epicondyle for traumatic ulnar neuritis. Journal of Bone and Joint Surgery 41B: 51–55

King R J, Motta G 1983 Iatrogenic spinal accessory nerve palsy. Annals of the Royal College of Surgeons of England 65: 35–37

King T T 1993 Clinical presentation and treatment of the cranial nerves and spinal roots. In: Dyck P J, Thomas P K (eds) Peripheral neuropathy, 3rd edn. W B Saunders, Philadelphia, p 1641–1672

Kinmonth J B 1952 The physiology and relief of traumatic arterial spasm. British Medical Journal 1: 59–64

Kinmonth J B, Hadfield G J, Connolly J E et al 1956 Traumatic arterial spasm. Its relief in man and in monkeys. British Journal of Surgery 44: 164–169

Kiricuta I 1963 L'emploi du grand épiploon dans la chirurgie du sein cancéreux. Presse Médicale 71: 15–17

Kirkup J R 1963 Major arterial injury complicating fracture of the femoral shaft. Journal of Bone and Joint Surgery 45B: 337–343

Kiss G, Komar J 1990 Suprascapular nerve compression at the spinoglenoid notch. Muscle and Nerve 13: 556–557

Kleinert H E, Kasdan H L, Romero J L 1963 Small blood vessel anastomosis for salvage of severely injured upper extremity. Journal of Bone and Joint Surgery 45A: 788–796

Klenerman L 1980 Tourniquet time – how long? The Hand 12: 231–234

Klenerman L, Biswas M, Hulands G H et al 1980 Systemic and local effects of the application of a tourniquet. Journal of Bone and Joint Surgery 62B: 385–388

Kline D G 1989 Civilian gun shot wounds to the brachial plexus. Journal of Neurosurgery 70: 166–174

Kline D G, Hudson A R 1995a Grading results. In: Nerve injuries. W B Saunders, Philadelphia, p 87–99

Kline D G, Hudson A R 1995b Operative care and techniques. In: Nerve injuries. W B Saunders, Philadelphia, p 117–145

Kline D G, Hudson A R 1995c Posterior approach to the brachial plexus. In: Nerve injuries. W B Saunders, Philadelphia, p 448–451

Kline D G, Hudson A R 1995d Injection injury. In: Nerve injuries. W B Saunders, Philadelphia, p 46–50

Kline D G, Hudson A R 1995e Operative approach to suprascapular nerve. In: Nerve injuries. W B Saunders, Philadelphia, p 456–458

Kline D G, Hudson A R 1995f Surgical exposure of the femoral nerve. In: Nerve injuries. W B Saunders, Philadelphia, p 334–335

Kline D G, Kott J, Barnes G et al 1978 Exploration of selected brachial plexus lesions by the posterior subscapular approach. Journal of Neurosurgery 49: 872–879

Kline D G, Donner T R, Happel L et al 1992 Intraforaminal repair of plexus spinal nerves by a posterior approach: an experimental study. Journal of Neurosurgery 76 (3): 459–470

Klumpke A 1885 Contribution a l'étude des paralysies radiculaires du plexus brachial: paralysies radiculaires totales. Revue de Medecine Interne (Paris) 5: 591–616

Knutsson B 1961 Comparative value of electromyographic, myelographic and clinical-neurological examinations in the diagnosis of lumbar root compression syndromes. Acta Orthopedica Scandinavica 49 (suppl): 1–135

Kocher T 1911 Operative surgery. Black, London

Kogelnik H D 1977 Einfluss der Dosis-Relation auf die Pathogenese der peripheren Neuropathie. Strahlentherapie 153: 467–469

Koka S R, Bonnici A V, Slater R N L et al 1996 Femoral neuropathy following total hip replacement: anatomical study and report of eight cases. Orthopaedics 4: 127–129

Koltzenburg M, Lundberg L E R, Torebjörk H E 1992 Dynamic and static components of mechanical hyperalgesia in human hairy skin. Pain 51: 207–220

Komatsu S, Tamai S 1968 Successful replantation of a completely cut off thumb. Plastic and Reconstructive Surgery 42: 374–377

Kon M, Bloem J 1987 The treatment of amputation neuromas in fingers with centrocentral nerve union. Annals of Plastic Surgery 18: 506–510

Kopell H P, Thompson W A L 1959 Pain and the frozen shoulder. Surgery, Gynecology and Obstetrics 109: 92–96

Korenman E M, Devor M 1981 Ectopic adrenergic sensitivity in damaged axons. Experimental Neurology 72: 63–81

Kori S H, Foley K M, Osner J B 1981 Brachial plexus lesions in patients with cancer. Neurology 31: 45–50

Kotani P T, Matsuda H, Suzuki T 1972 Trial surgical procedures of nerve transfers to avulsion injuries of the plexus brachialis. Excerpta Medica International Congress Series Number 291 (1973). Proceedings of the 12th Congress of SICOT, Tel Aviv, 9–12 October 1972, p 348–351

Kotani H, Miki T, Senzoku F et al 1995 Posterior interosseous nerve paralysis with multiple constrictions. Journal of Hand Surgery 20A: 15–17

Kozin F, Soin J S, Ryan L M et al 1981 Bone scintigraphy in the reflex sympathetic dystrophy syndrome. Radiology 138: 437–443

Kramis R C, Roberts W J, Gillette R G 1996 Post-sympathetic neuralgia: hypotheses on peripheral and central neuronal mechanisms. Pain 64: 1–9

Krarup C, Stewart J D, Sumner A S J et al 1990 A syndrome of asymmetric limb weakness with motor conduction block. Neurology 40: 118–127

Kratimenos G P, Crockard H A 1993 The far lateral approach for ventrally placed foramen magnum and upper cervical spine tumour. British Journal of Neurosurgery 7: 129–140

Kreel L, Thornton A 1992 Outline of medical imaging. Butterworth-Heinemann, Oxford, p 221

Kremer M, Gilliatt R W, Golding J S R, Wilson T G 1953 Acroparaesthesiae in the carpal-tunnel syndrome. Lancet ii: 590–595

Krikler S J, Grimer R J 1993 Pelvic chondrosarcoma presenting with meralgia paraesthetica. Hospital Update August: 460–464

Kühne W 1864 Über die Endigung der Nerven in den Nervenhügeln der Muskeln. Archiv fur Pathologische Anatomie und Physiologie und für Klinische Medicin (Virchow) 30: 187–220

Kulick M I, Gordello G, Javidi T et al 1986 Long term analysis of patients having surgical treatment for carpal tunnel syndrome. Journal of Hand Surgery 11A: 59–66

Kurer M H J, Regan M W 1990 Completely displaced supracondylar fracture of the humerus in children. A review of 1708 comparable cases. Clinical Orthopaedics and Related Research. 256: 205–214

Kux M 1978 Thoracic endoscopic sympathectomy in palmar and axillary hyperhidrosis. Archives of Surgery 113: 264–266

Kwan P, Lynch S, Davy A 1997 Munchausen's syndrome with concurrent neurological and psychiatric representations. Journal of the Royal Society of Medicine 90: 83–85

L'Episcopo J B, Brooklyn M D 1939 Restoration of muscle balance in the treatment of obstetrical paralysis. New York State Journal of Medicine 39: 357–363

La Banc J P, Gregg J M 1992 Trigeminal nerve injuries. Basic problems, historical perspectives, early successes and remaining challenges. Oral and Maxillofacial Surgery Clinics of North America: trigeminal nerve surgery: diagnosis and management. 4: 277–283

Laborde K J, Talisman M, Tsai T M 1982 Results of surgical treatments of painful neuromas of the hand. Journal of Hand Surgery 7: 190–193

Lagueny A, Diliac M M, Deliac P Durandeau A 1991 Diagnostic and prognostic value of electrophysiological tests in meralgia paraesthetica. Muscle and Nerve 14: 51–56

Laha R K, Panchal P 1979 Isolated accessory nerve palsy. Southern Medical Journal 72: 1005–1007

Laing J H E, Harrison D H 1991 Envenomation by the box-jellyfish – an unusual cause of ulnar nerve palsy. Journal of the Royal Society of Medicine 64: 115–116

Lalnandham T, Laurence W N 1984 Entrapment of the ulnar nerve in the callus of a supracondylar fracture of the humerus. Injury 16: 129–130.

Lam C R 1936 Nerve injury in fracture of the pelvis. Annals of Surgery 104: 945–951

Lam S J S 1962 A tarsal-tunnel syndrome. Lancet ii: 1354–1355

Lam S J S 1967 Tarsal tunnel syndrome. Journal of Bone and Joint Surgery 49B: 87–92

Lamb D 1970 Ulnar nerve compression at the wrist and hand. The Hand 2: 17–18

Lamb D W 1987a (ed) The paralysed upper limb. Churchill Livingstone, Edinburgh

Lamb D W 1987b The upper limb and hand in traumatic tetraplegia. In: The paralysed hand. Churchill Livingstone, Edinburgh, p 136–152

Lambrinudi C 1927 New operation on drop foot. British Journal of Surgery 15: 193–200

Lamerton A J, Bannister R, Withrington R et al 1983 Claudication of the sciatic nerve. British Medical Journal 286: 1785–1786

Lamotte R L, Thalhammer J G, Torebjörk H E et al 1982 Peripheral neural mechanisms of cutaneous hyperalgesia following mild injury by heat. Journal of Neuroscience 2: 765–781

Lamotte R H, Lundberg L E R, Torebjörk H E 1992 Pain, hyperalgesia and activity in nociceptive C units in humans after intradermal injection of capsaicin. Journal of Physiology 448: 749–764

Lampert P W, Davis R L 1964 Delayed effects of radiation on the human central nervous system. Neurology 14: 912–917

Lancet Leader 1988 How actively should shoulder dystocia be treated? Lancet January: 160

Landau W M 1953 The duration of neuromuscular function after nerve section. Neurosurgery 10: 64–68

Landi A, Copeland S 1979 Value of the Tinel sign in brachial plexus lesions. Annals of the Royal College of Surgeons of England 61: 470–471

Landi A, Copeland S A, Wynn-Parry C B et al 1980 The role of somatosensory evoked potentials and nerve conduction studies in the surgical management of brachial plexus injuries. Journal of Bone and Joint Surgery 62B: 492–496

Landi A, Schoenhuber R, Funicello R et al 1992 Compartment syndrome of the scapula. Annals of Hand Surgery 11: 383–388

Landon D N 1985 Structure and function of nerve fibres. In: Swash M, Kennard C (eds) Scientific basis of neurology. Churchill Livingstone, Edinburgh, p 375–389

Lange F 1900 Ueber periostale Schnenverpflanzungen bei Lähmungen Münchener Medizinische Wochenschrift 47: 486–470

Lange M 1951 Die Behandlung der Irreperablen Trapezius Lähmung. Langenbecks Archiv für Chirurgie 270: 437–439

Langley J N 1903 The autonomic nervous system. Brain 26: 1–26

Langley J N 1926 The autonomic nervous system. Cambridge, Heffer, part 1

Langley J N, Anderson H K 1904 The union of different kinds of nerve fibers. Journal of Physiology 31: 365–391

Langloh N D, Linschied R L 1972 Recurrent and unrelieved carpal-tunnel syndrome. Clinical Orthopaedics and Related Research 83: 41–47

Lanz U 1993 The carpal tunnel syndrome. In: Tubiana R(ed) The hand. W B Saunders, Philadelphia, vol IV, p 463–486

Lanz U, Wolter J 1975 Das akute Carpaltunnelsyndrom. Chirurgie 46: 33–35

Lapiere F, Maheut J 1986 Primary Tumour of the Main Sciatic Nerve. Peripheral Nerve Repair and Regeneration 4: 65–73.

Lascelles R G, Mohr P D, Neary D et al 1977 The thoracic outlet syndrome. Brain 100: 601–612

Lasek R J 1982 Translocation of the neuronal cytoskeleton and axonal locomotion. Philosophical Transactions of the Royal Society, London, Series B 299: 313–327

Lassa R, Shrewsbury M M 1975 A variation in the path of the deep motor branch of the ulnar nerve at the wrist. Journal of Bone and Joint Surgery 57A: 990–991

Lassen M, Krag C, Nielsen I M 1985 The latissimus dorsi flap. Scandinavian Journal of Plastic and Reconstructive Surgery 19: 41–52

Last R J 1949 Innervation of the limbs. Journal of Bone and Joint Surgery 31B: 452–464

Laurent J P, Lee R, Shenaq S et al 1993 Neurosurgical correction of upper brachial plexus birth injuries. Journal of Neurosurgery 79: 197–203

Laverick M D, Barros D'Sa A A B, Kirk S J et al 1990 Management of blunt injuries of the axillary artery and the neck of the humerus. Journal of Trauma 30: 360–361

Laviano M 1992/93 Il nervo accessorio spinale pro sovrascapolare nelle avulsioni del plesso brachiale. Tesi de Specializzazione, Universitá delgli studi di Roma "La Sapienza", Facolta di Medicina e Chirurgia

Lawson G M, Glasby M A 1995 A comparison of immediate and delayed nerve repair using autologous freeze-thawed muscle grafts in a large experimental animal. Journal of Hand Surgery 20B: 663–670

Learmonth J R 1933 The principles of decompression in the treatment of certain diseases of peripheral nerves. Surgical Clinics of North America 13: 905–913

Learmonth J R 1942 A technique for transplanting the ulnar nerve. Surgery, Gynecology and Obstetrics 75: 792–793

Leclerq D C, Carlier A J, Khuc T et al 1985 Improvement in the results in sixty-four ulnar nerve sections associated with arterial repair. Journal of Hand Surgery 10A (intl suppl 2): 997–999

Le Couer P 1967 Procédés de restoration de la flexion du coude paralytique pars transplantation du petit pectoral. Revue de Chirurgie Orthopedique (Paris) 53: 357–372

Lederman J R, Wilbourn A J 1984 Brachial plexopathy: recurrent cancer or radiation? Neurology 34: 1331–1335

Lederman R J, Paulson S M 1987 Brachial neuritis. In: Johnson R T (ed) Current therapy in neurological disease. B C Decker, p 320–322

Leffert R D 1985 Brachial plexus injuries. Churchill Livingstone, Edinburgh, p 91–120

Leffert R D 1972 Anterior submuscular transposition of the ulnar nerve by the Learmonth technique. Journal of Hand Surgery 7: 147–155

Leffert R D, Seddon H J 1965 Infraclavicular brachial plexus injuries. Journal of Bone and Joint Surgery 47B: 9–22

Lefrac B A 1976 Knee dislocation. Archives of Surgery 111: 1021–1024

Leijon G, Boivie J, Johannsen I 1989 Central post-stroke pain – a study of mechanisms through analysis of the sensory abnormalities. Pain 37: 173–185

Lele P P 1963 Effects of focused ultrasonic radiation on peripheral nerve with observations on local heating. Experimental Neurology 8: 47–83

Leonard M A 1972 Sciatic nerve paralysis following anticoagulant therapy. Journal of Bone and Joint Surgery 54B: 152–153

Le Quang C 1989 Post irradiation lesions of the brachial plexus. Hand Clinics 5: 23–32

Le Quesne P M 1993 Neuropathy due to drugs. In: Dyck P J, Thomas P K, Griffin J W, Low P A, Poduslo J F (eds) Peripheral neuropathy, 3rd edn. W B Saunders, Philadelphia, p 1571–1582

Leriche R 1916 De la causalgie envisagée comme une nevrite du sympathique et sur traitement par la dénudation et l'excision des plexus nerveux péri-artériels. Presse Médicale 24: 178–180

Letournel E, Judet R 1981 In: Elson R A (trans) Fractures of the acetabulum. Springer-Verlag, New York

Levi-Montalcini R 1987 The nerve growth factor 35 years later. Science 237: 1154–1162

Levi-Montalcini R, Angeletti P U 1968 Nerve growth factor. Physiological Review 48: 534–569

Levi-Montalcini R, Meyer H, Hamburger V 1954 In vitro experiments on the effects of mouse sarcomas 180 and 37 on the spinal and sympathetic ganglia of the chick embryo. Cancer Research 14: 49–57

Levin K H, Maggiano H J, Wilbourn A J 1996 Cervical radiculopathies: comparison of surgical and EMG localization of single-root lesions. Neurology 46: 1022–1025

Levine M G, Holroyde J, Woods J R et al 1984 Birth trauma: incidence and predisposing factors. Obstetrics and Gynaecology 63: 792–795

Lewis T 1936 Cutaneous hyperalgesia. Clinical Science 2: 373–4231

Lewis T, Pickering G W 1934 Observations upon maladies in which the blood supply to the digits ceases intermittently or permanently and upon gangrene of the digits: observations relevant to so-called "Raynaud's disease". Clinical Science 1: 327–366

Lewis T, Pickering G W 1936 Circulatory changes in the fingers in some diseases of the nervous system, with special reference to the digital atrophy of peripheral nerve lesions. Clinical Science 2: 149–183

Lewis T, Pickering G W, Rothschild P 1931a Centripetal paralysis arising out of arrested bloodflow to the limb. Heart 16: 1–32

Lewis T, Pickering G W, Rothschild P 1931b Observations on muscular pain in intermittent claudication. Heart 15: 359–383

Lexer E 1913 Ideale Aneurysmaoperation und Gefässtransplantation. Deutsche Medizinische Wochenschrift 39: 725

Light A R, Perl E R 1993 Peripheral sensory systems. In: Dyck P J, Thomas P K, Griffin J W, Low P A, Poduslo J F (eds) Peripheral neuropathy, 3rd edn. W B Saunders, Philadelphia, p 149–165

Lilla J A, Phelps D B, Boswick J A 1979 Microsurgical repair of peripheral nerve injuries in the upper extremity. Annals of Plastic Surgery 2: 24–31

Lim L T, Saletta J D, Flanagan D P 1979 Subclavian and innominate artery trauma. Surgery 86: 890–897

Lin L F H, Doherty D H, Lile J D et al 1993 GDNF: a glial cell line-derived neurotrophic factor for midbrain dopaminergic neurons. Science 260: 1130–1132

Linarte R, Gilbert A 1986 Trans-sacral approach to the sacral plexus. In: Peripheral nerve repair and regeneration. vol 4, p 17–20

Lindå H, Risling M, Shupliakov O et al 1993 Changes in the synaptic input to lumbar motorneurons after intermedullary axotomy in the adult cat. Thesis (Lindå H), Karolinska Institutet

Linderoth B, Gunasekera L, Meyerson B A 1991 Effects of sympathectomy on skin and muscle circulation during dorsal column stimulation: animal studies. Neurosurgery 29: 874–979

Lindsey D 1980 The idolatry of velocity, or lies, damn lies and ballistics. Journal of Trauma 20: 1068–1069 (editorial)

Linington C, Brostoff S W 1993 Peripheral nerve antigens. In: Dyck P J, Thomas P K, Griffin J W, Low P A, Poduslo J F (eds) Peripheral neuropathy, 3rd edn. W B Saunders, Philadelphia, p 404–417

Linscheid R L, Wheeler D K 1965 Elbow dislocation. Journal of the American Medical Association 194: 1171–1176

Linson M A, Leffert R, Todd D P 1983 The treatment of upper extremity reflex sympathetic dystrophy with prolonged continuous stellate ganglion blockade. Journal of Hand Surgery 8: 153–159

Linton S J 1986 Behavioral remediation of chronic pain: a status report. Pain 24: 125–141

Lipkin A F, Coker N J, Jenkins H A et al 1987 Intracranial and intratemporal facial neuroma. Otolaryngology – Head and Neck Surgery 96 (1): 71–79

Lipscomb P R, Sanchez J J 1961 Anterior transplantation of the posterior tibial tendon for persistent palsy of the common peroneal nerve. Journal of Bone and Joint Surgery 43A: 60–66

Lipton S 1968 Percutaneous electrical cordotomy in relief of intractable pain. British Medical Journal 2: 210–212

Lisney S J W 1989 Regeneration of unmyelinated axons after injury of mammalian peripheral nerve. Quarterly Journal of Experimental Physiology 74: 757–784

Lister G 1988 Emergency free flaps. In: Green D P (ed) Operative hand surgery, 2nd edn. Churchill Livingstone, Edinburgh, vol 2, p 1127–1149

Lister G D, Belsole R B, Kleinert H E 1979 The radial tunnel syndrome. Journal of Hand Surgery 4: 52–59

Littler E 1949 Tendon transfer and arthrodeses in combined median and ulnar nerve paralysis. Journal of Bone and Joint Surgery 31A: 225–234

Liveson J A 1984 Nerve lesions associated with electrodiagnostic study of 11 cases. Journal of Neurology, Neurosurgery and Psychiatry 47: 742–744

Livingstone E F, DeLisa J A, Halar E M 1984 Electrodiagnostic values through the thoracic outlet using C8 needle studies, F waves and cervical somatosensory potentials. Archives of Physical Medicine and Rehabilitation 65: 726–730

Loeser J D, Ward A A 1967 Some effects of deafferentation on neurons of the cat spinal cord. Archives of Neurology 17: 629–636

Loeser J D, Ward A, White L E 1968 Chronic deafferentation of human spinal cord neurons. Journal of Neurosurgery 29: 48–50

Loeser J D, Black R G, Christman A 1975 Relief of pain by transcutaneous stimulation. Journal of Neurosurgery 42: 308–314

Loh L, Nathan P W 1978 Painful peripheral states and sympathetic block. Journal of Neurology, Neurosurgery and Psychiatry 41: 664–671

London P S 1961 Simplicity of approach to treatment of the injured hand. Journal of Bone and Joint Surgery 43B: 454–464

London P S 1967 A practical guide to the care of the injured. E & S Livingstone, Edinburgh, p 664

Longo M F, Clagett T O, Fairbairn J F 1970 Surgical treatment of thoracic outlet compression. Annals of Surgery 171: 538–542

Lord J W 1971 Thoracic outlet syndromes. Annals of Surgery 173: 700–705

Lotem M, Fried A, Levy M et al 1971 Radial palsy following muscular effort. Journal of Bone and Joint Surgery 53B: 500–506

Louis D S, Greene T L, Noeller T R C 1985 Complications of carpal tunnel surgery. Journal of Neurosurgery 62: 352–356

Low P A, McLeod J G, Turtle J R et al 1974 Peripheral neuropathy in acromegaly. Brain 97: 139–152

Low P A, Wilson P R, Sandroni P et al 1996 Clinical characteristics of patients with reflex sympathetic dystrophy in the USA. Progress in Pain Research and Management 6: 49–77

Lowden I M R 1985 Superficial peroneal nerve entrapment. Journal of Bone and Joint Surgery 67B: 58–59

Luce E A, Griffen W O 1978 Shotgun injuries of the upper extremity. Journal of Trauma 18: 487–492

Luco J V, Eyzaguirre C 1955 Fibrillation and hypersensitivity to ACh in denervated muscle: effects of length on degenerated nerve fibers. Journal of Neurophysiology 18: 65–73

Lundberg A 1948 Potassium and the differential thermosensitivity of membrane potential, spike and negative after potential in mammalian A and C fibres. Acta Physiologica Scandinavica 15 (suppl 50): 1–67

Lundborg G 1979 The intrinsic vascularization of human peripheral nerves: structural and functional effects. Journal of Hand Surgery 4: 34–41

Lundborg G 1988a Intraneural microcirculation. Orthopaedic Clinics of North America 19: 1–12

Lundborg G 1988b Vascular systems. In: Nerve Injury and Repair. Churchill Livingstone, Edinburgh, p 32–63

Lundborg G 1988c Nerve regeneration. In: Nerve injury and repair. Churchill Livingstone, Edinburgh, p 149–195

Lundborg G 1988d The nerve trunk. In: Nerve injury and repair. Churchill Livingstone, Edinburgh, p 32–63

Lundborg G 1991 Neurotropism, frozen muscle grafts and other conduits. Journal of Hand Surgery 16B: 473–476

Lundborg G, Rydevik B 1973 Effects of stretching the tibial nerve of the rabbit: preliminary study of the intraneural circulation of the barrier function of the perineurium. Journal of Bone and Joint Surgery 55B: 390–401

Lundborg G, Dahlin L, Danielson N 1991 Ulnar nerve repair by the silicone chamber technique: case report. Scandinavian Journal of Plastic and Reconstructive Hand Surgery 25: 79–82

Lundborg G, Rosén B, Abrahamsson S O et al 1994a Reorganisation and orientation of regenerating nerve fibres, perineurium and epineurium in preformed mesothelial tubes. An experimental study on sciatic nerves in rats. Journal of Neuroscience Research 6: 265–281

Lundborg G, Rosén B, Abrahamsson S O et al 1994b Tubular repair of the median nerve in the human forearm: preliminary findings. Journal of Hand Surgery 19B: 273–276

Lundborg G, Rosén B, Dahlin L et al 1997 Tubular versus conventional repair of median and ulnar nerves in the human forearm: early results from a prospective, randomised clinical study. Journal of Hand Surgery 22A: 99–106

Lupi-Herrera E, Sanchez-Torres G, Marcushamer J, Mispireta J, Horwitz S 1977 Takayasu's arteritis – clinical study of 107 cases. American Heart Journal 93: 94–103

Lusk M D, Kline D G, Garcia C A 1987 Tumour of the brachial plexus. Neurosurgery 21: 439–453

Lynn B 1977 Cutaneous hyperalgesia. British Medical Bulletin 33: 103–108

McAllister R M R, Gilbert S E A, Calder J S et al 1996 The epidemiology and management of upper limb peripheral nerve injuries in modern practice. Journal of Hand Surgery 21B: 4–13

McAuliffe T B, Fiddian N J, Browett J P 1985 Entrapment neuropathy of the superficial peroneal nerve. Journal of Bone and Joint Surgery 67B: 62–63

McCleery A S, Kersterson J E, Kirtley J A 1951 Subclavius and anterior scalene muscle compression as a cause of intermittent obstruction of the subclavian vein. Annals of Surgery 133: 588–602

McClelland S J 1990 The couse of the superior gluteal nerve in the lateral approach to the hip. Journal of Bone and Joint Surgery 72A: 791

McComas A J, Sica R E P, Banarjee S 1978 Long-term effects of partial limb amputation in man. Journal of Neurology, Neurosurgery and Psychiatry 41: 425–432

McConachie I, McGeachie J 1995 Brachial plexus block. In: Healey T E J, Cohen P J (eds) Wylie and Churchill-Davidson's A Practice of Anaesthesia. Edward Arnold, London, Boston, Sydney etc, p 726–729

McCready R A, Procter C D, Hyde G L 1986 Subclavian axillary vascular trauma. Journal of Vascular Surgery 3: 24–31

McDonald W I 1963 The effects of experimental demyelination on conduction in peripheral nerves: a histological and electrophysiological study. Brain 86: 501–524

McDonald W I, Sears T A 1970 The effects of experimental demyelination on conduction in the central nervous system. Brain 93: 583–598

MacDonell R A L, Schwartz M S, Swash M 1990 Carpal tunnel syndrome: which finger should be tested? An analysis of sensory conduction in digital branches of the median nerve. Muscle and Nerve 13: 601–606

McFarland G B, Hoffer M M 1971 Paralysis of the intrinsic muscles of the hand secondary to lipoma in Guyon's canal. Journal of Bone and Joint Surgery 53A: 375–379

McGonagle T K, Levine S T, Donofrio P D et al 1990 Spectrum of patients with EMG features of polyradiculopathy without neuropathy. Muscle and Nerve 13: 63–69

McGregor I A, Jackson I T 1972 The groin flap. British Journal of Plastic Surgery 25: 3–16

Mackinnon S E 1996 Nerve allotransplantation following severe tibial nerve injury. Journal of Neurosurgery 84: 671–676

Mackinnon S E, Dellon A L 1985 Two point discrimination tester. Journal of Hand Surgery 10A: 906–907

Mackinnon S E, Dellon A L 1986 Experimental study of chronic nerve compression. Hand Clinics 2: 639–650

Mackinnon S E, Dellon A L 1988a Ischaemia of nerve. In: Surgery of the peripheral nerve. Thieme, New York, p 56

Mackinnon S E, Dellon A L 1988b Ischaemia of nerve: loss of vibration sensibility. In: Surgery of the peripheral nerve. Thieme, New York, p 57

Mackinnon S E, Dellon A L 1988c Injection injury. In: Surgery of the peripheral nerve. Thieme, New York, p 59–62

Mackinnon S E, Dellon A L, Hudson A R et al 1984 Chronic nerve compression – an experimental model in the rat. Annals of Plastic Surgery 13: 112–120

Mackinnon S E, Dellon A L, Hudson A R et al 1985 A primate model for chronic nerve compression. Journal of Reconstructive Surgery 1: 185–195

Mackinnon S E, Dellon A L, Hudson A R et al 1986 Chronic human nerve compression – a histological assessment. Neuropathology and Applied Neurobiology 12: 547–565

McLachlan E M, Janig W, Devor M et al 1993 Peripheral nerve injury triggers noradrenergic sprouting within dorsal root ganglia. Nature 363: 543–545

McLeod J G 1993a Para-neoplastic neuropathies. In: Dyck P J, Thomas P K (eds) Peripheral neuropathy, 3rd edn. W B Saunders, Philadelphia, vol III, p 1583–1590

McLeod J G 1993b Peripheral neuropathy associated with lymphomas, leukaemias and polycythaemia vera. In: Dyck P J, Thomas P K (eds) Peripheral neuropathy, 3rd edn. W B Saunders, Philadelphia, vol II, p 1591–1598

McManis P G, Low P A, Lagerlund T D 1993 Microenvironment of nerve: blood flow and ischaemia. In: Dyck P J, Thomas P K, Griffin J W, Low P A, Poduslo J F (eds) Peripheral neuropathy, 3rd edn. W B Saunders, Philadelphia, p 433–440

McQueen M M, Court-Brown C-M. 1996 Compartment monitoring in tibial fractures. Journal of Bone and Joint Surgery 78B: 99–104

McQueen M M, Christie J, Court-Brown C M 1996 Acute compartment syndrome in tibial diaphyseal fractures. Journal of Bone and Joint Surgery 78B: 95–98

Madrid R, Bradley W G 1975 The pathology of neuropathies with focal thickening of the myelin sheath (tomaculous neuropathy). Journal of Neurosurgical Sciences 25: 415–448

Magalon G, Lebreton E, Benaim L J 1993 Compression of the ulnar nerve at the elbow. In: Tubiana R (ed) The hand. W B Saunders, Philadelphia, vol IV, p 433–440

Magris C 1989 Danube. Tr Creagh P. Collins Harvill, p 204

Maher J 1995 Management of adverse effects following breast radiotherapy. Report of the Maher Committee, Royal College of Radiologists, London

Makins G H 1919 On gunshot injuries to the blood vessels: founded on experience during the Great War 1914–1918. Wright, London

Mallett J 1972 Paralysie obstétricale du plexus brachial. Revue de Chirurgie Orthopedique 58: 115–204

Malt R S 1964 Replantation of severed arms. Journal of the American Medical Association 189: 716

Manktelow R T 1988 Free muscle transfers. In: Green D P (ed) Operative hand surgery, 2nd edn. Churchill Livingstone, Edinburgh, vol 2, p 1215–1244

Manktelow R T 1993 Functional microsurgical muscle transplantation. In: Tubiana R (ed) The hand. W B Saunders, Philadelphia, vol IV, p 313–318

Manktelow R T, Mckee N H 1978 Free muscle transplantation to provide active finger flexion. Journal of Hand Surgery 3: 416–426

Manty H P W, Rogers S D, Honore P et al 1997 Inhibition and hyperalgesia by ablation of lamina 1 spinal neurons expressing the substance P receptor. Science 278: 275–279

Maor P, Levy M, Lotem M et al 1972 Iatrogenic Volkmann's ischaemia – a result of pressure transfusion. International Surgery 57: 415–416

Maran A G D 1994 Otorhinolaryngology. In: Powers M J, Harris N H (eds) Medical Negligence, 2nd edn. Butterworths, London, p 1022–1040

Marchettini P, Cline M, Ochoa J L 1990 Innervation territories for touch and pain afferents of single fascicles of the human ulnar nerve. Mapping through intraneural microrecording and microstimulation. Brain 113 (5): 1491–1500

Mariano A J 1992 Chronic pain and spinal cord injury. Clinical Journal of Pain 8: 87–92

Marie P, Foix C 1913 Atrophie isolée de l'éminence thénar d'origine nevritique. Role du ligament annulaire antérieur du carpe dans la pathogénie du lésion. Revue Neurologique 26: 647–649

Mark V H, Ervin F R, Hackett T P 1960 Clinical aspects of stereotactic thalamotomy in the human. Part 1. The treatment of chronic pain. Archives of Neurology 3: 351–367

Mark V H, Ervin F R, Yakovlev P I 1963 Stereotactic thalamotomy. Part 3. The verification of anatomical lesion sites in the human thalamus. Archives of Neurology 8: 528–538

Marmor L, Lawrence J F, Dubois E L 1967 Posterior interosseous nerve palsy due to rheumatoid arthritis. Journal of Bone and Joint Surgery 49A: 381–383

Marris H H, Peters B H 1976 Pronator syndrome: clinical and electrophysiological features in seven cases. Journal of Neurology, Neurosurgery and Psychiatry 39: 461–464

Marshall R W, de Silva R D 1986 Computerised tomography in traction lesions of the brachial plexus. Journal of Bone and Joint Surgery 68B: 734–738

Marshall R W, Williams D H, Birch R et al 1988 Operations to restore elbow flexion after brachial plexus injuries. Journal of Bone and Joint Surgery 70B: 577–582

Martin J, Tomkins G H, Hutchinson M 1983 Peripheral neuropathy in hypothyroidism – an association with spurious polycythaemia (Gaisbock's syndrome). Journal of the Royal Society of Medicine 76: 187–189

Martin W A, Kraft G H 1974 Shoulder girdle neuritis: a clinical and electrophysiological evaluation. Military Medicine 139: 21–25

Martini A, Fromm B 1989 A new operation for the prevention and treatment of amputation neuromas. Journal of Bone and Joint Surgery 71B: 379–382

Martini R, Schachner M 1986 Immunoelectron microscopic localization of neural cell adhesion molecules (L1, N-CAM and MAG) and their shared carbohydrate epitope and myelin basic protein in developing sciatic nerve. Journal of Cell Biology 103: 2439–2448

Maruyama Y, Mylrea M M, Logothetis J 1967 Neuropathy following radiation. American Journal of Roentgenology 101: 216–219

Mass D P, Ciano M C, Tortosa R et al 1984 Treatment of painful hand neuromas by their transfer into bone. Plastic and Reconstructive Surgery 74: 182–185

Masson P, Martin J F 1938 Rhabdomyomes des Nerfs. Bulletin de L'Association Française pour l'Etude de Cancer 27: 751–767

Match R M 1974 Radiation-induced brachial plexus paralysis. Archives of Surgery 110: 384–386

Mathes S J, Mathai F 1979 Clinical atlas of muscle and myocutaneous flaps. C V Mosby, St Louis

Matsen F A 1975 The compartmental syndrome: a unified concept. Clinical Orthopaedics and Related Research 113: 8–14

Matsen F A 1980 Compartmental syndromes. Grune & Stratton, New York

Matthews P B C 1981 Evolving views of the internal operation of and functional role of the muscle spindle. Journal of Physiology (London) 320: 1–30

Maudsley R H 1967 Fibular tunnel syndrome. Journal of Bone and Joint Surgery 49B: 384

May A G, Deweese J A, Rob C G 1969 Changes in sexual function following operation on the abdominal aorta. Surgery 65: 41–47

Mayer J H, Tomlinson D R 1983 Axonal transport of cholinergic transmitter enzymes in vagus and sciatic nerves of rats with acute experimental diabetes mellitus: correlation with motor nerve conduction velocity and effects of insulin. Neuroscience 9: 951–957

Maynard C W, Leonard R B, Coulter J D et al 1977 Central connections of ventral root afferents as demonstrated by the HRP method. Journal of Comparative Neurology 172: 601–608

Mayo-Robson A W 1917 Nerve grafting as a means of restoring function in limbs paralysed by gunshot or other injuries. British Medical Journal I: 117–118

Medical Research Council War Memorandum No. 13 1944 Arterial Injuries. Early diagnosis and treatment. The Vascular Sub-committee of the MRC War Wounds Committee. HMSO, London

Medical Research Council 1954 Seddon H J (ed) Peripheral nerve injuries. Special Report Series No 282. HMSO, London

Mehler W R, Feferman M E, Nauta W J H 1960 Ascending axon degeneration following anterolateral cordotomy: an experimental study in the monkey. Brain 83: 718–750

Mellgren S I, Conn D L, Stevens J C et al 1989 Peripheral neuropathy in primary Sjögren's syndrome. Neurology 39: 390–394

Melsaac G, Kiernan J A 1975 Acceleration of neuromuscular re-innervation by triiodothyronine. Journal of Anatomy 120: 551–560

Melville S, Sherburn T E, Coggeshall R E 1989 Preservation of sensory cells by placing stumps of transected nerve in an impermeable tube. Experimental Neurology 105: 311–315

Melzack R 1975 The McGill pain questionnaire. Pain 1: 277–299

Melzack R, Wall P D 1965 Pain mechanisms: A new theory. Science 150: 971–979

Mense S 1977 Nervous outflow from skeletal muscle following chemical noxious stimulation. Journal of Physiology (London) 267: 75–88

Mense S, Meyer H 1981 Response properties of group III and IV receptors in the achilles tendon of the cat. Pflügers Archiv 389: R25

Mense S, Schmidt R F 1974 Activation of group IV afferent units from muscle by algesic agents. Brain Research 72: 305–310

Merle D'Aubigné R, Postel M 1956 Traitement des séquelles de la retraction ischaemique des fléchisseurs. Maladie de Volkmann. Chirurgie Orthopédique des Paralysies. Masson et Cie, Paris

Merle d'Aubigné R, Ramadier J 1956 Paralysies du membre supérieur. Masson, Paris

Merle M, Amend P, Cour C et al 1986 Microsurgical repair of peripheral nerve lesions: a study of 150 injuries of the median and ulnar nerves. Peripheral Nerve Repair and Regeneration 2: 17–26

Merle M, Duprez K, Delandre D et al 1988 La neurolyse microchirurgicale des plexites brachiales postradiothérapiques. Chirurgie 114: 421–423

Merle M, Foucher G, Dap F et al 1993 Tendon transfer for treatment of the paralysed hand following brachial plexus injury. In: Tubiana R (ed) The Hand. W B Saunders, Philadelphia, vol IV, p 632–637 (English translation)

Merrington W R, Nathan P W 1949 A study of post-ischaemic paraesthesiae. Journal of Neurology, Neurosurgery and Psychiatry 12: 1–18

Merskey H M 1986 Classification of chronic pain: descriptions of chronic pain syndromes and definitions of pain terms prepared by the International Association for the Study of Pain Subcommittee on Taxonomy. Pain (suppl 3): 1–226

Merton P A 1953 Speculations on the servo control of movement. In: Wolstenholme E E W (ed) The spinal cord. Churchill, London, p 247–255

Mesgarzadeh M, Schenk C D, Bonakdarpoura A 1989a Carpal tunnel: MR imaging. Part 1. Normal anatomy. Radiology 171: 743–748

Mesgarzadeh M, Schenk C D, Bonakdarpoura A 1989b Carpal tunnel: MR imaging. Part II. Carpal tunnel syndrome. Radiology 171: 749–754

Messina A, Messina J C 1995 Transposition of the ulnar nerve and its vascular bundle for the entrapment syndrome at the elbow. Journal of Hand Surgery 20B: 638–651

Meyer M 1931 Paralysie obstétricale des membres inférieurs. Revue D'Orthopedique 18: 767–771

Meyer V E 1982 Langzeit result nach Nervenreconstrucktion Bereich des Plexus lumbalis – Ein Fallbericht. Hand Chirurgie Mikrochirurgie Plastische Chirurgie 14: 11–13

Meyer V E 1991 Major limb replantation and revascularisation. In: Meyer V E, Black M J M (eds) Microsurgical procedures. Vol 7. Hand and upper limb series. Churchill Livingstone, Edinburgh, p 37–68

Michelow B J, Clarke H M, Curtis C G et al 1994 The natural history of obstetrical brachial plexus palsy. Plastic and Reconstructive Surgery 93: 675–680

Mikami Y, Nagano A, Ochiai N, Yamamotos S 1997 Results of nerve grafting for injuries of the axillary and suprascapular nerves. Journal of Bone and Joint Surgery 79B: 527–531

Mikhail I K 1964 Median nerve lipoma of the hand. Journal of Bone and Joint Surgery 46B: 726–730

Millender L H, Nulebuff E A, Holdsworth D E 1973 Posterior interosseous nerve syndrome secondary to rheumatoid arthritis. Journal of Bone and Joint Surgery 55A: 753–757

Miller E M 1924 Late ulnar nerve palsy. Surgery, Gynecology and Obstetrics 38: 37–46

Miller R A 1939 Observations upon the arrangement of the axillary artery and brachial plexus. Journal of American Anatomy 64: 143–163

Miller R G 1979 The cubital tunnel syndrome: diagnosis and precise localisation. Annals of Neurology 6: 56–59

Miller R G 1991 Ulnar neuropathy at the elbow. Muscle and Nerve 14: 97–101

Millesi H 1977 Surgical management of brachial plexus injuries. Journal of Hand Surgery 2: 367–379

Millesi H 1968 Zum problem der Uberbrükung von Defecten peripheren nerven. Wiener Medizinische Wochenschrift 118: 182–187

Millesi H 1973 Microsurgery of peripheral nerves. Hand 5: 157–160

Millesi H 1980 Interfascicular nerve repair and secondary repair with nerve grafts. In: Jewitt D L, McCarroll H R Jr (eds) Nerve repair and regeneration. C V Mosby Company, St Louis, p 299–319

Millesi H 1981 Interfascicular nerve grafting. Orthopaedic Clinics of North America 12: 287–301

Millesi H 1987 Lower extremity nerve lesions. In: Terzis J (ed) Microreconstruction of nerve injuries. W B Saunders, Philadelphia, p 239–251

Millesi H 1988 Brachial plexus injuries. Clinical Orthopaedics and Related Research 237: 36–42

Millesi H 1991 Brachial plexus in adults: operative repair. In: Gelberman R H (ed) Operative nerve repair and reconstruction. J B Lippincott, Philadelphia, p 1285–1302

Millesi H, Zöch G, Rath T 1990 The gliding apparatus of peripheral nerve and its clinical significance. Annals of Hand Surgery 9: 87–97

Mills K R 1985 Orthodromic sensory action potentials from palmar stimulation in the diagnosis of carpal tunnel syndrome. Journal of Neurology, Neurosurgery and Psychiatry 48: 250–255

Mills W G 1949 A new neonatal syndrome. British Medical Journal 2: 464–466

Mixter W J, Barr J S 1934 Rupture of the intervertebral disc with involvement of the spinal canal. New England Journal of Medicine 211: 210–215

Miyauchi A, Ishikawa H, Matsusaka K et al 1993 Treatment of recurrent laryngeal nerve paralysis by several types of nerve suture. Journal of the Japanese Surgical Society 94: 550–555

Mizuguchi T 1976 Division of the pyriformis muscle for the treatment of sciatica. Archives of Surgery 111: 719–722

Mizuno K, Muratsu H, Kurosaka M et al 1990 Compression neuropathy of the suprascapular nerve as a cause of pain in palsy of the accessory nerve. Journal of Bone and Joint Surgery 72A: 938–939

Moberg E 1958 Objective methods for determining the functional value of sensibility in the hand. Journal of Bone and Joint Surgery 40B: 454–476

Moberg E 1975 Surgical treatment for absent single hand grip and elbow extension in quadriplegics. Journal of Bone and Joint Surgery 57A: 196–206

Moberg E 1976 Reconstructive hand surgery in tetraplegia, stroke and cerebral palsy. Some basic concepts in physiology and neurology. Journal of Hand Surgery 21: 29–34

Moberg E, Lamb D W 1980 Surgical rehabilitation of the upper limb in tetraplegia. Proceedings of the International Conference in Edinburgh. The Hand 12: 209–213

Molnar G E 1984 Brachial plexus injury in the newborn. Paediatrics Review 6: 110–115

Mondrup K, Olsen N K, Pfeiffer P et al 1990 Clinical and electro-diagnostic findings in breast cancer patients with radiation-induced brachial plexus neuropathy. Acta Neurologica Scandinavica 81: 153–158

Monforte R, Estrach R, Valls-Sole J et al 1995 Autonomic and peripheral neuropathies in patients with chronic alcoholism. Archives of Neurology 52: 45–51

Montgomery P Q, Goddard N J, Kemp H B S 1989 Solitary osteochondroma causing sural nerve entrapment neuropathy. Journal of the Royal Society of Medicine 82: 761

Moore J R 1971 Bone block to prevent posterior dislocation of the shoulder. In: Crenshaw A H (ed) Campbell's operative orthopaedics, 5th edn. C V Mosby, St Louis, p 1724

Moore M E, Berk S N, Nypaver J 1984 Chronic pain: in-patient treatment with small group effects. Archives of Physical Medicine and Rehabilitation 65: 356–361

Moossy J J, Nashold B S, Osborne D et al 1987 Conus medullaris root avulsions. Journal of Neurosurgery 66: 835–841

Morelli E, Raimondi P L, Saporiti E 1984 Il loro trattamento precoce. In: Pipino F (ed) Le paralisi ostetriche. Aulo Gaggi, Bologna, p 57–76

Morgan M H 1989 Nerve conduction studies. British Journal of Hospital Medicine 41: 22–36

Morley G H 1964 Intraneural lipoma of the median nerve in the carpal tunnel. Journal of Bone and Joint Surgery 46B: 734–735

Morley J 1913 Brachial plexus pressure neuritis due to a normal first thoracic rib: its diagnosis and treatment by excision of the rib. Clinical Journal 42: 461–463

Morris G C, Beall A C, Roof W R et al 1960 Surgical experience with 220 acute arterial injuries in civilian practice. American Journal of Surgery 99: 775–780

Morris J H, Hudson A H, Weddell G 1972 A study of degeneration and regeneration in the divided rat sciatic nerve based on electron microscopy. IV. Changes in fascicular microtopography. The perineurium and endoneurial fibroblasts. Zeitschrift für Zellforschung 124: 165–203

Morton T G 1876 A peculiar and painful affection of the fourth metatarsophalangeal articulations. American Journal of Medical Sciences 71: 37–45

Mountcastle V B 1980 In: Mountcastle V B (ed) Medical physiology, 14th edn. C V Mosby, St Lovis, p 61–63

Moxley R T 1991 Hereditary metabolic disorders in infancy and childhood. In: Swash M, Oxbury J (eds) Clinical Neurology. Churchill Livingstone, Edinburgh, p 1642–1643

Mubarak S J, Carroll N C 1979 Volkmann's contracture in children: aetiology and prevention. Journal of Bone and Joint Surgery 61B: 285–293

Mukherjee J J, Patel V, Dacie J E et al 1996 When imaging fails: pre-operative localization and treatment of a ganglioneuroma. Journal of the Royal Society of Medicine 89: 409–410

Mulder J D 1951 The causative mechanism in Morton's metatarsalgia. Journal of Bone and Joint Surgery 33B: 94–95

Mulder D S, Greenwood F A H, Brooks C E 1973 Post-traumatic thoracic outlet syndrome. Journal of Trauma 13: 705–715

Mulholland R C 1966 Non-traumatic progressive paralysis of the posterior interosseous nerve. Journal of Bone and Joint Surgery 48B: 781–783

Mumenthaler M 1964 Armplexus paresen in Anschluss an Röntgenbestrahlung. Mitteilung von 8 eigenen Beobachtungen. Schweizerische Medizinische Wochenschrift 94: 399–406

Munglani R, Hunt J P 1995 Molecular biology of pain. British Journal of Anaesthesia 75: 186–192

Murphy J B 1897 Resection of arteries and veins injured in continuity. End-to-end suture. Experimental and Clinical Research. Medical Record 51: 73–88

Murphy J B 1905 A case of cervical rib with symptoms resembling subclavian aneurysm. Annals of Surgery 41: 399–406

Murphy J J 1996 Current practice and complications of temporary transvenous cardiac pacing. British Medical Journal 312: 1134

Murphy T 1910 Brachial neuritis caused by pressure of first rib. Australian Medical Journal 15: 582–585

Murray G 1940 Heparin in surgical management of blood vessels. Archives of Surgery 40: 307–325

Murray I P C, Simpson J A 1958 Acroparaesthesia in myxoedema: a clinical and electromyographic study. Lancet i: 1360–1363

Mussad M, LoCicero J, Matano J et al 1991 Endoscopic thoracic sympathectomy. Lasers in Surgery and Medicine 11: 18–25

Myles M, Glasby M A 1992 The fate of muscle spindles after various methods of nerve repair in the rat. Neuroorthopaedics 13: 15–23

Naffziger H C, Grant W T 1938 Neuritis of the brachial plexus mechanical in origin. Surgery, Gynecology and Obstetrics 67: 722–730

Nagano A, Obinaga S, Ochiai N et al 1989a Shoulder arthrodesis by external fixation. Clinical Orthopaedics and Related Research 247: 97–100

Nagano A, Tsuyama N, Ochiai N et al 1989b Direct nerve crossing with the intercostal nerve to treat avulsion injuries of the brachial plexus. Journal of Hand Surgery 14A (b): 980–985

Nagano A, Ochiai N, Sugioka H et al 1989c Usefulness of myelography in brachial plexus injuries. Journal of Hand Surgery 14B: 59–64

Nagano A, Shibata K, Tokimura H et al 1996 Spontaneous anterior interosseous nerve palsy with hourglass-like fascicular constriction within the main trunk of the median nerve. Journal of Hand Surgery 21A: 266–270

Nahabidian M Y, Wittstadt E, Wilgis E F S 1995 Median nerve injury following YAG Laser carpal tunnel release. Journal of Hand Surgery 20A: 361–362

Nakano N K 1978 The entrapment neuropathies. Muscle and Nerve 1: 264–279

Napier J R 1995 The form and function of the carpa metacarpal joint at the thumb. Journal of Anatomy 89: 362–369

Narakas A O 1977 Indications et resultats du traitement chirurgicale dans les lésions par élongation du plexus brachial. Revue de Chirurgie Orthopédique et Réparatrice de l'Appareil Moteur 63: 44–45

Narakas A O 1978 Surgical treatment of traction injuries of the brachial plexus. Clinical Orthopaedics and Related Research 133: 71–90

Narakas A O 1981a Brachial plexus surgery. Orthopaedic Clinics of North America 12: 303–322

Narakas A O 1981b The effects on pain of reconstructive neurosurgery in 160 patients with traction and/or crush injury to the brachial plexus. In: Siegfried J, Zimmerman M (eds) Phantom and stump pain. Springer–Verlag, Berlin, p 126

Narakas A O 1984a Traumatic brachial plexus lesions. In: Dyck P J, Thomas P K, Lambert E H, Bunge R (eds) Peripheral neuropathy, 2nd edn. W B Saunders, Philadelphia, p 1394–1409

Narakas A O 1984b Operative treatment for radiation induced and metastatic brachial plexopathy in 45 cases, 15 having omentoplasty. Bulletin of the Hospital for Joint Diseases, Orthopaedic Institute 44: 354–375

Narakas A O 1985 Problems and challenges. Journal of Hand Surgery 10A: 992

Narakas A O 1986 Editorial "The Lumbosacral Plexus" Peripheral nerve repair and regeneration 4: 10

Narakas A O 1987a Obstetrical Brachial Plexus Injuries. In: Lamb D W (ed) The paralysed hand. Churchill Livingstone, Edinburgh, p 116–135

Narakas A O 1987b Thoughts on neurotization of nerve transfers in irreparable nerve lesions. In: Terzis J K (ed) Microreconstruction of nerve injuries. W B Saunders, Philadelphia, p 447–454

Narakas A O 1988 The use of fibrin glue in repair of peripheral nerves. Orthopaedic Clinics of North America 19: 187–199

Narakas A O 1991 Compression and traction neuropathies about the shoulder and arm. In: Gelberman R H (ed) Operative nerve repair and reconstruction. J B Lippincott, Philadelphia, p 1147–1176

Narakas A O 1987 Traumatic brachial plexus injuries. In: Lamb D W (ed) The Paralysed Hand. Churchill Livingstone, Edinburgh: p 100–115

Narakas A O 1989 Lésions du nerf axillaire et lésions associées du nerf suprascapulaire. Revue Médicale de la Suisse Romande 109: 545–556

Narakas A O 1993a Cervicobrachial compression. In: Tubiana R (ed) The hand. W B Saunders, Philadelphia, p 352–389

Narakas A O 1993b Multiple compressions. In: Tubiana R (ed) The hand. W B Saunders, Philadelphia, p 517–527

Narakas A O 1993c Paralytic disorders of the shoulder girdle. In: Tubiana R (ed) The hand. W B Saunders, Philadelphia, vol IV, p 112–125

Narakas A O, Bonnard C 1993 Epicondylalgia: conservative and surgical treatment. In: Tubiana R (ed) The hand. W B Saunders, Philadelphia, p 833–857

Narakas A O, Verdan C 1969 Les greffes nerveuses. Zeitschrift für Unfallchirurgie, Versicherungsmedizin und Berufskrankheiten 3: 137–152

Nashold B S 1981 Modification of lesion of DREZ technique. Journal of Neurosurgery 55: 1012

Nashold B S 1984 Current status of the DREZ operations 1984. Neurosurgery 15: 942–944

Nashold B S, Bullitt E 1981 Dorsal root entry zone lesions to control central pain in paraplegics. Journal of Neurosurgery 55: 414–419

Nashold B S, Friedman H 1972 Dorsal column stimulation for control of pain. Preliminary report on 30 patients. Journal of Neurosurgery 36: 590–597

Nashold B S, Ostdahl R H 1979 Dorsal root entry zone lesions for pain relief. Journal of Neurosurgery 51: 59–69

Nashold B S, Slaughter D G 1969 Effects of stimulating or destroying the deep cerebellar regions in man. Journal of Neurosurgery 31: 172–186

Nashold B S Jr, Wilson W P, Slaughter D G 1969a Sensation evoked by stimulation in the midbrain of man. Journal of Neurosurgery 30 (1): 14–24

Nashold B S, Wilson W P, Slaughter D G 1969b Stereotaxic midbrain lesions for central dysesthesia and phantom pain. Preliminary report. Journal of Neurosurgery 30 (2): 116–126

Natali J, Benhamou A C 1979 Iatrogenic vascular injuries: a review of 125 cases excluding angiographic injuries. Journal of Cardiovascular Surgery 20: 169–176

Nathan H 1960 Gangliform enlargement of the lateral cutaneous nerve of the thigh. Journal of Neurosurgery 17: 843–850

Nathan P A, Kenistin R C, Meadows K D 1995 Outcome study of ulnar nerve compression at the elbow treated with simple decompression and an early programme of physical therapy. Journal of Hand Surgery 20B: 628–637

Nathan P W 1947 On the pathogenesis of causalgia in peripheral nerve injuries. Brain 70: 145–171

Nathan P W 1977 Pain. British Medical Bulletin 33: 149–158

Nathan P W 1983 Pain and the sympathetic system. Journal of the Autonomic Nervous System 7: 363–370

Nathan P W, Smith M G 1987 The location of descending fibres to sympathetic preganglionic vasomotor and sudomotor neurons in man. Journal of Neurology, Neurosurgery and Psychiatry 50: 1257–1262

Nathaniel E J M, Nathaniel D R 1973 Regeneration of dorsal root fibers into the adult rat spinal cord. Experimental Neurology 40: 333–350

Neary D, Eames R A 1975 The pathology of ulnar nerve compression in man. Neuropathology and Applied Neurobiology 1: 69–88

Neary D, Ochoa J, Gilliatt R W 1975 Subclinical entrapment neuropathy in man. Journal of the Neurological Sciences 24: 283–298

Nelson K R, Bicknell J M 1987 Oblique pectoral crease and "scapular hump" in shoulder contour are signs of trapezius muscle weakness. Journal of Neurology, Neurosurgery and Psychiatry 50: 1082–1083

Nemni R, Bottachi E, Fazio R et al 1987 Polyneuropathy in hypothyroidism: clinical electrophysiological and morphological findings in four cases. Journal of Neurology, Neurosurgery and Psychiatry 50: 1454–1460

Nemoto K, Matsomoto N, Tazaki K et al 1987 An experimental study on the "double crush" hypothesis. Journal of Hand Surgery 12A: 552–559

Nercessian O A, Gonzalez E G, Stinchfield F E 1989 The use of somatosensory evoked potential during revision or reoperation for total hip arthroplasty. Clinical Orthopaedics and Related Research 243: 138–141

Newmark J, Levy S R, Hochberg F H 1985 Somatosensory evoked potentials in thoracic outlet syndrome. Archives of Neurology 42: 1036

Nicholas G G, Noone R B, Graham W P 1971 Carpal tunnel syndrome in pregnancy. The Hand 3: 80–83

Nichols J S, Lillehei K O 1988 Nerve injury associated with acute vascular trauma. Surgical Clinics of North America 68: 837–852

Nicholson D A 1991 Arterial injury following shoulder trauma: a report of two cases. British Journal of Radiology 64: 961–963

Nicholson M L, Hopkinson B R 1993 Endoscopic transthoracic sympathectomy of the upper limb. Hospital Update September: 500–505

Nicholson M L, Hopkinson B R, Dennis M J S 1994 Endoscopic transthoracic sympathectomy: successful in hyperhidrosis but can the indications be extended? Annals of the Royal College of Surgeons of England 76: 311–314

Nicoladoni C 1880 Ein Vorschlag zur Sehnennaht Wiener Medizinische Wochenschrift 30: 1413–1417

Nicoll E A 1952 Traumatic dislocation of the hip joint. Journal of Bone and Joint Surgery 34: 503–505

Nissen K I 1948 Planter digital neuritis. Journal of Bone and Joint Surgery 30B: 84–94

Nittner K 1976 Spinal meningeomas, neurinomas and neurofibromas and hour glass tumours. In: Vinken P J, Bruyn G W (eds) Handbook of Clinical Neurology. North Holland, Amsterdam, vol 20, p 177–322

Noordenbos W 1959 Pain. Problems pertaining to the transmission of nerve impulses which give rise to pain. Elsevier, Amsterdam

Noordenbos W, Wall P D 1981 Implications of the failure of nerve resection and graft to cure chronic pain produced by nerve lesions. Journal of Neurology, Neurosurgery and Psychiatry 44: 1068–1073

Nórden A 1946 Peripheral injuries to the spinal accessory nerve. Acta Chirurgica Scandinavica 94: 515–532

Norris A H, Shock N W, Wagman I H 1953 Age changes in the maximum conduction velocity of motor fibres of human ulnar nerves. Journal of Applied Physiology 5: 589–593

North R B, Ewend M G, Lawton M T et al 1991 Spinal cord stimulator for chronic, intractable pain: superiority of "multi-channel devices". Pain 44: 119–130

Notter G, Turesson I 1975 Strahlenbedingte Veränderungen im Bereich des peripheren Nervensystems. Deutscher Röntgen-Kongress, Berlin (unpublished)

Novak C B, Collins E D, Mackinnon S E 1995 Outcome following conservative management of thoracic outlet syndrome. Journal of Hand Surgery 20A: 542–548

Nulsen F E, Slade H W 1956 Recovery following injury to the brachial plexus. In: Woodhall B, Beebe G W (eds) Peripheral nerve regeneration. V A Medical Monograph, ch 9, p 389

Nunley J A, Gabel G 1991 Axillary nerve. In: Gelberman R H (ed) Operative Nerve Repair and Reconstruction. J B Lippincott, Philadelphia. p 437–452

Ober F R 1933 Tendon transplantation in the lower extremity. New England Journal of Medicine 209: 52–59

Ober W B 1992 Obstetrical events that shaped Western European history. The Yale Journal of Biology and Medicine 65: 201–210

Oberlin C, Alnot J Y 1986 Common peroneal nerve pedicle graft in repair of sciatic trunk. Peripheral Nerve Repair and Regeneration 4: 45–49

Oberlin C, Bastian D, Gréant P 1994 Les Lambeaux pédiculés pour couverture des membres. Expansion Scientifique Française, Paris

Oberlin C, Beal D, Bhatia A et al 1995 Nerf cubital (ulnaire), neurotisation du muscle biceps. In: Alnot J-Y, Narakas A (Eds) Les

paralysies du plexus brachial, 2nd edn. Monographie De La Société Française De Chirurgie De La Main, Paris, p 46–49

O'Brien B McC. 1975 Microsurgery in the treatment of injuries. In: McKibbin B (ed) Recent advances in orthopaedics. Churchill Livingstone, Edinburgh, p 235–279

Ochiai N, Nagano A, Akinaga S et al 1988 Brachial plexus injuries: surgical treatment of combined injuries of the axillary and suprascapular nerves. Journal of the Japanese Society of the Surgery of the Hand 5: 151–155

Ochiai N, Nagano A, Mikami Y, Yamamoto S 1997 Full exposure of the axillary and suprascapular nerves. Journal of Bone and Joint Surgery 79B: 532–533

Ochoa J, Mair W G P 1969 The normal sural nerve in man. II. Changes in the axons and Schwann cells due to ageing. Acta Neuropathologica (Berlin) 13: 217–239

Ochoa J, Marotte L 1973 The nature of the nerve lesion caused by chronic entrapment in the guinea-pig. Journal of the Neurological Sciences 19: 491–495

Ochoa J, Torebjörk H E 1983 Sensations evoked by intraneural microstimulation of single mechanoreceptor units innervating the human hand. Journal of Physiology 342: 633–654

Ochoa J, Torebjörk H E 1989 Sensations induced by intraneural microstimulation of C nociceptor fibres in human skin nerves. Journal of Physiology 415: 583–599

Ochoa J, Fowler T J, Gilliat R W 1972 Anatomical changes in peripheral nerves compressed by pneumatic tourniquet. Journal of Anatomy 113: 433–455

Ochs S, Barnes C D 1969 Regeneration of ventral root fibers into dorsal roots shown by axoplasmic flow. Brain Research 15: 600–603

Ochs S, Brimijoin W S 1993 Axonal transport. In: Dyck P J, Thomas P K, Griffin J W, Low P A, Poduslo J F (eds) Peripheral neuropathy, 3rd edn. W B Saunders, London, p 331–360

Ochsner A, Gage M, DeBakey M 1935 Scalenus anterior (Naffziger) syndrome. American Journal of Surgery 28: 699–695

Odling-Smee G W 1970 960 Civilian casualties in the Nigerian civil war. British Medical Journal 2: 592–596

O'Duffy J D, Randall R V, MacCarty C S 1973 Median neuropathy (carpal tunnel syndrome) in acromegaly. Annals of Internal Medicine 78: 379–383

Ogden J A 1972 An unusual branch of the median nerve. Journal of Bone and Joint Surgery 54A: 1779–1781

Oh S J, Thomas W A, Park K H et al 1991 Electrophysiological improvement following decompression surgery in tarsal tunnel syndrome. Muscle and Nerve 14: 407–410

Okutsu I 1987 Universal endoscope. Journal of Japanese Orthopaedic Association 61: 491–498

Olàrte M, Adams D 1977 Accessory nerve palsy. Journal of Neurology, Neurosurgery and Psychiatry 40: 1113–1116

Oleksak M, Edge A J 1992 Compression of the sciatic nerve by methylacrylate cement. Journal of Bone and Joint Surgery 74B: 729–730

Olsen N K, Pfeiffer P, Mondrup K, Rose C 1990 Radiation-induced brachial plexus neuropathy in breast cancer patients. Acta Oncologica 29: 885–895

Olsen N K, Pfeiffer P, Johannsen L et al 1993 Radiation-induced brachial plexopathy: neurological follow-up in 161 recurrence-free breast cancer patients. International Journal of Radiation, Oncology, Biology and Physics 26: 43–49

Olsen W L 1993 Reflex sympathetic dystrophy with tumour infiltration of the stellate ganglion. Journal of the Royal Society of Medicine 86: 482–483

Olson N D, Meng-Fong J, Quast J E et al 1978 Peripheral neuropathy in myotonic dystrophy. Archives of Neurology 35: 741–745

Omer G E 1974 Injuries to nerves of the upper extremity. Journal of Bone and Joint Surgery 56A: 1615–1624

Omer G E Jr 1980a The results of untreated traumatic injuries. In: Omer G E, Spinner M (eds) Management of peripheral nerve problems. W B Saunders, London, p 502–506

Omer G 1980b Range of conduction velocities. In: Omer E G, Spinner M (eds) Management of peripheral nerve problems. W B Saunders, Philadelphia p 6–7

Omer G E 1987 The management of pain. In: Lamb D W (ed) The paralysed hand. Churchill Livingstone, Edinburgh, p 216–231

Omer G E 1991 Nerve injuries associated with gunshot wounds of the extremities. In: Gelberman R H (ed) Operative nerve repair and reconstruction. J B Lippincott, Philadelphia, p 655–676

Omer G, Thomas S 1972 Treatment of causalgia: review of cases at Brooke General Hospital. Texas Medical Journal 67: 93–96

Orcutt M B, Levine B A, Root M D et al 1983 The continuing challenge of popliteal vascular injuries. American Journal of Surgery 146: 758–761

Orgel M G 1987 Epineurial versus perineurial repair of peripheral nerves. In: Terzis J K (ed) Microreconstruction of nerve injuries. W B Saunders, London, p 97–100

Osborne G V 1957 The surgical treatment of tardy ulnar neuritis. Journal of Bone and Joint Surgery 39B: 782

Osborne G V 1970 Compression neuritis of the ulnar nerve at the elbow. The Hand 2: 10–13

Osgaard O, Eskesen V, Rosenørn J 1987 Microsurgical repair of iatrogenic accessory nerve lesions in the posterior triangle of the neck. Acta Chirurgica Scandinavica 153: 171–173

Osterman A L 1988 The double crush syndrome. Orthopaedic Clinics of North America 19: 147–155

Osterman A L 1991 The double crush syndrome. In: Gelberman R H (ed) Operative nerve repair and reconstruction. J B Lippincott, Philadelphia, p 1211–1229

Ottolenghi C E 1971 Prophylaxie du syndrome de Volkmann dans les fractures supracondyliennes du coude chez l'enfant. Revue Chirurgie Orthopedique 57: 517–525

Oudot J, Cormier J B 1953 La localisation la plus fréquente de l'artérite segmentaire: celle de la fémorale superficielle. Presse Médicale 67: 1361–1364

Ovelmen-Levitt J, Blumenkopf B, Sharpe R et al 1982 Electrical activity and neuropeptide localization in the lumbar dorsal horn after dorsal root avulsion and rhizotomy in the cat. Society of Neuroscience Abstracts 8: 94

Ovelmen-Levitt J, Johnson B, Bedenbaugh P et al 1984 Dorsal root rhizotomy and avulsion in the cat: a comparison of long term effects on dorsal horn neuronal activity. Journal of Neurosurgery 15 (6): 921–927

Owen R, Tsimboukis B 1967 Ischaemia complicating tibial and fibular shaft fractures. Journal of Bone and Joint Surgery 49B: 268–275

Owen-Smith M S 1981 High velocity missile wounds. Edward Arnold, London

Pace J B, Nagle 1976 Piriform syndrome. The Western Journal of Medicine 124: 435–439

Pagni C A 1989 Central pain due to spinal cord and brain stem damage. In: Wall P D, Melzack R (eds) Textbook of pain. Churchill Livingstone, Edinburgh, p 634–655

Palande D D 1973 A review of twenty-three operations on the ulnar nerve in leprous neuritis. Journal of Bone and Joint Surgery 55A: 1457–1464

Pallis C M 1966 The neuropathies of rheumatoid arthritis. Journal of the Royal College of Physicians of London 1: 19–28

Pallis C M, Scott J J 1965 Peripheral neuropathy in rheumatoid arthritis. British Medical Journal 1: 1141–1147

Palumbo L T 1956 Anterior transthoracic approach for upper thoracic sympathectomy. Archives of Surgery 72: 659–666

Panas 1878 Sur une cause peu connue de paralysie du nerf cubital. Archives Générale de Médicine 2: 5–22

Panegyres P K, Moore N, Gibson R et al 1993 Thoracic outlet syndromes and magnetic resonance imaging. Brain 116: 823–841

Paradiso G, Grañana N, Maza E 1997 Prenatal brachial plexus injury. Neurology 49: 261–262

Parkes A R 1945 Traumatic ischaemia of peripheral nerves, with some observations of Volkmann's ischaemic contracture. British Journal of Surgery 32: 403–414

Parkes A R 1951 The treatment of established Volkmann's contracture by tendon transplantation. Journal of Bone and Joint Surgery 33B: 359–362

Parkes A R 1959 Treatment of traumatic ischaemia of muscle and nerve. Journal of Bone and Joint Surgery 41B: 628–629

Parkes A R 1961 Intraneural ganglion of the lateral popliteal nerve. Journal of Bone and Joint Surgery 43B: 784–790

Parkhouse N, Le Quesne P 1988 Quantitative objective assessment of peripheral nociceptive C fibre function. Journal of Neurology, Neurosurgery and Psychiatry 51: 28–34

Parks B J 1973 Postoperative peripheral neuropathies. Surgery 74: 348–357

Parry E W, Eastcott H H G 1992 Cervical rib and thoracic outlet syndrome. In: Eastcott H H G (ed) Arterial surgery, 3rd edn. Churchill Livingstone, Edinburgh, p 333–353

Parsonage M T, Turner J W A 1948 Neuralgic amyotrophy. Lancet i: 973–978

Pasila M, Kivikioto O, Jaroma H et al 1980 Recovery from primary shoulder dislocation and its complications. Acta Orthopaedica Scandinavica 51: 257–262

Patel A N, Lalitha V S, Dastur D K 1968 The spindle in normal and pathological muscle. Brain 91: 737–750

Patey D W, Campbell M J, Hughes D 1974 Carcinomatous neuropathy: immunological studies. Journal of Neurology, Neurosurgery and Psychiatry 37: 142–151

Patrick J 1946 Fracture of the medial epicondyle with displacement into the elbow joint. Journal of Bone and Joint Surgery 28: 143–147

Patterson F P, Morton K S 1973 Neurological complications of fractures and dislocations of the pelvis. Journal of Trauma 12: 1013–1024

Patterson M, Dunkerton M, Birch R et al 1990 Reinnervation of the suprascapular nerve in brachial plexus injuries. Journal of Bone and Joint Surgery 72B: 993

Patterson V H, Boddie H G 1977 Anterior tibial compartment syndrome with alcohol abuse. British Medical Journal 1: 269–270

Paul R L, Goodman H, Merzenich M 1972 Alterations in mechanoreceptor input to Brodmann's areas 1 and 3 of the postcentral area of Macaca mulatta after nerve section and regeneration. Brain Research 39: 1–19

Payan J 1969 Electrophysiological localization of ulnar nerve lesions. Journal of Neurology, Neurosurgery and Psychiatry 32: 208–220

Payan J 1970 Anterior transposition of the ulnar nerve: an electrophysiological study. Journal of Neurology, Neurosurgery and Psychiatry 33: 157–165

Payan J 1986 An electromyographer's view of the ulnar nerve. Journal of Bone and Joint Surgery 68B: 13–15

Payan J 1987 Nerve injury. In: Taylor T H, Major E (eds) Hazards and complications of anaesthesia. Churchill Livingstone, Edinburgh, p 392–400

Pearce J M S 1996 Tinel's sign of formication. Journal of Neurology, Neurosurgery and Psychiatry 61: 61

Pecina M 1979 Contribution to the aetiologic explanation of the piriformis syndrome. Acta Anatomica 105: 181–7

Peet R M, Henriksen J D, Anderson P T et al 1956 Thoracic outlet syndrome: evaluation of a therapeutic exercise program. Proceedings of Staff Meetings of the Mayo Clinic 31: 281–287

Pellegrini V D, McCollister Evarts C 1991 Compartment syndromes. In: Rockwood A C, Green D P, Bucholz R W (eds) Fractures, 3rd edn. J B Lippincott, Philadelphia, vol 1, p 390–416

Peltonen J, Jaakola S, Lebwohl M et al 1988 Cellular differentiation and expression of matrix genes in type 1 neurofibromatosis. Laboratory Investigation 59: 760–771

Penfield W, Boldrey E 1937 Somatic motor and sensory representation in the cerebral cortex of man as studied by electrical stimulation. Brain 60: 389–443

Penfield W, Rasmussen T 1950 The cerebral cortex of man. Macmillan, New York

Perry M O, Thal E R, Shires G T 1971 Management of arterial injuries. Annals of Surgery 173: 403–408

Pert C B, Snyder S H 1979 Opiate receptors: demonstration in nervous tissue. Science 179: 1011–1014

Peterson G W, Will A D 1988 Newer electrical techniques in peripheral nerve injuries. Orthopedic Clinics of North America 19: 13–25

Petrera J E 1991 Neuralgic amyotrophy. A clinical and electrophysiological study. Doctorate of Medicine Thesis, University of Copenhagen

Petrera J E, Trojaborg W 1984 Conduction studies of the long thoracic nerve in serratus anterior palsy of different etiology. Neurology 34: 1033–1037

Petrucci F S, Morelli A, Raimondi P L 1982 Axillary nerve injuries: 21 cases treated by nerve graft and neurolysis. Journal of Hand Surgery 7: 271–278

Peyron R, Garcia-Larrea L, Deiter M P et al 1995 Electrical stimulation of precentral cortical area in the treatment of central pain: electrophysiological and positron emission tomography study. Pain 62: 275–286

Pfeffer G, Osterman A L, Chow J 1986 Double crush syndrome: cervical radiculopathy and carpal tunnel syndrome. Journal of Hand Surgery 11A: 766

Phalen G S 1966 The carpal-tunnel syndrome. Journal of Bone and Joint Surgery 48A: 211–228

Phalen G S 1972 The carpal-tunnel syndrome. Clinical Orthopaedics and Related Research 83: 29–40

Phalen G S 1981 The birth of a syndrome, or carpal-tunnel revisited. Journal of Hand Surgery 6: 109–110

Phillips L H, Park T S 1991 Electrophysiological mapping of the segmental anatomy of the muscles of the lower extremity. Muscle and Nerve 14: 1213–1218

Pho R W H 1991 Vascularised bone grafts in upper extremity reconstruction. In: Meyer V E, Black M J M (eds) Microsurgical procedures. The hand and upper limb series No 7. Churchill Livingstone, Edinburgh, p 158–171

Pierquin B, Mazeron J J, Glaubiger D 1986 Conservative treatment of breast cancer in Europe: report of the Groupe Européen De Curiethérapie. Radiotherapy and Oncology 6: 187–198

Pike J, Hollingsworth R 1995 Audit of post-operative auto-transfusion of shed blood in arthroplasty. Journal of the Royal Society of Medicine 88: 522P–523P

Platt H 1928 On the peripheral nerve complications of certain fractures. Journal of Bone and Joint Surgery 10: 402–414

Platt H 1973 Obstetrical paralysis: a vanishing chapter in orthopaedic surgery. The Bulletin of the Hospital of Joint Diseases 34: 4–21

Po B T, Hansen R 1969 Iatrogenic brachial plexus injury. Anaesthesia and Analgesia 48: 915–922

Poggio G F, Mountcastle V B 1963 The functional properties of ventrobasal thalamic neurons studies in unanaesthetized monkeys. Journal of Neurophysiology 26: 775–806

Politis M J, Spencer P S 1983 An in vivo assay of neurotropic activity. Brain Research 278: 229–231

Pollard J D 1993 Neuropathy in diseases of the thyroid and pituitary glands. In: Dyck P J, Thomas P K, Griffin J W, Low P A, Poduslo J F (eds) Peripheral neuropathy, 3rd edn. W B Saunders, Philadelphia, p 1266–1274

Pollock L J, Golseth J G, Arieff A J 1946 The response of muscle to electrical stimuli during degeneration, denervation and regeneration. Military Neuropsychiatry 25: 236–257

Pomeranz B, Wall P D, Weber W W 1968 Cord cells responding to fine myelinated afferents from viscera, muscle and skin. Journal of Physiology 199: 511–532

Pomeranz B, Mullen M, Markus H 1984 Effect of applied electrical fields on sprouting of intact saphenous nerve of rabbit. Brain Research 303: 331–336

Porter M F 1967 Arterial injuries in an accident unit. British Journal of Surgery 54: 100–105

Posniak H V, Olson M C, Dudiak C M et al 1993 MR imaging of the brachial plexus. American Journal of Roentgenology 161: 373–379

Post M, Hashell S S 1974 Reconstruction of the median nerve following entrapment in supracondylar fracture of the humerus. Journal of Trauma 14: 252–264

Powell R J 1996 New roles for thalidomide. British Medical Journal 313: 377–378

Power C 1994 National trends in birth weight. British Medical Journal 308: 1270–1271

Preston D C, Logigan E L 1992 Lumbrical and interossei recording in carpal tunnel syndrome. Muscle and Nerve 15: 1253–1257

Price D D, Mayer D J 1974 Physiological laminar organization of the dorsal horn of M Mulatta. Brain Research 79: 321–325

Pringle J A S 1996 Osteosarcoma: the experiences of a specialist unit. Current Diagnostic Pathology 3: 127–136

Pringle J H 1913 Two cases of vein grafting for the maintenance of a direct arterial circulation. Lancet i: 1795

Privat J M, Mailhe D, Allieu Y et al 1982 Precoce hemilaminectomie cervicale exploratrice et neurotisation du plexus brachial. In: Simon L (ed) Plexus brachiale et medecine de ré-éducation. Masson, Paris, p 66–73

Proctor H 1973 Dislocations of the hip joint (excluding "central" dislocations) and their complications. Injury 5: 1–12

Pulvertaft R G 1964 Unusual tumours of the median nerve. Journal of Bone and Joint Surgery 46B: 731–733

Pulvertaft R G 1983 Report of the committee on paralytic diseases including leprosy. Paralytic Diseases Committee of the International Federation of Societies for Surgery of the Hand. Journal of Hand Surgery 8: 745–748

Purcell S M, Dixon S L 1989 Schwannomatosis. An unusual variant of neurofibromatosis or a distinct clinical entity. Archives of Dermatology 125: 390–393.

Puri R, Clark J, Corkery P H 1985 Axillary artery damage following closed fracture of the neck of the humerus. Injury 16: 426–427

Putnam J J 1880 A series of cases of paraesthesia, mainly of the hand, of periodical recurrence, and possibly of vaso-motor origin. Archives of Medicine (New York) 4: 147–162

Putti V 1932 Analisi della triada radiosintomatica degli stati di prelussazione. Chirurgia degli Organi di Movimento XVII: 453–459

Raaf J 1955 Surgery for cervical rib and scalenus anticus syndrome. Journal of the American Association 157: 219–223

Räf L 1966 Double vertical fractures of the pelvis. Acta Chirurgica Scandinavica 131: 298–305

Raimondi P 1993 Evaluation of results in obstetric brachial plexus palsy. The hand. Paper read to the International Meeting on Obstetric Brachial Plexus Palsy, Heerlen 1993

Rajashekter R P, Herbison G J 1974 Lumbosacral plexopathy caused by retroperitoneal haemorrhage: report of two cases. Archives of Physical Medicine and Rehabilitation 55: 91–93

Raji A R M, Bowden R E M 1983 Effects of high-peak electromagnetic field on the degeneration and regeneration of the common peroneal nerve in rats. Journal of Bone and Joint Surgery 65B: 478–493

Raju S 1979 Shotgun arterial injuries of the extremities. American Journal of Surgery 138: 421–425

Ramon y Cajal S 1928a Late conditions shown by the nerve sprouts of the central stump and of the scar. In: May R M (trans, ed) Degeneration and regeneration in the nervous system. Oxford University Press, London, p 198–222

Ramon y Cajal S 1928b Neurotrophic action of distal stump. In: May R M (trans, ed) Degeneration and regeneration in the nervous system. Oxford University Press, London, p 196

Ramon y Cajal S 1928c Regeneration from the proximal stump. In: May R M (trans, ed) Degeneration and regeneration in the nervous system. Oxford University Press, London, p 194

Ramon y Cajal S 1928d Historical notes concerning degeneration and regeneration of the nerves. In: May R M (trans, ed) Degeneration and regeneration in the nervous system. Oxford University Press, London, p 3–26

Ramon y Cajal S 1954 In: Purkiss W U, Fox CA (trans) Neuron theory or reticular theory? Consejo Superior de Investigaciones Cientificas Instituto "Ramon y Cajal", Madrid

Rang H P, Urban L 1995 New molecule in analgesia. British Journal of Anaesthesia 75: 145–156

Ransford A O, Hughes S P F 1977 Complete brachial plexus lesions. Journal of Bone and Joint Surgery 59B: 417–442

Ranson S W 1915 Unmyelinated nerve fibres as conductors of protopathic sensation. Brain 38: 381–389

Rao S B, Crawford A H 1995 Median nerve entrapment after dislocation of the elbow in children. Clinical Orthopaedics and Related Research 312: 232–237

Rapoport S, Blair D N, McCarthy S M et al 1988 Brachial plexus: correlation of MR Imaging with CT and pathological findings. Radiology 167: 161–165

Rasminsky M 1985 Conduction in normal and pathological nerve fibres. In: Swash M, Kennard C (eds) Scientific basis of clinical neurology. Churchill Livingstone, Edinburgh, p 390–399

Ratliff A H C 1984 Neurological complications. In: Ling R S M (ed) Complications of total hip replacement. Churchill Livingstone, Edinburgh p 23–29

Rate J A, Parkinson R W, Meadows T H et al 1992 Acute carpal tunnel syndrome due to pseudo-gout. Journal of Hand Surgery 17B: 217–218

Redler M, Ruland L J, McCue F C 1986 Quadrilateral space syndrome in a throwing athlete. American Journal of Sports Medicine 14: 511–513

Redmond M D, Rivner M H 1988 False positive electrodiagnostic tests in carpal tunnel syndrome. Muscle and Nerve 11: 511–517

Reis N S 1980 Anomalous triceps tendon as a cause for snapping elbow and ulnar neuritis: a case report. Journal of Hand Surgery 5: 361–362

Renaut J 1881a Récherches sur quelques points particuliers de l'histologie des nerfs. Archives de Physiologie Normale et Pathologique 8: 161–190

Renaut J 1881b Système hyalin de soutinement des centres nerveux et de quelques organes des sens. Archives de Physiologie Normale et Pathologique 8: 845–860

Retif J, Brihaye J, Vander Haegen J J 1967 Syndrome douloureux "thalamique" et lésion pariétale. A propos de trois observations de tumeur à localisation pariétale, étant accompagnés de douleurs spontanées de l'hemicorps contralatéral. Neurochirurgie 13: 375–384

Rexed B 1952 The cytoarchitectonic organisation of the spinal cord in the cat. Journal of Comparative Neurology 96: 415–495

Rexed B 1954 A cytoarchitectonic organization of the spinal cord in the cat. Journal of Comparative Neurology 100: 297–379

Rexed B 1964 Some aspects of the cytoarchitectonics and synaptology of the spinal cord. Progress in Brain Research 11: 58–92

Reynolds D V 1969 Surgery in the rat during electrical analgesia induced by focal brain stimulation. Science 164: 444–445

Reynolds R R, McDowell H A, Diethelm A G 1979 The surgical treatment of arterial injuries in the civilian population. Annals of Surgery 189: 700–707

Riccardi V M 1990 Neurofibromatosis. Recent Advances in Clinical Neurology 6: 186–208

Rich K M, Alexander T D, Pryor J C, Hollowell J P 1989 Nerve growth factor enhances regeneration through silicone chambers. Experimental Neurology 105: 162–170

Rich N M, Spencer F C 1978 Vascular trauma. W B Saunders, Philadelphia

Rich N M, Baugh J H, Hughes C W 1970 Acute arterial injuries in Vietnam: 1000 cases. Journal of Trauma 10: 359–369

Rich N M, Jarstfer B S, Greer T M 1974 Popliteal artery repair failure: causes and possible intervention. Journal of Cardiovascular Surgery 13: 340–351

Rich N M, Hobson R W, Collins G J 1975 Traumatic arteriovenous fistulae and false aneurysms: a review of 558 lesions. Surgery 78: 817–828

Richards B M 1989 Interosseous transfer of tibialis posterior for common peroneal palsy. Journal of Bone and Joint Surgery 71B: 834–837

Richards P, Kennedy I M, Woolf H 1996 Managing medical mishaps. British Medical Journal 313: 243–244

Richards R L 1967 Causalgia. A centennial review. Archives of Neurology 16: 339–350

Richardson D E, Akill H 1977 Pain reduction by electrical brain stimulation in man. Journal of Neurosurgery 47: 178–183

Richardson P M, Thomas P K 1979 Percussive injury to peripheral nerve in rats. Journal of Neurosurgery 51: 178–187

Richter H P, Sertz K 1984 Dorsal root entry zone lesions for the control of deafferentation pain: experiences in ten patients. Neurosurgery 15: 956–959

Richter H P, Schachenmayr W 1984 Is the substantia gelatinosa the target in dorsal root entry zone lesions? An autopsy report. Neurosurgery 15: 913–916

Riley D A, Lang D H 1984 Carbonic anhydrase activity of human peripheral nerves: a possible histochemical aid to nerve repair. Journal of Hand Surgery 9A: 112–120

Riley D A, Ellis S, Bain J L W 1984 Ultrastructural cytochemical localization of carbonic anhydrase activity in rat peripheral sensory and motor nerves, dorsal root ganglia and dorsal column nuclei. Neuroscience 13: 189–206

Rinaldi P C, Young R F, Albe-Fessard D et al 1991 Spontaneous neuronal hyperactivity in the medial intralaminar thalamic nuclei of patients with deafferentation pain. Journal of Neurosurgery 74: 415–421

Risling M, Culheim S, Hildebrand C 1983 Reinnervation of the ventral root L7 from ventral horn neurons following intramedullary axotomy in adult cats. Brain Research 280: 15–23

Risling M, Fried K, Lindå H et al 1993 Regrowth of motor axons following spinal cord lesions. Distribution of laminin and collagen in the CNS scar tissue. Brain Research Bulletin 30: 405–411

Rivner M H, Swift T R, Crout B O et al 1990 Toward more rational nerve conduction interpretations: the effect of height. Muscle and Nerve 13: 232–239

Roaf R 1963 Lateral flexion injuries of the cervical spine. Journal of Bone and Joint Surgery 45B: 38

Rob C G, Standeven A 1956 Closed traumatic lesions of the axillary and brachial arteries. Lancet i: 597–599

Rob C G, Standeven A 1958 Arterial occlusion complicating thoracic outlet compression syndrome. British Medical Journal 2: 709–712

Robert R, Labat J J, Lehar P A et al 1989 Réflexions cliniques, neurophysiologiques et thérapeutiques à partir des donnes anatomiques sur le nerf pudendal (honteux interne) lors de certaines algies périnéales. Chirurgie 115: 515–520

Roberts W J 1986 A hypothesis on the physiological basis for causalgia and related pains. Pain 24: 297–311

Robertson D P, Simpson R K, Rose J E et al 1993 Video-assisted endoscopic thoracic sympathectomy. Journal of Neurosurgery 79: 238–240

Robinson D R 1947 Piriformis syndrome in relation to sciatic pain. American Journal of Surgery 73: 355–358

Robinson P 1994 Raw nerves. British Journal of Oral and Maxillofacial Surgery 32: 69–70

Rockwood C A, Thomas S C, Matsen P A 1991 Subluxations and dislocations about the gleno-humeral joint. In: Rockwood C A, Green D P, Bucholz R W (eds) Fractures. J B Lippincott, Philadelphia, vol 1, p 1021–1179

Rodeo S A, Forster R A, Weiland A J 1993 Neurological complications due to arthroscopy. Journal of Bone and Joint Surgery 75A: 917–926

Roles N C, Maudsley R H 1972 Radial tunnel syndrome. Journal of Bone and Joint Surgery 54B: 499–508

Rolfsen L 1970 Snapping triceps tendon with ulnar neuritis. Report on a case. Acta Orthopaedica Scandinavica 41: 74–76

Romanes G J 1946 Motor localization and the effects of nerve injury on the ventral horn cells of the spinal cord. Journal of Anatomy 80: 117–131

Rongioletto I F, Drago F, Renora A 1989 Multiple cutaneous plexiform schwannomas with tumour of the central nervous system. Archives of Dermatology 125: 431–432

Roos D B 1966 Transaxillary approach for first rib resection to relieve thoracic outlet syndrome. Annals of Surgery 163: 354–358

Roos D B 1971 Experience with first rib resection for thoracic outlet syndrome. Annals of Surgery 173: 429–442

Roos D B 1979 New concepts of thoracic outlet syndrome which explain etiology, symptoms, diagnosis and treatment. Vascular Surgery 13: 313–321

Roos D B 1981 Essentials and safeguards of surgery for thoracic outlet syndrome. Angiology 32: 187–192

Roos D B 1982 The place for scalenectomy and first-rib resection in thoracic outlet syndrome. Surgery 92: 1077–1085

Roos D B 1984 Axillary–subclavian vein occlusion. In: Rutherford R B (ed) Vascular surgery, 2nd edn. W B Saunders, Philadelphia, p 1385–1393

Roos D B 1987 Thoracic outlet syndrome: update 1987. American Journal of Surgery 154: 568–573

Roos D B 1995 Quoted by Earnshaw J J in conference report. Hospital Update 21: 422–423

Roos D B, Owens J C 1966 Thoracic outlet syndrome. Archives of Surgery 93: 71–74

Roos D B, Byars L T, Ackerman L V 1958 Neurilemmomas of the facial nerve presenting as parotid gland tumours. Annals of Surgery 144: 258–262

Rose D S C, Wilkins M J, Birch R et al 1992 Malignant peripheral nerve sheath tumour with rhabdomyoblastic and glandular differentiation. Immunohistochemical features. Histopathology 21: 287–290

Rosen I, Werner C O 1980 Neurophysiological investigation of posterior interosseous nerve entrapment causing lateral elbow pain. Electroencephalography and Clinical Neurophysiology 50: 125–133

Rosenbaum R B, Ochoa J L 1993a Carpal tunnel syndrome and other disorders of the median nerve. Butterworth-Heinemann, Oxford, p 71–125

Rosenbaum R B, Ochoa J L 1993b Carpal tunnel syndrome and other disorders of the median nerve. Butterworth-Heinemann, Oxford, p 127–175

Rosental J J, Gaspar M R, Gjerdrum T C et al 1976 Vascular injuries associated with fractures of the femur. Archives of Surgery 110: 494–499

Rosfors S, Eriksson M, Hoglund N et al 1993 Duplex ultrasound in patients with suspected aorto-iliac occlusive disease. European Journal of Vascular Surgery 7: 513–517

Rosin D 1993 Thoracoscopic cervicothoracic sympathectomy. In: Rosin D (ed) Minimal access medicine and surgery. Radcliffe Memorial Press, Oxford, p 250–252

Ross A, Birch R 1993 Reconstruction of the paralysed shoulder after brachial plexus injuries. In: Tubiana R (ed) The hand. W B Saunders, Philadelphia, vol 4, p 126–133 (English translation)

Ross D A, Schaffer K 1992 A case of malignant epithelioid schwannoma arising on the face. Journal of the Royal Society of Medicine 85: 237–238

Rossi L N, Vassella F, Mumenthaler M 1982 Obstetrical lesions of the brachial plexus. European Journal of Neurology 21: 1–7

Rosson J W 1987 Disability following closed traction lesions of the brachial plexus sustained in motor cycle accidents. Hand Surgery 12B: 353–355

Rosson J W 1988 Closed traction lesions of the brachial plexus – an epidemic among young motor cyclists. Injury 19: 4–6

Roth G, Magistris M R, Le Fort D et al 1988 Plexopathies post-radique. Bloc de conduction persistant. Décharges myokimiques et crampes. Revue Neurologique 144: 173–180

Roth W K 1895a Meralgia paraesthetica. S Karger, Berlin

Roth W K 1895b Meralgia paraesthetica. Meditsinskoye Obozrenie Sprimona 43: 678

Rousso T, Wexler M R 1988 Burns of the upper limb; medical and surgical treatment. In: Tubiana R (ed) The hand. W B Saunders, Philadelphia, vol III, p 794–818

Rowntree T 1949 Anomalous innervation of the hand muscles. Journal of Bone and Joint Surgery 31B: 505–510

Rubin A 1964 Birth injuries: incidence, mechanics and end results. Obstetrics and Gynaecology 23: 218–221

Rudge P 1974 Tourniquet paralysis with prolonged conduction block. Journal of Bone and Joint Surgery 56B: 716–720

Rudge P R, Ochoa J, Gilliatt R W 1974 Acute peripheral nerve compression in the baboon. Journal of Neurological Science 23: 403–420

Ruffini A 1897 Observations on sensory nerve-endings in voluntary muscle. Brain 20: 367–374

Rydevik B, McLean W G, Sjostrand J et al 1980 Blockage of axonal transport indiced by acute graded compression of the rabbit vagus nerve. Journal of Neurology, Neurosurgery and Psychiatry 43: 690–698

Rydevik B, Lundborg G, Bagge U 1981 Effects of graded compression on intraneural blood flow. Journal of Hand Surgery 6: 3–12

Sabour M S, Fadel H E 1970 The carpal tunelsyndrome as a new complication ascribed to the "pill". American Journal of Obstetrics and Gynecology 107: 1270

Saeed M A, Gatens P F 1982 Accessory nerve palsy: a hazard of lymph node biopsy. Military Medicine 147: 586–588

Saghal V, Morgan C A 1976 Histochemical and morphological changes in human muscle spindle in upper and lower motor neuron lesion. Acta Neuropathologica 34: 41–46

Salah S, Horcojada J, Perneczky A 1975 Spinal neurinomas – a comprehensive clinical and statistical study on 47 cases. Neurochirurgia 18: 77–84

Salsbury R E, Dingeldein G P 1988 The burnt hand and upper extremity. In: Green D P (ed) Operative hand surgery 2nd edn. Churchill Livingstone, Edinburgh, vol II, p 2135–2164

Sallström J, Celegin Z 1983 Physiotherapy in patients with thoracic outlet syndrome. Vasa 12: 257–261

Salner A L, Botnik L E, Herzog A G et al 1981 Reversible brachial plexopathy following primary radiation therapy for breast cancer. Cancer Treatment Reports 65: 797–802

Salob S P, Atherton D J, Kiely E M 1991 Thoracic endoscopic sympathectomy for palmar hyperhidrosis in an adolescent female. Journal of the Royal Society of Medicine 84: 114–115

Salzberg C A, Salisbury R E 1991 Thermal injury of peripheral nerve. In: Gelberman R H (ed) Operative nerve repair and reconstruction. J B Lippincott, Philadelphia, p 671–678

Samii M 1980 Repair of the facial nerve. In: Omer G E, Spinner M (eds) Management of peripheral nerve problems. W B Saunders, Philadelphia, p 527–533

Samii M, Moringane J R 1984 Thermocoagulation of the dorsal root entry zone for the treatment of intractable pain. Neurosurgery 15: 953–955

Samii M, Migliori M M, Tatgiba M, Babu R 1995 Surgical treatment of trigeminal schwannomas. Journal of Neurosurgery 82: 711–718

Sampaio E P, Sarno E N, Galilly R et al 1991 Thalidomide selectively inhibits tumour necrosis factor a production by stimulated human monocytes. Journal of Experimental Medicine 173: 699–703

Samson R, Pasternak B M 1980 Traumatic arterial spasm – rarity or nonentity. Journal of Trauma 20: 607–609

Sanders F K 1942 The repair of large gaps in the peripheral nerves. Brain 65: 281–337

Sanders F K, Young J Z 1946 The influence of peripheral connections on the diameter of regenerating nerve fibres. Journal of Experimental Biology 22: 203–212

Sanders R J, Haug C 1990 Subclavian vein obstruction and thoracic outlet syndrome: a review of etiology and management. Annals of Vascular Surgery 4: 397–410

Sanders R J, Haug C E 1991 Etiology. In: Thoracic outlet syndrome. A common sequela of neck injuries. J B Lippincott, Philadelphia, p 21–31

Sanders R J, Monsour J W, Gerber W F et al 1979 Scalenectomy versus first rib excision for treatment of the thoracic outlet syndrome. Surgery 85: 109–121

Sandmire H F, O'Halloin T J 1988 Shoulder dystocia: its incidence and associated risk factors. International Journal of Gynaecology and Obstetrics 26: 65–73

Sanjuanbenito L, Esteban A, Gonzalez-Martinez E 1976 Regeneration of the spinal ventral roots. Acta Neurochirurgica 34: 203–214

Santa M, Sulla I, Fagula J 1991 Verlagerungsoperation des N. ulnaris. Zentralblatt für Neurochirurgie 52: 127–129

Sapega A A, Heppenstall R B, Chance B et al 1985 Optimizing tourniquet application and release times in extremity surgery. Journal of Bone and Joint Surgery 67A: 303–314

Sargent P 1921 Lesions of the brachial plexus associated with rudimentary ribs. Brain 44: 95–124

Sato J, Perl E R 1991 Adrenergic excitation of cutaneous pain receptors induced by peripheral nerve injury. Science 251: 1608–1610

Savala P K, Nishihara T, Oh S J 1979 Meralgia paraesthetica: electrophysiological study. Archives of Physical Medicine and Rehabilitation 60: 30–31

Scadding J W 1981 Development of ongoing activity. Mechanosensitivity and adrenaline sensitivity in severed peripheral nerve axons. Experimental Neurology 73: 345–364

Scadding J W 1984 Ectopic impulse generation in damaged peripheral axons in abnormal nerves and muscles as impulse generators. In: Ochoa J, Culp W (eds) Abnormal nerves and muscles as impulse generators. Oxford University Press, Oxford

Scaglietti O 1938 The obstetrical shoulder trauma. Surgery, Gynecology and Obstetrics 66: 868–877

Schady W, Ochoa J L, Torebjörk H E 1983 Peripheral projections of fascicles in the human median nerve. Brain 106: 745–760

Scher L A, Veith F J, Haimovici H et al 1984 Staging of arterial complications of cervical rib: guidelines for surgical management. Surgery 95: 644–649

Schiller J C von 1801 Das Mädchen von Orléans. akt III, szene 2

Schmalzried T P, Amstutz H C 1991 Nerve injury and total hip arthroplasty. In: Gelberman R H (ed) Operative nerve repair and reconstruction. J B Lippincott, Philadelphia, p 1245–1254

Schoenen J 1973 Organisation cytoarchitectonique de la moelle épinière de différents mammifères et de l'homme. Acta Neurologiques (Belgium) 73: 348–358

Schott G D 1994 Visceral afferents: their contribution to "sympathetic-dependent" pain. Brain 117: 397–413

Schottstaedt E R, Larsen L J, Bost F C 1955 Complete muscle transposition. Journal of Bone and Joint Surgery 37A: 897–919

Schröder J M 1974a The fine structure of de- and re-innervated muscle spindles. I. The increase, atrophy of intrafusal muscle fibres. Acta Neuropathologica 30: 109–128

Schröder J M 1974b The fine structure of de- and re-innervated muscle spindles. II. Regenerated sensory and motor nerve terminals. Acta Neuropathologica 30: 129–144

Schröder J M, Kemme P T, Scholz L 1979 The fine structure of denervated and reinnervated muscle spindles: morphometric study of intrafusal nerve fibres. Acta Neuropathologica 46: 95–106

Schuind F A, Goldschmidt D, Bastin C et al 1995 A biomechanical study of the ulnar nerve at the elbow. Journal of Hand Surgery 20B: 623–627

Schulze F 1893 Ueber Akroparästhesie. Deutsche Zeitschrift für Nervenheilkunde 3: 300–318

Schwann T 1839 Mikroskopische Untersuchungen über die Übereinstimmung in der Struktur und dem Wachstum der Tiere und Pflanzen. Sander, Berlin

Schwartzmann J R, Crego C H 1948 Hamstring tendon transplantation for relief of quadriceps femoris paralysis in residual poliomyelitis. A follow up study of 134 cases. Journal of Bone and Joint Surgery 30A: 541–549

Seddon H J 1943 Three types of nerve injury. Brain 66: 237–288

Seddon H J 1947 The use of autogenous grafts for the repair of large gaps in peripheral nerves. British Journal of Surgery 35: 151–167

Seddon H J 1952 Carpal ganglion as a cause of paralysis of the deep branch of the ulnar nerve. Journal of Bone and Joint Surgery 34B: 386–390

Seddon H J (ed) 1954 Peripheral nerve injuries. MRC Special Report No. 222. HMSO, London

Seddon H J 1956 Volkmann's contracture. Treatment by excision of the infarct. Journal of Bone and Joint Surgery 38B: 152–174

Seddon H J 1963 Nerve grafting. Journal of Bone and Joint Surgery 45B: 447–461

Seddon H J 1964 Volkmann's ischaemia. British Medical Journal 1: 1587–1592

Seddon H J 1975a Preface to the first edition. Surgical disorders of the Peripheral Nerves, 2nd edn. Churchill Livingstone, Edinburgh, p ix

Seddon H J 1975b Mobilization of the nerve. Ibid, p 267–270

Seddon H J 1975c Ancillary examinations. Ibid, p 55–56

Seddon H J 1975d Loop suture. Ibid, p 279–280

Seddon H J 1975e Ganglion of common peroneal nerve. Ibid, p 125–126

Seddon H J 1975f Plantar digital neuroma. Ibid, p 126–129

Seddon H J 1975g Radiation neuropathy. Ibid, p 137–138

Seddon H J 1975h Ulnar nerve entrapment. Ibid, p 114–117

Sedel L 1977 Traitement palliatif d'une série de 103 paralysies par élongation du plexus brachial. Evolution spontanée et résultats. Revue de Chirurgie Orthopédique 63: 651–666

Sedel I 1987 Surgical management of lower extremity nerve lesions. In: Terzis JK (ed) Microreconstruction of nerve injuries. W B Saunders, Philadelphia, p 253–265

Sedel L 1988 Repair of severe traction lesion of the brachial plexus. Clinical Orthopaedics and Related Research 237: 62–63

Sedel L, Nizard R R 1993 Nerve grafting for traction injuries of the common peroneal nerve. A report of 17 cases. Journal of Bone and Joint Surgery 75B: 772–774

Sedel L, Alnot J Y, Raimondi P L et al 1989 Les tumeurs du plexus brachial. In: Alnot J Y, Narakas A (eds) Les paralysies du plexus brachial. Monographies du Groupe pour l'étude de la Main No 15. Expansion Scientifique Française, Paris

Seigel D B, Gelberman R H 1991 Peripheral nerve injuries associated with fractures and dislocations. In: Gelberman R H (ed) Operative nerve repair and reconstruction. J B Lippincott, Philadelphia, p 619–633

Seizinger B R, Martuza R L, Gusella J F 1986 Loss of genes on chromosome 22 in tumorigenesis of human acoustic neuroma. Nature 322: 644–647

Seltzer Z, Devor M 1979 Ephaptic transmission in chronically damaged peripheral nerves. Neurology 29: 1061–1064

Semple J C, Cargill A O 1969 Carpal tunnel syndrome. Results of surgical decompression. Lancet i: 918–919

Sen C N, Sekhar C N 1990 An extreme lateral approach to intradural lesions of the cervical spine and foramen magnum. Neurosurgery 28: 197–204

Sendtner M, Kreutzberg G W, Thoenen H 1990 Ciliary neurotrophic factor prevents the degeneration of motor neurons after axotomy. Nature 345: 440–441

Seradge H, Jia Y C, Owens W 1995 In vivo measurement of carpal tunnel pressure in the functioning hand. Journal of Hand Surgery 20A: 855–859

Seror P 1996 Anterior interosseous nerve lesions. Journal of Bone and Joint Surgery 78B: 238–241

Sever J W 1925 Obstetrical paralysis. Report of eleven hundred cases. JAMA 85: 1862–1865

Seyffarth H 1951 Primary myosis in the m. pronator teres as cause of lesion of the n. medianus (the pronator syndrome). Acta Psychiatrica et Neurologica Scandinavica 74 (suppl): 251–254

Shanghai Sixth People's Hospital 1976 Free muscle transplantation by microvascular neurovascular anastomoses. Chinese Medical Journal 2: 47–50

Sharma B S, Bannerjee A K, Kak V K 1989 Malignant schwannoma of the brachial plexus presenting as spinal cord compression. Neurochirurgia 32: 189–191

Sharpe W 1916 The operative treatment of brachial plexus paralysis. Journal of American Medical Association 66: 876

Sharrard W J W 1955 The distribution of the permanent paralysis in the lower limb in poliomyelitis. Journal of Bone and Joint Surgery 37B: 540–558

Sharrard W J W 1966 Posterior interosseous injuries. Journal of Bone and Joint Surgery 48B: 777–780

Sharrard W J W 1968 Anterior interosseous neuritis. Journal of Bone and Joint Surgery 50B: 804–806

Sharrard W J W 1971a Paediatric orthopaedics and fractures, 2nd edn. Blackwell, Oxford

Sharrard W J W 1971b Paediatric orthopaedics and fractures, 2nd edn. Blackwell, Oxford, p 904–908

Shaw J L, Sakellarides H 1967 Radial nerve paralysis. Journal of Bone and Joint Surgery 49A: 899–902

Shea J D, McClain E J 1969 Ulnar nerve compression syndromes at and below the wrist. Journal of Bone and Joint Surgery 51A: 1095–1105

Shealy C N, Mortimer J T, Reswick J B 1967 Electrical inhibition of pain by stimulation of the dorsal columns. Anaesthesia and Analgesia 46: 489–491

Sheean G L, Houser M K, Murray N M F 1995 Lumbrical–interosseous latency comparison in the diagnosis of carpal tunnel syndrome. Electroencephalography and Clinical Neurophysiology 97: 285–289

Sheehan K H 1987 Caesarean section for dystocia. A comparison of practices in two countries. Obstetrics and Gynaecology 59: 340–346

Shepard G H 1980 High-energy low velocity close range shotgun wounds. Journal of Trauma 20: 1065–1067

Sherrill J G 1913 Direct suture of brachial artery following rupture, result of traumatism. Annals of Surgery 58: 534–536

Sherrington C 1979 In: Denny-Brown D (ed) Selected writings of Sir Charles Sherrington. Oxford University Press, Oxford, p 158

Sherrington C S 1894 On the anatomical constitution of nerves of skeletal muscles: with remarks on recurrent fibres in the ventral spinal nerve-root. Journal of Physiology 17: 211–258

Sherrington S C 1903 Selectivity for a certain quality of stimulus. Journal of Physiology 30: 39

Shimpo T, Gilliatt R W, Kennet R P et al 1987 Susceptibility to pressure neuropathy distal to a constricting ligature in the guinea pig. Journal of Neurology, Neurosurgery and Psychiatry 50: 1625–1632

Shumacker H B 1990 Weglowski and what might have been. Australian and New Zealand Journal of Surgery 60: 219–224

Sidaway vs Board of Governors of the Bethlem Royal Hospital and the Maudsley Hospital 1984 Law Society Gazette Report 899

Siegel D B, Gelberman R G 1991 Peripheral neve injuries associated with fractures and dislocations. In: Gelberman R H (ed) Operative nerve repair and reconstruction. J B Lippincott, Philadelphia, p 619–633

Siegel D B, Kuzma G, Eakins D 1995 Anatomic investigation of the role of the lumbrical muscles in carpal tunnel syndrome. Journal of Hand Surgery 20A: 860–863

Silverton J S, Nahai F, Jurkiewicz M J 1978 The latissimus dorsi myocutaneous flap to replace a defect of the upper arm. British Journal of Plastic Surgery 31: 29–31

Simeone J F, Robinson F, Rothman S L G et al 1977 Computerised tomographic demonstration of a retroperitoneal haematoma causing femoral neuropathy. Report of two cases. Journal of Neurosurgery 47: 946–948

Simpson J A 1956 Electrical signs in the diagnosis of carpal tunnel and related syndromes. Journal of Neurology, Neurosurgery and Psychiatry 19: 275–280

Sinclair D C 1955 Cutaneous sensation and the doctrine of specific energy. Brain 78: 584–614

Sindou M 1972 Étude de la jonction radiculo-médullaire postérieure. La radicellotomie postérieure sélective dans la chirurgie de la douleur. Thèse, Lyons

Sindou M, Daher A 1988 Spinal cord ablative procedures for pain. In: Dubner R, Gebhart G F, Bond M R (eds) Proceedings of the 5th World Congress in Amsterdam. Elsevier, Amsterdam, p 477

Sindou M, Keravel Y 1980 Analgésie par la méthode d'électrostimulation transcutanée: résultats dans les douleurs neurologiques à propos de 180 cas. Neurochirurgie 26: 153–157

Sindou M, Mertens P 1993 Neurosurgical treatment of pain in the upper limb. In: Tubiana R (ed) The hand. W B Saunders, Philadelphia, vol IV, p 858–870

Sindou M, Quoex O, Baleydier C 1974 Fibre organisation at the posterior spinal cord rootlet junction in man. Journal of Comparative Neurology 153: 15–26

Singh N, Behse F, Buchthal F 1974 Electrophysiological study of peroneal palsy. Journal of Neurology, Neurosurgery and Psychiatry 37: 1202–1213

Sjöstrom L, Mjöberg B 1992 Suprascapular nerve entrapment in an arthrodesed shoulder. Journal of Bone and Joint Surgery 74B: 470–471

Slamon D J, Boone T C, Seeger R C et al 1986 Identification and characterisation of the protein encoded by the human N-myc oncogene. Science 232: 768–???

Slingluff C L, Terzis J K, Edgerton M T 1987 The quantitative microanatomy of the brachial plexus. In: Terzis J K (ed) Microreconstruction of nerve injuries. W B Saunders, Philadelphia, p 285–324

Slooff A C J 1993 Obstetric brachial plexus lesions and their neurosurgical treatment. Clinical Neurology and Neurosurgery 95 (suppl.) 573–577

Slooff A C J, Blauuw G 1995 Aspects particulaires. In: Alnot J Y, Narakas A (eds) Les paralysies du plexus brachial, 2nd edn. Monographie De La Société Française de Chirurgie de la Main. Expansion Scientifique Française, Paris, p. 282–284

Smaje J C 1983 Serial stimulation of the ulnar nerve. Electroencephalography and Clinical Neurophysiology 56: 19P

Smellie W 1764 Collection of Preternatural cases and observations in Midwifery, compleating (sic) the design of illustrating his first volume on that subject. Vol III p 504–505 London

Smellie W 1768 A collection of cases and observations in Midwifery Ed Wilson and Durham 4th edition. Volume 2 pp 446 and quoted by E W Johnson. International Abstracts of Surgery 1950 3: 409

Smith I C 1995 Multiple cranial nerve palsies in a motorcyclist caused by the helmet. Injury 26: 405–406

Smith J R, Gomez N H 1970 Local injection therapy of neuromata of the hand with triamcinolone acetamide. A preliminary study of twenty-two cases. Journal of Bone and Joint Surgery 52A: 71–83

Smith K F 1979 The thoracic outlet syndrome: a protocol of treatment. Journal of Orthopaedic and Sport Physical Therapy 1: 89–99

Smith K J, Kodoma R T 1991 Reinnervation of denervated skeletal muscle by central neurons regenerating via ventral roots implanted into the spinal cord. Brain Research 551: 221–229

Smith P J, Mott G 1986 Sensory threshold and conductance testing in nerve injuries. Journal of Hand Surgery 11B: 157–162

Smith R W 1849 Treatise on the pathology of diagnosis and treatment of neuroma. Hodges and Smith, Dublin

Smith S J M 1996 The role of neurophysiological investigation in traumatic brachial plexus injuries in adults and children. Journal of Hand Surgery 21B: 145–148

Smyth E H J 1969 Major arterial injury in closed fracture of the neck of the humerus. Journal of Bone and Joint Surgery 51B: 508–510

Snyder C C 1981 Epineurial repair. Orthopedic Clinics of North America 12: 267–276

Soares D 1996 Tibialis posterior transfer for the correction of foot drop in leprosy. Journal of Bone and Joint Surgery 78B: 61–62

Soferman W, Weissman S L, Haimar M 1964 Acroparaesthesiae in pregnancy. American Journal of Obstetrics and Gynecology 89: 528–531

Sogaard I 1983 Sciatic nerve entrapment neuropathy. Journal of Neurosurgery 45: 216–217

Solheim L F, Hagen R 1980 Femoral and sciatic neuropathies after total hip arthroplasty. Acta Orthopaedica Scandinavica 51: 531–534

Solheim L F, Siewers P, Paus B 1981 The piriformis muscle syndrome secondary to pseudogout. Acta Orthopaedica Scandinavica 52: 73–75

Sonck W A, Francx M M, Engels H L 1991 Innervation anomalies in upper and lower extremities: potential clinical implications. Electromyography and Clinical Neurophysiology 31: 67–80

Sordillo P P, Helson L, Hajdu S L et al 1981 Malignant schwannoma – clinical characteristics, survival and response to therapy. Cancer 47: 2503–2509

Sorensen S A, Mulvihill J J, Neilson A 1986 Nationwide follow up of Recklinghausen neurofibromatosis survival and malignant neoplasms. New England Journal of Medicine 314: 1010–1015

Sorrel E, Sorrel-Déjerine M M E 1938 Les lésions nerveuses dans les fractures fermées récentes de l'extrémité inférieure de l'humérus. Revue Orthopédique 25: 609–647

Specht D D 1975 Brachial plexus palsy in the newborn: incidence and prognosis. Clinical Orthopaedics and Related Research 110: 32–34

Spiegel P G, Ginsberg M, Skosey J L et al 1976 Acute carpal tunnel syndrome secondary to pseudo-gout. Clinical Orthopaedics and Related Research 120: 185–187

Spiess H 1972 Schädigungen am peripheren Nervensystem durch ionisierende Strahlen. In: Schriftenreihe Neurologie, Band 10. Springer-Verlag, New York

Spillane J D 1943 Localised neuritis of the shoulder girdle. Lancet ii: 532–535

Spilsbury J, Birch R 1996 Some lesions of the circumflex and suprascapular nerves. Journal of Bone and Joint Surgery 73B (suppl 1): 59 (abstract)

Spindler H A, Dellon A L 1982 Nerve conduction studies and sensibility during testing in carpal tunnel syndrome. Journal of Hand Surgery 7: 260–263

Spindler H A, Dellon A L 1990 Nerve conduction studies in the superficial radial entrapment syndrome. Muscle and Nerve 13: 1–5

Spinner M 1968 The arcade of Frohse and its relationship to posterior interosseous nerve paralysis. Journal of Bone and Joint Surgery 50B: 809–812

Spinner M 1970 The anterior interosseous-nerve syndrome. Journal of Bone and Joint Surgery 52A: 84–94

Spinner M 1993 Nerve compression lesions of the forearm, elbow and hand. In: Tubiana R (ed) The hand. W B Saunders, Philadelphia, vol IV, p 400–432

Spinner M, Spencer P S 1974 Nerve compression lesions of the upper extremity. Clinical Orthopaedics and Related Research 104: 46–67

Spinner R J, Lins R E, Collins A J et al 1993 Posterior interosseous nerve compression due to an enlarged bicipital bursa confirmed by MRI. Journal of Hand Surgery 18B: 753–756

Spittle M F 1995 Brachial plexus neuropathy after radiotherapy for breast cancer. British Medical Journal 311: 1516–1517

Sprague J M, Ha H C 1964 The terminal fields of dorsal root fibres in the lumbosacral spinal cord of the cat, and the dendritic organisation of the motor nuclei. Progress in Brain Research 11: 120–154

Spurling R G 1930 Causalgia of the upper extremity: treatment by dorsal sympathetic ganglionectomy. Archives of Neurology and Psychiatry 23: 784–788

Srinavasan H, Mukherjee S M, Supramanian R A 1968 Two tail transfer of tibialis posterior for correction of dropped foot in leprosy. Journal of Bone and Joint Surgery 50B: 623–628

Srinivasan R, Rhodes J 1981 The median-ulnar anastomosis (Martin Gruber) in normal and congenitally abnormal fetuses. Archives of Neurology 38: 418–419

Stableforth P G 1984 Four part fractures of the neck of the humerus. Journal of Bone and Joint Surgery 66B: 104–108

Stacey M J 1969 Free nerve endings in the skeletal muscle of the cat. Journal of Anatomy 105: 231–254

Stack R E, Bianco A J, MacCarty C S 1965 Compression of common peroneal nerve by ganglion cysts. Journal of Bone and Joint Surgery 17A: 773–778

Stamford J A 1995 Descending controls of pain. British Journal of Anaesthesia 75: 217–227

Stanton-Hicks M, Jänig W, Hassenbusch S et al 1995 Reflex sympathetic dystrophy: changing concepts and taxonomy. Pain 63: 127–133

Starr C L 1922 Army experience with tendon transference. Journal of Bone and Joint Surgery 4: 3–21

Steindler A 1918 A muscle plasty for the relief of flail elbow in infantile paralysis. Interstate Medical Journal 35: 235–241

Steindler A 1939 Tendon transplantation in the upper extremity. American Journal of Surgery 44: 260–271

Steiner R C, Fallet G H, Moody J F et al 1971 Lésions du plexus brachial survénant apres radiothérapie pour cancer du sein. Schweizerische Medizinische Wochenschrift 101: 1846–1848

Stevens J H 1934 Brachial plexus paralysis. In: Codman E A (ed) The Shoulder. IG Miller, Brooklyn, New York

Stewart F W, Copeland M M 1931 Neurogenic Sarcoma. American Journal of Cancer 15: 1235–1320

Stewart J D 1987 The variable clinical manifestations of ulnar neuropathies at the elbow. Journal of Neurology, Neurosurgery and Psychiatry 50: 252–258

Stewart J D 1993 Compression and entrapment neuropathies. In: Dyck P J, Thomas P K, Griffin J W, Low P A, Poduslo J F (eds) Peripheral neuropathy, 3rd edn. W B Saunders, Philadelphia, p 961–979

Stewart M, Birch R 1996 Penetrating injuries of the brachial plexus. Journal of Bone and Joint Surgery 73B (suppl II/III): 165

Stewart M P M, Kinninmonth A 1993 Shotgun wounds of the limbs. Injury 10: 667–670

Still J M, Kleinert H E 1973 Anomalous muscles and nerve entrapment in the wrist and hand. Plastic and Reconstructive Surgery 52: 394–400

Stoehr M 1978 Traumatic and postoperative lesions of the lumbosacral plexus. Archives of Neurology 35: 757–760

Stoker D J, Cobb J D, Pringle J A S 1991 Needle biopsy of musculo skeletal lesions. A review of 208 procedures. Journal of Bone and Joint Surgery 73B: 498–500

Stoll B A, Andrews J T 1966 Radiation-induced peripheral neuropathy. British Medical Journal 1: 834–837

Stoll G, Griffin J W, Li C Y, Trapp B D 1989 Wallerian degeneration in the peripheral nervous system: participation of both Schwann cells and macrophages in myelin degradation. Journal of Neurocytology 18: 671–683

Stookey B 1928 Meralgia paresthetica. Journal of the American Medical Association 90: 1705–1707

Stopford J B, Telford E D 1919 Compression of the lower trunk of the brachial plexus by a first dorsal rib. With a note on the surgical treatment. British Journal of Surgery 7: 168–177

Stout A P, 1937 The malignant tumour of peripheral nerves. Cancer 25: 1–36

Stout A P 1947 Ganglioneuroma of the sympathetic nervous system. Surgery, Gynecology and Obstetrics 84: 101–110

Strange F G St C 1947 An operation for pedicle nerve grafting. British Journal of Surgery 34: 423–425

Strange F G St C 1950 Case report on pedicled nerve graft. British Journal of Surgery 37: 331–333

Struthers J 1848 On a peculiarity of the humerus and humeral artery. Monthly Journal of Medical Science 9: 264–267

Struthers J W 1903 The anatomy of the long thoracic nerve, with special reference to paralysis of the serratus magnus. Review of Neurology and Psychiatry 1: 731–736

Subbotitch V 1913 Military experiences of traumatic aneurysms. Lancet ii: 720–721

Subbotitch V 1914 Kriegschirurgie erfahrungen Uber traumatische aneurysmen. Deutsche Zeitschrift für Chirurgie 127: 446–472

Suber D A, Massey E W 1979 Pelvic mass presenting as meralgia paraesthetica. Obstetrics and Gynecology 53 (2): 257–258

Sudeck P 1902 Über die akute (troponeurotische) Knochenatrophie nach Entzündungen und Traumen der Extremitäten. Deutsch Medizinische Wochenschrift 28: 336–342

Sugioka H 1984 Evoked potentials in the investigation of traumatic lesions of peripheral nerves and the brachial plexus. Clinical Orthopaedics and Related Research 184: 852–892

Sugioka H, Nagano A 1989 Électrodiagnostic dans l'évaluation des lésions par élongation du plexus brachial. In: Alnot J Y, Narakas A (eds) Les paralysies du plexus brachial. Monographies du Groupe d'Étude de la Main No 15. Expansion Scientifique, Paris, p 123–129

Sugiura Y, Terui N, Hosoya Y 1989 Difference in distribution of central terminals between visceral and somatic unmyelinated (C) primary afferent fibres. Journal of Neurophysiology 62: 834–840

Sumner D S 1993 Evaluation of noninvasive testing procedures: data analysis and interpretation. In: Bernstein EF (ed) Vascular diagnosis, 4th edn. C V Mosby, St Louis, p 39–63

Sumner D S, Eastcott H H G, Rich N M 1992 Arteriovenous fistulae In: Eastcott H H G (ed) Arterial surgery, 3rd edn. Churchill Livingstone, Edinburgh, p 521–559

Sunderland S 1951 A classification of peripheral nerve injuries producing loss of function. Brain 74: 491–516

Sunderland S 1976 The nerve lesion in the carpal tunnel syndrome. Journal of Neurology, Neurosurgery and Psychiatry 39: 615–626

Sunderland S 1978a Nerves and nerve injuries, 2nd edn. Churchill Livingstone, Edinburgh

Sunderland S 1978b Thermal injury of nerves. In: Nerves and nerve injuries, 2nd edn. E&S Livingstone, Edinburgh, p 164

Sunderland S 1981 The anatomic foundation of peripheral nerve repair techniques. Orthopedic Clinics of North America 12: 245–266

Sunderland S 1968 Intraneural topography. In: Nerves and nerve injuries. E & S Livingstone, Edinburgh. Median nerve, p 758–769; ulnar nerve, p 816–825; radial nerve, p 905–914; sciatic nerve, p 1029–1046

Sunderland S 1991a Nerve injury and sensory function. In: Nerve injuries and repair. A critical appraisal. Churchill Livingstone, Edinburgh, p 305–331

Sunderland S 1991b Conversion hysteria. In: Nerve injuries and repair. A critical appraisal. Churchill Livingstone, Edinburgh, p 327

Sunderland S, Bradley K 1949 The cross sectional area of peripheral nerve trunks devoted to nerve fibres. Brain 72: 428–449

Sunderland S, Ray L J 1947 The selection and use of autografts for bridging gaps in injured nerves. Brain 70: 75–92

Sunderland S, Lavarack J O, Ray L J 1949 The caliber of nerve fibers in human cutaneous nerves. Journal of Comparative Neurology 91: 87–101

Sunderland S, McArthur R A, Nam D A 1993 Repair of a transected sciatic nerve. Journal of Bone and Joint Surgery 75A: 911–914

Swanson A B, Boeve N R, Lumsden R M 1977 The prevention and treatment of amputation neuromata by silicone capping. Journal of Hand Surgery 2: 70–78

Swash M, Fox P 1974 The pathology of the human muscle spindle: effect of denervation. Journal of Neurological Sciences 22: 1–24

Sweet W H 1984 Deafferentation pain after posterior rhizotomy, trauma to a limb, and herpes zoster. Neurosurgery 15: 928–932

Sweet W H 1991 Deafferentation pain syndromes. In: Nashold B S, Ovelman-Levitt (eds) Advances in Pain Research and Therapy Vol 19. Raven Press, New York, p 264

Sweet W H, Poletti C E 1985 Causalgia and sympathetic dystrophy. In: Aronoff G M (ed) Evaluation and treatment of chronic pain. Urban & Schwarzenberg, Baltimore, p 149–165

Symeonides P P 1972 The humerus supracondylar spur syndrome. Clinical Orthopaedics and Related Research 82: 141–143

Symeonides P P, Paschaloglue C, Pagalides T 1975 Radial nerve enclosed in the callus of a supracondylar fracture. Journal of Bone and Joint Surgery 57B: 523–524

Symonds C P 1927 Cervical rib: thrombosis of subclavian artery, contralateral hemiplegia of sudden onset, probably embolic. Proceedings of the Royal Society of Medicine 20: 1244–1245

Synek V M 1987 The piriformis syndrome: review and case presentation. Clinical and Experimental Neurology 23: 31–37

Szabo R M, Gelberman R H, Williamson R V et al 1984 Vibratory sensory testing in acute peripheral nerve compression. Journal of Hand Surgery 9A: 104–109

Szentágothai J 1975 The "module concept" in cerebral cortex architecture. Brain Research 95: 475–496

Tackmann W, Kaeser H E, Magun H G 1981 Comparison of orthodromic and antidromic sensory nerve conduction velocity measurements in the carpal tunnel syndrome. Journal of Neurology 224: 257–266

Tahmoush A J, Alonso R J, Tahmoush G P et al 1991 Cramp-fasciculation syndrome: a treatable hyper-excitable nerve disorder. Neurology 41: 1021–1024

Tait G R, Danton M 1991 Contralateral sciatic nerve palsy following femoral nailing. Journal of Bone and Joint Surgery 73B: 689–690

Takahura Y, Kitada C, Sugimoto K et al 1991 Tarsal tunnel syndrome. Journal of Bone and Joint Surgery 73B: 125–126

Taleisnik J 1973 The palmar cutaneous branch of the median nerve and the approach to the carpal tunnel. Journal of Bone and Joint Surgery 55A: 1212–1217

Tamai S, Komatsu S, Sakamoto H et al 1970 Free muscle transplants in dogs with microsurgical neurovascular anastomoses. Journal of Plastic and Reconstructive Surgery 46: 219–225

Tan K L 1973 Brachial palsy. Journal of Obstetrics and Gynaecology of the British Commonwealth 80: 60–62

Tansini I 1906 Sopra il mio nuovo processo di amputazione della mammela. Riformi Medica 12: 757. Gazzetta Medica Italiana 57: 141

Tarlov I M 1944 Autologous plasma clot suture of nerves. Journal of the American Medical Association 126: 741–748

Tasaki I, Takeuchi T 1941 Der am Ranvierschen Knoten entstehende Aktionström und seine Bedeutung für die Erregungsleitung. Pflügers Archiv 244: 696–711

Tasaki I, Takeuchi T 1942 Weitere Studien über den Aktionsström der markhältigen Nervenfäser und über die elektrosaltatorische Uberträgung des Nervenimpulses. Pflügers Archiv 245: 764–782

Tasker R, DeCarralto G T C 1989 Intractable central pain of cord origin – clinical features and implication for surgery. Journal of Neurosurgery 70: 316A–317A

Tassin J L 1983 Paralysies obstétricales du plexus brachial: évolution spontanée, résultats des interventions réparatrices précoces. Thèse, Université de Paris VII

Tatsumi Y, Okuda H 1970 Free muscle transplants in dogs with microsurgical neurovascular anastomoses. Journal of Plastic and Reconstructive Surgery 46: 219–225

Tavernier 1936, Dechaume J, Pouzet F 1936 Infarctes musculaires et lésions nerveuses dans le syndrome de Volkmannn. Journal de Médecine (Lyon) 12: 815

Taylor A S 1920 Brachial birth palsy and injuries of a similar type in adults. Surgery, Gynecology and Obstetrics 30: 494–502

Taylor G I, Miller G D H, Ham F J 1975 The free vascularised bone graft. A clinical extension of microvascular techniques. Journal of Plastic and Reconstructive Surgery 55: 533–544

Taylor I G, Ham F J 1976 The free vascularized nerve graft. Plastic and Reconstructive Surgery 57: 413–426

Taylor P E 1962 Traumatic intradural avulsion of the nerve roots of the brachial plexus. Brain 85: 579–602

Taylor P K 1984 Non-linear effects of age on nerve conduction in adults. Journal of the Neurological Sciences 66: 223–234

Taylor T E, Wills B A, Kazembe P et al 1993 Magnetic resonance neurography Lancet 341: 659–661

Teot L, Montoya P, Dimeglio A et al 1986 Uncommon neonatal sciatic palsy. Peripheral Nerve Repair and Regeneration 4: 51–53

Terzis J K, Breidenbach W C 1987 The anatomy of free vascularised nerve grafts. In: Terzis J K (ed) Microreconstruction of nerve injuries. W B Saunders, London, p 101–116

Terzis J K, Strauch B 1978 Microsurgery of the peripheral nerve: a physiological approach. Clinical Orthopaedics and Related Research 133: 39–48

Theodorides T, de Keyzer G 1977 Injuries of the axillary artery caused by fractures of the neck of the humerus. Injury 8: 120–123

Thoburn W 1900 Secondary suture of the brachial plexus. British Medical Journal 1: 1073–1075

Thomas C, Merle M, Gilbert A 1993 Endoscopic treatment of carpal tunnel syndrome. In: Tubiana R (ed) The hand. W B Saunders, Philadelphia, vol IV, p 487–498

Thomas D G T, Jones S J 1984 Dorsal root entry zone lesions (Nashold's procedure) in brachial plexus avulsion. Neurosurgery 15: 966–968

Thomas D G T, Kitchen N D 1994 Long term follow up of dorsal root entry zone lesions in brachial plexus avulsion. Journal of Neurology, Neurosurgery and Psychiatry 57: 737–738

Thomas D G T, Sheehy J P R 1983 Dorsal root entry zone lesions (Nashold's procedure) for pain relief following brachial plexus avulsion. Journal of Neurology, Neurosurgery and Psychiatry 46: 924–928

Thomas J E, Colby M Y 1972 Radiation-induced or metastatic brachial plexopathy. Journal of the American Medical Association 222: 1392–1395

Thomas J E, Cascino T L, Earle J D 1985 Differential diagnosis between radiation and tumor plexopathy of the pelvis. Neurology 35: 1–7

Thomas M, Smibert J G, Morley T R 1992 Management of neurological compression due to spinal malignancy. Journal of Bone and Joint Surgery 74B: 277 (abstract)

Thomas M, Stirratt A, Birch R et al 1994 Freeze thawed muscle grafting for painful cutaneous neuromas. Journal of Bone and Joint Surgery 76B: 474–476

Thomas P K 1963 The connective tissue of peripheral nerve; an electron microscope study. Journal of Anatomy 97: 35–42

Thomas P K 1964 Changes in the endoneurial sheaths of peripheral myelinated nerve fibres during Wallerian degeneration. Journal of Anatomy 98: 175–182

Thomas P K 1966 The cellular response to nerve injury. 1. The cellular outgrowth from the distal stump of a transected nerve. Journal of Anatomy 100: 287–303

Thomas P K, Claus D, Jaspert A, Workman J M, King R H M, Larner A J et al 1996 Focal upper limb demyelinating neuropathy. Brain 119: 765–774

Thomas P K, Fullerton P M 1963 Nerve fibre size in the carpal tunnel syndrome. Journal of Neurology, Neurosurgery and Psychiatry 26: 520–527

Thomas P K, Holdorff B 1993 Neuropathy due to physical agents. In: Dyck P J, Thomas P K, Griffin J W, Low P A, Poduslo J F (eds) Peripheral neuropathy, 3rd edn. W B Saunders, Philadelphia, p 990–1013

Thomas P K, Jones D G 1967 The cellular response to nerve injury. 2. Regeneration of the perineurium after nerve section. Journal of Anatomy 101: 45–55

Thomas P K, Lascelles R G 1996 The pathology of diabetic neuropathy. Quarterly Journal of Medicine 35: 489–502

Thomas P K, Ochoa J 1993 Clinical features and differential diagnosis. In: Dyck P J, Thomas P K, Griffin J W, Low P A, Poduslo J F (eds) Peripheral neuropathy, 3rd edn. W B Saunders, London, p 749–774

Thomas P K, Berthold C-H, Ochoa J 1993a Microscopic anatomy of the peripheral nervous system. In: Dyck P J, Thomas P K, Griffin J W, Low P A, Poduslo J F (eds) Peripheral neuropathy, 3rd edn. W B Saunders, London, p 38

Thomas P K, Berthold C-H, Ochoa J 1993b Age changes in peripheral nerve fibres. In: Dyck P J, Thomas P K, Griffin J W, Low P A, Poduslo J F (eds) Peripheral neuropathy, 3rd edn. W B Saunders, London, p 605

Thomas P K, Scaravilli J, Belai A 1993c Pathological alterations in cell bodies of peripheral neurons in neuropathy. In: Dyck P J, Thomas P K, Griffin J W, Low P A, Poduslo J F (eds) Peripheral neuropathy, 3rd edn. W B Saunders, London, p 476–513

Thompson V P, Epstein H C 1951 Traumatic dislocation of the hip: a survey of 204 cases covering a period of 21 years. Journal of Bone and Joint Surgery (Am) 33: 746–778

Thornes J J 1909 Nerve involvement in the ischaemic paralysis and contracture of Volkmann. Annals of Surgery 49: 330

Thyayagarajan D, Cascino T, Harms G 1995 Magnetic resonance imaging in brachial plexopathy of cancer. Neurology 45: 421–427

Tile M 1984 Fractures of the pelvis and acetabulum. Williams & Wilkins, Baltimore

Tinel J 1915 Le signe du "fourmillement" dans les lésions des nerfs périphériques. Presse Médicale 47: 388–399

Tinel J 1916 Les blessures des nerfs. Masson, Paris

Tinel J 1917a The formication sign. In: Rothwell R (trans), Joll C A (rev and ed). Nerve wounds. Baillière, Tindall & Cox, London, p 34–35 and 75–76

Tinel J 1917b Nerve grafting. *Ibid*, p 203 and p 304–305

Tobin S M 1967 Carpal tunnel syndrome in pregnancy. American Journal of Obstetrics and Gynecology 97: 493–498

Todd T E 1912 "Cervical rib": factors controlling its presence and its size. Its bearing on the morphology and development of the shoulder (with four cases). Journal of Anatomy and Physiology 46: 244–288

Tohgi H, Tsukagoshi H, Toyokura Y 1977 Quantative changes with age in normal sural nerves. Acta Neuropathologica (Berlin) 38: 213–220

Topliss E 1993 Social and economic aspects of disablement. In: Greenwood R, Barnes M P, McMillan T M, Ward C D (eds) Neurological rehabilitation. Churchill Livingstone, Edinburgh, p 51–58

Torebjörk H E, Hallin R G 1973 Perceptual changes accompanying controlled preferential blocking of A and C fibres in intact human nerves. Experimental Brain Research 16: 321–332

Torebjörk H E, Hallin R G 1979a Microneurographic studies of peripheral pain mechanisms in man. Advances in Pain Research and Therapy 3: 121–131

Torebjörk H E, Hallin R G 1979b Perceptual changes accompanying controlled preferential blocking of A and C fibre responses in intact human skin nerves. Experimental Brain Research 16: 321–332

Torebjörk H E, Ochoa J L 1980 Specific sensations evoked by activity in single identified sensory units in man. Acta Physiological Scandinavica 110: 445–447

Torebjörk H E, Ochoa J L 1983a Selective stimulation of sensory units in man. In: Bonica J J, Lundblom H, Iggo A (eds). Advances in Pain Research and Therapy. Vol 2. Raven Press, New York, p 99–104

Torebjörk H E, Lundberg L E R, Lamotte R H 1992 Central changes in processing of mechanoreceptor input in capsaicin induced sensory hyperalgesia in humans. Journal of Physiology (London) 448: 765–780

Torebjörk E, Wahren L K, Wallin G et al 1995 Noradrenaline evoked pain in neuralgia. Pain. 63: 11–20

Tower S S 1932 Atrophy and degeneration in the muscle spindles. Brain 55: 77–90

Tower S S 1943 Regenerative capacity of ventral roots after avulsion from the spinal cord. Archives of Neurology and Psychiatry 49: 1–12

Treavor W J, Lambert E H, Herrick J F 1953 Block of conduction in bullfrog nerve fibres by heat. American Journal of Physiology 175: 258–262

Treede R D, Davis K D, Campbell J N et al 1992 The plasticity of cutaneous hyperalgesia during sympathetic ganglion blockade in patients with neuropathic pain. Brain 115: 607–621

Triche T, Cavazzana A 1988 Round cell tumour of bone. In: Krishnan U (ed) Bone tumours. Churchill Livingstone, New York, p 199–224

Triffitt P D, Konig D, Harper W M et al 1992 Compartment pressures after closed fracture of the tibia. Journal of Bone and Joint Surgery 74B: 195–198

Trojaborg W 1976 Motor and sensory conduction in the musculocutaneous nerve. Journal of Neurology, Neurosurgery and Psychiatry 39: 889–899

Trojaborg W 1977 Prolonged conduction block with axonal degeneration. An electrophysiological study. Journal of Neurology, Neurosurgery and Psychiatry 40: 50–57

Trombetta A 1880 Sullo stiramento dei nervi. Fratelli D'Angelo, Messina

Trumble T E, Kahn U, Vanderhooft E et al 1995 A technique to quantitate motor recovery following nerve grafting. Journal of Hand Surgery 20A: 367–372

Tsubokawa T, Katayama Y, Yamamoto T et al 1993 Chronic motor cortex stimulation in patients with thalamic pain. Journal of Neurosurgery 78: 393–401

Tsuyama N, Hara T 1972 Intercostal nerve transfer in the treatment of brachial plexus injury of root-avulsion type. Proceedings of the SICOT, Tel Aviv, 9–12 October 1972. Excerpta Medica International Congress Series No 291. Excerpta Medica, Amsterdam, p 348–351

Tubiana R 1988 Burns. In: Tubiana R (ed) The hand. W B Saunders, Philadelphia, vol III

Tubiana R 1993a Paralysis of the thumb. In: Tubiana P (ed) The hand. W B Saunders, Philadelphia, vol IV, p 182–253 (English translation)

Tubiana R 1993 The hand. Volume 4. W B Saunders. Philadelphia (English translation)

Tubiana R 1993b Paralysis of the extensors of the wrist, thumb and proximal phalanges. In: Tubiana R (ed) The hand. Vol IV. W B Saunders, Philadelphia, p 147–181 (English translation)

Tubiana R, Brockman R 1993 General considerations in carpal tunnel syndrome In: Tubiana R (ed) The hand. Vol IV. W B Saunders, Philadelphia, p 441–449

Tubiana R, McCullough C J 1984 Paralysis of the intrinsic muscles of the hand. In: Brooks D M, Birch R (eds) Rob and Smith's, operative surgery. The hand, 4th edn. Butterworths, London, p 318–343

Tupper J W, Crick J C, Mattich L R 1988 Fascicular nerve repairs. Orthopaedic Clinics of North America 19: 57–69

Tupper J 1980 Fascicular nerve repair. In: Jewett J L, McCarroll H R Jr (eds) Nerve repair and regeneration. Its clinical and experimental basis. C V Mosby, St Louis, p 320

Turner J W, Cooper R R 1972 Anterior transfer of the tibialis posterior through the interosseous membrane. Clinical Orthopaedics and Related Research 83: 241–244

Turner O A, Taslitz N, Ward S 1990 Handbook of peripheral nerve entrapments. Humana Press, Clifton, New Jersey

Tuttle H 1912 Exposure of the brachial plexus with nerve transplantation. Journal of the American Medical Association 61: 15–17

Tyrer P 1989 Conversion hysteria. In: Classification of neuroses. Wiley, New York, p 106–107, 111–112

Uhlschmid G, Clodius L 1978 Eine Neue Anwendung des freien Transplantation Omentums. Der Chirurg 49: 714–718

Ungley C C, Blackwood D W 1942 Peripheral vasoneuropathy after chilling. Lancet ii: 447–451

Ungley C C, Channell G B, Richards R L 1945 The immersion foot syndrome. British Journal of Surgery 33: 17–31

Upton A R M, McComas A J 1973 The double crush in nerve entrapment syndrome. Lancet ii: 359–361

Upton A R M, Durracott J, Bianchi F A 1978 Ulnar neuropathies in rheumatoid arthritis. The Hand 10: 77–81

Urich H 1993 Pathology of tumours of cranial nerves, spinal nerve roots and peripheral nerves. In: Dyck P J, Thomas P K (eds) Peripheral neuropathy, 3rd edn. W B Saunders, Philadelphia, p 1641–1672

Urschel H C, Razzuk M A 1972 Management of the thoracic-outlet syndrome. New England Journal of Medicine 286: 1140–1143

Urschel H C, Razzuk M A, Wood R E et al 1971 Objective diagnosis (ulnar nerve conduction velocity) and current therapy of thoracic outlet syndrome. Annals of Thoracic Surgery 12: 608–620

Vallbo Å B, Hagbarth K E 1968 Activity from skin mechanoreceptors recorded percutaneously in awake human subjects. Experimental Neurology 21: 270–289

Vallbo Å B, Hulliger M 1981 Independence of skeletomotor and fusimotor activity. Brain Research 223: 176–180

Vallbo Å B, Hagbarth K E, Torebjörk H E et al 1979 Somatosensory, proprioceptive and sympathetic activity in human peripheral nerve. Physiological Reviews 59: 919–957

Valtonen E J, Lilius H J 1974 Late sequelae of iatrogenic spinal accessory nerve injury. Acta Chirurgica Scandinavica 140: 453–455

Vandeput J, Tanner J C, Huypens L 1969 Electrophysiological orientation of the cut ends in primary peripheral nerve repair. Plastic and Reconstructive Surgery 44: 378–383

Van der Molen A, Evans D M 1996 Results of transfer of the extensor indicis for restoration of adduction of the thumb. Presented at the combined meeting of Hellenic and British Societies for Surgery of the Hand

Vanderpool D W, Chalmers J, Lamb D W et al 1968 Peripheral compression lesions of the ulnar nerve. Journal of Bone and Joint Surgery 50B: 793–803

Van Heest A, Waters P, Simmons B et al 1995 A cadaveric study of the single-portal endoscopic carpal tunnel release. Journal of Hand Surgery 20A: 362–366

Varro A, Green T, Holmes S et al 1988 Calcitonin gene-related peptide in visceral afferent nerve fibres: quantification by radioimmunoassay and determination of axonal transport rated. Neuroscience 26: 927–932

Vasili L R 1988 Diagnosis of vascular injury in children with supracondylar fractures of the humerus. Injury 19: 11–13

Vastamäki M, Solonen K A 1984 Accessory nerve injury. Acta Orthopaedica Scandinavica 55: 296–299

Vazquez-Burquero A, Pascual J, Quintana F et al 1994 Cervical schwannoma presenting as a spinal subdural haematoma. British Journal of Neurosurgery 8: 739–741

Veilleux M, Steven J C, Campbell J K 1988 Somatosensory evoked potentials: lack of value for diagnosis of thoracic outlet syndrome. Muscle and Nerve 11: 571–575

Velchik M S, Alavi A, Kressel H Y et al 1989 Localisation of phaechromocytomas: MIBG, CT and MRI correlation. Journal of Nuclear Medicine 30: 328–336

Venna M, Bielawski M, Spatz E M 1991 Sciatic nerve entrapment in a child. Journal of Neurosurgery 75: 652–654

Verbiest H 1988 Tumours involving the cervical spine. In: The Cervical Spine. The Cervical Spine Research Society, J B Lippincott, Philadelphia, p. 430–476

Verdugo R, Ochoa J 1994 Sympathetically maintained pain. I. Phentolamine block questions the concept. Neurology 44: 1003–1010

Verghese J P, Bradley W G, Mitsumoto H et al 1982 A blind controlled trial of adrenocorticotrophic and cerebral gangliosides in nerve regeneration in the rat. Experimental Neurology 77: 455–460

Verola O, Dallot A, Audebaud G et al 1985 Sarcomes neurogéniques survenant au cours de la maladie de Von Recklinghausen. Archives d' Anatomie et de Cytologie Pathologiques 33: 5–16

Vertu M J, Applebaum E L, McClusky D A et al 1977 Cranial nerve injury during carotid endarterectomy. Annals of Surgery 185: 192–195

Viard H, Sautreux J L, Haas O et al 1989 Tumeurs nerveuses en sablier. Chirurgie 115: 521–525

Vichare N A 1968 Spontaneous paralysis of the anterior interosseous nerve. Journal of Bone and Joint Surgery 50B: 806–808

Villar R H 1992 Hip arthroscopy. British Journal of Hospital Medicine 47: 763–766

Vincent C, Clements R V 1995 Clinical risk management – why do we need it? Clinical Risk 1: 1–4

Vizoso A D, Young J Z 1948 Internode length and fibre diameter in developing and regenerating nerves. Journal of Anatomy 82: 110–134

Volkmann R von 1881 Die ischaemische Muskellähmungen und Kontrakturen. Zentralblatt für Chirurgie 8: 801–803

Volkmann R von 1882. Verletzungen und Krankheiten der Bweengungs organe. Die Krankheiten der Muskeln und Sehne. In: Pitha F, von Billroth T (eds) Handbuch der allgemeinen und speziellen chirurgie. Verlag von Ferdinand Enke, Stuttgart, Band 2; Abt 2, Erstl Hälfte p 845–920

Von Frey M 1894 Beitrage zur physiologie der Schmerzsinns. Berichte der Königliche Sächsische Gesellschaften der Wissenschaften 46: 185–196

Von Frey M 1895 Beitrage zur Sinnesphysiologie der Haut. Berichte der Königliche Sächsische Akademie der Wissenschaften 47: 166–184

Von Frey M 1896 Untersuchungen über die Sinnesfunktionen der menschlichen Haut. 1.1. Druckempfindung und Schmerz. Berichte der Königliche Sächsische Gesellschaft der Wissenschaften 48: 175–264

Vosburgh L F, Finn W F 1961 Femoral nerve impairment subsequent to hysterectomy. American Journal of Obstetrics and Gynecology 82: 931–937

Vredeveld J W, Rozeman C A M, Slooff A C J 1994 Obstetric brachial plexus lesion: only a peripheral lesion? Journal of Neurology, Neurosurgery and Psychiatry 57: 1299 (abstract)

Vulpius O 1904 Der Heutige Stand der Sehnenplastik. Zeitschrift für Orthopädische Chirurgie 1

Wadsworth T G 1972 Injuries of the capitular (lateral humeral condylar) epiphysis. Clinical Orthapaedics and Related Research 85: 127–142

Wadsworth T G 1977 The external compression syndrome of the ulnar nerve at the cubital tunnel. Clinical Orthopaedics and Related Research 124: 189–204

Wadsworth T G 1982 The elbow, 1st edn. Churchill Livingstone, Edinburgh

Wadsworth T G 1984a In: Birch R, Brooks D M (eds) Operative surgery. The hand. Butterworth, Oxford, p 472

Wadsworth T G 1984b In: Birch R, Brooks D M (eds) Operative surgery. The hand. Butterworth, London, p 481

Wadsworth T G, Brooks D M 1982 Neurological disorders. In: Wadsworth T G (ed) The elbow. Churchill Livingstone, Edinburgh, p 71

Wahle H, Tönnis D 1958 Familiäre Anfälligkeit gegenuber Druckschädigungen peripherer Nerven. Fortschritte der Neurologie Psychiatrie 26: 371–376

Wahren L K, Torebjörk E, Nyström B 1991 Quantitative sensory testing before and after regional guanethidine block in patients with neuralgia in the hand. Pain 46: 23–30

Wahren L K, Goroh T, Torebjörk E 1995 Effects of regional intravenous guanethidine in patients with neuralgia in the hand; a follow up study over a decade. Pain 62: 379–385

Walker A E, Nulson F 1948 Electrical stimulation of the upper thoracic portion of the sympathetic chain in Man. Archives of Neurology and Psychiatry 59: 559–560

Wall P D 1970 The sensory and motor role of impulses travelling in the dorsal columns towards the cerebral cortex. Brain 93: 505–524

Wall P D 1978 The gate control theory of pain mechanisms. A re-examination and re-statement. Brain 101: 1–18

Wall P D 1985 In: Swash M, Kennard C (eds) Scientific basis of clinical neurology. Churchill Livingstone, Edinburgh, p 163–171

Wall P D 1988 The prevention of postoperative pain. Pain 33: 289–290

Wall P D, Devor M 1981 The effect of peripheral nerve injury on dorsal root potentials and on transmission of afferent signals into the spinal cord. Brain Research 209: 95–111

Wall P D, Gutnick M 1974a The properties of afferent nerve impulses originating from a neuroma. Nature 248: 740–742

Wall P D, Gutnick M 1974b Ongoing activity in peripheral nerves: the physiology and pharmacology of impulses arising from a neuroma. Experimental Neurology 43: 580–593

Wall P D, Sweet W H 1967 Temporary abolition of pain in man. Science 155: 108–109

Waller A 1850 Experiments on the section of the glossopharyngeal and hypoglossal nerves of the frog, and observations of the alterations produced thereby in the structure of their primitive fibres. Philosophical Transactions of the Royal Society of London 140: 423–429

Walsh J C, Low P A, Allsopp J L 1976 Localised sympathetic activity: an uncommon complication of lung cancer. Journal of Neurology, Neurosurgery and Psychiatry 39: 93–95

Walsh J F 1877 The Anatomy of the brachial plexus. American Journal of Medical Science 74: 387–399

Walshe F M R 1942 The anatomy and physiology of cutaneous sensibility. Brain 65: 48–112

Walshe F M R, Jackson Fi, Wyburn-Mason R 1944 On some pressure effects associated with cervical rib and with rudimentary and "normal" first rib. Brain 67: 141–177

Walters A 1959 The differentiation of causalgia and hyperpathia. Canadian Medical Association Journal 80: 105

Watkins E S, Koeze T H 1993 Spinal cord stimulation and pain relief. British Medical Journal 307: 462

Watkins M B, Jones J B, Ryder C T et al 1954 Transplantation of the posterior tibial tendon. Journal of Bone and Joint Surgery 36A: 1181–1189

Watson B V, Brown W F 1992 Quantitation of axon loss and conduction block in acute radial nerve palsies. Muscle and Nerve 15: 768–773

Watson B V, Merchant R N, Brown W F 1992 Early postoperative ulnar neuropathies following coronary artery bypass surgery. Muscle and nerve 15: 701–705

Watson–Jones R 1930 Primary nerve lesions in injuries of the elbow and wrist. Journal of Bone and Joint Surgery 12: 121–140

Watson-Jones R 1931 Styloid process of the fibula in the knee joint with peroneal palsy. Journal of Bone and Joint Surgery 13: 258–260

Watson-Jones R 1936 Dislocation of the shoulder joint. Proceedings of the Royal Society of Medicine 29: 1060–1062

Watson-Jones R 1949 Leri's pleonosteosis, carpal canal compression of the median nerves and Morton's metatarsalgia. Journal of Bone and Joint Surgery 46B: 736

Watson-Jones R 1957 Fractures and Joint Injuries Vol. 1. 4th edn.

Watson-Jones R 1964 Encapsulated Lipoma of the Median Nerve at the Wrist. Journal of Bone and Joint Surgery 46B: 736

Watt J 1995 Bolam versus Friern Barnet H M C. Clinical Risk 1: 84–85

Weale P E 1980 Upper thoracic sympathectomy by transthoracic electrocoagulation. British Journal of Surgery 67: 71–72

Webber R H 1961 Some variations in the lumbar plexus of nerves in man. Acta Anatomica 44: 336–345

Weber E R, Daube J R, Coventry M B 1976 Peripheral Neuropathies associated with total hip arthroplasty. Journal of Bone and Joint Surgery 58A: 66–69

Webster D R, Woolhouse F M, Johnson J L 1942 Immersion foot. Journal of Bone and Joint Surgery 24: 785–794

Webster H deF 1993 Development of peripheral nerve fibers. In: Dyck P J, Thomas P K, Griffin J W, Low P A, Poduslo J F (eds) Peripheral neuropathy, 3rd edn. W B Saunders, p 243–266

Weddell G 1941 The pattern of cutaneous innervation in relation to cutaneous sensibility. Journal of Anatomy 75: 346–366

Weddell G 1955 Somesthesis and the chemical senses. Annual Review of Psychology 6: 119–135

Weddell G, Harpman J A, Lambley D G et al 1940 The innervation of the musculature of the tongue. Journal of Anatomy 74: 255–267

Weddell G, Feinstein B, Pattle R E 1944 The electrical activity of voluntary muscle in man under normal and pathological conditions. Brain 67: 178–252

Wedel D J 1994 Interscalene block. In: Miller R D (ed) Anaesthesia, 4th edn. Churchill Livingstone, p 1536–1538

Weglowski R 1925 Uber die Gefässtransplantation. Centralblutt für Chirurgie 52: ii: 2241–2243

Weigert M 1920 As quoted by Gjörup. Obstetrical lesions of the brachial plexus: Acta Neurologica Scandinavica 1965, 4–2 (suppl 18): 9–38

Weiland A J, Russell Moore J 1988 Vascularised bone grafts. In: Green D P (ed) Operative Hand Surgery, 2nd edn. Churchill Livingstone, Edinburgh, vol 2, p 1245–1269

Weinstein J D, Dick H M, Grantham S A 1968 Pseudo-gout, hypoparathyroidism and carpal tunnel syndrome. Journal of Bone and Joint Surgery 50A: 1669–1674

Weisl H, Osborne G V 1964 The pathological changes in rats' nerves subject to moderate compression. Journal of Bone and Joint Surgery 45B: 297–306

Weiss J W, Langloss J M, Enzinger F M 1983 Value of S-100 protein in the diagnosis of soft tissue tumour with particular reference to benign and malignant schwann cell tumours. Laboratory Investigations 49: 299–308

Weiss P, Hiscoe H B 1948 Experiments on the mechanism of nerve growth. Journal of Experimental Zoology 107: 315–395

Wertsch J J 1992 Anterior interosseous nerve syndrome. Muscle and Nerve 15: 977–983

West J G, Haymor D R, Goodkin R et al 1994 Magnetic resonance imaging signal changes in denervated muscle after peripheral nerve injury. Neurosurgery 35: 1077–1086

Wetmore C, Eide R 1991 Detection and characterization of a sensory microganglion associated with the spinal accessory nerve: a scanning laser confocal microscopic study of the neurons and their processes. Journal of Comparative Neurology 305: 148–163

Wetzel N, Arief A, Tunchbay E 1963 Retroperitoneal lumbar and pelvic malignancies simulating the "disc" syndrome. Archives of Surgery 86: 1069–1071

Wey J M, Guinn G A 1985 Ulnar nerve injury with open heart surgery. Annals of Thoracic Surgery 39: 358–360

Whiston R, Wheeler J, Lewis M 1995 An unusual cause of malnutrition. Hospital Update July: 338–339

White J C, Scoville W B 1945 Trench foot and immersion foot. New England Journal of Medicine 232: 415–422

White J C, Sweet W H 1969 Pain and the neurosurgeon: A forty year experience. C C Thomas, Springfield, IL, p 895–896

White J S, Goodfellow J W, Mowat A 1988 Posterior interosseous nerve palsy in rheumatoid arthritis. Journal of Bone and Joint Surgery 70B: 468–471

Whitelaw G P, Smithwick R H 1951 Some secondary effects of sympathectomy. New England Journal of Medicine 245: 1212–1230

Whiteley M S, Fox A D, Harris R A et al 1995 Iso-osmotic bowel preparation improves the accuracy of iliac artery colour flow duplex examination. Journal of the Royal Society of Medicine 88: 657P–660P

Whitesides T E, Haney T C, Morimoto K et al 1975 Tissue pressure measurements as a determinant for the need for fasciotomy. Clinical Orthopaedics and Related Research 113: 43–51

Whitworth I H, Brown R A, Dore C et al 1995 Orientated mats of fibronectin as a conduit material for use in peripheral nerve repair. Journal of Hand Surgery 20B: 429–436

Whitworth I H, Brown R A, Dore C J et al 1996 Nerve growth factor enhances nerve regeneration through fibronectin grafts. Journal of Hand Surgery 21B: 514–522

Wick M R, Swanson P E, Scheithauer B W et al 1987 Malignant peripheral nerve sheath tumour. An immunohistochemical study of 62 cases. American Journal of Clinical Pathology 87: 425–433

Wickham J E A, Martin P 1962 Aneurysm of the subclavian artery in association with cervical abnormality. British Journal of Surgery 50: 205–209

Wickstrom J 1960 Birth injuries of the brachial plexus. Journal of Bone and Joint Surgery 42A: 1448–1449

Wickstrom J 1962 Birth injuries of the brachial plexus: treatment of defects in the shoulder. Clinical Orthopaedics and Related Research 23: 187–196

Wiggins H E 1975 The anterior tibial compartment syndrome. Clinical Orthopaedics and Related Research 113: 90–94

Wilbourn A J 1982 True neurogenic thoracic outlet syndrome: case report. American Association of Electromyography and Electrodiagnosis, Rochester, Minnesota, p 3–10

Wilbourn A J 1985 Electrodiagnosis of plexopathies. Neurologic Clinics 3: 511–529

Wilbourn A J 1988 Thoracic outlet syndrome surgery causing severe brachial plexopathy. Muscle and Nerve 11: 66–74

Wilbourn A J 1993 Brachial plexus disorders. In: Dyck P J, Thomas P K (eds) Peripheral neuropathy, 3rd edn. W B Saunders, Philadelphia, p 911–950

Wilbourn A J, Hulley W 1977 Monomelic ischemic neuropathies. Neurology 27: 363 (abstract)

Wilbourn A J, Lederman R J 1984 Evidence for conduction delay in thoracic-outlet syndrome is challenged. New England Journal of Medicine 310: 1052–1053 (letter)

Wilde J, Moss T, Thrush D 1987 X linked bulbo-spinal neuronopathy: a family study of three patients. Journal of Neurology, Neurosurgery and Psychiatry 50: 279–284

Wilde O 1890 The picture of Dorian Gray. Lippincott's Monthly Magazine July 1990: 3–100

Wilhelm A 1993 The proximal radial nerve compression syndrome. In: Tubiana R (ed) The hand. W B Saunders, Philadelphia, vol IV, p 390–399

Wilkins K E 1984 Fractures and dislocation of the elbow region. In: Rockwood C A, Wilkins K E, King R E (eds) Fractures in children. J P Lippincott, Philadelphia, p 363–576

Wilkins K E 1991 Fractures and dislocations of the elbow region. In: Rockwood C A, Wilkins K E, King R E (eds) Fractures in children, 3rd edn. J B Lippincott, Philadelphia, p 509–828

Wilkinson H A 1984 Percutaneous radiofrequency upper thoracic sympathectomy: a new technique. Neurosurgery 15: 811–813

Wilkinson M C P, Clarke J A 1992 Burns to the Brachial Plexus. Injury 23: 341–342

Wilkinson M 1960 The carpal-tunnel syndrome in pregnancy. Lancet i: 453–454

Wilkinson M C P, Birch R 1995 Repair of the common peroneal nerve. Journal of Bone and Joint Surgery 77B: 501–503

Wilkinson M C P, Birch R, Bonney G 1993 Brachial plexus injuries: when to amputate. Injury 24 (9): 603–605

Williams L F, Geer T 1963 Acute carpal tunnel syndrome secondary to pyogenic infection of the forearm. Journal of the American Medical Association 185: 409–410

Williams P H, Trzil K P 1991 Management of meralgia paraesthetica. Journal of Neurosurgery 74: 76–80

Williams P L, Warwick R, Dyson M et al 1989 Neurochemical transmission. In: Gray's anatomy, 37th edn. Churchill Livingstone, Edinburgh, p 886–892

Williams W, Unwin A, Smith D 1995 Fibre content of the accessory nerve. Presented at the Reading Shoulder Course

Williams W W, Twyman R S, Donell S T et al 1996a The posterior triangle and the painful shoulder – spinal accessory nerve injury. Journal of Bone and Joint Surgery 73B (suppl 1): 60

Williams W W, Twyman R S, Donell S T 1996b The posterior triangle and the painful shoulder: spinal accessory nerve injury. Annals of the Royal College of Surgeons 78: 521–525

Willis W D, Coggeshall R E 1991 Sensory mechanisms of the spinal cord, 2nd edn. Plenum Press, New York

Willis W D, Kenshalo D R, Leonard R B 1979 The cells of origin of the primate spinothalamic tract. Journal of Comparative Neurology 188: 543–574

Willshire W H 1860 Supernumerary first rib. Lancet ii: 633

Wilson D L, Stone G C 1979 Axoplasmic transport of proteins. Annual Review of Biophysics and Bioengineering 8: 27–45

Wilson G R 1985 A simple device for the objective evaluation of peripheral nerve injuries. Journal of Hand Surgery 10B: 324–330

Wilson J N 1960 The management of fracture dislocations of the hip. Proceedings of the Royal Society of Medicine 53: 941–945

Wilson P 1945 Reflex sympathetic dystrophy: changing concepts and taxonomy. Pain 63: 127–133

Wilson S A K 1913 Some points in the symptomatology of cervical rib, with especial reference to muscle wasting. Proceedings of the Royal Society of Medicine 6: 133–141

Wilson S A K 1954 Cervical rib. In: Bruce A N (ed) Neurology (Kinnear Wilson), 2nd edn. Butterworth, Oxford, vol 2, p 1203–1213

Wilson-Macdonald J, Caughey M A 1984 Diurnal variation in nerve conduction, hand volume and grip strength in the carpal tunnel syndrome. British Medical Journal 289: 1042

Windebank A J 1993 Neuronal growth factors in the peripheral nervous system. In: Dyck, P J, Thomas P K, Griffin J W, Low P A, Poduslo J F (eds) Peripheral neuropathy, 3rd edn. W B Saunders, Philadelphia, p 377–388

Winkelman N W 1958 Femoral nerve complications after pelvic surgery. American Journal of Obstetrics and Gynecology 75: 1063–1065

Winnie A P 1970 Interscalene brachial plexus block. Anesthesia and Analgesia … Current Researches 49: 455–466

Wise M P, Blunt S, Lane R J M 1995 Neurological presentations of hypothyroidism: the importance of slow-relaxing reflexes. Journal of the Royal Society of Medicine 88: 272–274

Withrington R N, Wynn-Parry C B 1984 The management of pain in peripheral nerve disorders. Journal of Bone and Joint Surgery 9B: 24–28

Woltmann H W, Learmonth J R 1934 Progressive paralysis of the nervus interosseus dorsalis. Brain 57: 25–31

Wood M B 1991 Peripheral nerve injuries to the lower extremity. In: Gelberman R H (ed). Operative nerve repair and reconstruction. J B Lipincott, Philadelphia, p 489–504

Wood V E, Frykman G K 1980 Winging of the scapula as a common complication of first rib resection. Clinical Orthopaedics and Related Research 149: 160–163

Wood V E, Twito R, Verska J M 1988 Thoracic outlet syndrome. Orthopedic Clinics of North America 19: 131–146

Woodhall B, Beebe G W (eds) 1956 Peripheral nerve regeneration. V A Medical Monograph. US Government Printing Office, Washington, DC

Woodruff J M, Chernik N L, Smith M C et al 1973 Peripheral nerve tumours with rhabdomyosarcomatous differentiation. (Malignant "triton" tumours). Cancer 32: 426–439

Woodruff R E 1898 The causes of the explosive effects of modern small calibre bullets. New York Medical Journal 67: 593–601

Woolf C J 1995 Somatic pain – pathogenesis and prevention. British Journal of Anaesthesia 75: 169–176

Woolf C J 1996 Windup and central sensitization are not equivalent. Pain 66: 105–108

Woolf C J, Shortland P, Coggleshall R E 1992 Peripheral nerve injury triggers central sprouting of myelinated afferents. Nature 355: 75–77

Woolf H 1996 Access to justice: final report to the Lord Chancellor on the civil justice system in England and Wales. HMSO, London

Woolsey C N 1964 Cortical localization as defined by evoked potential and electrical stimulation studies. In: Schaltenbrand G, Woolsey C N (eds) Cerebral localization and organization. University of Wisconsin Press Madison, p 17–32

Wright A 1942 Pathology and treatment of war wounds. Heinemann, London, p 175

Wright A, Bradford R 1995 Management of acoustic neuroma. British Medical Journal 311: 1141–1144

Wulff C H, Gilliatt R W 1979 F waves in patients with hand wasting caused by a cervical rib and band. Muscle and Nerve 2: 452–457

Wyburn-Mason R 1941 Brachial neuritis occurring in epidemic form. Lancet ii: 662–663

Wyeth J A, Sharpe W 1917 The field of neurological surgery in a general hospital. Surgery, Gynecology and Obstetrics 24: 29–36

Wynn Parry C B, Frampton V, Monteith A 1987 Rehabilitation of patients following traction lesion of the brachial plexus. In: Terzis J K (ed) Microreconstruction of nerve injuries. W B Saunders, Philadelphia, p 483–495

Wynn Parry C B 1953 Electrical methods in diagnosis and prognosis of peripheral nerve injuries. Brain 76: 229–265

Wynn Parry C B 1980 Pain in avulsion lesions of the brachial plexus. Pain 9: 41–53

Wynn Parry C B 1981 Rehabilitation of the hand, 4th edn. Butterworths, London

Wynn Parry C B 1984 Review of splint usage.

Wynn Parry C B 1989 Pain in avulsion of the brachial plexus. Neurosurgery 15: 960–965

Wynn Parry C B, Salter R M 1976 Sensory re-education after median nerve lesions. British Journal of Hand Surgery 8: 250–257

Wynn Parry C B, Withrington R H 1984 Painful disorders of peripheral nerves. Postgraduate Medical Journal 60: 869–875

Xu D, Pollock M 1994 Experimental nerve thermal injury. Brain 117: 375–384

Xu H 1996 Motor and sensory fibres in C7. Intra-operative studies by acetyl cholinesterase staining. Paper read to the Shanghai International Brachial Plexus Symposium. Shanghai. 1996

Yarnitsky D, Ochoa J L 1991 Warm and cold specific somatosensory systems. Brain 114: 1819–1826

Yeoman P 1964 Fatty infiltration of the median nerve. Journal of Bone and Joint Surgery 46B: 737–739

Yeoman P M 1968 Cervical myelography in traction injuries of the brachial plexus. Journal of Bone and Joint Surgery 50B: 253–260.

Yeoman P M 1984 Quoted by Narakas A O. Traumatic brachial plexus lesion. In: Dyck P J, Thomas P K, Lambert E H, Bunge R (eds) Peripheral neuropathy, 2nd edn. W B Saunders, Philadelphia, p 1394

Yeoman W 1928 The relation of arthritis of the sacroiliac joint to sciatica. Lancet ii: 1119–1120

Ygge J 1989 Neuronal loss in lumbar dorsal root ganglia after proximal as apposed to distal sciatic nerve resection: a quantitative study in the rat. Brain Research 478: 193–195

Yoshikawa H, Dyck P J 1991 Uncompacted inner myelin lamellae in inherited tendency to pressure palsy. Journal of Neuropathological and Experimental Neurology 50: 649–657

Young J N, Nashold B S, Cosman E R 1989 A new insulated caudalis nucleus DREZ electrode. Journal of Neurosurgery 70: 283–284

Young J Z 1942 Functional repair of nervous tissue. Physiological Reviews 22: 318–374

Young J Z 1945 The history of the shape of a nerve fibre. In: Le Gros Clark W E, Medawar P B (eds) Essays on growth and form. Oxford University Press, Oxford, p 41

Young J Z 1949 Factors influencing the regeneration of nerves. Advances in Surgery 1: 165–220

Young J Z 1993 First evidence of axonal transport. In: Dyck P J, Thomas P K, Griffin J W et al (eds) Peripheral neuropathy, 3rd edn. W B Saunders, Philadelphia, p 2

Young J Z, Holmes W 1940 Nerve regeneration. Lancet ii: 128–130

Young J Z, Medawar P B 1940 Fibrin suture of peripheral nerves. Lancet ii: 126–128

Young R R, Henniman E 1961 Reversible block of nerve conduction by ultrasound. Archives of Neurology 4: 83–89

Yu Y L, Murray N M F 1984 A comparison of concentric needle electromyography, quantitative EMG and single fibre EMG in the diagnosis of neuromuscular diseases. Electroencephalography and Clinical Neurophysiology 58: 220–225

Yuen E C, Olney R K, So Y T 1994 Sciatic neuropathy: clinical and prognostic features in 73 patients. Neurology 44: 1669–1674

Yuen E C, Yuen T S, Olney R K 1995 The electrophysiologic features of sciatic neuropathy in 100 patients. Muscle and Nerve 18: 414–420

Yunshao H, Shizhen Z 1988 Acetylcholinesterase: a histochemical identification of motor and sensory fascicles in human peripheral nerve and its use during operation. Plastic and Reconstructive Surgery 82: 125–132

Zachary R B 1945 Thenar palsy due to compression of the median nerve in the carpal tunnel. Surgery Gynecology and Obstetrics 81: 213–217

Zachary R B 1946 Tendon transplantation for radial paralysis. British Journal of Surgery 33: 358–364

Zachary R B 1947 Transplantation of teres major and latissimus dorsi. Lancet ii: 757–758

Zancolli E A 1957 Claw hand caused by paralysis of the intrinsic muscles. A simple surgical procedure for its correction. Journal of Bone and Joint Surgery 39A: 1076–1080

Zancolli E 1979 Structural and dynamic basis of hand surgery, 2nd edn. J B Lippincott, Philadelphia

Zancolli E, Mitre H 1973 Latissimus dorsi transfer to restore elbow flexion. Journal of Bone and Joint Surgery 55A: 1265–1275

Zancolli E A, Zancolli E R 1993 (Eng trans) Palliative surgical procedures in sequelae of obstetrical palsy. In: Tubiana R (ed) The hand. W B Saunders, Philadelphia, vol IV p 602–623

Zorub D S, Nashold B S, Cook W A 1974 Avulsion of the brachial plexus. 1. A review with implications on the therapy of intractable pain. Surgery and Neurology 2: 347–353

Zu J G 1996 The histochemical study of C7 nerve root and its clinical significance. Shanghai International Brachial Plexus Symposium, Autumn

Index

Page numbers in **bold** indicate figures and tables.

Abdomen and pelvis, exposure of nerves 114–115
Accessory
  deep peroneal nerve, anomalous innervation 475
  insertion, trick movements 453
  nerve *see* Spinal accessory nerve
Acetylcholine 28, 36
Acoustic neurofibromas 339–340
Acromegaly 85
Acute carpal tunnel syndrome 267
Acute nerve injury
  associated signs 71–72
  compression 46
  demyelinating conduction block 37–38, 46
  early symptoms 72
  examination 72
  ischaemia 47, 49
Adduction contraction of thumb 423
Adjustment to daily living 464
Adrenaline 36
Afferent
  cutaneous pathways 16
  fibres
    in anterior roots 28
    entering spinal cord 17, **20**
    unmyelinated 17
Age and outcome
  peripheral nerve trunk repairs 237
  vascularised ulnar nerve grafts 197, **198**
Ageing, changes in nerves 25
Alcock's canal syndrome 288
Alcoholic neuropathy 84–85
Allodynia 374, 380
Allografts 101
Alpha-cells, motor neurons 27
Amputation
  gas gangrene, early wound closure 124
  MPNST 363
  neuroma 396
  neurovascular brachial plexus injury 175
  phantom limb pain 377
  revascularisation 139–143
  for severe pain 455–456
  and sympathectomy, plexus pain 399
Anaesthesia 88
  local, conduction block 38
Analgesics, plexus pain 399
Aneurysm 174, 175
  see also False aneurysm
Angiography *see* Arteriography

Anhidrosis 73, 74
Ankle and foot
  see also Foot
  equinovarus deformity 420–**421**
  flexors, motor function testing 79
  multiple schwannomas **347**
Ansa hypoglossi 5
Anterior
  horn cell disorders, electrodiagnosis 489
  interosseous nerve entrapment syndromes 284–285
  roots 5–14, 17, 28, **29**
  shoulder dislocation, operative treatment, iatropathic injury 314–315
  supraclavicular thoracic outlet approach 262, 263–264, 265–266
  ulnar nerve subcutaneous transposition 278–279
Antibiotics
  prophylactic 94
  wound treatment 123
Anticoagulants, iatropathic nerve injury 295–296
Approaches to individual nerves 106–121
  abdomen and pelvis
    femoral nerve 115
    lumbosacral plexus 114
  arm and axilla
    median and ulnar nerves 111–112
    radial nerve 112–**113**
  foot and ankle
    plantar nerves 118, **120**
    tibial nerve 117–118
  forearm
    median nerve 113–114
    posterior interosseous nerve 113, **114**
  hip, sciatic nerve 115–**117**
  neck 106–111
    see also Brachial plexus exposure
    brachial plexus 106–110
    circumflex nerve 110
    spinal accessory nerve 111
    suprascapular nerve 110–**111**
  popliteal fossa and below, tibial and peroneal nerves 117
  wrist and hand, ulnar nerve 114
Arcade of Frohse, simple entrapment at 283
Arcuate ligament, inadequate, ulnar neuritis 275
Arm
  median and ulnar nerve approaches 111–112
  penetrating missile injuries 137, 138
  radial nerve approach 112–**113**

Arterial
  injection
    accidental 301
    producing bleeding 299–300
  injuries
    1975–1996 **127**
    brachial plexus trauma 173–175
    lower limb 241–242
  lesions associated with fractures 300–301
  ligation 126
  repair
    access and control of vessels 175–181
    failure, causes 179, 181
    shunts 126
  spasm 126, 128, 173, 300
Arterial thoracic outlet syndrome 248, 254–258
  appearance at operation **257**, **258**
  imaging 255–256
  operative treatment 256–258
  results 266
  signs 254–255
Arteriography
  arterial thoracic outlet syndrome 255, **256**
  bleeding into fascial sheath following 299, 300
Arteriovenous fistulae and false aneurysm 130–**132**, 174, 175
Arthrodesis 430–431
  triple, foot and ankle 445
  wrist 437
Arthroplasty of hip
  foot drop following, electrodiagnosis 480–481
  iatropathic nerve injury 317, 319, 320–323
    femoral nerve 320
    gluteal nerves 320, 323
    primary or secondary arthroplasty **322**
    sciatic nerve 50, 296, 325, 389
  motor function testing 79
Arthroscopy, neurological injury secondary to 304
Ascending tracts, cord, brainstem and cortex **35**
Askin tumour of chest wall 338, 339
Auditory nerve 1
Autogenous cable grafts 95, 97
Autonomic nervous system 1, 15–16
Avulsion, spinal nerves **159**, **160**, 164, **166**, **168**, **169**, **170–171**
  see also Brachial plexus: injury: closed traction lesions
  bruising and swelling **71**
  classification **158**

Avulsion (cont'd)
  electrodiagnostic triad 473
  OBPP intraoperative appearance 216, **217**
  pain 381–382, 398–403
  reimplantation 201–207
    Bonney 201–203
    Carlstedt 203–204, **206, 207**
    outcomes **205**
Axillary
  artery
    circumferential rupture of intima **174**
    exposure 109–**110**
    false aneurysm, case report 174
    occlusion, displaced fracture **127**
    rupture, closed lesions **142**
    rupture of intima **174**
    transected **125**
  median and ulnar nerve approaches
    111–112
  nerve lesions, electrodiagnosis 482
Axolemma 17
Axon-myelin sheath-Schwann cell complexes
    18, 20
Axonal
  degeneration see Wallerian degeneration
  sprouts, regeneration 60
  transport 24–25
    entrapment neuropathy 246
Axonotmesis 41, **44**
  recovery after 64
Axonotomy
  death of neurones following 380–381
  regeneration after 64
Axons 17
  entrapment neuropathy 246, 247
  myelinated **20, 22, 24, 36**, 162
  reimplantation regeneration, animal studies
    203, **204, 205**
  unmyelinated **22, 24, 30, 36**
Axoplasm 14

Benign tumours, peripheral nerves 336
  see also Neurofibromatosis
  benign schwannoma **337**, 338
  in NF1 **340**
  or tumour-like conditions 354, 356–**358**
Bernard-Horner sign 121, 165, 167–168, **169**,
    213, 311
Beta-endorphins 36
Biopsy
  lymph node, iatropathic injury 313–314,
    318, 482
  needle, iatropathic injury 307, 309
  peripheral nerve tumours, diagnosis 339
Birth
  lesions, brachial plexus see Obstetric
    brachial plexus palsy (OBPP)
  weight, OBPP 210–211
Blood supply, nerves 25, **26**
Bloodless field 301–302
Bomb fragments, injury from 71
Bone
  fragments, nerve lesions 143
  grafts, limb reconstruction 448
  and joint injuries 143–150
  spike, causing neurostenalgia 397–398
Bonney, reimplantation of spinal nerves
    201–203
Brachial artery
  elbow trauma 128
  false aneurysm case report 131, **132**
  supracondylar fracture of humerus
    149–150, **301**

Brachial plexus 5, **6**
  see also Obstetric brachial plexus palsy
    (OBPP); Traumatic lesions, brachial
    plexus
  adult lesions and OBPP, differences 222
  anatomical considerations 157–164
    blood supply 162
    course in neck 160–162
    divisions 161
    functional distribution 162
    individual variations 8–9, 162, **163**
    microanatomy 162
    relation to axial skeleton **6**
  aponeurotic fibromatosis **357**
  electrodiagnosis of plexopathies 482–487
  iatropathic injury
    closed pressure and traction from within
      304
    external pressure during GA 303–304
    operations on sympathetic chain 311–312
    tumour excision 307, 308–**309**, 316, **317**
  infiltration, malignant tumours 335
  injury 181–200
    closed traction lesions 174–175, 381–382
    electrodiagnosis, adult traumatic lesions
      483
    infraclavicular closed traction lesions
      184–185
    late changes **80**
    open 181–183
    penetrating missile 136–138, **139**
    severe, CSF release 88
    spinal cord atrophy following 55
    supraclavicular closed traction lesions
      183–184
  intradural injury 44, 46, 83
    see also Avulsion, spinal nerves
    central pain 381–382, 398–403
    classification **58, 157, 159–160**
    regeneration after 62
  MPNST 359–360, **362, 365**
  neurofibroma, solitary malignant **355**
  neurotisation 102
  paralysis, causes **415**
  radiation neuropathy 326, **329**
  rupture, operative diagnosis
    early 88–89, **90**
    late 89, **91**
  schwannoma, upper trunk **307, 348, 349**
  splints 460–462
  supraclavicular lesions
    admission for rehabilitation, usefulness
      462
    return to work or study **463**
    time off work **463**
    use of splint and TENS **462**
Brachial plexus exposure **181**
  see also Fiolle-Delmas exposure
  anterior approaches 106, 262
    infraclavicular 109–110, **178**
    supraclavicular 175–177, 216, 263–264
    transaxillary 262–263, 264–265
    transclavicular 177, 179, **180**
  intradural lesions 106
  posterior approach 263, 265
  posterolateral approach 106–109
Brain derived neurotrophic factor (BDNF)
    63, **65**
Brand's transfer 442
Breast cancer, neuropathy 86
Breech deliveries, OBPP 210, 211–212
Brown-Séquard syndrome 164
Burns, compound nerve injuries 155

Cable grafts 95, 97
Callus, pressure causing neurostenalgia
    397–398
Cannabis, plexus pain 399
Carcinomatous neuropathy and myopathy
    86
Carlstedt, spinal nerve reimplantation
    203–204, **206–207**
Carpal tunnel, anatomy 268–269
Carpal tunnel syndrome 46, 266–275
  associated conditions 85, 266, 267
  classes 266–267
  clinical features 269–270
  differential diagnosis 270
  electrodiagnosis 475–477
  operation 271–275
    difficulties, dangers and complications
      273–274
    endoscopic division 273
    iatropathic injury 273–274, 310–311
    indications 270, 477
    open exposure 271, **272**
    restricted exposure 271, 273
    results 274–275, 477
  proximal lesion 268
  treatment, non-operative 270–271
  vascular mechanisms 246
Cauda equina 1
Causalgia 374, 388–393
  CRPS type 2 387
  location of lesion 383
  lumbar sympathetic block 391–393
  MRC definition 383
  penetrating missile injuries 139, 388–389
  spontaneous resolution of pain 389
  sympathetic ganglion block 389, **390**, 391
  treatment, response to 389, **390**
Causalgia-reflex sympathetic dystrophy
    386
Cell body and proximal stump, degenerative
    lesion 40–41
Central
  analysis, sensory impulses 406
  connections, sensory receptors 33–36
  nervous system 1
  neurofibromatosis see Neurofibromatosis:
    NF1
  projections, nociception 377
  sensitisation 375, 377
    abnormal 386
Central pain 403–404
  brachial plexus injury 381–382, 398–403
    amputation and sympathectomy 399
    interventions on spinal cord 401–403
    non-operative 398–399
    reinnervation of limb 399–401
  poststroke 403
Cerebral cortex, direct stimulation 377
Cervical
  plexus 5
  primary rami
    anterior 5–10
    posterior 14
  radiculopathy, carpal tunnel syndrome 268
  spinal cord 1
Cervicothoracic
  (stellate) ganglion
    relations **16**
    sympathetic block 382
  sympathectomy 118, 121
Chemical
  blockade 382
  sympathectomy 383

Chemotherapy and radiotherapy,
    neuropathy 328
    see also Radiation neuropathy
Children, fixed deformities 417–**418**
'Chinese cracker' vascularised nerve graft
    100, 101
Chronic
    ischaemia 49
    nerve compression 46–47
        see also Entrapment syndromes;
            Radiation neuropathy
    pain programme 456–458
Ciliary neurotrophic factor (CNTF) 64
Circumflex nerve
    bone and joint injuries 145–147
    exposure 110
    ruptures **78**, 145
    and suprascapular nerves, repair results 238
Classical neurogenic thoracic outlet syndrome
    259–261
Clinical aspects, nerve injury *see* Nerve injury:
    clinical aspects
Closed
    injuries, associated signs 71–72
    traction injury, brachial plexus 174–175,
        183–184
        history of treatment 164–166
        natural history 165
Cold
    exaggerated reaction 82, 374, 454
    injury 49–50
    vasodilation response 169
Colles fracture, reflex sympathetic dystrophy
    complicating 394
Common peroneal nerve
    assessment of recovery **242**
    entrapment at knee 289–290
    exposure 117
    external pressure during GA 304
    fixed deformity after untreated lesion **418**
    haemangiopericytoma **365**
    intraneural ganglion 289, 356
    knee injuries, traction rupture 154,
        154–155
    nerve action potential (NAP) **480**
    palsy
        dropped foot 445–447
        transfer for **446**
    repair, multistrand free graft **100**
    results of repairs **243**
    untreated lesion, fixed deformity resulting
        418
Compartment syndrome 133–134
    iatropathic 301
    indications for decompression 134
Compartmental pressure, interoperative
    monitoring 134
Compensation claims 333, 463, 466
Complex regional pain syndrome (CPRS)
    type 1 (reflex sympathetic dystrophy) 386
    type 2 (causalgia) 387
Complex repetitive discharges, EMG 470
Compound muscle action potentials
    (CMAPs) 468
    conduction block 468
Compound nerve injury 123–155
    see also Traumatic lesions, brachial plexus
    burns 155
    lumbosacral plexus 150–155
    nerve, bone and joint injuries 143–150
    neurovascular injuries 139–143
    penetrating missile injuries *see* Penetrating
        missile injuries

skin lesions 135
    vascular lesions 125–**132**
        technical comments 132–134
    wound 123–124
Compression
    acute, demyelination 246
    axonal transport 246
Conduction
    nerve fibres 24, 25
        changes with ageing 25
    and resistance, sensory testing 407
    sensory pathway 36
Conduction block 37, 37–38, 72
    acute demyelinating 37–38, 46
    classification **41**
    conduction velocity 472
    electrophysiological changes 472–473
    local anaesthetic 38
    recovery 64
    signs 82
    tourniquet paralysis 302
    in ulnar neuropathy **478**
Congenital insensitivity to pain 373
Congenital lesion, OBPP 212
Connective tissue, entrapment neuropathy
    247
Contralateral C7 transfer 188
Conversion hysteria 465
Coracoid overgrowth 224, **225**, 231
Cortical evoked potentials, determining level
    of lesion 170
Costoclavicular compression 248
Cranial nerves 1, 4–5, 16
    iatropathic injury 324–325
    tumours 343
CT
    brachial plexus lesions 171, **172**
    peripheral nerve tumours, diagnosis 339
    radiation neuropathy and metastases,
        distinguishing between 327
Cubital tunnel 275
    syndrome, electrodiagnosis 478–479
Cutaneous
    nerves
        foot 24
        forearm **9**, 92
        hand **9**, 74–75, **92**, **93**, 269
        iatropathic damage 323–324
        lower limb **14**, 75, **93**, **94**
        neck **92**
    sensibility 30
    sensory receptors 31, 405–406
        following denervation **54**, 66
Cytoskeleton, nerve cell 17

Day case operations and iatropathic injury
    295, 305, 333
Deep
    musculoaponeurotic fibromatosis 356–**357**
    sensibility 30–32, 405
    sensory receptors **32**
Deformities in OBPP 214–215, 222–224
    causation 224–**228**
    elbow 222, 223, 231
    shoulder
        complex subluxation/dislocation
            225–226, **227**
        inferior glenohumeral angle 226, **228**
        medial rotation contracture 223–224
        posterior dislocation, simple 224–225,
            226
        posterior glenohumeral contracture
            226, **228**

posterior subluxation, simple 224
    treatment 228–**233**
        analysis of treatment, systems for
            228–229
        complex dislocation 231, **232, 233**
        dislocation/subluxation, simple 230
        elbow flexion deformity 231
        subscapularis slide 229–**230**
Deformity, correction
    see also Fixed deformity
    reconstruction 417–424
        elbow 431–**437**
        foot and ankle 445–447
        forearm flexors and intrinsic muscles,
            hand 440–444
        hip 444
        knee 444–445
        shoulder girdle 424, 428–431
        wrist and hand 437–440
    rehabilitation 454, **455**
    serial splinting results **426, 427**
Degenerative lesions *see* Wallerian
    degeneration
Degenerative and non-degenerative injury,
    distinguishing between 72
Delay, effect on vascularised ulnar nerve grafts
    197, 198
Deltoid
    motor function testing 77
    shoulder elevation in complete paralysis **145**
Demyelination 24
    conduction block 37–38, 46, 472
    entrapment neuropathy 246
    neuropathic processes, electrophysiological
        changes 471
Denervation
    EMG findings **471**
    MRI appearance **83**
    peripheral effects 54–55, 66, 80
Dental operations, risk to cranial nerves
    324–325
Depth of injury 37, 72
Descending pathways, pain 377, 379
Diabetic
    amyotrophy 482
    neuropathy 85, 381
Digital nerves, results of repairs 240–241
Direct
    muscular neurotisation 102
    substitution, trick movements 453
Distal stump
    degenerative lesion 41, 44, 46
    regeneration **57, 58**
Distraction from pain 398
Dorsal
    horn, changes, nerve injury 380
    root entry zone
        coagulation 402–403
        selective posterior rhizotomy 401–402
Double-crush syndrome 245, 487–488
    cervical nerve affection, carpal tunnel
        syndrome 268
Drains, wound, general principles 91
Drugs
    causing iatropathic injury 295–296
    central pain, brachial plexus injury 399
Duchenne's lesion 209, **210**
Dynamic sensibility 405
Dysaesthesiae 374

Echo-planar functional MRI, cerebral activity,
    repetitive stimulation 379
Efferent fibres 17, 20

Elbow
    active reconstruction 431–437
        extension 436
        flexorplasty 432, 433, **434**
    bony injury, nerves involved 147–150
        displayed at operation **148**
    deformity, OBPP 222, 223, 231
        Gilbert and Raimondi classification, recovery **220**
    dislocation, closed reduction 149, **150**
    lock splint 460
    vascular injury 128
Electric shock 50
    burns 155
Electrodiagnosis 82, 467–490
    carpal tunnel syndrome 270
    diffuse problems 489–490
    entrapment neuropathies 475–482
    historical aspects 467
    innervation, normal variants 475
    localisation of lesion 473–**475**
    plexopathies 482–487
    radiculopathies 487–489
    techniques 468–471
    thoracic outlet syndrome 260–261
Electrodiagnostic correlates, Seddon's classification, nerve injuries 473
Electromyography (EMG) 469–471
    OBPP 215, 216
    safety 481
Electrophysiological changes, pathophysiological correlates 471–473
Employers' attitudes to disabled applicants 463
Employment Advisor 464
Encapsulated lipomas 354, 356
End-organs, injury and regeneration 64–67, 406
Endoneurium 22, **23**
Endoscopic techniques, iatropathic injury
    carpal tunnel decompression 311
    sympathetic chain 311
Enkephalins 36, 401
Ensheathment 102–103
Enteric nervous system 15
Entrapment syndromes 46, 245–291
    carpal tunnel syndrome see Carpal tunnel syndrome
    causes 245
    clinical features 247
    definition 245
    electrodiagnosis 475–482
    iatropathic damage during operations for 309–311
    neural pathology 246–247
    thoracic outlet syndrome see Thoracic outlet syndrome
    ulnar nerve at elbow 275–279
    uncommon
        pelvis and lower limb 287–291
        upper limb 280–286
Entubation 102–103
Envenomation 52, 54
Ephapses 380
Epidermal growth factor (EGF) 64
Epineurectomy 103
Epineurial suture 96, 97, **98**
Epineurium 22, **23**
Epineurotomy 103
Equinovarus deformity of ankle and foot 420–**421**
Erb's palsy
    see also Duchenne's lesion
    electrodiagnosis 483

Ewing's tumour 338–339, **369**
Exercises
    OBPP 214–215, 228
    rehabilitation 454
Expert evidence, medical negligence cases 293
Extensor origin of forearm, proximal advancement 432
External
    neurolysis 103
    pressure, vulnerability during GA 303
Extra-abdominal desmoid 356–**357**
Extrafascicular injection **297**
Extrapyramidal tracts 27

F response, nerve conduction studies 468
Facial nerve 1
    iatropathic injury 324
False aneurysm 173–174
    and arteriovenous fistulae 130–**132**
Fascial compartment, infusion into 301
Fascicular
    alignment, regeneration 62
    suture 96–97, **97–98**
    vascular units 246
Fasciculations, EMG 470
Fasciocutaneous flaps 135
Fasciotomy 181
Femoral artery thrombosis **125**
Femoral nerve 11–12
    course and distribution **13**
    exposure 115
    intraoperative iatropathic injury 320
    neuropathies, electrodiagnosis 481–482
    results of repairs 242, **243**
Femoral plexus **10**
Femoral and tibial fractures, popliteal artery rupture 129–130
Fibrillation potentials, EMG 470
    conduction block 472
Fibroblast growth factors (FGF-1 and -2) 64
Fibroblasts **358**
Fibromatosis, extra-abdominal 356–**357**
Fibronectin mats, graft material 101–102
Fibula fracture, anterior tibial artery rupture **129**
First rib 251
    fracture dislocation 175
    and relations **249**
    removal 263, 265
Fixed deformity
    see also Deformity, correction
    chief causes 417
    children 417–418
    postischaemic contracture 419–424
Flail arm splint 460, **461–462**
Flexion and pronation deformity, elbow 222
Flexor digitorum superficialis and profundus, motor function testing 77, **79**
Flexor muscle slide **420**, 423, 424, **425**
Flexor origin of forearm, proximal advancement 433, **434**
Flexor retinaculum **269**
    incomplete division 274
Flexor to extensor transfer, splint for **417**
Fiolle-Delmas exposure 109, **110**, 175, **177**
Fontana, spiral bands of 47
Foot
    see also Ankle and foot
    cutaneous nerves **94**
    dropped
        and ankle reconstruction 445–447
        common peroneal palsy 445–447
        splints for **460**

growing, progressive deformities 447
    plantar nerves, exposure **120**
Forearm
    cutaneous nerves **92**
    ischaemic contracture, flexor muscles **423**
    median nerve approach 113–114
    posterior interosseous nerve approach 113, **114**
Foreign body, neurostenalgia 397
Fos protein 377
Fractures
    associated arterial lesions 125, 127–128, 129–130, 300–301
    nerves injured by 143–144
Free functioning muscle transfers 448–450
Free nerve endings 30, 33
Freeze-thawed muscle graft 395
Froment's sign **79**
Function, assessment 408
Functional splints **458–459**

Gamma-cells, motor neurons 27
Ganglia 15
    cervicothoracic (stellate) ganglion **16**
    common peroneal nerve 289
    posterior root ganglion 17
Ganglioneuroma 371
Ganglionic sympathetic block 382
Gangrene
    following arterial ligation 126
    gas 123, 124
Gate theory, Melzack and Wall 387–388
Gauntlet splint 460
General anaesthesia (GA)
    closed pressure and traction during 303–304
    manipulation under 304–305
Genitofemoral nerve 11
Giant nerves 356
Gilbert classification, shoulder paralysis 219–220
Gilbert and Raimondi, elbow recovery classification **220**
Gilbert and Tassin grading, OBPP 212–213
    1986–1995, lesions by **214**
Glabrous skin
    cutaneous sensory receptors **31**
    mechanoreceptors 30
Glenohumeral arthrodesis 430–431, **432**
Glial derived neurotrophic factor (GDNF) 64, 65
Glossopharyngeal nerve 4
Gluteal nerves 13
    iatropathic injury 320, 323
Glutei, motor function testing 79
Grafts
    nerve 97, 99–102
        allograft 101
        cable 95, 97
        length required 97, 99
        multistrand free graft **100**
        non-neural material 101–102
        regeneration through 66, 67, **68–69**
        sandwich 100–101
        standard 186
        techniques 99–100
        vascularised **68–69**, 100, **101**, 186–187, 195–198
    vascular 133
        arterial repair, historical aspects 125–126
Great occipital nerve 14
Grey rami 15
Grip and pinch, measurement 451, **452**

Growth cone, regeneration 62
Guanethidine 384
  block 392–393
Gunshot injuries 71
  see also Shotgun injuries
  axilla, false aneurysm and arteriovenous
    fistula 130–131
  brachial plexus 173
  causalgia 388–389
  civilian 137
  upper limb **137**
Guyon's space, ulnar nerve entrapment 285,
  286, 479

H reflex 468, **469**
Haemangioma 356
Haemangiopericytoma **365**
Haemodialysis, carpal tunnel syndrome
  associated 267
Haemostasis, general principles 90
Hairy skin
  cutaneous sensory receptors **31**
  mechanoreceptors 30
Hamstrings, anterior transfer for knee
  extension 444–445
Hand
  see also Wrist and hand
  digital nerves, results of repairs 240–241
  evaluation scale, Raimondi **220**
  fixed flexion deformity, serial splinting **426**
  innervation 7–8
    anomalous 475
    cutaneous **10, 92, 93, 269**
  intrinsic muscles
    contracture **419, 423**
    paralysis, transfers for 442, **443**
    release 421, 423
    wasting **261**
  replantation after amputation 140
  ulnar nerve approach 114
  ulnar nerve entrapment in 285–286
Head and neck
  electrode placement, sensory evoked
    potentials **89**
  sympathetic supply 15
Heat injury 50, **51–52**
Henry, exposure
  posterior interosseous nerve 113
  sciatic nerve **115–117**
Heparin, iatropathic nerve injury 296
High median and ulnar palsies 441–443
  combined paralysis 442–443
Hip
  bone and joint injuries, compound nerve
    injuries 152–154
  fracture dislocation 152–154
  intraoperative iatropathic injury
    see also Arthroplasty of hip
    innominate osteotomy, sciatic nerve **418**
    operations other than arthroplasty **323**
    pain from 397
  knee and ankle, flexion deformity **418**
  reconstruction 444
Histamine test, brachial plexus lesions 169
Home births, OBPP 211–212
Hormonal changes, carpal tunnel syndrome
  associated 267
Horner syndrome *see* Bernard-Horner
  syndrome
Hospital Employment Advisor 463–464
Hourglass constriction, traction injury **44**
Humerus
  closed fracture, radial nerve rupture **147**

proximal closed fracture, ruptured axillary
  artery and radial nerve **142**
proximal fractures, vascular injury 127–128
Hydrocortisone injection, carpal tunnel
  syndrome 271
Hyperaesthesia 374
  digital nerve repairs 240
Hyperalgesia 374, 386
Hyperpathia 374, 383, 385
  guanethidine blocks 392–393
Hypoglossal nerve 5
Hypothyroidism 85

Iatropathic injury 293–333
  see also Arthroplasty of hip; Hip:
    intraoperative iatropathic injury;
    Lymph node biopsy: iatropathic injury
  cranial nerves 324–325
  drugs causing 295–296
  failure to recognise acute 323, 325–326,
    333
  health service reforms 293–294
    day case operations 295, 305, 333
    indemnification 294
  injection injury 296–297
    interscalene block 298
    intra-arterial 301
    intraneural 73, 296–297, 298–299
    producing arterial bleeding 299–300
  intraoperative 305–309, 313–324
    arthroplasty of hip *see* Arthroplasty of hip
    chest and abdomen 316–317
    cutaneous nerves 323–324, 394–395
    entrapment syndromes 273–274,
      309–311
    GA, closed pressure and traction during
      303–304
    lower limb 317
    manipulation under GA 304–305
    for neoplastic disease 312
    open heart surgery 303–304
    pacemaker insertion 314
    sympathetic chain 311–312
    thyroid surgery 325
    tourniquet paralysis, bloodless field
      301–303
  ischaemia 300–303
  legal aspects 325
    expert evidence 293
    medical negligence claims 294–295,
      333, 395
    record keeping, necessity 294, 295
  radiation neuropathy *see* Radiation
    neuropathy
  risk management 332–333
Iliac thrombectomy after anterior lumbosacral
  fusion 268–259
Iliohypogastric nerve 11
Ilioinguinal nerve 11
Iliopsoas transfer, spina bifida 444
Immobilisation, postoperative 104–105
Immune disorders 86
Incisions, general principles 90
Incisures of Schmidt-Lanterman 20
Indemnification, responsibility for 294
Indications for surgical intervention 87
Inferior
  glenohumeral angle, diminished 226, **228**
  glenohumeral contracture 224
Inflammatory muscle disorders, EMG
  findings 489
Infraclavicular lesions 142, 166, **173**, 239
  closed 141–143, 174, **175**, 184–185

Infraclavicular lesions, median and ulnar
  nerves 239
Infraspinatus, motor function testing 77
Injection injury 296–297
  interscalene block 298
  intra-arterial 301
  intraneural 296–297, 298–299
  producing arterial bleeding 299–300
Innervation, normal variants 475
Innominate osteotomy, iatropathic sciatic
  nerve injury **418**
Instruments and apparatus 88, **89, 90**
Intercostal nerve transfers 189, 200, 400
Intercostobrachial nerve 11
Interfascicular neurolysis 103
Internal neurolysis 103
Interscalene block, iatropathic injury 298
Intra-arterial injection, accidental 301
Intradural extramedullary tumour 344, **345,**
  346
Intradural injury 44, 45, 46
  see also Avulsion, spinal nerves
  regeneration after 62–63
  rupture **158, 160**, 164, 382, 400
Intrafascicular injection **297**
Intraneural
  bleeding, anticoagulants 295–296
  changes, entrapment neuropathy 245
  ganglion 289, 356
  haemorrhage 73
  injection 73, 296–297
    treatment 298–299
Intraoperative evoked potentials, determining
  level of lesion 170
Intrinsic muscles of hand *see* Hand: intrinsic
  muscles
Irradiation neuropathy *see* Radiation
  neuropathy
Ischaemia 133
  acute 47, 49
  carpal tunnel syndrome 46
  chronic 49
  iatropathic injury 300–303
  postischaemic contracture 419–424
  signs 73
  unrecognised 300–301

Job Centres, Disablement Resettlement
  Officers 463
Jugular foramen syndrome 343

Kiloh-Nevin syndrome 284
Kline and Hudson, grading systems of
  measurement **236**
Klumpke's lesion, OBPP 209, **210**, 213, 483
Knee
  bone and joint injuries, compound nerve
    injuries 154–155
  dislocation, popliteal artery rupture **129**
  flexors, motor function testing 79
  muscle transfer for active extension
    444–445
  vascular injury 128–130
Kneecapping injury 126
'Knuckle duster' and opposition spring splints
  458–459
Kyphoscoliosis, neurofibromatosis 343–343

Lambrinudi's operation 445
Laminae of grey matter, posterior horn
  34, **35**
Lateral genicular artery, false expanding
  aneurysm 131, **132**

Latissimus dorsi
  motor function testing 77
  transfers
    for elbow flexion 432, 434, 436, 449
    for lateral shoulder rotation 429–**430**
    to supra and infraspinatus muscles 223
Legal aspects, iatropathic injury *see*
      Iatropathic injury: legal aspects
Leprosy
  correction of dropped foot 447
  neurolysis 104
  ulnar neuropathy 276
Leukaemia inhibitory factor-cholinergic
      differentiation factor (LIF/CDF) 64
Levator scapulae
  motor function testing 77
  and rhomboids, transfer for trapezius
      paralysis 428
Level of injury and outcome, nerve trunk
      repairs 237
    median and ulnar nerve repairs 239–240
    spinal accessory nerve 237–238
Light touch, sensory testing 408
Limb
  length, disparity in OBPP 213
  lengthening, iatropathic injury 305, 320
Lipomas, encapsulated 354, 356
'Lively splint' **459**
Local hypertrophic neuropathy 356
Localisation, re-education 410
  testing 408, **409**, **412–413**
Long flexors of fingers, motor function tests
      77, 79
Louisiana State University Medical Center
      grading systems **236**
Low threshold mechanoreceptors 30
Lower limb
  see also Ankle and foot; Foot
  active reconstruction 444–447
  compound nerve injuries 150–155
  conduction velocity 469
  entrapment syndromes 287–291, 480–482
  functional splints **460**
  innervation 14, 15, **93**, **94**
    cutaneous 14, **93**, **94**
    sympathetic supply 15
  intraoperative iatropathic injury 317
  lower tibial and plantar nerves, approaches
      117–118, **120**
  motor function testing 79
  penetrating missile injuries with nerve
      lesions 137
  radiation neuropathy in 328–329
  tibial and common peroneal nerves,
      approaches 117, **118–119**
  trunk nerves, results of repairs 241–243
Lower motor neuron disorders, causes of
      paralysis 415
Lumbar
  canal stenosis 488
  plexus *see* Lumbosacral plexus
  posterior primary rami 14–15
  and sacral anterior primary rami 11–14
  sympathectomy 121
    intraoperative iatropathic injury 312
  sympathetic block 391–393
    complications 391
    warning and preparation 391–392
Lumbosacral plexus **10**, **11**
  compound nerve injuries 150–155
  electrodiagnosis, neuropathies 487
  exposure 114
  infiltration, malignant tumours 335–336

intradural injury 44
  regeneration 62
lesions
  infancy 152
  pelvic fractures 150, **151**
Lumbosacral trunk 12
Lung cancer, neuropathy 86
Lymph node biopsy, iatropathic injury
  brachial plexus 314
  femoral nerve **318**
  spinal accessory nerve 237–238, 313–314,
      482
Lymph node clearance, radical in neck 312

Macrophages
  degenerative lesions 41
  regeneration **57**
Macrosomia 211
Magnetic resonance imaging *see* MRI
Magnification, surgery 88
Malignant disease 358–370
  infiltration by disseminated 335
Malignant peripheral nerve sheath tumours
      (MPNST) 336, 338, 358–360
  biopsy 360
  brachial plexus **365**
  clinical features 360
  five year survival or disease-free interval **358**
  NF1 341, 358, **359**, 362, **363**, **364**, **366**
  pathology 360–362
  solitary 359, **363**, **367**
  treatment 363–364
Malignant transformation
  benign schwannoma 350, 352
  solitary neurofibroma 352, 353–354
Malingering 466
Mallet system, shoulder function
      measurement 219
Manipulation under anaesthesia, iatropathic
      injury 304–305
Martin-Gruber anastomosis 9, **10**, 475
  entrapment, EMG findings 477–478
Medial
  gastrocnemius free muscle transfer **449**
  lemniscus 35
  rotation contracture, shoulder 222, **223**,
      224, **225**
Medial rotation contracture, shoulder 222,
      223–224, **225**
  high paralysis 442–443
Median nerve 7–8
  cutaneous distribution **74–75**, **269**
  electrodiagnosis, neuropathies 475–478
  encapsulated lipomas 356
  entrapment
    carpal tunnel *see* Carpal tunnel syndrome
    in forearm 284
    fracture, distal humerus **426**
  exposure
    in arm and axilla 111–112
    lower part 113–114
  graft, failure of regeneration through **67**
  high palsy, transfer for 441, **442**
  injury
    closed reduction, elbow dislocation
        149–**150**
    iatropathic 273–274, **297**
    late changes 80
  motor function testing 77
  pain following decompression 396–397
  primary suture, recognition and localisation
      following 410, **411**, **412**
  primitive neuroectodermal tumour **370**

repairs in axilla, results **240**
rupture, closed injury **185**
schwannoma, enucleation **306**
sensory and motor fibres, organisation
      22, 24
thermal injury **51–52**
Median and ulnar nerves
  reconstruction 442–443
  results of repairs 239–240
    distal lesions 240, **241**
    high lesions 239–240
    infraclavicular lesions 239
    method of grading **241**
Medical negligence claims 294–295, 333, 395
Medical Research Council (MRC)
  measures of outcomes **235**
  1954 peripheral nerve injuries report 164
  scale, recording sensibility 407–408
  War Memorandum No 13 126
Meissner corpuscles 30
Melzack and Wall, gate theory 387–388
Meningioma, thoracic spinal canal **345**
Meralgia paraesthetica 287–288, 482
Merkel cells 30
Metacarpophalangeal
  fixed extension 421
  release **422**
Microscopic structure, nervous system
      17–26
  ageing, changes 25
  axonal transport 24–25
  blood supply 25, **26**
  nervi nervorum 25
Minifascicles 60
  remyelination **61**
Missile wounds *see* Penetrating missile
      injuries
Mixed parotid tumour, schwannoma of
      mistaken for 309, 324
Moberg's pick-up test 408, 451
Morphine binding sites 379
Morton's metatarsalgia 290–291
Motor
  end-plates 27–28
    following denervation 65–66
  fibres 162
  function testing 74
    long flexors of fingers 77, 79
    lower limb 79
    recording 81
    thoracoscapular, thoracohumeral and
        scapulohumeral muscles 76–77
  nerve cell unit **18**
  neurones, cell bodies 27
  response after nerve section 39–40
  and sensory
    fibres, distinguishing between 95–96
    function, grading system **326**
    nerves, terminology 33, **34**, 144
    pathways 27–36
  symptoms, entrapment neuropathy 247
  system 27–**29**
  Unit Potentials (MUPs), EMG 470
MRI 83–84
  brachial plexus lesions 171, **172**
  knife track, stab wounds **183**
  OBPP 215
  peripheral nerve tumours, diagnosis 339
  radiation neuropathy and metastases,
      distinguishing between 327
Mucopolysaccharidosis, carpal tunnel
      syndrome associated 267
Munchausen syndrome 465–466

Muscle
  examination
    see also Motor: function testing
      determining level of lesion 169, 170
    nerve and main root supply used, EMG
      474–475
  relaxant, peripheral nerve surgery 88
  spindles 30–31, **32**
    denervation, reaction to 54–55
  transfers 223, 448–450
    latissimus dorsi see Latissimus dorsi
      transfers
Musculocutaneous nerve
  isolated lesions, electrodiagnosis 482
  results of repairs 238
  upper limb **8**
Myelin sheath 18, 20, **21**
  entrapment neuropathy 246
Myelinated fibres **20, 22**
  alpha-delta 374, 375
  brachial plexus microanatomy 162
  calibre 24
  conductance 24, 36
  nociceptors innervated by 30
Myelography 83
  brachial plexus lesions 170, **171, 172**
  OBPP 215
Myokymia 327
  EMG discharges 470
Myopathic disorders, EMG findings
  471, 489
Myotonic discharges, EMG 470

Narakas' score chart **192–193**
National Health Service reforms 293–294
Nauta-Laidlaw technique, degeneration of
  nerve fibres and their terminals **378**
Neck
  brachial plexus approaches 106–110
  brachial plexus, course in 160–162
  circumflex nerve approach 110
  cutaneous nerves **92**
  lump, needle biopsy 307, 309
  spinal accessory nerve approach 111
  suprascapular nerve approach 110–**111**
Neoplastic conditions
  benign 354, 356–**357**
  iatropathic injury during operation for
    305–309, 3122
  infiltration, pressure and distortion
    335–336
  malignant 358–**370**
  neuropathy secondary to 335
  peripheral nerve tumours 336–354
    cranial nerve tumours 343
    malignant tumours 358–**370**
    neurofibromatosis see Neurofibromatosis
    schwannoma see Schwannoma
    solitary neurofibroma 352–354, **355**
    spinal nerve tumours 343–346
    sympathetic chain 371
Nerve
  cell 17, **18**
  compression, chronic 46–47
  conduction studies 468–469
    conduction velocity 468–469
    safety 471
  fibres
    fascicular arrangement **23**
    function and topographical segregation
      22, 24
    myelinated **20, 22,** 24, 36, 162
    unmyelinated **22,** 24, 30, 36

Nerve growth factor 63–64
  see also Brain derived neurotrophic factor
    (BDNF); Glial derived neurotrophic
    factor (GDNF)
  immuno-reactivity, dorsal root ganglion and
    distal stump **69**
  maintenance of pain 381
Nerve injury
  see also Traumatic lesions, brachial plexus
  with arterial injury **127,** 173–175, 241–242
  avulsion see Avulsion, spinal nerves
  birth injury, brachial plexus see Obstetric
    brachial plexus palsy (OBPP)
  clinical aspects 71–86
    abnormal susceptibility, conditions
      causing 84–86
    conditions causing susceptibility 84–86
    see also Double-crush syndrome
    depth of injury 72
    diagnosis, aids to 82–84
    late signs 79–80
    motor function testing 74, 76–77, 79, 81
    reinnervation, signs 81–82
    signs 71–72, 73–82
  differential affection of fibres 73
  electrodiagnostic features 471, **473**
  events after 379–382
    central pain, preganglionic injury
      381–382
    neuromuscular function 38–40
    regeneration see Regeneration
    release of chemical agents 379–380
    spinal cord changes 380–381
  reactions to 37–55
    acute compression 46
    acute ischaemia 47, 49
    causes 37
    cell body and proximal stump 40–41,
      59, 60, 61
    chronic compression 46–47
    see also Entrapment syndromes
    chronic ischaemia 49
    degenerative lesions see Wallerian
      degeneration
    denervation, peripheral effects 54–55
    distal stump 41, 44, 46, **57, 58**
    electric shock 50
    envenomation 52, 54
    percussion 50
    pressure effects 37–38, 46–47
    radiation see Radiation neuropathy
    stretch injury 47
    thermal injury 49–50, **51–52,** 155
    ultrasound 52
  repair
    grafts see Grafts: nerve
    primary, general contraindications 123
    regeneration, factors for 414
    and relief of pain 399–401
    sensibility, recovery of 404–414
    suture 96–97, **97–98,** 99–100
  rupture
    infraclavicular lesions 141, **142,** 143
    intradural **158, 160,** 164, 382, 400
  types of 46–55
Nerve transfer 187–**190**
  brachial plexus trauma, case study
    185–186
  OBPP, results of late 221, **222**
  reinnervation, pain relief 400
  results 198–200
  technical consideration 188–**190**
Nervi nervorum 25

Neural thoracic outlet syndrome 248,
  259–261
Neuralgia, post-traumatic 139
Neuralgic amyotrophy 310
Neurapraxia 37–38, 64
Neurilemmoma see Solitary benign
  schwannoma
Neurinoma see Solitary benign schwannoma
Neuroblastoma 371
Neuroepithelioma 338–339, **370**
Neurofibroma 338
  intradural extramedullary **345**
  plexiform, of lumbosacral plexus **418**
  solitary 352–354, **355**
Neurofibromatosis 306, 336, 336–337,
  339–343
  localised forms of 342
  malignant tumours arising in 358
  NF1 340–342
    benign tumours **340**
    diagnostic criteria **340**
    four categories of complications 341
    MPNST in **341, 359,** 362, **363, 364, 366**
    outcome of treatment 363–364
    paraspinal neurofibroma 341
    risk of 341–342
  NF2 339–340
    diagnostic criteria **340**
  pathological features of tumours 342
  spine in 342–343
Neurogenic EMG pattern **470**
Neurolysis 103–104
  and revascularisation, radiation neuropathy
    330
Neuroma
  amputation 396
  extent of recovery through 89–90
  painful, of cutaneous sensory nerves **394**
  resection of terminal 104
Neuromodulation 36
Neuromuscular
  function, following nerve injury 38–40
  junction, electrodiagnosis of disorders 490
Neuropathic pain 373
Neuropathy, conditions causing 84–86
  see also Double-crush syndrome
  secondary to malignant disease 335
Neuropeptide modulators 36
Neurostenalgia 139, 397–398
Neurotisation 102
Neurotmesis 41, **44,** 72
Neurotoxic drugs 295
Neurotransmitters 36
  descending pathway 379
  in dorsal horn 375
Neurotrophic factors 60
Neurotrophin-3 (NT-3) 63
Neurotrophin-4 (NT-4) 63
Neurotropic
  effect 60, 62
  factors 60
Neurovascular
  bundle, injection beneath sheath 297
  injuries, amputation revascularisation
    139–143
Nociception, definition of terms 374
Nociceptors 30
  fibres 374–375
  segregation within nerve trunks 375
Nocicipient 374
Node of Ranvier 17–18, **21**
Non-degenerative lesions 37–38
  recovery, signs 82

Non-freezing cold injury 50
Nonmetastatic carcinomatous neuropathy
    335
Nonmyelinated C-fibres 374, 375
Noradrenaline 36
    hypersensitivity 386
    regenerating sprouts, response to 379, 380
    sensitivity, causalgia 384
Nucleus ventralis posterolateralis (VPL) 377

Oberlin's operation 24, 200
Object recognition
    re-education 410–414
    sensory testing 408
Obstetric brachial plexus palsy (OBPP) 80,
        209–233, 305
    classification 212–213
    deformities in 222–224
        causation 224–**228**
        treatment 228–**233**
    diagnosis 214
        electrodiagnosis 215, 216, 483–486
        neurophysiological examination,
            preoperative 215–216
        other investigations 215–216
    epidemiology 210–212
    late reinnervation 221–222
    measurement of outcome 219–221
    natural history 212–**214**
    outcomes after spinal cord reimplantation
        203, **204**
    paralysis, evolution of 215
    physiotherapy 214–215
    surgical intervention
        appearance 216–217
        exposure 216
        indications 214
        late reinnervation 221–222
        the nerve lesions 216–217, **218**
        nerve repair 216–219, 221–222
        neurophysiological intraoperative findings
            217–218
        the operation 216–219
        repair, technique 218–219
        results 219, **221**
        shoulder deformity 228–**233**
Obturator nerve 12
Occipital nerve, cervical spine **14**
Occupational therapy and functional splinting
    458–463
Olfactory nerve 1
Oligohydramnios, OBPP 212
Omentoplasty 329, 330
Open
    exploration, diagnosis at 88–89
    heart surgery
        brachial plexus damage 304
        pressure on ulnar nerve at elbow 303
    nerve injuries 181–183
Operating on peripheral nerves 87–121
    apparatus and instruments 88, **89, 90**
    conditions for 87–88
    general principles 90, 94, 95
    indications 87
    methods of repair 94–106
    postoperative immobilisation 104–105
Operating on peripheral nerves, objectives
    88–90
Opponens, motor function testing 77
Opposition
    splint **458**
    of thumb, motor function testing 77, **79**
Optic nerve 1

Pacemaker insertion, iatropathic brachial
    plexus injury 314
Pacinian corpuscles 30
Pain 373–404
    acute nerve injury 72
    central projections, nociception 377
    classification 388
        causalgia 388–393
        central 403–404
        central, brachial plexus injury 398–403
        neurostenalgia 397–398
        post-traumatic neuralgia 394–397
        reflex sympathetic dystrophy 393–394
    definition 373
    descending pathways 377, 379
    diagnostic description, preganglionic
        brachial plexus lesions 167
    the gate theory 387–388
    management programme 456–458
    mechanisms and pathways 374–377
    nerve injury, events after 379–382
    OBPP 222
    relief or abatement, rehabilitation 454–458
    sensory testing 408
    spinal nerve tumours 344
    and sympathetic nervous system 382–387
Palmar nerves section, signs **73**
Paraldehyde, iatropathic nerve injury 297
Paralysis, causes **415**
    not physically determined 464–466
Paraesthesiae 374
Parasympathetic nervous system 15, 16
Parotid gland
    intraoperative iatropathic injury to facial
        nerve 324
    schwannoma, facial nerve mistaken for
        tumour 309
Pectoralis major transfers
    elbow flexion 432, 434
    serratus palsy 428–429
Pectoralis minor transfers
    elbow flexion 432, 432–433
    to biceps **223**
Pelvic
    fractures, severe 150–151
        crush injury case report **152, 153**
    splanchnic nerves 16
Pelvis
    fracture-dislocation, lumbosacral plexus
        injury 150, **151**
    and lower limb, entrapment syndromes
        287–291
Penetrating brachial plexus injuries,
        incidence, open and vascular **173**
Penetrating missile injuries 123, 135–139,
        171
    see also Gunshot wounds; Shotgun wounds
    brachial plexus 173
    case reports 130–131
    causalgia 383–384, 388–389
    neurostenalgia 139
    pain 139
    spontaneous recovery 136
Percussion injury 50
Percutaneous cordotomy 401
Perineal paralysis of the cyclist 288
Perineural suture 96
Perineurioma 337, 338
Perineurium 22, **23**
Peripheral
    nervous system 1
    neurofibromatosis see Neurofibromatosis:
        NF1

Peripheral nerve tumours see Neoplastic
    conditions
Peroneal division of sciatic nerve 481
Peroneal nerves
    common, course and distribution **13**
    deep and superficial 13
    electrodiagnosis 480–481
Phantom limb pain 377
Phrenic nerve 5
    iatropathic damage, potential for 264
    in OBPP surgery 216
    transfer, ipsilateral 187–188
Physical therapy
    OBPP 214–215, 228
    rehabilitation 454
Physiological tests, brachial plexus trauma
    169–170
Pinch grip, restoration 442, **443**
Piriformis syndrome 288–289, 481
Pisoretinacular space, ulnar nerve entrapment
    285, **286,** 479
Plantar nerves
    digital nerve entrapment 290–291
    exposure 117–118, **120**
Plasma clot suture 99–100
Platelet derived growth factor (PDGF) 64
Plexopathies, electrodiagnosis 482–487
PNI Unit system **194–195**
Polymerising cement
    extrusion, nerve damage 320, **321–322**
    thermal injury
        arthroplasty of hip 50, 320
        median nerve **51–52**
Popliteal
    artery, vascular injury 128–130
    fossa, tibial and common peroneal nerve
        approaches 117
Position sense, sensory testing 408
Post-traumatic neuralgia 139, 394–397
    after injury to minor nerves 394–395
    after trunk nerve injury 396–397
Posterior
    approach, thoracic outlet 263, 265
    column stimulators 401, 402
    dislocation/subluxation, shoulder 224–225,
        226
    glenohumeral contracture 224, 226, **228,**
        231
    horn, grey matter 34, **35**
    primary rami 14–15
    roots 17
        avulsion **19**
Posterior interosseous nerve 479–480
    entrapment syndromes 283–284
    exposure 113, **114**
    results of repairs **239**
Postirradiation tumours 358–359
Postischaemic contracture 419–424
    cases requiring operative treatment,
        1977–1995 **419**
Pouting bundles 94, **96**
Preganglionic injuries 400
    see also Avulsion, spinal nerves; Intradural
        rupture
    brachial plexus, classifications **157, 158**
Pregnancy, MPNST in 360
Pressure effects on nerve **37**
Pressure injury
    pressure paralysis, inherited susceptibility
        84
    prolonged 37–38
    vibratory thresholds 73
Pressure, sensory testing 408

Primary rami 1, **4**
Primary repair of nerves
    general contraindications 123
    grafts *see* Grafts
    plasma clot suture 99–100
    suture 96–97, 97–98
Primitive neuroectodermal tumours
    bone 338–339
    nerves 364, **368**, **369**, **370**
Propriospinal fibres 33
Protein synthesis, nociceptor activity 377
Proximal stump
    injury and regeneration 40–41, **59**, **60**, **61**
    remyelination **61**
Pseudomyotonic discharges, EMG 470
Pudendal nerve 13
    entrapment 288

Quadrilateral space syndrome 281–282

Radial nerve 8
    cutaneous distribution **75**
    electrodiagnosis of lesions 479–480
    entrapment 282–283
    exposure 112–**113**
    iatropathic injury
        external pressure during GA 303
        fixation of humerus fracture 314, **315**
    MPNST **363**
    palsy, functional splint **459**
    results of repairs 239
    rupture, closed fracture of humerus **142**,
        147
    schwannoma **350**
    superficial, pure lesions 480
Radiation neuropathy 50, 52, **53**, 162,
        326–332
    Bates and Evans independent review 328
    differentiation from metastases 326–327
    incidence 327–328
    in lower limb 328–329
    pathology and natural course 328
    sex distribution and diagnoses of **332**
    treatment 329–332
        indications for operation 331
        results of operation 331–332
Radiculopathies, electrodiagnosis 487–489
Radius, rotation osteotomy 223
Raimondi, hand evaluation scale **220**
Reactions to injury *see* Nerve injury:
        reactions to
Rebound, assessment 453
Receptor organs, deep sensibility 30
Recognition, sensory testing, charts **412–413**
Reconstruction 415–450
    fixed deformity 417–424
    methods of active
        lower limb 444–447
        upper limb 424–444
        vascularised bone and muscle transfer
            448–450
    operations 1977–1995 **415**
    requirements 416–417
Record keeping 94, **95**
    iatropathic injury 294, 295
    tourniquet use, duration of 303
Recurrent laryngeal nerve, thyroid surgery
        325
Red Cross Wound Classification **124**
Reflex sympathetic dystrophy 385–387,
        393–394
Regeneration 57–69
    acceleration 105–106

after intradural injury 62–63
after repair, factors for 414
electrophysiological changes 471
end-organs 64–67
failure of through graft **67**
nerve growth factor 63–64
pain 396
predictors of recovery 64
process 57–62
rate of peripheral outgrowth 62
through graft, rat **66**
Rehabilitation 451–466
    adjustment to daily living 464
    after nerve suture 410
    assessment 451–453
    correction of deformity 454, **455**
    functional training and splinting 458–463
    objects 451
    pain relief or abatement 454–458
    return to work 463–464
    treatment 453–464
        measuring effects 451, **452**
        physical therapy 454
Reinnervation
    EMG findings 470–471
    factors influencing 66
    of limb, plexus pain 399–401
    signs 81–82
        imperfect recovery 82
Remyelination 60, **61**
Repetitive strain injury 268
Resection 91
    general principles 91
    pouting bundles 94, **96**
Results
    obstetric brachial plexus palsy (OBPP)
        219–221
    peripheral nerve trunk repairs 235–243
        systems of measurement 235–237
Retraining 464
Retroclavicular lesions, brachial plexus 166,
        167, 184
Return to work following brachial plexus
        injury 463–464
Rheumatoid arthritis, neuropathy 86
Rhomboids, motor function testing 76–77
Risk
    disclosure of 293
    management, iatropathic injury 332–333
Rotation osteotomy of radius 223
Rotator cuff
    latissimus dorsi transfer 420–**430**
    rupture 146, 147, 238
Round cell tumours of bone 338–339
Ruffini's corpuscle 30

S-100 staining of Schwann cells 338
Sacral and lumbar anterior primary rami
        11–14
Sacral plexus **10**, 12
    cutaneous distribution **76**
    relations **11**
Sacral posterior primary rami 15
Saltatory conduction 24, 36
`Sandwich' grafts 100–101
Sarcoma
    arising from nerves **368**
    and radiation neuropathy 328
Scalenus
    anticus syndrome 248
    medius band, removal 263
    minimus **250**, 251
    sickle 248, **250**, **261**

Scapulohumeral muscles, motor function tests
        76–77
Schwann cells 17–18, **23**
    immunohistochemistry 338
    in regeneration 57, **58**, 62
    Wallerian degeneration 39, **40**, 41, **43**
Schwannoma 337, 338
    ancient changes **348**
    cranial nerves 343
    dumb-bell tumour, cervical region, case
        report 344, 346
    enucleation 306, 307, **308**
    intradural extramedullary schwannoma
        345
    malignant change 309, 350, 352
    misdiagnosis 306, 309, 324
    multiple benign, 15 cases 351
    multiple, foot and ankle **347**
    solitary benign 347–350, **351**
    upper trunk, brachial plexus **348**, **349**
    removed with **307**
Sciatic nerve 12
    distribution **13**, **75**
    electrodiagnosis 481
    exposure 115–**117**
    hip fracture dislocations 152–153
    iatropathic injury
        anticoagulant use 296
        arthroplasty of hip 50, 296, 317, 320,
            321, **321–322**, 323, 325, 389
        external pressure during GA 304
        innominate osteotomy **418**
        medullary nail removal **319**
        recognition and action 343
    longitudinal section **48**
    neuroepithelioma **370**
    penetrating missile injuries 138–139
    position in protrusio acetabuli 320
    repair, results 242
    rupture and sepsis **48–49**
    solitary MPNST **362**
Seddon
    classification of nerve injuries,
        electrodiagnostic correlates 473
    penetrating missile injuries 136–137
Segmental innervation, upper limb **9**
Sensibility, recovery after repair 415–414
    assessment of function 408
    re-education 408, 410–414
    testing 406–408
Sensory
    action potentials 169, 468, 473
    cells, avulsed posterior root ganglion **19**
    chart 453
    conduction block 473
    derivation, electrodiagnosis **474**
    evoked potentials, intraoperative 218
    fibres, microanatomy 162
    function testing, recording 81
    nerve cell units 18
    neuroma, tethering 395
    symptoms, entrapment neuropathy 247
    testing 406–408
Sensory system 30–36
    central analysis of impulses 406
    central connections 33–36
    conduction of impulses 36
    deep sensibility 30–33
    receptors
        cutaneous end-organs 405–406
        deep **32**
        nociceptors 30
        thermoreceptors 30

Serial
   plasters 454, **455**
   splinting 424, **426**
   results **426–427**
Serotonin 379
Serratus anterior
   motor function testing 76
   nerve to
      entrapment syndrome 280
      iatropathic injury 310
      results of repair 238
   palsy, pectoralis muscle transfer 428–429
   reinnervation 188, 198
Seventh cervical rib 251–**253**, 254, **254**, **255**
   arterial affection, four stages of 257–258
   associated with arterial affection **254**
   removal 263, 265
   variations 252–**253**
Shotgun injuries 135–136, 137–138
Shoulder
   see also Deformities in OBPP
   dislocation
      anterior, brachial plexus injury 185
      arterial lesions 127
      circumflex palsies 146
   dystocia, OBPP 211
   Gilbert's classification, paralysis 219–220
   Mallet system, measuring function 219
   medial rotation contracture 222, 223–224,
      225
   shoulder girdle
      dropping 248, 259
      and glenohumeral injuries, nerve injuries
         associated 144–145
      reconstruction 424, 428–431
Shunts, intraluminal, arterial repair 126
Sibson's fascia **250**, 251
Silicone entubation, divided nerves 102–103
Skin
   flaps, general principles 90
   lesions, compound nerve injuries 135
Small nerve fibre function, assessment 469
Solitary
   benign schwannoma 347–350, **351**
   MPNST **361**, **362**, **367**
   neurofibroma 352–354
      malignant transformation 352, 353–354,
      355
Somatic
   motor system 27–**29**
   sensory system 30–36
Specialisation and iatropathic injury 333
Spina bifida, iliopsoas transfer 444
Spinal accessory nerve 4, 144
   exposure 111
   iatropathic injury
      lymph node biopsy in neck 482
      section **144**
   isolated paralysis 314
   lesions and recovery **144**
      classification 237
   operations **237**
   results of repairs 237–238
   to suprascapular transfer 188, **189**, **190**,
      196, 221
   results 198, **199**
Spinal column, metastatic disease 336
Spinal cord
   afferent and efferent pathways 17, **20**
      autonomic 15
      major descending tracts **27**
   changes, following nerve damage 55,
      380–381

grey matter, longitudinal section **376**
interventions, central pain 401–403
and roots, causes of paralysis 415
Spinal nerves 1, 5–15
   nerve roots, relation to spinal cord 3
   primary rami **2**, **4**
      anterior 5–14
      posterior 14–15
   reimplantation, avulsed 201–207
   tumours 343–346
Spinothalamic system 377
Spiral bands of Fontana 47
Splanchnic nerves 16
Splints
   for flexor to extensor transfer **417**
   lower limb **460**
   serial 424, **426**
   upper limb, functional **458**, **459**
Stab wounds
   axilla, artery, median and ulnar nerve suture
      140, **141**
   brachial plexus 181–183
   infraclavicular 140
   sciatic nerve repairs 242
Static sensibility 405
Stellate (cervicothoracic) ganglion **16**
   sympathetic block 382
Stimulating and recording apparatus, surgery
   88, **89**
Stretch injury 47
Subclavian artery
   arteriovenous fistula **131**
   avulsion 174–175
   rupture **125**
   saccular aneurysm, bullet wound **132**
Subclavian vein
   acute thrombosis, thoracic outlet syndrome
      258
   behind clavicle, iatropathic damage 264
Subscapularis
   motor function testing 77
   slide, OBPP shoulder deformity 229–**230**
Supraclavicular
   brachial plexus injury 166
      closed traction lesion 174, 183–184
      iatropathic section **144**
      incidence of open **173**
      injuries to individual spinal nerves **183**
      patterns of intradural injury **183**
      stab wound 181–183
   exposure, vascular lesions 175–177,
      256–257
Supracondylar
   fracture, brachial artery injury 149–150
   spur 282
Suprapleural membrane **250**, 251
Suprascapular closed lesions, results of
   operated (1975–1984) **191**
Suprascapular nerve 144
   bone and joint injuries 145–147
   and circumflex nerves, results of repairs
      238
   entrapment syndromes 280–281
      electrodiagnosis 482
   exposure 110–**111**
   ruptures 145
Supraspinatus, motor function testing 77, **78**
Sural nerve 12–13
   graft, failure of regeneration **68–69**
Surface anatomy and iatropathic injury
   332–333
Surgical intervention *see* Operating on
   peripheral nerves

Sutures
   arteries 133, 179, 181
   nerves, methods 96–97, 97–**98**
      plasma clot 99–100
Sweating test 84
Sympathectomy 382
   causalgia 384, 389
   pain arising after 385
Sympathetic
   block 382–383
      acute limb ischaemia 126–127
      and causalgia 383–384, 389, **390**, 391
      cutaneous hyperalgesia 386
      indications for sympathectomy 391
      reflex sympathetic dystrophy 393
      sympathetically maintained pain 385, 386
   chain
      extraosseous Ewing's tumour **369**
      iatropathic injury 311–312
      tumours of 371
   ganglionectomy 118, 121
   nervous system 15–16
      and pain 382–387
      sympathetically determined pain 34, 36
      sympathetically maintained pain 385, 386

Tarsal tunnel syndrome 290, 482
Temperature, sensory testing 408
Tennis elbow, resistant 283
Tenodesis action 453
Teres major and minor, motor function
   testing 77
Tetraplegia
   with C5/C6 sparing, reconstruction 440–441
   reconstruction for elbow extension 436
Thalamic syndrome 403
Thalidomide 295
Thenar muscles, motor function testing 77
Thermal injury 49–50, **51–52**, 155
Thermoreceptors 30
Thoracic
   anterior primary rami 11
   duct, iatropathic injury 264
   posterior primary rami 14
   spinal canal, meningioma **345**
Thoracic outlet
   iatropathic damage 309–310
   routes of access 262–265
      anterior 262, 263–264
      posterior 263, 265
      transaxillary 262–263, 264–265
Thoracic outlet syndrome 247–266
   aetiology, symptoms and treatment 254–261
   anatomy 248–**253**
   arterial syndrome 248, 254–258
      imaging 255–256
      operative treatment 256–258
      signs 254–255
   association with carpal tunnel syndrome 268
   neurological syndrome 259–261
      classical 259–261
      electrodiagnosis 486–487
      operation 262–265, 265–266
      without plain motor signs 261–262
Thoracohumeral muscles, motor function
   tests 76–77
Thoracoscapular
   arthrodesis 430, **431**
   muscles, motor function tests 76–77
Thumb
   adduction contracture 423
   paralysis, reconstruction 443–444
   restoration of pinch grip 442, **443**

Thyroid operations, iatrophatic injury 325
Tibia, and femur, open fractures with arterial
    rupture 129–130
Tibial artery, rupture, fractured neck of fibula
    129
Tibial nerve 13
    assessment of results **242**
    at ankle **290**
    course and motor distributions 13
    exposure 117–118, **118–119**
    multinodular schwannoma 350
    posterior, results of repairs **243**
Tibialis posterior, forward transfer by
    superficial route 445–446
Tinel sign 81–82, 168–169
Tomaculous neuropathy 84
Tourniquet
    duration of use, record keeping 303–304
    guidelines for use 302–303
    paralysis 301–303
Transaxillary
    approach, thoracic outlet and neurovascular
        bundle 262, 263, 264–265
    removal, first rib 258
Transclavicular exposure, vascular lesions,
    brachial plexus trauma 177, 179, **180**
Transcutaneous stimulation 398–399, 456
    post-traumatic neuralgia **396**
    use of TENS, supraclavicular plexus lesions
        462
Transient ischaemia, nerve damage 37
Transitional zone 17, **19**, 157
    preganglionic injury 164, 381, 382
Trapezius
    motor function testing 76
    paralysis, levator scapulae and rhomboids
        transfer 428
Traumatic lesions, brachial plexus 157–207
    see also Brachial plexus: injury
    diagnosis
        clinical features 166–169
        special investigations 169–172, 483
    epidemiology
        incidence 165
        major types 166
        mechanism of injury 165–166
        natural history 165
    history of treatment 164–166
    operation, indications and techniques
        173–190
        avulsed spinal nerves, reimplantation
            201–207
        nerve injury 181–200
        vascular lesion 173–181
    surgical intervention
        results 191–200
        strategies of repair 185
Trench foot 50
Triceps to biceps transfer, elbow flexion 432,
    434, **435**, **437**
Trick movements, assessment 451, 453
Trigeminal nerve 1
Triple arthrodeses, foot and ankle 445
Tumours, peripheral nerves see Neoplastic
    conditions
Two-point discrimination 406–407, 408

Ulnar and median nerves
    paralysis, high 442–443
    results of repairs 239–240
        grading results **241**
        high lesions 239–240
        infraclavicular lesions 239

Ulnar nerve 7, 8
    at elbow **275**
    compression syndromes, definition
        according to level 286
    decompression, pain after 396–397
    entrapment
        elbow 275–279, 311
        Guyon's space 285, 286, 479
        medial condyle fracture reduction
            148–149
        wrist and hand 285–286
    epineurial vessels **26**
    exposure
        in arm and axilla 111–112
        in wrist and hand 114
    external compression syndrome 275
    F response, nerve conduction study **468**
    flexor muscle slide **420**
    grafts
        regeneration through **68**
        single strand **101**
        vascularised 186–187, 195–198
    high palsy 441–442
    iatrophatic injury
        above elbow fracture fixation 314
        external pressure during GA 303
        venepuncture, mechanisms **299**
    injury
        adult elbow dislocation **150**
        distal stump changes at 3 weeks **39, 40**
        late changes **80**
    medial epicondylar lesions, electrodiagnosis
        478
    motor function testing 77, **458**
    neuropathies
        electrodiagnosis 478–479
        lateral condylar physis fracture in
            childhood 148
    reconstruction for high palsy 441–442
    simple decompression 278
    transposition 278–279
        common mistakes associated 311
Ulnar to biceps transfer (Oberlin's operation)
    189, **190**
Ultrasound injury 52
Unmyelinated fibres 17, **22**
    C fibres 374
    conductance 24, 36
    nociceptors innervated by 30
Upper limb
    conduction velocity 468–469
    cutaneous supply 7
    entrapment syndromes 280–286
        see also Carpal tunnel syndrome;
            Thoracic outlet syndrome; Ulnar
            nerve: entrapment
    functional splinting **458, 459**
    gunshot wounds **137**
    innervation 5, **6**, 7, **7, 8, 9**
        elbow and upper forearm **9**
        hand, cutaneous supply **10**
        segmental supply **9**
        sympathetic supply 15
    motor distribution 7, **8**
    nerve injuries complicated by arterial
        injuries (1977–1995) **141**
    neurovascular injuries 139–143
    splints for extensive paralysis 460,
        461–462
Upper motor neuron disorders, causes of
    paralysis **415**
Uraemia, carpal tunnel syndrome associated
    267

Vagus nerve 4, 16
Varicose vein procedures, iatrophatic injuries
    317, **319**, 356
Vascular
    mechanisms, entrapment neuropathy 246
    prostheses 126, 133, 175, 179
Vascular lesions 125–**132**
    historical perspectives 125–127
    intra-arterial injection 299–300, 301
    proximal humerus, fractures 127–128
    shoulder dislocation 127
    surgical intervention 173–181
        access and control of vessels 175
        open 173–174
        suprascapular exposure 175–177
        technical details 132–134, 179–181
        transclavicular exposure 177, 179, **180**
Vascularised bone and muscle transfer
    448–450
Vascularised grafts 100, **101**, 186–187,
    195–198
Venepuncture, iatrophatic injury **299**
Venous syndrome, thoracic outlet syndrome
    258–259, 266
    costoclavicular compression 248
Ventral primary rami see Anterior primary rami
Visceral
    afferents 34, 36, 384–385
    plexuses 15–16
    reflexes 16
Visual analogue scales, pain measurement 373
Volkmann's contracture see Postischaemic
    contracture
von Recklinghausen's disease see
    Neurofibromatosis: NF1

Wallerian degeneration 38–40
    cell body and proximal stump 40–41
    distal stump 41, 44, 46
    eighth cervical nerve root at six weeks **42**
    electrophysiological changes 471–472
    late changes **43**
    late signs 79–80
    reinnervation, signs 82
White rami 15
Whole-nerve injury, Louisiana State
    University Medical Center grading
    system **236**
Wind up 375, 377
Wound
    compound nerve injury 123–124
        categories **124**
        early closure 123, 124
    infection
        surgery, antibiotic cover 94
        trauma 123, 124
Wrist
    arthrodesis 437
    hyperextension deformity after wrist flexor
        transfer **437**
    ulnar nerve
        approach 114
        entrapment in 285–286
Wrist and hand
    flexor to extensor transfers 438, **439–440**
    reconstruction 437–440
        flexor muscle paralysis with extensor
            preservation 440–444

X-rays 83
    effects on peripheral nerves 326

Zancolli's dynamic lasso procedure 442